Osteoporosis in Men

Osteoporosis in Men

The Effects of Gender on Skeletal Health

Edited by

Eric S. Orwoll

Oregon Health Sciences University
Portland VA Medical Center
Portland, Oregon

ACADEMIC PRESS

San Diego   London   Boston   New York   Sydney   Tokyo   Toronto

Front cover photograph: Histological section of the vertebral body edge from an 82-year-old woman. For more details, see Figure 4 (color insert) in Chapter 16.

This book is printed on acid-free paper.

Academic Press
a division of Harcourt Brace & Company
525 B Street, Suite 1900, San Diego, California 92101-4495, USA
http://www.apnet.com

Academic Press
24-28 Oval Road, London NW1 7DX, UK
http://www.hbuk.co.uk/ap/

Library of Congress Catalog Card Number: 99-83125

International Standard Book Number: 0-12-528640-6

PRINTED IN THE UNITED STATES OF AMERICA
99 00 01 02 03 04 EB 9 8 7 6 5 4 3 2 1

Contents

Chapter 3

Hip and Vertebral Fractures

Frazer H. Anderson and Cyrus Cooper

Chapter 7
Aging and Changes in Cortical Mass and Structure

R. Bruce Martin

Chapter 8

Skeletal Effects of Exercise in Men

Belinda Beck and Robert Marcus

Chapter 9

Insulin-like Growth Factors and Bone: Implications for the Pathogenesis and Treatment of Osteoporosis

Clifford J. Rosen

Chapter 13

Androgens and Bone: Clinical Aspects

Eric S. Orwoll

Chapter 14

Estrogens and Bone Health

Patrick M. Doran, Russell T. Turner, B. Lawrence Riggs, and Sundeep Khosla

Chapter 15

Age-Related Changes in Bone Remodeling

Torben Steiniche and Erik F. Eriksen

Chapter 16
Trabecular Microarchitecture and Aging
Lis Mosekilde

Chapter 17
Risk Factors for Low Bone Mass in Men
Tuan V. Nguyen and John A. Eisman

Chapter 18

Risk Factors for Fractures in Men

Jane A. Cauley and Joseph M. Zmuda

Chapter 19

Idiopathic Osteoporosis in Men

John P. Bilezikian, Etah S. Kurland, and Clifford J. Rosen

Chapter 20
Glucocorticoids and Osteoporosis

Ian R. Reid

Chapter 21
Alcohol

Robert F. Klein

Chapter 22

Hypercalciuria and Bone Disease

Joseph E. Zerwekh

Chapter 23

Secondary Causes of Osteoporosis

Peter R. Ebeling

Chapter 24

The Assessment of Bone Mass in Men

Philip D. Ross, Antonio Lombardi, and Debra Freedholm

Chapter 25

The Clinical Evaluation of Osteoporosis in Men

Eric S. Orwoll

Chapter 26

The Prevention and Therapy of Osteoporosis in Men

Eric S. Orwoll

Contributors

Numbers in parentheses indicate the pages on which the authors' contributions begin.

Frazer Anderson (29) Department of Geriatric Medicine, Southampton General Hospital, Southampton SO16 6YD, United Kingdom

Belinda Beck (129) Musculoskeletal Research Laboratory, Veterans Affairs Medical Center, Palo Alto, California 94304

Daniel D. Bikle (179) Department of Medicine, University of California, San Francisco; and Division of Endocrinology, Veterans Affairs Medical Center, San Francisco, California 94121

John P. Bilezikian (395) Division of Endocrinology, College of Physicians and Surgeons, Columbia University, New York, New York 10032

Jane A. Cauley (363) Department of Epidemiology, University of Pittsburgh, Pittsburgh, Pennsylvania 15261

Cyrus Cooper (29) Medical Research Council Environmental Epidemiology Unit, University of Southampton, Southampton General Hospital, Southampton SO16 6YD, United Kingdom

Bess Dawson-Hughes (197) Calcium and Bone Metabolism Laboratory, USDA Nutrition Center at Tufts University, Boston, Massachusetts 02111

Patrick M. Doran (275) Endocrine Research Unit, Division of Endocrinology and Metabolism, Mayo Clinic and Mayo Foundation, Rochester, Minnesota 55905

Peter R. Ebeling (483) Department of Diabetes and Endocrinology, The Royal Melbourne Hospital, Parkville 3050, Victoria, Australia

John A. Eisman (335) Bone and Mineral Research Division, Garvan Institute of Medical Research, St. Vincent's Hospital, Sydney 2010, New South Wales, Australia

Erik Fink Eriksen (299) University Department of Endocrinology, Aarhus Amtssygehus, University Department of Pathology, Aarhus Kommunehospital, Aarhus DK-7000, Denmark

Debra Freedholm (505) Merck & Co., Inc., Rahway, New Jersey 07065

Vicente Gilsanz (65) Radiology Department, Children's Hospital Los Angeles, Los Angeles, California 90027

Deborah T. Gold (51) Departments of Psychiatry and Behavioral Sciences, Sociology, and Psychology, Duke Aging Center, Duke University Medical Center, Durham, North Carolina 27710

Bernard P. Halloran (179) Department of Medicine, University of California, San Francisco; and Division of Endocrinology, Veterans Affairs Medical Center, San Francisco, California 94121

Sundeep Khosla (275) Endocrine Research Unit, Division of Endocrinology and Metabolism, Mayo Clinic and Mayo Foundation, Rochester, Minnesota 55905

Robert F. Klein (437) Oregon Health Sciences University, Portland VA Medical Center, Portland, Oregon 97201

Etah S. Kurland (395) College of Physicians and Surgeons, Columbia University, New York, New York 10032

Antonio Lombardi (505) Merck & Co., Inc., Rahway, New Jersey 07065

Robert Marcus (129) Stanford University School of Medicine, Veterans Affairs Medical Center, Palo Alto, California 94304

R. Bruce Martin (111) Orthopaedic Research Laboratories, University of California at Davis Medical Center, Sacramento, California 95817

L. Joseph Melton III (1) Mayo Clinic and Mayo Foundation, Rochester, Minnesota 55905

Lis Mosekilde (313) Department of Cell Biology, Institute of Anatomy, University of Aarhus, DK-8000 Aarhus, Denmark

Tuan V. Nguyen (335) Wright State University School of Medicine, Yellow Springs, Ohio 45387

Eric S. Orwoll (211, 247, 527, 553) Bone and Mineral Unit, Department of Medicine, Oregon Health Sciences University, Portland VA Medical Center, Portland, Oregon 97207

Ian R. Reid (417) Department of Medicine, University of Auckland, Auckland, New Zealand

B. Lawrence Riggs (275) Endocrine Research Unit, Division of Endocrinology and Metabolism, Mayo Clinic and Mayo Foundation, Rochester, Minnesota 55905

Clifford J. Rosen (157, 395) Maine Center for Osteoporosis Research and Education, St. Joseph Hospital, Bangor, Maine 04401

Philip D. Ross (505) Scientific Communications Group, Merck & Co., Inc., Rahway, New Jersey 07065

Ego Seeman (87) Department of Endocrinology, Austin and Repatriation Medical Center, University of Melbourne, Heidelberg, Melbourne 3084, Victoria, Australia

Torben Steiniche (299) University Department of Endocrinology, Aarhus Amtssygehus, University Department of Pathology, Aarhus Kommune-hospital, Aarhus DK-7000, Denmark

Anna N. A. Tosteson (15) Clinical Research Section, Department of Medicine, and Center for the Evaluative Clinical Sciences, Department of Community and Family Medicine, Dartmouth Medical School, Lebanon, New Hampshire 03756

Russell T. Turner (275) Department of Orthopedics, Mayo Clinic and Mayo Foundation, Rochester, Minnesota 55905

Kristine M. Wiren (211) Bone and Mineral Research Unit, Portland VA Medical Center, Department of Medicine, Oregon Health Sciences University, Portland, Oregon 97201

Joseph E. Zerwek (463) Center for Mineral Metabolism and Clinical Research, University of Texas Southwestern Medical School, Dallas, Texas 75235

Joseph M. Zmuda (363) Department of Epidemiology, University of Pittsburgh, Pittsburgh, Pennsylvania 15261

Preface

The recognition that osteoporosis is a huge public health problem came recently, but it rapidly stimulated the emergence of a major new province in biology and medicine. Professional meetings devoted to bone metabolism and metabolic bone disorders have blossomed, new journals have emerged, and the pioneering careers of dedicated early investigators have inspired the vigor of a new generation of scientists. All this research interest is already yielding substantial benefit for patients as new diagnostic methods and effective preventative and therapeutic approaches promise to dramatically reduce the personal and economic burden of osteoporosis. Even as the care of osteoporosis is becoming a routine part of clinical medicine, there is eminent promise of even more impressive breakthroughs.

Clearly, postmenopausal women bear the brunt of osteoporosis. That demographic has driven research, and the foundations of knowledge of osteoporosis are to be found in studies of older women. Every effort directed toward that part of the problem has been welcome and appropriate, but it is now starkly apparent to clinicians that little information exists to direct the evaluation and therapy of men with osteoporosis. In response to that realization, and because its study may provide a broader scientific insight, eminent investigators have turned their attention to the issue. A rapid expansion in the understanding of osteoporosis in men has begun, and this volume is devoted to that knowledge.

The goal for the volume was twofold—to summarize the current state of the art and to identify directions for needed research. Of special importance was an attempt to examine bone biology and osteoporosis in men in light of how they differ from similar events in women. It may be through that prism that accomplishments in this area can be most remarkable.

Though much remains to be done, the insights presented here should help to form the foundation for subsequent basic and clinical investigation and for the translation of existing data to the clinical environment. It is also my hope that this summary of the emerging coherence of the field will encourage its further growth and maturation. It is critically important that a better comprehension of osteoporosis in men has the potential to be of huge benefit to patients. By understanding the influence of gender, the general science of bone biology may be dramatically enriched as well.

It is important to note that this work would have been impossible without marvelous support from Academic Press. Jasna Markovac, Jennifer Wrenn, and Hazel Emery were all encouraging, patient, and extremely competent.

Eric S. Orwoll
Portland, Oregon

Chapter 1

L. Joseph Melton III

Section of Clinical Epidemiology
Department of Health Sciences Research
Mayo Clinic and Mayo Foundation
Rochester, Minnesota

Epidemiology of Fractures

I. Introduction

Osteoporosis has long been considered synonymous with vertebral fractures in postmenopausal women. Only in the past few decades has it been shown that men account for about 20% of all hip fractures and, more recently still, that vertebral fractures may be as common in men as in women (see Chapter 3). The lifetime risk of any fracture of the hip, spine, or distal forearm in men has been estimated at 13%, compared to 40% in women, and is similar to the lifetime risk of prostate cancer (Melton *et al.*, 1992). Even though it is recognized that diaphyseal fractures of arms, legs, hands, and feet are more common among men, there has been little interest in these injuries which are generally attributed to severe trauma. However, these same fractures in elderly women are due in part to low bone mineral density (BMD) levels (Seeley *et al.*, 1991). There is a similar relationship between bone density and fractures in men (Nguyen *et al.*, 1996), and a panel of

1

experts judged that osteoporosis might account for 60–85% of hip fractures in men, depending on age, along with 70–90% of vertebral fractures,
40–45% of distal forearm fractures, and 15–45% of fractures at other skeletal sites (Melton *et al.*, 1997). These osteoporotic fractures in men account
for annual expenditures of $2.7 billion, or one-fifth of the total cost of osteo-
porotic fractures in the United States each year (Ray *et al.*, 1997). Interest
has also grown with the advent of potent drugs that can be used to treat
osteoporosis in men (see Chapter 26) and with the realization that there is a
large population of men at risk. For example, data from the Third National
Health and Nutrition Examination Survey (NHANES III) indicate that 7, 5,
and 3%, respectively, of white, African-American, and Hispanic men currently have osteoporosis of the hip (Looker *et al.*, 1997). This chapter provides an overview of fracture epidemiology in men and provides a basis for
more detailed exploration of these issues in the subsequent chapters.

II. Effects of Age

Overall fracture incidence in the community is bimodal (Figure 1).
Among adolescents and young adults, fractures are more common among
males than females and usually result from significant trauma (Melton,
1995). Fractures of the shafts of long bones typify this pattern of occurrence.

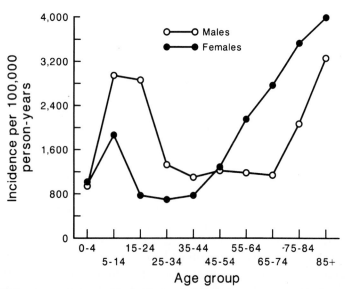

FIGURE I   Age- and sex-specific incidence of all limb fractures among Rochester, Minnesota, residents. From Garraway *et al.* (1979), with permission.

Distal forearm fractures are more frequent among males than females below age 35 years, but over this age they become more frequent in women (Owen *et al.*, 1982), as do the other fractures that have been associated with osteoporosis. These traditionally include fractures of the hip and spine (Melton, 1995) but, as mentioned earlier, essentially all fractures in elderly women are associated with low bone density. Men also lose bone with aging (see Chapter 18). Moreover, most limb fractures are the result of falls, and the risk of falling increases with aging in men as well as women (Winner *et al.*, 1989). Consequently, there are age-related increases not only for hip and spine fractures in men but also for fractures of the proximal humerus (Baron *et al.*, 1996; Bengnér *et al.*, 1988; Donaldson *et al.*, 1990; Knowelden *et al.*, 1964; Kristiansen *et al.*, 1987; Rose *et al.*, 1982), pelvis (Baron *et al.*, 1996; Knowelden *et al.*, 1964; Lüthje *et al.*, 1995; Melton *et al.*, 1981; Ragnarsson and Jacobsson, 1992), patella (Baron *et al.*, 1996) and, in some studies, the ankle (Daly *et al.*, 1987).

III. Effects of Gender

Fractures are actually more frequent among men than women at most skeletal sites (Donaldson *et al.*, 1990). Fractures of the hands and feet, for example, are nearly three times more common among men (Garraway *et al.*, 1979); over a third of these fractures are incurred during recreational and sporting activities, whereas another fifth are related to crush injuries, often occupational. Only for fractures of the proximal humerus, distal forearm, pelvis, and proximal femur are rates greater among women (Table I). For these four sites combined, the incidence was over 60% greater among women, and, because there are many more elderly women than men, the female excess in the actual number of cases is even higher. The greater risk of these fractures in women has been attributed both to lower average bone mass compared to men as well as a greater risk of falling (see Chapter 18). Data from NHANES III show that total hip BMD is 12–13% greater in white, African-American, and Hispanic men compared to women of the same ethnicity (Looker *et al.*, 1995), whereas the risk of falling at any age above 65 years is 10–70% greater among women (Winner *et al.*, 1989). This may not be true in all populations, however. Among the Maori in New Zealand, men and women have similar hip fracture incidence rates (Stott and Gray, 1980), whereas hip fracture rates are higher among Bantu men in South Africa (Solomon, 1968) and Chinese and Malay men in Singapore (Wong, 1964). Most studies show that prevalence rates for vertebral fractures are similar in women and men (see Chapter 3), but prevalence rates were higher in men in two surveys in rural North Dakota, where farming was the primary occupation (Bernstein *et al.*, 1966). When all fractures are

TABLE I   Average Annual Incidence (per 100,000 population) of Fractures at Different Sites among Men and Women in Leicestershire, England

Fracture sites	Males	Females	Ratio male:female
Radius and ulna (lower end)	182	243	0.8
Neck of femur	39	121	0.3
Ankle	87	65	1.3
Humerus (other than upper end)	36	36	1.0
Metacarpals	117	19	6.2
Tarsals and metatarsals	73	52	1.4
Radius and ulna (upper end and shaft)	61	55	1.1
Clavicle	67	32	2.1
Skull	69	23	3.0
Tibia and fibula (shaft)	58	24	2.4
Carpals	44	19	2.3
Femoral shaft	34	29	1.2
Tibia and fibula (upper end)	34	19	1.8
Chest	25	11	2.3
Spine	19	12	1.6
Pelvis	16	18	0.9
Patella	14	8	1.8
Phalanges of foot	15	7	2.1
Scapula	8	2	4.0
Humerus (upper end)	22	40	0.6
All other sites	170	60	2.8
All sites	1002	810	1.2

Modified from Donaldson *et al.* (1990), with permission.

considered, however, the actual number in men exceeds that in women by 10–20% (Donaldson *et al.*, 1990; Garraway *et al.*, 1979).

IV. Effects of Race

Within each gender, fracture rates are usually highest for whites and lower for other ethnic groups, as illustrated for hip fractures in Figure 2. Rates are high among persons of northern European extraction whether they live in North America, Scandinavia, New Zealand, or South Africa (Melton, 1991). Conversely, hip fracture incidence is very low among the Maori people in New Zealand (Stott and Gray, 1980) and the Bantu in South Africa (Solomon, 1968). The lower incidence among African-Americans (Farmer *et al.*, 1984; Griffin *et al.*, 1992; Jacobsen *et al.*, 1990a; Rodriguez *et al.*, 1989; Silverman and Madison, 1988), has been explained on the basis of their greater bone mass. In NHANES III, for example, total hip BMD was 10% greater in African-Americans compared to whites of each sex (Looker *et al.*,

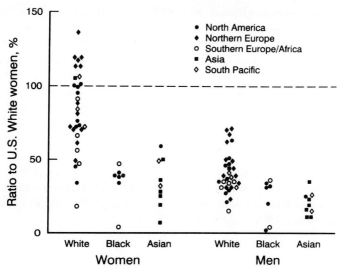

FIGURE 2   Hip fracture incidence around the world as a ratio of the rates observed to those expected for United States white women of the same age. From Melton (1991), with permission.

1995). The South African Bantu, on the other hand, have the lowest hip fracture incidence of any population, yet have metacarpal bone density lower than Johannesburg whites (Solomon, 1979). Similar observations have been made for women in Gambia (Aspray *et al.*, 1996). Likewise, the incidence of hip fractures among men and women of Asian ancestry is about half that of their white counterparts (Ho *et al.*, 1993; Lau *et al.*, 1990; Lauderdale *et al.*, 1997; Ross *et al.*, 1991; Silverman and Madison, 1988) even though their bone mass is somewhat lower. However, racial comparisons of bone density are confounded by differences in bone size, and, when these are taken into account, there is little difference between white and Asian women (Bhudhikanok *et al.*, 1996; Cundy *et al.*, 1995; Ross *et al.*, 1996; Russell-Aulet *et al.*, 1993). Alternatively, the lower risk of hip fracture in nonwhites could be due to a lower risk of falling (Lipsitz *et al.*, 1994; Nevitt *et al.*, 1989; Tinetti *et al.*, 1988) or to other risk factors like decreased hip axis length or femoral neck angle (Cummings *et al.*, 1994; Nakamura *et al.*, 1994; Villa *et al.*, 1995).

The prevalence of vertebral fractures among Asians is about as high as in whites (Lau *et al.*, 1996; Ross *et al.*, 1995), despite their lower hip fracture rates. For example, hip fracture incidence rates are lower among Japanese women than among Japanese-Americans, whose rates in turn are lower than those of whites (Ross *et al.*, 1991). Vertebral fracture prevalence, on the other hand, was almost twice as high among women in Hiroshima compared to Hawaiian women of Japanese descent but was also 20–80% greater than rates for white women (Ross *et al.*, 1995). Few data are available for other ethnic groups. Hospital discharge rates for vertebral fractures in the United States are about four times greater for elderly whites than for African-American men and women (Jacobsen *et al.*, 1992). Likewise, the prevalence of vertebral fractures is lower among Mexican-American as compared to non-Hispanic white women (Bauer and Deyo, 1987). Forearm fractures are less frequent in African-American (Anonymous, 1996; Baron *et al.*, 1994; Griffin *et al.*, 1992) and Japanese populations (Hagino *et al.*, 1989), but there is still a substantial female excess. In Africa and Southeast Asia, however, distal forearm fractures are even less common and rates for women are little more than those for men (Adebajo *et al.*, 1991; Wong, 1965). Lower rates for African-Americans than whites have also been reported for fractures of the proximal forearm, humerous, ribs, pelvis, patella, ankle, hands, and feet (Anonymous, 1996; Griffin *et al.*, 1992).

V. Effects of Geography

Fracture rates at different sites tend to correlate within a population (Table II). Thus, forearm fracture rates in the United Kingdom are around 30% lower than those in the United States, as are hip fracture rates (Melton, 1995). More difficult to explain is the variation in fracture incidence within populations. For example, hip fracture rates vary more than sevenfold from

TABLE II   Age-Adjusted[a] Incidence (per 100,000 per year) of Distal Forearm Fractures Compared to Hip Fractures in Different Populations of Persons 35 Years of Age or Older

Geographic locality	Distal forearm		Proximal femur	
	Women	Men	Women	Men
Oslo, Norway	767	202	421	230
Malmö, Sweden	732	178	378	241
Stockholm, Sweden	637	145	340	214
Rochester, Minnesota	410	85	320	177
Trent, United Kingdom	405	97	294	169
Oxford-Dundee, United Kingdom	309	73	142	69
Yugoslavia				
High calcium area	228	95	44	44
Low calcium area	196	110	105	94
Tottori, Japan	149	59	108	54
Singapore	59	63	42	73
Adebajo, Nigeria	3	4	1	3

[a]Age-adjusted to the population structure of United States whites ≥ 35 years old in 1985.
From Melton (1995), with permission.

one country to another within Europe (Elffors *et al.*, 1994; Johnell *et al.*, 1992), and comparable variation has been observed for vertebral fractures (Johnell *et al.*, 1997; O'Neill *et al.*, 1996). Five of the six lowest hip fracture rates for white women in Figure 2 are from the Middle East or Southern Europe or for American women of Hispanic origin. Although the latter data mostly reflect the experience of Mexican-Americans, hip fracture incidence is comparable in Madrid, Seville, Barcelona, and Salamanca (Diez *et al.*, 1989; Elffors *et al.*, 1994; Ferrandez *et al.*, 1992) even though the American "Hispanic" and Spanish populations are not genetically comparable (Hanis *et al.*, 1991). Likewise, hip fracture incidence (Ross *et al.*, 1991) and bone mass (Sugimoto *et al.*, 1992) differ among Asian populations. An important role for environmental factors is also suggested by the marked variation in fracture incidence seen even within specific countries. Although the higher incidence of fractures in urban as opposed to rural districts has been explained on the basis of lower bone mass among urban residents (Gärdsell *et al.*, 1991), studies in America indicate that the problem is more complex. In over 2000 countries nationwide, hip fracture rates in white women were higher in the South than the North (Jacobsen *et al.*, 1990b), whereas the incidence of distal forearm and proximal humerus fractures was higher in the East and lower in the Western United States (Karagas *et al.*, 1996). More detailed studies are needed to identify the environmental factors responsible for such regional differences.

VI. Secular Trends

Osteoporosis and its attendant fractures impose a formidable burden on the medical system now (see Chapter 2), but increases in hip fracture incidence are occurring in many regions of the world (Melton *et al.*, 1987), as shown in Figure 3. In Rochester, hip fracture incidence rates increased dramatically among women between 1928 and 1950 only to fall slowly thereafter, whereas rates in men rose steadily until 1980 but have since declined (Melton *et al.*, 1996). Overall age- and sex-adjusted hip fracture incidence rates fell by almost 8% between 1963 to 1972 and 1983 to 1992 (Melton *et al.*, 1998a), and rates now appear to be stabilizing for women in Sweden (Naessén *et al.*, 1989), Great Britain (Spector *et al.*, 1990) and Australia (Lau, 1993). However, a sharp increase in hip fracture incidence in some parts of the Far East in recent decades is bringing rates there closer to those in Northern Europe (Lau *et al.*, 1990; Ling *et al.*, 1996). Rochester rates for Colles' fracture have also been relatively stable (Melton *et al.*, 1998b), but the incidence of distal forearm fractures, ankle fractures, proximal humerus fractures, proximal tibia fractures, and possibly vertebral fractures appears to be increasing in other areas (Obrant *et al.*, 1989). Detailed studies have found no evidence of an increase in vertebral fracture incidence

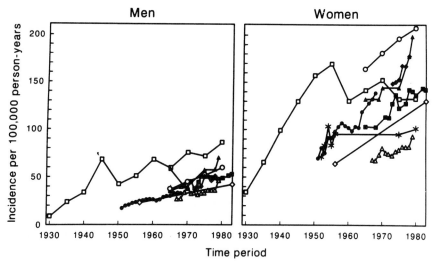

FIGURE 3   Incidence of hip fractures over time as reported from various studies: □—□ Rochester, Minnesota; ■—■ United States; ◇—◇ Oxford, England; ◆—◆ Funen County, Denmark; Δ—Δ Holland; ▲—▲ Göteborg, Sweden; ○—○ Uppsala, Sweden; ■—■ New Zealand; *—* Dundee, Scotland. From Melton *et al.* (1987), with permission.

in more recent years (Cooper *et al.,* 1992a; Hansen *et al.,* 1992), but the incidence of tibia and ankle fractures was found to have increased by 72% and 272%, respectively, in Rochester between 1969 to 1971 and 1989 to 1991 (Melton *et al.,* 1999).

VII. Public Health Implications

With continued aging of the population, the annual number of fractures is expected to rise dramatically in coming decades. In the United States, for example, the number of individuals aged 65 years and over is expected to rise from 32 million to 69 million between 1990 and 2050, and the number aged 85 years and over will grow from 3 million to 15 million. As a consequence, the number of hip fractures and their associated costs could triple by 2040 (Schneider and Guralnik, 1990), and other estimates are comparable (Cummings *et al.,* 1990). Likewise, hip fractures might increase in the United Kingdom from 46,000 in 1985 to 60,000 in 2016 (Anonymous, 1989) and in Australia from 10,150 in 1986 to 18,550 in 2011 (Lord and Sinnett, 1986). Health authorities in Finland anticipate a 38% increase in the number of hip fractures between 1983 and 2010 with a 71% increase in resulting hospital bed-days (Simonen, 1988). On a worldwide basis, the 323 million individuals who are 65 years of age and over will grow to an estimated 1.555

billion by the year 2050 with the greatest increase, from 190 million in 1990 to 1.271 billion in 2050, in Asia, Latin America, the Middle East and Africa (Cooper *et al.*, 1992b). Because hip fracture incidence rates rise exponentially with aging, these demographic trends could cause the number of hip fractures worldwide to increase from an estimated 1.7 million in 1990 to a projected 6.3 million in 2050 (Cooper *et al.*, 1992b). Any rise in incidence rates, over and above that due to population aging, will increase future fractures still further. Indeed, taking this into account, the number of hip fractures worldwide in 2050 could be as high as 21.3 million (Gullberg *et al.*, 1997). It is clear, therefore, that large numbers of individuals will experience the pain, expense, disability, and decreased quality of life caused by osteoporotic fractures (Melton, 1995). If the enormous costs associated with osteoporotic fractures are to be reduced, increased attention must be given to the design and implementation of effective control programs. The chapters that follow provide more insight into the pathophysiology of bone loss and fractures in men, and they provide essential clinical guidance with respect to osteoporosis prevention, diagnosis and treatment.

Acknowledgments

This work was supported in part by research grants AG-04875 and AR-30582 from the National Institutes of Health, U.S. Public Health Service.

References

Adebajo, A. O., Cooper, C., and Evans, J. G. (1991). Fractures of the hip and distal forearm in West Africa and the United Kingdom. *Age Ageing* 20, 435–438.

Anonymous (1989). Fractured neck of femur: Prevention and management: Summary and recommendations of a report of the Royal College of Physicians. *J. R. Coll. Physicians London* 23, 8–12.

Anonymous (1996). Incidence and costs to Medicare of fractures among Medicare beneficiaries aged ≥ 65 years—United States, July 1991–June 1992. *Morbid. Mortal. Wkly. Rep.* 45, 877–883.

Aspray, T. J., Prentice, A., Cole, T. J., Sawo, Y., Reeve, J., and Francis, R. M. (1996). Low bone mineral content is common but osteoporotic fractures are rare in elderly rural Gambian women. *J. Bone Miner. Res.* 11, 1019–1025.

Baron, J. A., Barrett, J., Malenka, D., Fisher, E., Kniffin, W., Bubolz, T., and Tosteson, T. (1994). Racial differences in fracture risk. *Epidemiology* 5, 42–47.

Baron, J. A., Karagas, M., Barrett, J., Kniffin, W., Malenka, D., Mayor, M., and Keller, R. B. (1996). Basic epidemiology of fractures of the upper and lower limb among Americans over 65 years of age. *Epidemiology* 7, 612–618.

Bauer, R. L., and Deyo, R. A. (1987). Low risk of vertebral fracture in Mexican American women. *Arch. Intern. Med.* 147, 1437–1439.

Bengnér, U., Johnell, O., and Redlund-Johnell, I. (1988). Changes in the incidence of fracture of the upper end of the humerus during a 30-year period: A study of 2125 fractures. *Clin. Orthop.* **231**, 179–182.

Bernstein, D. S., Sadowsky, N., Hegsted, D. M., Guri, C. D., and Stare, F. J. (1966). Prevalence of osteoporosis in high- and low-fluoride areas in North Dakota. *J. Am. Med. Assoc.* **198**, 499–504.

Bhudhikanok, G. S., Wang, M. C., Eckert, K., Matkin, C., Marcus, R., and Bachrach, L. K. (1996). Differences in bone mineral in young Asian and Caucasian Americans may reflect differences in bone size. *J. Bone Miner. Res.* **11**, 1545–1556.

Cooper, C., Atkinson, E. J., Kotowicz, M., O'Fallon, W. M., and Melton, L. J., III (1992a). Secular trends in the incidence of postmenopausal vertebral fractures. *Calcif. Tissue Int.* **51**, 100–104.

Cooper, C., Campion, G., and Melton, L. J., III (1992b). Hip fractures in the elderly: A world-wide projection. *Osteoporosis Int.* **2**, 285–289.

Cummings, S. R., Rubin, S. M., and Black, D. (1990). The future of hip fractures in the United States: Numbers, costs, and potential effects of postmenopausal estrogen. *Clin. Orthop.* **252**, 163–166.

Cummings, S. R., Cauley, J. A., Palermo, L., Ross, P. D., Wasnich, R. D., Black, D., and Faulkner, K. G. (1994). Racial differences in hip axis lengths might explain racial differences in rates of hip fracture. Study of Osteoporotic Fractures Research Group. *Osteoporosis Int.* **4**, 226–229.

Cundy, T., Cornish, J., Evans, M. C., Gamble, G., Stapleton, J., and Reid, I. R. (1995). Sources of interracial variation in bone mineral density. *J. Bone Miner. Res.* **10**, 368–373.

Daly, P. J., Fitzgerald, R. H., Jr., Melton, L. J., and Ilstrup, D. M. (1987). Epidemiology of ankle fractures in Rochester, Minnesota. *Acta Orthop. Scand.* **58**, 539–544.

Diez, A., Puig, J., Martinez, M. T., Diez, J. L., Aubia, J., and Vivancos, J. (1989). Epidemiology of fractures of the proximal femur associated with osteoporosis in Barcelona, Spain. *Calcif. Tissue Int.* **44**, 382–386.

Donaldson, L. J., Cook, A., and Thomson, R. G. (1990). Incidence of fractures in a geographically defined population. *J. Epidemiol. Commun. Health* **44**, 241–245.

Elffors, I., Allander, E., Kanis, J. A., Gullberg, B., Johnell, O., Dequeker, J., Dilsen, G., Gennari, C., Lopes Vaz, A. A., Lyritis, G., Mazzuoli, G. F., Miravet, L., Passeri, M., Perez Cano, R., Rapado, A., and Ribot, C. (1994). The variable incidence of hip fracture in southern Europe: The MEDOS Study. *Osteoporosis Int.* **4**, 253–263.

Farmer, M. E., White, L. R., Brody, J. A., and Bailey, K. R. (1984). Race and sex differences in hip fracture incidence. *Am. J. Public Health* **74**, 1374–1380.

Ferrandez, L., Hernandez, J., Gonzalez-Orus, A., Devesa, F., and Ceinos, M. (1992). Hip fracture in the elderly in Spain: Incidence 1977–88 in the province of Salamanca. *Acta Orthop. Scand.* **63**, 386–388.

Gärdsell, P., Johnell, O., Nilsson, B. E., and Sernbo, I. (1991). Bone mass in an urban and a rural population: A comparative, population-based study in southern Sweden. *J. Bone Miner. Res.* **6**, 67–75.

Garraway, W. M., Stauffer, R. N., Kurland, L. T., and O'Fallon, W. M. (1979). Limb fractures in a defined population. I. Frequency and distribution. *Mayo Clin. Proc.* **54**, 701–707.

Griffin, M. R., Ray, W. A., Fought, R. L., and Melton, L. J., III (1992). Black-white differences in fracture rates. *Am. J. Epidemiol.* **136**, 1378–1385.

Gullberg, B., Johnell, O., and Kanis, J. A. (1997). World-wide projections for hip fracture. *Osteoporosis Int.* **7**, 407–413.

Hagino, H., Yamamoto, K., Teshima, R., Kishimoto, H., Kuranobu, K., and Nakamura, T. (1989). The incidence of fractures of the proximal femur and the distal radius in Tottori prefecture, Japan. *Arch. Orthop. Trauma Surg.* **109**, 43–44.

Hanis, C. L., Hewett-Emmett, D., Bertin, T. K., and Schull, W. J. (1991). Origins of U.S. Hispanics: Implications for diabetes. *Diabetes Care* **14**, 618–627.

Hansen, M. A., Overgaard, K., Nielsen, V.-A. H., Jensen, G. F., Gotfredsen, A., and Christiansen, C. (1992). No secular increase in the prevalence of vertebral fractures due to postmenopausal osteoporosis. *Osteoporosis Int.* **2**, 241–246.

Ho, S. C., Bacon, W. E., Harris, T., Looker, A., and Maggi, S. (1993). Hip fracture rates in Hong Kong and the United States, 1988 through 1989. *Am. J. Public Health* **83**, 694–697.

Jacobsen, S. J., Goldberg, J., Miles, T. P., Brody, J. A., Stiers, W., and Rimm, A. A. (1990a). Hip fracture incidence among the old and very old: A population-based study of 745,435 cases. *Am. J. Public Health* **80**, 871–873.

Jacobsen, S. J., Goldberg, J., Miles, T. P., Brody, J. A., Stiers, W., and Rimm, A. A. (1990b). Regional variation in the incidence of hip fracture: U.S. white women aged 65 years and older. *J. Am. Med. Assoc.* **264**, 500–502.

Jacobsen, S. J., Cooper, C., Gottlieb, M. S., Goldberg, J., Yahnke, D. P., and Melton, L. J., III (1992). Hospitalization with vertebral fracture among the aged: A national population-based study, 1986–1989. *Epidemiology* **3**, 515–518.

Johnell, O., Gullberg, B., Allander, E., and Kanis, J. A. (1992). The apparent incidence of hip fracture in Europe: A study of national register sources. MEDOS Study Group. *Osteoporosis Int.* **2**, 298–302.

Johnell, O., Gullberg, B., and Kanis, J. A. (1997). The hospital burden of vertebral fracture in Europe: A study of national register sources. *Osteoporosis Int.* **7**, 138–144.

Karagas, M. R., Baron, J. A., Barrett, J. A., and Jacobsen, S. J. (1996). Patterns of fracture among the United States elderly: Geographic and fluoride effects. *Ann. Epidemiol.* **6**, 209–216.

Knowelden, J., Buhr, A. J., and Dunbar, O. (1964). Incidence of fractures in persons over 35 years of age: A report to the M.R.C. Working Party on fractures in the elderly. *Br. J. Prev. Soc. Med.* **18**, 130–141.

Kristiansen, B., Barfod, G., Bredesen, J., Erin-Madsen, J., Grum, B., Horsnaes, M. W., and Aalberg, J. R. (1987). Epidemiology of proximal humeral fractures. *Acta Orthop. Scand.* **58**, 75–77.

Lau, E. M. C. (1993). Admission rates for hip fracture in Australia in the last decade: The New South Wales scene in a world perspective. *Med. J. Aust.* **158**, 604–606.

Lau, E. M. C., Cooper, C., Wickham, C., Donnan, S., and Barker, D. J. P. (1990). Hip fracture in Hong Kong and Britain. *Int. J. Epidemiol.* **19**, 1119–1121.

Lau, E. M. C., Chan, H. H. L., Woo, J., Lin, F., Black, D., Nevitt, M., and Leung, P. C. (1996). Normal ranges for vertebral height ratios and prevalence of vertebral fracture in Hong Kong Chinese: A comparison with American Caucasians. *J. Bone Miner. Res.* **11**, 1364–1368.

Lauderdale, D. S., Jacobsen, S. J., Furner, S. E., Levy, P. S., Brody, J. A., and Goldberg, J. (1997). Hip fracture incidence among elderly Asian-American populations. *Am. J. Epidemiol.* **146**, 502–509.

Ling, X., Aimin, L., Xihe, Z., Xiaoshu, C., and Cummings, S. R. (1996). Very low rates of hip fracture in Beijing, People's Republic of China: The Beijing Osteoporosis Project. *Am. J. Epidemiol.* **144**, 901–907.

Lipsitz, L. A., Nakajima, I., Gagnon, M., Hirayama, T., Connelly, C. M., Izumo, H., and Hirayama, T. (1994). Muscle strength and fall rates among residents of Japanese and American Nursing homes: An International Cross-Cultural Study. *J. Am. Geriatr. Soc.* **42**, 953–959.

Looker, A. C., Wahner, H. W., Dunn, W. L., Calvo, M. S., Harris, T. B., Heyse, S. P., Johnston, C. C., Jr., and Lindsay, R. L. (1995). Proximal femur bone mineral levels of U.S. adults. *Osteoporosis Int.* **5**, 389–409.

Looker, A. C., Orwoll, E. S., Johnston, C. C., Jr., Lindsay, R. L., Wahner, H. W., Dunn, W. L., Calvo, M. S., Harris, T. B., and Heyse, S. P. (1997). Prevalence of low femoral bone density in older U.S. adults from NHANES III. *J. Bone Miner. Res.* **12**, 1761–1768.

Lord, S. R., and Sinnett, P. F. (1986). Femoral neck fractures: Admissions, bed use, outcome and projections. *Med. J. Aust.* **145**, 493–496.

Lüthje, P., Nurmi, I., Kataja, M., Heliövaara, M., and Santavirta, S. (1995). Incidence of pelvic fractures in Finland in 1988. *Acta Orthop. Scand.* **66**, 245–248.

Melton, L. J., III, (1991). Differing patterns of osteoporosis across the world. *In* "New Dimensions in Osteoporosis in the 1990s" (C. H. Chesnut, III, ed.), Proc. 2nd Asian Symp. Osteoporosis, 1990, Asia Pac. Congr. Ser. No. 125, pp. 13–18. Excerpta Medica, Hong Kong.

Melton, L. J., III (1995). Epidemiology of fractures. *In* "Osteoporosis: Etiology, Diagnosis, and Management" (B. L. Riggs and L. J. Melton, III, eds.), 2nd ed., pp. 225–247. Lippincott-Raven, Philadelphia.

Melton, L. J., III, Sampson, J. M., Morrey, B. F., and Ilstrup, D. M. (1981). Epidemiologic features of pelvic fractures. *Clin. Orthop.* **155**, 43–47.

Melton, L. J., III, O'Fallon, W. M., and Riggs, B. L. (1987). Secular trends in the incidence of hip fractures. *Calcif. Tissue Int.* **41**, 57–64.

Melton, L. J., III, Chrischilles, E. A., Cooper, C., Lane, A. W., and Riggs, B. L. (1992). Perspective. How many women have osteoporosis? *J. Bone Miner. Res.* **7**, 1005–1010.

Melton, L. J., III, Atkinson, E. J., and Madhok, R. (1996). Downturn in hip fracture incidence. *Public Health Rep.* **111**, 146–150.

Melton, L. J., III, Thamer, M., Ray, N. F., Chan, J. K., Chesnut, C. H., III, Einhorn, T. A., Johnston, C. C., Raisz, L. G., Silverman, S. L., and Siris, E. S. (1997). Fractures attributable to osteoporosis: Report from the National Osteoporosis Foundation. *J. Bone Miner. Res.* **12**, 16–23.

Melton, L. J., III, Therneau, T. M., and Larson, D. R. (1998a). Long-term trends in hip fracture prevalence: The influence of hip fracture incidence and survival. *Osteoporosis Int.* **8**, 68–74.

Melton, L. J., III, Amadio, P. C., Crowson, C. S., and O'Fallon, W. M. (1998b). Long-term trends in the incidence of distal forearm fractures. *Osteoporosis Int.* **8**, 341–348.

Melton, L. J., III, Crowson, C. S., and O'Fallon, W. M. (1999). Fracture incidence in Olmsted County, Minnesota: Comparison of urban with rural rates and changes in urban rates over time. *Osteoporosis Int.* (in press).

Naessén, T., Parker, R., Persson, I., Zack, M., and Adami, H.-O. (1989). Time trends in incidence rates of first hip fracture in the Uppsala health care region, Sweden, 1965–1983. *Am. J. Epidemiol.* **130**, 289–299.

Nakamura, T., Turner, C. H., Yoshikawa, T., Slemenda, C. W., Peacock, M., Burr, D. B., Mizuno, Y., Orimo, H., Ouchi, Y., and Johnston, C. C., Jr. (1994). Do variations in hip geometry explain differences in hip fracture risk between Japanese and white Americans? *J. Bone Miner. Res.* **9**, 1071–1076.

Nevitt, M. C., Cummings, S. R., Kidd, S., and Black, D. (1989). Risk factors for recurrent nonsyncopal falls: A prospective study. *J. Am. Med. Assoc.* **261**, 2663–2668.

Nguyen, T. V., Eisman, J. A., Kelly, P. J., and Sambrook, P. N. (1996). Risk factors for osteoporotic fractures in elderly men. *Am. J. Epidemiol.* **144**, 255–263.

Obrant, K. J., Bengnér, U., Johnell, O., Nilsson, B. E., and Sernbo, I. (1989). Increasing age-adjusted risk of fragility fractures: A sign of increasing osteoporosis in successive generations? *Calcif. Tissue Int.* **44**, 157–167.

O'Neill, T. W., Felsenberg, D., Varlow, J., Cooper, C., Kanis, J. A., and Silman, A. J. (1996). The prevalence of vertebral deformity in European men and women: The European Vertebral Osteoporosis Study. *J. Bone Miner. Res.* **11**, 1010–1018.

Owen, R. A., Melton, L. J., III, Johnson, K. A., Ilstrup, D. M., and Riggs, B. L. (1982). Incidence of Colles' fracture in a North American community. *Am. J. Public Health* **72**, 605–607.

Ragnarsson, R., and Jacobsson, B. (1992). Epidemiology of pelvic fractures in a Swedish county. *Acta Orthop. Scand.* **63**, 297–300.

Ray, N. F., Chan, J. K., Thamer, M., and Melton, L. J., III (1997). Medical expenditures for the treatment of osteoporotic fractures in the United States in 1995: Report from the National Osteoporosis Foundation. *J. Bone Miner. Res.* **12**, 24–35.

Rodriguez, J. G., Sattin, R. W., and Waxweiler, R. J. (1989). Incidence of hip fractures, United States, 1970–83. *Am. J. Prev. Med.* **5,** 175–181.

Rose, S. H., Melton, L. J., III, Morrey, B. F., Ilstrup, D. M., and Riggs, B. L. (1982). Epidemiologic features of humeral fractures. *Clin. Orthop.* **168,** 24–30.

Ross, P. D., Norimatsu, H., Davis, J. W., Yano, K., Wasnich, R. D., Fujiwara, S., Hosoda, Y., and Melton, L. J., III (1991). A comparison of hip fracture incidence among native Japanese, Japanese Americans, and American Caucasians. *Am. J. Epidemiol.* **133,** 801–809.

Ross, P. D., Fujiwara, S., Huang, C., Davis, J. W., Epstein, R. S., Wasnich, R. D., Kodama, K., and Melton, L. J., III (1995). Vertebral fracture prevalence in women in Hiroshima compared to Caucasians or Japanese in the U.S. *Int. J. Epidemiol.* **24,** 1171–1177.

Ross, P. D., He, Y., Yates, A. J., Coupland, C., Ravn, P., McClung, M., Thompson, D., and Wasnich, R. D. (1996). Body size accounts for most differences in bone density between Asian and Caucasian women. The EPIC Study Group. *Calcif. Tissue Int.* **59,** 339–343.

Russell-Aulet, M., Wang, J., Thornton, J. C., Colt, E. W., and Pierson, R. N., Jr. (1993). Bone mineral density and mass in a cross-sectional study of white and Asian women. *J. Bone Miner. Res.* **8,** 575–582.

Schneider, E. L., and Guralnik, J. M. (1990). The aging of America: Impact on health care costs. *J. Am. Med. Assoc.* **263,** 2335–2340.

Seeley, D. G., Browner, W. S., Nevitt, M. C., Genant, H. K., Scott, J. C., and Cummings, S. R. (1991). Which fractures are associated with low appendicular bone mass in elderly women? The Study of Osteoporotic Fractures Research Group. *Ann. Intern. Med.* **115,** 837–842.

Silverman, S. L., and Madison, R. E. (1988). Decreased incidence of hip fracture in Hispanics, Asians, and Blacks: California Hospital Discharge Data. *Am. J. Public Health* **78,** 1482–1483.

Simonen, O. (1988). Epidemiology and socio-economic aspects of osteoporosis in Finland. *Ann. Chir. Gynaecol.* **77,** 173–175.

Solomon, L. (1968). Osteoporosis and fracture of the femoral neck in the South African Bantu, *J. Bone Jt. Surg., Br. Vol.* **50-B,** 2–13.

Solomon, L. (1979). Bone density in ageing Caucasian and African populations. *Lancet* **2,** 1326–1330.

Spector, T. D., Cooper, C., and Lewis, A. F. (1990). Trends in admissions for hip fracture in England and Wales, 1968–85. *Br. Med. J.* **300,** 1173–1174.

Stott, S., and Gray, D. H. (1980). The incidence of femoral neck fractures in New Zealand. *N.Z. Med. J.* **91,** 6–9.

Sugimoto, T., Tsutsumi, M., Fujii, Y., Kawakatsu, M., Negishi, H., Lee, M. C., Tsai, K.-S., Fukase, M., and Fujita, T. (1992). Comparison of bone mineral content among Japanese, Koreans, and Taiwanese assessed by dual-photon absorptiometry. *J. Bone Miner. Res.* **7,** 153–159.

Tinetti, M. E., Speechley, M., and Ginter, S. F. (1988). Risk factors for falls among elderly persons living in the community. *N. Engl. J. Med.* **319,** 1701–1707.

Villa, M. L., Marcus, R., Ramirez Delay, R., and Kelsey, J. L. (1995). Factors contributing to skeletal health of postmenopausal Mexican-American women. *J. Bone Miner. Res.* **10,** 1233–1242.

Winner, S. J., Morgan, C. A., and Evans, J. G. (1989). Perimenopausal risk of falling and incidence of distal forearm fracture. *Br. Med. J.* **298,** 1486–1488.

Wong, P. C. (1964). Femoral neck fractures among the major racial groups in Singapore. Incidence patterns compared with non-Asian communities. No. II. *Singapore Med. J.* **5,** 150–157.

Wong, P. C. (1965). Epidemiology of fractures in the aged, its application in Singapore, *Singapore Med. J.* **6,** 62–70.

Chapter 2

Anna N. A. Tosteson
Clinical Research Section
Department of Medicine and Center for the Evaluative Clinical Sciences
Department of Community and Family Medicine
Dartmouth Medical School
Hanover, New Hampshire

Economic Impact of Fractures

I. Introduction

In recent years, constrained health care budgets have fueled interest in the economic aspects of disease. Osteoporosis, which affects a large proportion of the elderly population, results in fractures that have costly human and economic consequences. In 1994, ten-year projections for white women age 45 years and older in the United States estimated that 5.2 million osteoporotic fractures would result in 2 million person-years of fracture-related functional impairment at a cost of more than $45 billion (Chrischilles *et al.,* 1994). These projections, which did not include nonwhite female or male populations, reflect only a portion of the human and economic costs of osteoporosis. This is of concern because, in the United States alone, there are already 1 million to 2 million men with osteoporosis and 8 million to 13 million with osteopenia (Looker *et al.,* 1997). As the elderly U.S. population grows from approximately 34 million age 65 and older in 1998 to 62 million in 2025, the total number of men and women affected by osteoporosis will increase (U.S. Census Bureau, 1996).

Osteoporosis is also recognized as an international health care problem (Avioli 1988, 1991; Melton, 1993). In England, the number of hip fractures is projected to increase by 22% over the next 15 years solely because of population changes (Hollingworth *et al.,* 1996). Worldwide, it is estimated that the number of men affected by hip fracture will increase from 463,028 in 1990 to 1,793,677 in the year 2050 (Melton, 1993). The worldwide annual cost of hip fractures among men is expected to exceed $14.2 billion by the year 2050 (Randell *et al.,* 1995).

From a public health and policy perspective, these projections make it imperative that we understand the overall costs of osteoporosis and identify economically sound approaches to osteoporosis prevention and treatment. In the next section, two forms of economic evaluation that may assist public health decision makers in establishing research and spending priorities are briefly introduced. Subsequent sections include a definition of costs to consider when assessing the economic burden of osteoporosis and a review of studies that address economic aspects of osteoporosis. Emphasis is given to the cost of osteoporosis in male populations.

II. Economic Evaluation

A. Cost of Illness Studies

Cost of illness studies estimate the overall economic burden of disease in a defined population (Hodgson and Meiners, 1982). Estimates of total costs, which may be based on prevalent or incident cases, are the primary outcome of such studies. Prevalence-based cost of illness studies are helpful for drawing attention to the overall economic impact of a disease and for identifying patterns of resource consumption. Incidence-based cost of illness studies are required to assess the economic impact of interventions that affect disease incidence. Most cost of illness studies of osteoporosis and fractures have been based on prevalent cases.

B. Cost-Effectiveness Analysis

In contrast to cost of illness studies, cost-effectiveness analyses (Gold *et al.,* 1996) estimate the relative value of alternative health interventions and identify interventions that provide good value for the resources invested. The cost-effectiveness ratio, which is defined as the net change in cost divided by the net change in effectiveness, is the primary outcome for such studies. Quality-adjusted life years (QALYs), an effectiveness measure that accounts for both length and quality of life, are recommended for assessing the cost-effectiveness of interventions in health and medicine (Gold *et al.*, 1996). Although the cost-effectiveness of interventions that affect osteoporosis and fracture incidence in women have been assessed (Torgerson and Reid, 1997), such studies have not addressed male populations.

III. Definition of Costs

The costs that are included in an economic evaluation depend on the purpose of the study and the perspective from which it is executed. Common perspectives include those of society, the patient, and the payor (e.g., insurer). The societal perspective, which includes all costs regardless of the payor, is often most compelling and relevant for informing public policy decision makers. In this section, the direct, indirect, and intangible costs that have been estimated in osteoporosis are introduced.

A. Direct Costs

Direct costs are those associated with goods and services and are often identified as transactions in the marketplace. Direct costs may include both medical and nonmedical goods and services. Broad categories of direct medical cost often include inpatient, outpatient, and nursing home care. To facilitate cost estimation for each category, costs are further disaggregated into discrete units, such as physician visits, and an average price is assigned to each unit. Direct costs are estimated by multiplying the average price per unit by the number of units consumed. Summing costs across categories (e.g., inpatient, outpatient, long-term care) provides an estimate of total direct medical cost.

To demonstrate how cost estimation is implemented, consider the direct medical outpatient costs of treating osteoporotic fractures as estimated in a recent study (Ray *et al.*, 1997). Outpatient costs included the following components: emergency room encounters, physician visits, hospital encounters, physical therapy sessions, diagnostic radiology, medications, home health care visits, ambulance encounters, and orthopedic and other supplies. To estimate component costs, average costs per unit and the number of units consumed were multiplied together. For example, the cost of emergency room encounters was estimated at \$106.4 million by multiplying the number of encounters by the average price per encounter ($219,815 \times \$484$). An estimate of total outpatient cost was obtained by adding the cost of emergency room encounters to the costs of other components.

B. Indirect Costs

In contrast to direct costs, indirect costs are more difficult to identify and measure. Indirect costs of an illness are those costs associated with a loss in productivity resulting from morbidity and mortality. One approach to the valuation of indirect costs, which has been applied to assessing the cost of fractures (Holbrook *et al.*, 1984; Praemer *et al.*, 1992), is known as the human capital approach (Hodgson and Meiners, 1982). Under this approach, lost productivity is valued based on losses in projected earnings. For example, indirect costs of fracture are estimated based on the amount of time lost from work. The human capital approach tends to underestimate the costs of diseases, such as osteoporosis, that affect a disproportionate share of nonworking persons (e.g., elderly retired persons). Although several studies have estimated the indirect cost of osteoporosis based on productivity losses of fracture subjects, these studies have not accounted for lost productivity of others who may be affected. For example, the indirect costs of hip fracture may also include time lost from work by a family member to care for a parent who is convalescing following a hip fracture.

An alternative approach to estimating the indirect costs of an illness is to assess society's willingness to pay to avoid the morbidity and mortality associated with a disease. Estimates may be made using revealed preferences or the technique of contingent valuation (O'Brien and Viramontes, 1994). These methods have not been implemented for osteoporosis health outcomes.

C. Intangible Costs

In addition to productivity losses due to morbidity and mortality that result from osteoporotic fractures, human costs of pain and suffering must be considered. In cost-effectiveness evaluations, the intangible costs of disease may be included by using quality-adjusted life years as the effectiveness measure. When estimating QALYs, each year of life is assigned a preference weight ranging from 1 to 0, where 1 represents perfect health and 0 represents death. Preference weights (e.g., utilities) reflect how health states are valued relative to perfect health and death. An accurate assessment of the intangible costs of osteoporosis requires data on preference weights for health outcomes associated with fracture (Tosteson, 1997; Gabriel *et al.*, 1999). Such data are not yet available for male populations.

IV. Review of Studies

Studies of the economic costs of osteoporosis have focused primarily on the direct medical costs of fractures and have sometimes been limited to female populations. Although our focus is on the cost of osteoporosis in male populations, no studies have focused exclusively on men. In this section, studies that have addressed the cost of osteoporosis in either male and/or female populations are reviewed. To allow for comparison between cost estimates made in different years, estimates were inflated to 1998 U.S. dollars using the general medical care component of the U.S. consumer price index (U.S. Bureau of Labor Statistics, 1998).

A. Cost of Illness Studies

Several prevalence-based cost of illness studies have addressed osteoporosis and/or fractures (Table I). Caution is required when making comparisons in cost estimates between studies. Studies differ in the populations considered, fractures evaluated, and costs included. Even though some studies assess the indirect costs of lost productivity due to the morbidity and mortality of fractures, others do not. Furthermore, although most studies include inpatient, outpatient, and nursing home costs as identifiable components of direct cost, additional components are sometimes included. Despite differences in methodology between studies, one consistent finding is the overall importance of hip fracture and nursing home costs as substantial direct costs of osteoporosis.

In 1984, a comprehensive cost of illness study for selected musculoskeletal conditions included costs associated with fractures and osteoporosis (Holbrook *et al.*, 1984). This was the first study to address the cost of osteoporosis explicitly in a defined population. This report, which was based on 1977 prevalence data, estimated the average annual number of hospital discharges in the United States with a first-listed diagnosis of osteoporosis at 26,000, with men comprising 20% of these discharges (Holbrook *et al.*, 1984). Costs associated with all fractures, hip fractures, and osteoporosis were made separately and included direct medical, direct nonmedical, and indirect costs. The latter were estimated using the human capital approach. The costs associated with all fractures in men and women in the United States were estimated at $18.1 billion ($41.2 billion in 1998 U.S. dollars). All hip fractures, not just those occurring in the elderly, were estimated to cost $7.3 billion in 1984 ($16.5 billion in 1998 U.S. dollars). Thus, hip fractures comprised 40% of all fracture-related costs. The annual costs of osteoporosis were estimated at $6.1 billion ($13.9 billion in 1998 U.S. dollars).

The first prevalence-based cost of illness study to focus exclusively on osteoporosis was limited to direct medical costs incurred among women age 45 years and older (Phillips *et al.*, 1988). Phillips *et al.* estimated that $5.2 billion ($10.3 billion in 1998 U.S. dollars) in direct medical costs were attributable to osteoporosis in 1986 (Phillips *et al.*, 1988). Age- and diagnosis-specific attribution weights, which were developed by an expert panel, were used to identify costs associated with osteoporosis. This study highlighted the magnitude of the direct costs associated with nursing home stays ($2.1 billion for nursing home compared with $2.8 billion for inpatient care, Table I) but did not explicitly value the human pain and suffering costs of osteoporosis (Norris, 1992). Although hip fractures were not costed separately, fractures of the upper femur comprised substantial proportions of all osteoporosis-related

TABLE I Summary of U.S. Cost-of-Illness Studies That Estimate the Costs of Fractures

	Includes men	Study year	Estimated total cost (U.S. $ billions)		Indirect costs as percent of total costs[a]	Percent of direct costs comprising:				Hip fracture cost per case[e]
			Study year	1998		In-patient	Out-patient	Nursing home	Other	
All Fractures										
Holbrook et al. (1984)	yes	1984	18.1	41.2	4	35	23	26	16	
Praemer et al. (1992)	yes	1988	20.1	35.2	18	50	16	17	17	
Osteoporotic Fractures										
Holbrook et al. (1984)[b]	yes	1984	6.1	13.9	7	46	4	40	10	
Phillips et al. (1988)[c]	no	1986	5.2	10.3	—	55	4	41	—	
Ray et al. (1997)[d]	yes	1995	13.8	15.2	—	63	9	28	—	
Hip Fractures										
Owen et al. (1980)	yes	1976	0.9	4.1	—	100	—	—	—	$26,400[f]
Holbrook et al. (1984)	yes	1984	7.3	16.5	1	26	2	56	16	$36,800
Praemer et al. (1992)	yes	1988	8.7	15.3	19	49	12	22	17	$36,300
OTA Study (1995)	yes	1990	5.4	8.1	—	49	14	37	—	$28,600
Ray et al. (1997)	yes	1995	8.7	9.6	—	64	4	32	—	$34,000

Table adapted from (Ray et al., 1997) with permission from the American Society for Bone and Mineral Research.
—not estimated.

[a] Estimated using the human capital approach.
[b] Includes fractures of the vertebrae, upper femur, and forearm.
[c] Includes fractures of the vertebrae, upper femur, forearm, humerus, tibia, and fibula.
[d] Includes fractures of the vertebrae, upper femur, forearm, humerus, pelvis, skull, ribs, and other sites.
[e] Inflated to 1998 from reference (Ray et al., 1997) based on incident hip fracture population of 281,423 persons derived from the 1992 National Hospital Discharge Survey.
[f] Estimate not provided by reference (Ray et al., 1997).

costs including 37% of hospitalization costs, 74% of nursing home costs, and 10% of outpatient services in women age 45 and older.

In 1988, the estimated costs of selected musculoskeletal conditions in the United States were updated (Praemer *et al.*, 1992). The projected total cost of all fractures in the United States was estimated at $20.1 billion ($35.2 billion in 1998 U.S. dollars), and the indirect costs of morbidity and mortality comprised 18% of total costs (Praemer *et al.*, 1992). The two largest components of direct medical cost were hospitalizaton and nursing home costs (Table I). Hip fractures, which were estimated to cost $8.7 billion ($15.3 billion in 1998 U.S. dollars), comprised 43% of overall fracture costs. Estimates were not made for men and women separately. Although estimated rates of hospitalization for fracture were 35–55% lower in men than in women, rates were substantial at 71.4 per 10,000 for all fractures and 41.1 per 10,000 for fractures of the neck of femur in men age 65 and older. Fractures were also estimated to result in a substantial number of restricted activity days and bed disability days for both men and women.

More recently, a prevalence-based cost of illness study estimated the direct medical cost of treating osteoporotic fractures in adults age 45 and older in the United States (Ray *et al.*, 1997). To estimate direct medical costs, allowed payment amounts for health care goods and services were used as a surrogate for costs. Indirect costs were not estimated. This study is notable because direct medical costs for hospitalization, nursing home stays, and outpatient services were estimated separately for men and women. Furthermore, expenditures for many fracture types, not just fractures of the hip, spine, and forearm, were included according to the proportion deemed attributable to osteoporosis based on expert panel criteria (Ray *et al.*, 1997). In 1995, $13.8 billion ($15.2 billion 1998 U.S. dollars) were spent on treatment of osteoporosis-related fractures (Ray *et al.*, 1997). Approximately 20% of these costs, or $2.7 billion ($3 billion in 1998 U.S. dollars), were attributed to osteoporotic fractures in men. Direct medical costs for inpatient, outpatient, and nursing home services were 66, 11, and 23% of total direct costs in men and 62, 9, and 29% of total direct costs in women, respectively. Compared with women, men had a 4% higher expenditure for inpatient services and a 7% lower expenditure for nursing home services. Further examination of the distribution of total expenditures within genders showed that expenditures were more common in 45–64 year old men than in women (21.1% versus 10.3%) and less common in men age 85 and older than in women (28% versus 36.5%). Hip fractures accounted for a larger proportion of total expenditures in men than in women (72.7% versus 60.7%). Overall, 22.6% of hip fracture expenditures occurred in men.

Estimates of the cost of incident fracture may be made in prospective cohort studies. Costs in men accounted for 21.9% of fracture costs in the prospective Australian Dubbo Osteoporosis Epidemiology Study (DOES), which began in 1989 (Randell *et al.*, 1995). This is remarkably similar to the proportion of overall costs attributable to men reported by Ray *et al.* (1997) who used administrative rather than prospective cohort data. In contrast to the recent U.S. estimate that hip fractures comprise approximately 60% of total expenditures for osteoporotic fractures (Ray *et al.*, 1997), this Australian study (Randell *et al.*, 1995) found that hip fractures accounted for only 53.5% of total direct medical expenditures for fracture. The largest components of cost were noted as in-hospital rehabilitation and out-of-hospital community service costs. No differences were found between men and women in the direct cost of incident fractures.

Another alternative to prevalence-based cost of illness studies is to estimate longitudinal population costs and health effects of diseases using mathematical models (Beck and Pauker, 1983; Sonnenberg and Beck, 1993). Such models facilitate estimates of the net economic impact of fracture prevention (Ross *et al.*, 1988; Levy, 1989; Chrischilles *et al.*, 1991; Clark and Schuttinga, 1992). One model estimated the remaining lifetime direct medical costs and health consequences of proximal femur, vertebra, and distal forearm fractures in five age cohorts (50, 60, 70, 80, and 90 years) of 10,000 women (Chrischilles *et al.*, 1994). These fractures were estimated to cost $45.2 billion ($57.7 billion in 1998 U.S. dollars) among U.S. white women age 45 and older over the next 10 years, with long-term-care costs comprising 37% of total costs. Hip fractures were projected to account for most of the fracture-related dependent function (67–79%), fracture-related nursing home placement (87–100%) and short-term costs (87–96%).

Because hip fractures are the most acutely devastating of the common osteoporotic fractures, several studies have focused exclusively on estimating hip fracture costs [Owen *et al.*, 1980; Office of Technology Assessment (OTA), 1995; Brainsky *et al.*, 1997]. These studies have identified nursing home costs as a substantial component of direct medical cost (Table I). This is not surprising given the identified role of hip fracture as a leading cause of incident disability in a recent prospective population-based cohort study (Ferrucci *et al.*, 1997). Among subjects with incident catastrophic disability (72 men and 154 women), hip fracture was among the six most frequent principal discharge diagnoses and had a prevalence of 5.6% in men compared with 11% in women. Hip fracture was also a common principal diagnosis among those with progressive disability (67 men and 145 women) occurring in 1.5% of men and 9.7% of women. One study found that men were significantly less likely to recover walking ability at one year postfracture than were women (Magaziner *et al.*, 1990). Although male sex has not been identified as a significant predictor of prolonged nursing home residence following hip fracture (Steiner *et al.*, 1997), one study reported that 45% of men admitted to nursing home following hip fracture remain there at one year (Poór *et al.*, 1995). These data support the view that hip fracture is a common and costly cause of disability in both men and women.

One of the first studies to address the national costs of acute hip fracture care addressed the cost of hip fractures (Owen *et al.*, 1980) and estimated the median cost of hip fracture in 1976 at $5,655 ($26,400 in 1998 U.S. dollars). Although use of medical services associated with hip fracture changed substantially in the United States after implementation of the prospective payment system (Fitzgerald *et al.*, 1988; Palmer *et al.*, 1989; Ray *et al.*, 1990), this study's estimate of the cost of hip fracture is remarkably consistent with more recent estimates (Table I) (OTA, 1995).

The U.S. Office of Technology Assessment (OTA) estimated that the average per-patient expenditure for hip fracture was $19,335 in 1990 ($28,883 in 1998 U.S. dollars) for persons age 50 and older (OTA, 1995). The OTA estimates of average hip fracture costs were lower than most previous estimates (Table I) but did not include indirect costs and only included the costs of nursing home stays that occurred in the year following hip fracture.

A study of community dwelling men and women age 65 and older with hip fracture assessed the costs associated with hip fracture in the year following fracture and was based on incident hip fractures between October 1, 1984, and September 30, 1986 (Brainsky *et al.*, 1997). Although costs were not estimated separately for men and women, men comprised 20.6% of the sample. This cohort study provided an estimate of the incremental costs of hip fracture, which ranged from $16,322 to $18,727 ($19,617 to $22,508 in 1998 U.S. dollars) in the year following the fracture. Thirty-three percent of the increment in costs in the first 6 months after the fracture was the result of nursing home stays. An understanding of the *incremental* impact of fractures on health care utilization, such as that provided by this study, is critical for assessing the economic value of interventions that prevent fracture.

B. Cost-Effectiveness Studies

Several studies provide model-based estimates of the cost-effectiveness of osteoporosis interventions targeted at women at highest risk of fracture (Tosteson *et al.*, 1990; Geelhoed *et al.*, 1994; Jönsson *et al.*, 1995; OTA, 1995; Torgerson and Kanis, 1995; Garton *et al.*, 1997; Torgerson and Reid, 1997; Visentin *et al.*, 1997). One study, which estimated components of costs for hip fracture prevention in 50-year-old white women, indicated that savings from nursing home stays prevented would exceed savings from acute hip fracture care (Tosteson *et al.*, 1990). Studies that estimate the cost per life year and per QALY saved have highlighted the impact that quality of life considerations have on the overall value of interventions in osteoporosis (Tosteson *et al.*, 1990; Jönsson *et al.*, 1995; Tosteson, 1997). They also have identified intervention costs and side effects of treatment as important determinants of cost-effectiveness. To date, however, cost-effectiveness studies have not focused on male populations.

V. Summary of Findings

Prevalence-based cost-of-illness studies have estimated the cost of osteoporotic fractures at between $10.3 billion and $15.2 billion in the United States annually (Table I). These estimates vary in part because of the methods used and the populations studied. The low estimate of $10.3 billion was from a study that included only white women ages 45 and older (Phillips *et al.*, 1988). Although the high estimate of $15.2 billion was not limited to white women and included most osteoporotic fractures, the indirect costs of morbidity and mortality that result from osteoporotic fractures were not included (Ray *et al.*, 1997). Thus, the true costs of osteoporosis have probably been underestimated.

Few studies have estimated costs in male populations separately, but those that have indicate that the costs of osteoporosis in men are substantial. Two recent studies indicate that approximately 20% of all fracture-related costs are incurred by men (Randell *et al.*, 1995; Ray *et al.*, 1997). In view of the finding that the largest expenditures for osteoporosis-related fractures occurred at younger ages in men (45–64 year olds) than in women (Ray *et al.*, 1997), it is possible that the proportion of all fracture-related costs that are incurred by men would increase if the indirect costs of morbidity and mortality were included.

Cost-of-illness studies in osteoporosis have found that hip fractures comprise a substantial proportion of the overall osteoporosis costs, with nursing home care representing a large component of direct costs. This is not surprising given that hip fracture has been identified as one of the top six conditions for which both men and women are hospitalized in the year in which they become catastrophically or progressively disabled (Ferrucci *et al.*, 1997).

Hip fractures have been estimated to cost between $4.1 billion and $16.5 billion annually in the United States (Table I). The low estimate of $4.1 billion assessed only acute hip fracture costs and did not include costs of nursing home care (Owen *et al.*, 1980), which account for a substantial proportion of direct costs (Table I). In contrast, the high estimate of $16.5 did not limit the age range and included the indirect costs of fracture using the human capital approach (Holbrook *et al.*, 1984). The only study to estimate costs of osteoporosis separately for both men and women (Ray *et al.*, 1997) noted that hip fractures comprised a larger proportion of total costs in men than in women (72.7% versus 60.7%, respectively).

Cost-effectiveness evaluations of osteoporosis treatment and prevention have been successful in identifying important determinants of cost-effectiveness in female populations. No studies have assessed the cost-effectiveness of interventions in male populations.

VI. Directions for Future Research

Cost-of-illness studies in osteoporosis have helped establish osteoporosis as a public health priority. Both epidemiological and economic evidence that highlights osteoporosis as an important public health problem among men as well as women is growing. To prevent the morbidity, mortality, and economic costs that result from complications of osteoporosis, it is imperative that cost-effective approaches to osteoporosis prevention and treatment be identified for both men and women. To accomplish this, additional data on the longitudinal impact of fractures on both health care expenditures and quality of life are required. Even though several studies have identified cost-effective approaches to osteoporosis among women, interventions among men have not yet been evaluated. Further research into the epidemiology, economic, and quality-of-life impact of osteoporosis in men is an important area for future research.

Acknowledgment

This work was supported by a grant from the National Institute on Aging (AG 12262).

References

Avioli, L. (1988). Socio-economic costs of osteoporosis and changing patterns. *Ann. Chir. Gynaecol.* **77**, 168–172.

Avioli, L. (1991). Significance of osteoporosis: A growing international health care problem. *Calcif. Tissue Int.* **49** (Suppl.), S5–S7.

Beck, J., and Pauker, S. (1983). The Markov model of medical prognosis. *Med. Decis. Making* **3**, 419–458.

Brainsky, A., Glick, H., Lydick, E., *et al.* (1997). The economic cost of hip fractures in community-dwelling older adults: A prospective study. *J. Am. Geriatr. Soc.* **45**, 281–287.

Chrischilles, E., Butler, C., Davis, C., and Wallace, R. (1991). A model of the lifetime osteoporosis impact. *Arch. Intern. Med.* **151**, 2026–2032.

Chrischilles, E., Shireman, T., and Wallace, R. (1994). Costs and health effects of osteoporotic fractures. *Bone* **15**, 377–387.

Clark, A., and Schuttinga, J. (1992). Targeted estrogen/progestogen replacement therapy for osteoporosis: Calculation of health care cost savings. *Osteoporosis Int.* **2**, 195–200.

Ferrucci, L., Guralnik, J., Pahor, M., Corti, M., and Havlik, R. (1997). Hospital diagnoses, medicare charges, and nursing home admissions in the year when older persons become severely disabled. *J. Am. Med. Assoc.* **277**(9), 728–734.

Fitzgerald, J., Moore, P., and Dittus, R. (1988). The care of elderly patients with hip fracture: Changes since implementation of the prospective payment system. *N. Engl. J. Med.* **319,** 1392–1397.

Gabriel, S., Kneeland, T., Melton, L., *et al.* (1999). Health-related quality of life in economic evaluations for osteoporosis: Whose values should we use? *Med. Decis. Making,* in press.

Garton, M., Cooper, C., and Reid, D. (1997). Perimenopausal bone density screening—will it help prevent osteoporosis. *Maturitas* **26,** 35–43.

Geelhoed, E., Harris, A., and Prince, R. (1994). Cost-effectiveness analysis of hormone replacement therapy and life-style intervention for hip fracture. *Aust. J. Public Health* **18,** 153–160.

Gold, M., Siegel, J., Russell, L., and Weinstein, M. (1996). "Cost-Effectiveness in Health and Medicine." Oxford University Press, New York.

Hodgson, T., and Meiners, M. (1982). Cost-of-illness methodology: A guide to current practices and procedures. *Milbank Meml. Fund Q./Health Soc.* **60**(3), 429–462.

Holbrook, T., Grazier, K., Kelsey, J., and Sauffer, R. (1984). The frequency of occurrence, impact, and cost of musculoskeletal conditions in the United States. *Am. Acad. Orthop. Surg.,* pp. 1–187.

Hollingworth, W., Todd, C., and Parker, M. (1996). The cost of treating hip fractures in the Twenty-First Century: Short report. *Osteoporosis Int.* **2,** S13–S15.

Jönsson, B., Christiansen, C., Johnell, O., and Hedbrandt, J. (1995). Cost-effectiveness of fracture prevention in established osteoporosis. *Osteoporosis Int.* **5,** 136–142.

Levy, E. (1989). Cost analysis of osteoporosis related to untreated menopause. *Clin. Rheum.* **8**(2), 76–82.

Looker, A. C., Orwoll, E. S., Johnston, C. C., Jr., Lindsay, R. L., Wahner, H. W., Dunn, W. L., Calvo, M. S., Harris, T. B., and Heyse, S. P. (1997). Prevalence of low femoral bone density in older U.S. adults from NHANES III. *J. Bone Miner. Res.* **12**(11), 1761–1768.

Magaziner, J., Simonsick, E., Kashner, T., *et al.* (1990). Predictors of functional recovery one year following hospital discharge for hip fracture: A prospective study. *J. Gerontol.* **45**(3), M101–M107.

Melton, L. (1993). Hip fractures: A worldwide problem today and tomorrow. *Bone* **14,** S1–S8.

Norris, R. (1992). Medical costs of osteoporosis. *Bone* **13,** S11–S16.

O'Brien, B., and Viramontes, J. (1994). Willingness-to-pay: A valid and reliable measure of health state preference. *Med. Decis. Making* **14,** 289–297.

Office of Technology Assessment (OTA) (1995). "Effectiveness and Costs of Osteoporosis Screening and Hormone Replacement Therapy," Vol. 2. U.S. Govt. Printing Office, Washington, DC.

Owen, R., Melton, L., III, Gallagher, J., and Riggs, B. (1980). The national cost of acute care of hip fractures associated with osteoporosis. *Clin. Orthop. Relat. Res.* **150,** 172–176.

Palmer, R., Saywell, R., Jr., Zollinger, T., *et al.* (1989). The impact of the prospective payment system on the treatment of hip fractures in the elderly. *Arch. Intern. Med.* **149,** 2237–2241.

Phillips, S., Fox, N., Jacobs, J., *et al.* (1988). The direct medical cost of osteoporosis for American women aged 45 and older. *Bone* **9,** 271–279.

Poór, G., Atkinson, E. J., Lewallen, D. G., O'Fallon, W. M., and Melton, L. J., III (1995). Age-related hip fractures in men: Clinical spectrum and short-term outcomes. *Osteoporosis Int.* **5,** 419–426.

Praemer, A., Furner, S., and Rice, D. (1992). "Musculoskeletal Conditions in the United States." American Academy of Orthopaedic Surgeons, Washington, DC.

Randell, A., Sambrook, P., Nguyen, T., *et al.* (1995). Direct clinical and welfare costs of osteoporotic fractures in elderly men and women. *Osteoporosis Int.* **5,** 427–432.

Ray, N., Chan, J., Thamer, M., and Melton, L. J., III (1997). Medical expenditures for the treatment of osteoporotic fractures in the United States in 1995. *J. Bone Miner. Res.* **12,** 24–35.

Ray, W., Griffin, M., and Baugh, D. (1990). Mortality following hip fracture before and after implementation of the prospective payment system. *Arch. Intern. Med.* **150,** 2109–2114.

Ross, P., Wasnich, R., Maclean, C., Hagino, R., and Vogel, J. (1988). A model for estimating the potential costs and savings of osteoporosis prevention strategies. *Bone* **9**, 337–347.

Sonnenberg, F., and Beck, J. (1993). Markov models in medical decision making: A practical guide. *Med. Decis. Making* **13**, 332–338.

Steiner, J., Kramer, A., Eilertsen, T., and Kowalsky, J. (1997). Development and validation of a clinical prediction rule for prolonged nursing home residence after hip fracture. *J. Am. Geriatr. Soc.* **45**, 1510–1514.

Torgerson, D., and Kanis, J. (1995). Cost-effectiveness of preventing hip fracture in the elderly using vitamin D and calcium. *Q. J. Med.* **88**, 135–139.

Torgerson, D., and Reid, D. (1997). The economics of osteoporosis and its prevention: A review. *Pharmacoeconomics* **11**, 126–138.

Tosteson, A. (1997). Quality of life in the economic evaluation of osteoporosis prevention and treatment. *Spine* **22**(24S), 58S.

Tosteson, A., Rosenthal, D., Melton, L. J., and Weinstein, M. C. (1990). Cost-effectiveness of screening perimenopausal white women for osteoporosis: Bone densitometry and hormone replacement therapy. *Ann. Intern. Med.* **113**, 594–603.

U.S. Bureau of Labor Statistics (1998). "1998 Consumer Price Index—All Urban Consumers." U.S. Department of Labor, Washington, DC.

U.S. Census Bureau (1996). "Population Projections of the United States by Age, Sex, Race and Hispanic Origin 1995 to 2050," p. 131. U.S. Govt. Printing Office, Washington, DC.

Visentin, P., Ciravegna, R., and Fabris, F. (1997). Estimating the cost per avoided hip fracture by osteoporosis treatment in Italy. *Maturitas* **26**, 185–192.

Chapter 3

Frazer H. Anderson[*]
Cyrus Cooper[†]

*University of Southampton
Southampton General Hospital
Southampton, United Kingdom

†Medical Research Council Environmental Epidemiology Unit
Southampton General Hospital
Southampton, United Kingdom

Hip and Vertebral Fractures

I. Introduction

Osteoporosis is an asymptomatic condition, which exists only as a pathological or (disputably) radiological entity until and unless structural mechanical failure under loading leads to fracture of one or more bones. The epidemiology of male osteoporosis has been little studied until quite recently (Dennison and Cooper, 1996; Melton *et al.*, 1992; Kannus *et al.*, 1996), and there are only a small number of studies addressing the clinical and social consequences of fracture in men. In this chapter we will review the evidence available on the global epidemiology, clinical impact, and outcome of the two fracture types most clearly associated with skeletal fragility in men—vertebral compression fractures and femoral neck fractures.

29

II. Demographic Factors _____

    The incidence of femoral neck fracture in men is rising in all countries for which data are available, and the rate of increase is itself accelerating in many countries (Obrant *et al.*, 1989; Cooper *et al.*, 1992a). A similar though less marked pattern is seen in the incidence of symptomatic vertebral fracture in most countries, although for reasons discussed later the trend appears to be leveling off in some developed nations. The most powerful force driving these increases is undoubtedly the extension of average lifespan which has occurred in all parts of the developed world and in many developing nations (Lau and Cooper, 1996; Kalache, 1996) during the last hundred years. Not only has average life expectancy risen by decades in this time, but the age structure of populations has also undergone qualitative change (Figure 1). This effect is especially marked in countries which are in transition from "less developed" status to a social and economic structure more in line with the Western industrialized nations. These countries, of which Singapore is a good example, typically see a slowing of overall population growth accompanied by a rapid increase in the proportion of their society composed of older people (Kalache, 1996). It is often asserted that the "dependency ratio" of such a society is increasing (i.e., the ratio of economically dependent adults to economically productive adults), and this perception underlies recent efforts in many developed countries to control health care expenditure.

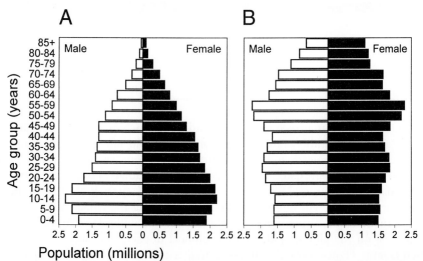

FIGURE 1   Age structure of developing and post-industrial societies. (A) The age distribution of a typical developing nation. Children are numerous but life expectancy is short and adults over 70 years of age are few. (B) The age-distribution pattern in a post-industrial society, where the proportion of children has fallen below the replacement rate and the number of elderly people is much larger, both in absolute and relative terms. Data from Kalache (1996).

However, if one takes a broader view of the relevant population demographics by including children, it can be seen that the ratio of dependent *citizens* to productive adults is changing in a less straightforward way, and may even be falling in some countries (Figure 2). This effect is associated with a redistribution of the disease burden in a given society, from infectious diseases affecting predominantly children and younger adults to degenerative diseases of old age.

Insofar as the slow decrease in bone mineral density (BMD) from the fourth decade onward can be regarded as an age-related change rather than a pathological event, the rising absolute number of osteoporotic fractures in late life is inextricably though not exclusively linked to the absolute number of older people in a population. However, large changes in the *relative* prevalence of such conditions will occur only in the context of the change in age structure described previously, and it is this relative change which is of social and economic consequence to a society.

III. Gender-Specific Factors

The incidence and prevalence of femoral and vertebral fractures in men differ appreciably from that in women in most populations studied. There is a particularly striking pattern in prevalence of vertebral deformity, with reversal of the sex ratio with increasing age (O'Neill *et al.*, 1996) (Figure 3). Gender-specific reasons for this disparity fall into three main categories: differences in skeletal growth in childhood, differences in the hormonal milieu during adult life, and differences in exposure to major trauma.

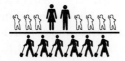

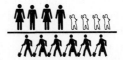

Less developed   Post-industrial
societies   societies

FIGURE 2   Dependency ratios in developing and post-industrial societies. Dependency ratios are a measure of the ratio of economically productive adults to those who are economically inactive. If the definition of the "inactive" group is restricted to older adults, then dependency ratios fall sharply as a society moves to the post-industrial model. On the other hand, if children are included in the ratios, then there is no major change. This is critical to understanding of the economic impact of aging on society.

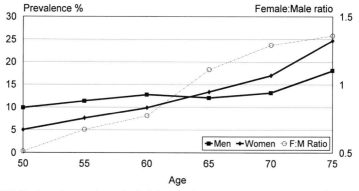

FIGURE 3   Prevalence of vertebral deformity by age in European men and women. The prevalence of radiological vertebral deformation in men and women aged 50–75 years is shown by five-year age groupings (left scale). As the sex ratio changes with advancing age (right scale) show, men have nearly twice as many vertebral deformities as women in middle age but only two-thirds as many in the eighth decade. Data from Dennison and Cooper (1996) and O'Neill et al. (1996).

A. Skeletal Growth

The attainment of peak bone mass in both sexes is almost certainly controlled both directly by genetic factors and indirectly by genetic control of hormones and their receptors (Smith *et al.,* 1994; Morishima *et al.,* 1995; Kasperk *et al.,* 1997). Skeletal size is clearly a heritable characteristic, but it is not clear whether the larger size of the average male skeleton is a result of specific habitus-determining genes (which would have to be on the Y chromosome) or whether men are constitutionally larger because of the effect of sex hormones on the agents of bone growth. The general observation that childhood growth is roughly comparable in boys and girls before the onset of puberty suggests the latter. Prevalent vertebral deformation is more common in young men than in young women, probably mainly as a result of trauma, but it may be that the axial skeleton of men in their early twenties is more sensitive to traumatic damage than women's skeletons. In eugonadal men, growth of the vertebral bodies continues for about five years longer than in women, and active haematopoietic (red) marrow is present in regions of trabecular bone formation, giving rise to a rich supply of bone cell precursors in proximity to active growth plates. There is fairly good evidence from trials of antiresorptive drugs in osteoporosis that bone turnover rates and the proportion of total bone volume participating in remodeling are risk factors for vertebral fracture independent of measured bone density (Ravn *et al.,* 1997; Riggs *et al.,* 1996), and it seems reasonable to speculate that resistance to trauma is lower in the spines of men than in women during a period of a few years in early adult life when injuries are fairly common. This might lead to a greater accumulation of minor vertebral deformations than in women of the same age whose epiphyses have closed, which are then detected in radiographic surveys many years later as prevalent deformities (O'Neill *et al.*, 1996).

The effect on peak bone mass of defects at any point in the pathways by which sex hormones act is clear, with testosterone deficiency leading to late epiphyseal closure, increased height, and low bone mass (Horowitz *et al.*, 1992). Recently it has become apparent that "female" sex hormones are also necessary for normal skeletal growth in men (Smith *et al.*, 1994; Selby *et al.*, 1996), a role mediated by stochastic conversion of testosterone to oestradiol by the cytochrome P-450 enzyme aromatase. Failure of this pathway, either because of aromatase inactivation or oestrogen receptor deficiency, leads to a physical and skeletal appearance similar to that seen in hypoandrogenic states, with delay of epiphyseal closure, low peak bone mass, and vertebral fractures (Morishima *et al.*, 1995; Soule *et al.*, 1995; Carani *et al.*, 1997).

Risk factors other than bone mass and density are heritable; skeletal structure at the gross level is clearly under genetic control, as shown by variations in hip axis length according to race and family history (Nelson *et al.*, 1995; Cummings *et al.*, 1994a).

B. Hormonal Influences in Adult Life

Skeletal growth is complete by the middle of the third decade, and after a few years of balanced bone turnover men enter a state of net bone resorption which persists for the rest of their lives. This bone loss may be an inevitable and direct consequence of skeletal aging, or it may plausibly be a result of reducing physical activity with advancing years (Silman *et al.*, 1997). There is considerable debate over whether the rate of bone loss is more rapid in hormonally replete women than in men during this period, and there appears to be more variation between individuals than between the sexes. What is not in doubt is that once women enter the perimenopause they begin to lose bone mass—and also bone microstructure—at a rate which rapidly and permanently increases their fracture risk, both absolute and relative to men.

Gonadal failure in men is uncommon until late life and is not a normal consequence of aging even then. The absence of a universal "male menopause" is the dominant factor associated with the lower incidence of fragility fracture in men of all cultures and races studied. Nonetheless, gonadal failure for any reason is associated with a deterioration in bone quality (Štepán *et al.*, 1989), and some degree of gonadal dysfunction is commonly detected in men with both hip (Jackson and Spiekerman, 1989; Stanley *et al.*, 1991) and vertebral (Baillie *et al.*, 1992) fractures. The degree of hypogonadism is often not otherwise clinically apparent, and appropriate endocrine assessment is a necessary part of the investigation of any man with vertebral fracture and is at least advisable in all but the most elderly men with hip fracture.

C. Trauma

The prevalence of vertebral fracture is greatly influenced by the appreciably higher risk of traumatic fracture in men of most societies studied. Because the radiological techniques used in many epidemiological studies offer no insight into the causation of a vertebral abnormality, it has been difficult to distinguish between fragility-related and traumatic fracture with confidence. However, some much-needed light is being shed on this area by results from recent research such as the European vertebral osteoporosis study (EVOS) (O'Neill *et al.*, 1996), although there are inevitably problems of recall bias, survivor effects, and all the usual hazards of retrospective analysis. It not only appears fairly clear that the risk attributable to trauma varies according to the fracture site studied, but it also seems much higher in studies of prevalent vertebral deformity than with clinical vertebral fracture or appendicular fractures at any site (Silman *et al.*, 1997; Cooper *et al.*, 1992b, 1993a; Melton *et al.*, 1993). Societal influences on the risk of trauma are discussed later.

IV. Factors Affecting Case Definition

There is at present no universally agreed upon definition of a vertebral fracture, which might be expected to hinder any attempt to assess incidence or prevalence.

A. Radiological—Morphometric

Prevalent vertebral deformity, assessed by spinal radiography, has been the main outcome measure of international epidemiological studies (O'Neill *et al.*, 1996; Cooper *et al.*, 1993a; Melton *et al.*, 1993) and offers a useful comparative measurement for studies across populations, but only if exactly the same technique is used to interpret the radiographs in all the groups studied. Two techniques for quantitative assessment of vertebral deformity using standardized lateral thoracolumbar radiographs have been used in population studies including men, that of McCloskey *et al.* (1993) and Eastell *et al.* (1991). Differences in techniques for reading the radiographs mean that results obtained using the two techniques are not identical and that of Eastell generally gives higher prevalences. This may account for some part of the differences in prevalent vertebral deformity between European countries and the United States.

B. Radiological—Densitometric

The task of accurately measuring the structural strength of a complex, irregularly shaped, partially hollow object of nonuniform composition which is exposed to loading in a variety of planes is one to give any materials scientist nightmares; in practical terms, it simply cannot be done. Fracture risk assessment is therefore based on indirect measures of bone strength, principally radiological measurement of bone density. In developed countries, the peak skeletal mass of men is 20–40% greater than in women, but "true" bone density is much the same when calculated by measurement of ash weight and bone volume in cadaveric specimens (Nielsen *et al.*, 1980). This indicates that much of the difference between bone mineral content in men and women is associated with systematic differences in bone size. The relationship between bone size and bone density is neither simple nor linear, and fracture risk prediction in men cannot rely too heavily on a technique which has been validated mainly in women without taking this into account. There are particular problems in the interpretation of BMD results obtained by dual energy X-ray absorptiometry (DXA), which is vulnerable to systematic differences in bone size because results are expressed as "areal density" (mineral content per unit area), which does not adjust for bone size in the long axis of measurement. An additional problem with DXA measurements in anteroposterior lumbar spine views is the presence of calcification outside the vertebral bodies but within the radiological "region of interest." This "irrelevant" calcium is mainly associated with osteophyte formation at intervertebral joints with a small contribution from calcification in the aorta, both of which are more prevalent in men than in women (Liu *et al.*, 1997). Both factors elevate measured BMD and thus interfere with attempts to generate risk ratios. Although authoritative working parties have proposed a classification of DXA results in men with the aim of allowing risk stratification in the same way as with women (Miller *et al.*, 1996), the link with fracture risk is not nearly as well supported from research evidence. DXA measurement forms the basis of the World Health Organization risk classification for osteoporosis in women, but there is no equivalent statement in relation to men. DXA measurements at the hip can, however, validly be used in men to assess change in density over time. Of the other techniques available, only quantitative computed tomography (QCT) routinely estimates true volumetric density, but the extra information obtained on bone size has not generally been incorporated into fracture risk assessment because of lack of evidence regarding the nature of the relationship. In any case, the relatively large radiation dosage associated with QCT has proved a barrier to widespread acceptance of the technique in lower risk subjects.

C. Clinical

It is estimated that only about 30% of incident vertebral deformations are diagnosed contemporaneously (Ross, 1997). This does not necessarily mean that the other 70% of events are asymptomatic; many of those afflicted probably resort to self-medication and rest and an unknown proportion are

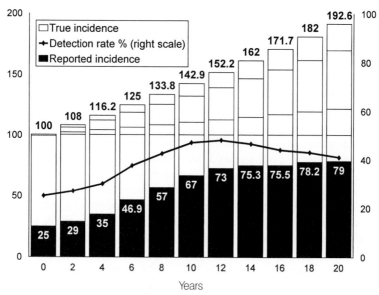

FIGURE 4 A model of the effect of physician awareness of vertebral osteoporosis on reported rates of osteoporotic vertebral fracture. Increasing awareness of a condition affects its
reported incidence. If the rate of vertebral fracture increases annually as a result of population
growth (1%), relative increase in the elderly (2%), and rising age-specific incidence (1%), the
true incidence would increase steadily as shown. If awareness of the condition improved quickly
over a short period, the detection rate could change nonlinearly, leading to a rapid rise in
reported rates followed by a leveling-off.

misdiagnosed by their medical practitioners as having a lesion of the spinal
ligaments or intervertebral discs. The proportion of those with back pain
who present to a doctor and the proportion whose lesion is correctly diagnosed at presentation are both highly likely to vary according to social factors and medical knowledge. The increasing awareness among the health
care professions and their patients of osteoporosis as a condition relevant to
men has very probably affected the reported incidence of clinical vertebral
fractures, although the size of this effect is by definition impossible to judge.
If a point is reached where most medical practitioners are aware of osteoporosis, there will be a leveling-off of reported rates regardless of the underlying
incidence (Figure 4). Data on clinical vertebral fractures, particularly on secular trends in incidence, must therefore be viewed with considerable caution.

V. Social and Economic Factors

Many aspects of the structure of a society affect the risk of fracture,
acting at various points on the pathway from risk of trauma to skeletal

fragility. Most of these effects are at least partly gender-specific; occupation, diet, exercise and risk behaviors are all influenced by social attitudes to gender roles. Economic conditions prevailing during the working lifetime of a typical male citizen may have interacting influences on the risks of vertebral fracture; for example, in recessionary conditions, unemployment reduces the risk of exposure to trauma but reduces activity levels and increases the likelihood of poor dietary intake of important nutrients.

A. Occupation

The aetiology of trauma of sufficient severity to cause vertebral deformation in men with "normal" bone mineral density and no other conditions detrimental to bone quality is very poorly understood. A review of the literature would suggest that most of these injuries are a result of playing hazardous sports, but this clearly reflects publication bias. Among the factors which are capable of accounting for the very large numbers of vertebral deformities detected in EVOS, the strongest contender is occupational injury, particularly among workers in the classic heavy industries of steelmaking, shipbuilding and mining, the construction industry, and agriculture. This kind of personal history will probably be familiar to many clinicians who see male patients with vertebral deformities, but the evidence is sparse to nonexistent. Road traffic accidents may also be a significant factor. There are therefore significant social and demographic influences on the prevalence of traumatic vertebral fracture between populations depending on the size of the labor force in "at risk" occupations within each country. There is evidence in the results from the EVOS study (O'Neill *et al.*, 1996) that European countries which have undergone a transition to an economy based on value-additive manufacture and service industries have a lower total prevalence and a different age distribution of male vertebral deformation when compared to countries whose economies still rely primarily on extractive industries and heavy engineering (Figure 5), but the association with occupation is not proven as yet. One unavoidable gap in the EVOS data is that it tells us relatively little about vertebral fracture prevalence in predominantly agrarian societies because none of the participating centers were based in countries with a substantial proportion of the workforce employed in agriculture— the agricultural workforce within countries studied ranging from less than 1% of the total up to a maximum of 22% in Greece (Anonymous, 1998). In a given economy farm workers will benefit from sunlight exposure, regular physical exercise, and possibly better diet than an office or factory worker. This is partially offset by lower socioeconomic status for agricultural workers in most cultures and by a greater risk of trauma. Data on fracture prevalence and BMD collected from agrarian populations in less developed countries (Lau and Cooper, 1996; Solomon, 1979; Bloom and Pogrund, 1982; Aspray *et al.*, 1996) cannot be compared directly either to nonwhite urban popula-

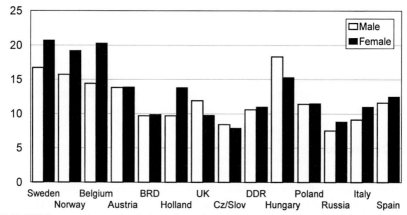

FIGURE 5   Prevalence of radiological vertebral deformation in men and women aged 50 to 75 years, selected from the general population in the European vertebral osteoporosis study. BRD, former West Germany; DDR, former East Germany; UK, United Kingdom; Cz/Slov, Czech and Slovak republics. Data from O'Neill *et al.* (1996).

tions (Daniels *et al.*, 1995; Cummings *et al.*, 1994b) or to European or U.S. data because there are invariably large differences in ethnic composition or social structure of the populations studied. Direct comparisons could perhaps be made where ethnically concordant populations have been exposed to discordant social and environmental influences—one example would be Chinese citizens of Hong Kong island and of Guangdong province on the mainland—but there are too many other factors involved for this to be a straightforward undertaking.

B. Diet

The dietary components which are relevant to skeletal health—calcium, vitamin D, and protein—are obtained from a variety of sources. There are large variations among societies in the availability of these nutrients, and within a society there are often culturally determined gender-specific differences in their distribution, particularly in times of hardship. Although severe protein-energy malnutrition is now rare in developed countries, this has not always been the case during the lifespan of our older citizens. Whether the nutritional needs of males or females were given priority at such times may have affected skeletal health, especially in those who were peripubertal at the time. However, the effect of a given set of adverse circumstances may be unpredictable and even counter-intuitive, for example, the average British diet during the period of food rationing during and after the Second World War was appreciably better in nutritional terms than in the preceding years because of a more equitable distribution of supplies and the national implementation of nutritional guidelines. Serving military personnel (mostly young men) were favored in food distribution, as is often the case in times of conflict. However, women who contributed to the war effort by becoming agricultural workers (the "Land Army") had opportunities to supplement their rations which were not available to those working in manufacture.

It is clear that cross-sectional dietary surveys must be limited by the complex interplay of cultural factors within and among societies during the lifespan of older adults.

C. Exercise

Exercise is important for skeletal growth and maintenance, and in Western societies this century, men have had a greater average level of physical exercise than women. Physical labor as part of an occupation has been much more important than recreational activity until recently, but the number of men engaged in physically taxing employment has been falling for a generation, and the gender difference is narrowing (Cooper *et al.*, 1990). However, this observation cannot be generalized to other cultures; in many societies, particularly those reliant on subsistence agriculture, women perform much more physical work than men (Anonymous, 1998). Continuing physical activity in late life is consistently shown to be negatively correlated with fracture risk, but causality is difficult to establish for this association because of the potential for confounding by poor general physical health (Grisso *et al.*, 1997; Nguyen *et al.*, 1996; Jaglal *et al.*, 1993).

D. Leisure Activities

Smoking and excessive alcohol consumption are important risk factors for osteoporosis and fracture (Kiel *et al.*, 1996; Diaz *et al.*, 1997). Both activities are more prevalent in men in all societies where they are permitted.

Sporting and other outdoor leisure activities are also pursued more frequently by men and would generally be expected to have a favorable effect on bone health as a result of exercise and sunlight exposure. Unfortunately, this benefit is probably at least partially offset by an increased risk of fracture as a result of trauma (Silman *et al.*, 1997).

VI. Falls

The vast majority of osteoporosis-related fractures occur as a result of a fall. Factors which influence the likelihood of falling are therefore important contributors to overall fracture risk, especially in older patients and those who have already sustained a nonvertebral fracture. Separately, factors associated with protective responses and with force transmission from the im-

TABLE I   Risk Factors for Hip Fracture in Men[a]

Risk factor	Unit[b]	Odds ratio	Adjusted odds ratio[c]	Mechanism		
				Frailty	Falls	Bone quality
Femoral neck BMD	−1 s.d.	1.4–2.4	—	±	—	+++
Previous fracture	+/−	1.2–2.0	1.4–2.2	±	++	++
Body sway	+1 s.d.	1.16–1.7	1.13–2.0	+	++	—
Quads strength	−1 s.d.	1.23–2.2	1.14–1.7	++	++	—
Walking speed	−1 s.d.	1.4	1.3	++	+	—
Activity score	−1 s.d.	1.4–1.7	1.16–1.7	+	+	+
Activity—strenuous	+/−	0.2	0.4	+	±	+
Previous falls	+/−	1.1	1.2	+	+++	+
Visual acuity	−1 s.d.	1.5–2.0	1.3–2.2	±	++	+
Impaired activities of daily living (ADL)	+/−	4.2	n/a	++	+	—
Current weight	quintile	2.2–3.8	2.4–3.7	+	±	+
Psychotropic drugs	+/−	1.6–2.2	n/a	+	++	—
Multiple illness	>2	2.5	1.5	++	+	+
Cognitive	[d]	1.7–2.7	n/a	++	++	—
impairment	+/−	1.6–3.2	1.7–3.3	+	—	+
Smoking—current	+/−	1.4	1.4			
former	mid/low	1.1–2.0	—			
Composite scores[e]	high/low	3.7–7.2	—			

[a]Risk factors for fracture are a combination of falls risk, general frailty and bone quality. Those factors which have been associated with fracture risk in men are shown, indicating the odds ratio and making a tentative allocation of mechanism to each risk. Data are mainly from Grisso *et al.* (1997) and Nguyen *et al.* (1996) with supporting information from other studies (Dargent-Molina *et al.*, 1996; Poor *et al.*, 1995a; Cummings *et al.*, 1995; Jacobsen *et al.*, 1995; Ranstam *et al.*, 1996).
[b]Unit of difference from the mean/median, or categorical label.
[c]Crude O.R. adjusted for BMD where available.
[d]Cognitive impairment; values shown are mid-range versus normal.
[e]Composite scores for multiple risk factors; values are middle category and highest two categories versus lowest two categories.

pact site are highly relevant to femoral fracture risk (Table I). Studies have shown an increased risk in association with markers of frailty such as use of a walking aid and use of medications which impair neuromuscular coordination (Grisso *et al.*, 1997; Nguyen *et al.*, 1996; Dargent-Molina *et al.*, 1996; Poor *et al.*, 1995a; Cummings *et al.*, 1995; Jacobsen *et al.*, 1995; Ranstam *et al.*, 1996). Force transmission is influenced by height and weight independently of BMD (Grisso *et al.*, 1997; Nguyen *et al.*, 1996; Cummings *et al.*, 1995), and the geometry of bone affects the likelihood of structural failure in response to a given force, the best documented example being hip axis length (Karlsson *et al.*, 1996). By comparison with vertebral fractures, the incidence of most types of nonvertebral fracture is more sensitive to falls risk and rather less affected by factors acting on BMD.

VII. Consequences of Osteoporotic Vertebral and Femoral Fracture

Of all the consequences of osteoporosis, proximal femoral fracture is associated with the greatest morbidity, mortality, and economic consequences (Barrett-Connor, 1995). About 20–25% of proximal femoral fractures occur in men (Cooper *et al.*, 1992a; McColl *et al.*, 1998), and these fractures account for more than 85% of the total economic impact of osteoporosis in both sexes (Ray *et al.*, 1997). Although some proximal femoral fractures are associated with major trauma, there is a consensus that the vast majority occur in the context of clinically important loss of skeletal integrity due to osteoporosis (Melton *et al.*, 1997). The clinical consequences of proximal femoral fracture are early mortality and long-term morbidity. Mortality in the first six months after fracture is 18–34%, which is to 10 to 20 percentage points higher than in age-matched controls, and men appear to have a significantly higher mortality than age-matched women (Poor *et al.*, 1995b,c; Sembo and Johnell, 1993). However, in both personal and economic terms, the morbidity of femoral fracture is perhaps even more daunting than the mortality. Six months after the event, more than half of patients are still in pain and require assistance with walking (Sernbo and Johnell, 1993). Loss of independence is nearly universal because of both decreased mobility and loss of confidence (Jensen and Bagger, 1982), with one-third of patients moving into residential care or living permanently with relatives (Poor *et al.*, 1995c; Jensen and Bagger, 1982). The economic impact of femoral fracture in men can be calculated from available data as approximately one-fifth of the total cost of osteoporosis, or about $2.75 billion annually in the United States alone (Ray *et al.*, 1997; Dolan and Torgerson, 1998).

Vertebral fractures are associated with a much smaller proportion of the economic costs of osteoporosis, but morbidity is considerable (Ross, 1997; Kanis *et al.*, 1992; Burger *et al.*, 1997; Scane *et al.*, 1994). In a study from the United Kingdom of men questioned at least six months after a symptomatic vertebral fracture (Scane *et al.*, 1994), three-quarters reported sleep disturbance by pain and half were still using analgesics every day (Figure 6). No figures are available for loss of earnings. There are few deaths attributed directly to vertebral osteoporosis, but survival curves show a continuing excess of mortality during follow-up after incident fracture, which is probably due mainly to underlying disease to which the patient's vertebral osteoporosis is secondary or incidental (Cooper *et al.*, 1993b). Nonetheless, death from vertebral osteoporosis is not rare in male sufferers and is usually a result

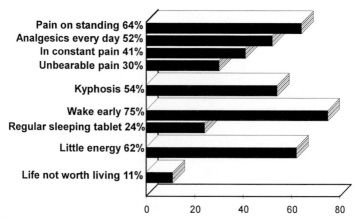

FIGURE 6   Responses to a questionnaire among 63 men with one or more symptomatic vertebral fractures of McCloskey Grade II or above, attending a metabolic bone disease clinic in Newcastle upon Tyne, United Kingdom. Data from Scane *et al.* (1994).

of a combination of elements such as respiratory compromise, toxicity from prescribed and other medications, and/or depression.

VIII. Intervention

Specific pharmacological therapy for male osteoporosis is discussed in Chapter 26, but in many patients with clinically important disease, drug therapy for osteoporosis is experimental, inappropriate, or ineffective. In almost all cases, antiresorptive therapy is reserved until the patient has been thoroughly investigated and other appropriate measures have been taken.

A. Pain Control

Analgesia is the cornerstone of the early management of osteoporotic fracture. Almost all patients require pain relief, and, in the initial stages after any fracture, strong opiates are usually indicated. The WHO "ladder of analgesia" is a reasonable guide to systemic treatment in the acute phase, and the administration of epidural, spinal, or regional anaesthesia can be of great benefit. In patients with chronic pain after vertebral fracture, the same initial approach is followed, but pain relief will be inadequate in a significant minority of patients. There is little evidence to support the use of different analgesics in combination or adjunctive agents such as tricyclic antidepressants, and polypharmacy may do more harm than good. Nonetheless, most practitioners who regularly see osteoporosis sufferers have their own empirical approach, often including combinations such as opiates and nonsteroidal anti-inflammatory drugs. The antiresorptive agent calcitonin appears to have analgesic properties when used for the acute treatment of vertebral fracture (Ljunghall *et al.*, 1991), but evidence of its superiority over other analgesics is limited, and it is costly. The role of nonpharmacological therapy for pain relief is unclear and somewhat controversial, but a trial of transcutaneous electrical nerve stimulation (TENS) will be of benefit to some. Physiotherapy, particularly hydrotherapy, may be of considerable value where there is a large component of secondary muscle spasm. Acupuncture and complementary medicines have their advocates, but proof of efficacy is even more sparse than for "conventional" therapies. Osteopathic and chiropractic manipulation would seem likely on the face of it to be actively harmful, but in fact there is no convincing evidence either way.

B. Surgery

Assessment of the risks and benefits of surgical intervention is appropriate for all nonvertebral fractures as soon as immediate analgesia has been given. In the case of proximal femoral fractures, the choice is stark: operative fixation of the fracture or nurse the patient in bed until their death, which is unlikely to be long delayed. The effective delivery of immediate care requires cooperation among specialties and among professions, with important roles for emergency room staff, physicians with acute elderly care experience, anaesthetists, orthopaedic surgeons, and nursing staff. The patient's condition should be optimized for surgery as quickly as possible, and repair of the fracture should follow at the earliest opportunity. There is compelling evidence that the steps taken in the first 48 hours after a hip fracture have a significant effect on longer-term morbidity and resource usage (Millar and Hill, 1994; Parker and Pryor, 1992; Audit Commission, 1995). However, no effect on early mortality has been demonstrated, suggesting that there is a subgroup of patients whose other morbidities may be too great to overcome no matter how optimal their care. After surgery, if analgesia is carefully titrated to the patient's needs, it should be possible to begin mobilization on the second postoperative day. Length of stay, after plunging dramatically in the 1970s, has continued to fall steadily in recent years with the appreciation that early repair and mobilization shortens recovery time in survivors (Millar and Hill, 1994).

C. Reduction of Falls Risk

Multiprofessional assessment of factors contributing to the risk of falls is an essential part of the management of patients who have sustained a low-trauma fracture (Tinetti *et al.*, 1994; Clemson *et al.*, 1996; Parker *et al.*, 1996). In the case of older patients, components of this would typically include physician review of medications, physiotherapy training to improve muscle tone and gait, occupational therapy assessment of safety in the home, and liaison with primary care workers in the community for monitoring of events after discharge from hospital. Where risk of further misadventure is high, it may be appropriate to consider moving the patient to a more pro-tected environment such as residential care or a relative's home; however, among the many problems with this course of action is obtaining consent from all involved parties. Older people place an extremely high value on their home environment (Sixsmith, 1986) and may lose the will to live if displaced—any change of address is associated with a significant early mortality.

D. Reduction of Forces Acting at the Impact Site

It is well recognized that factors affecting the impact force associated with a fall onto the hip have a major influence on fracture rates (Hayes *et al.,* 1993; Maitland *et al.,* 1993; Einhorn, 1992). Since the introduction of hip protectors in the late 1980s, there has been considerable interest in the use of strategies to minimize the likelihood of fracture in the event of a completed fall. Lauritzen *et al.* (1993) showed that in residents of nursing homes the wearing of hip protectors conferred almost complete immunity from proximal femoral fracture; unfortunately, there are practical difficulties with this ap-proach, not the least of which is persuading at-risk older people to wear their hip protectors consistently enough to derive benefit (Villar *et al.,* 1998; Ekman *et al.,* 1997). Compliance with this intervention is in the range 30–50%, although it is fair to say that long-term compliance with most pharmaceuti-cal therapies is no better.

IX. Future Trends

The enormous increase in the incidence of osteoporosis-related femoral and vertebral fractures in men is a problem which is extremely likely to get worse before it gets better. There are probably several distinct phenomena underlying the rising fracture rates seen in men in most developed countries. First, and most influentially, aging of the population brings more "low-risk" men into the osteoporotic range of bone density, which has a disproportion-ate effect on femoral fractures. Secondly, the rising age-specific rates reflect a composite of various factors influencing bone health and trauma risk whose importance we cannot easily judge; these include dietary, occupational, and social trends. Finally, increasing awareness of osteoporosis in men, coupled with universal access to health care in many developed countries (except perhaps the United States, where high-risk low-paid workers are most likely to be uninsured), is probably resulting in enhanced detection of vertebral fracture. The leveling-off of vertebral fracture incidence rates which has re-cently begun to emerge (Melton *et al.,* 1996) may represent a true effect on osteoporosis (such as dietary improvement in the last 50 years), an effect on trauma caused by occupational change or the reaching of a "steady state" of diagnostic accuracy. Most probably it reflects all of these plus other factors which are as yet unknown.

Management of vertebral fracture depends on good analgesia and the prevention of further fracture by appropriate treatment. There is scope for great progress in this area, mainly because of our lack of existing knowledge as much as the current intensity of interest in male osteoporosis. Antiresorptive agents such as bisphosphonates are likely to become established, and new drugs acting by unrelated mechanisms will probably emerge.

Proximal femoral fracture will continue to kill a large number of elderly men, and in those in whom it occurs simply as a terminal event in a process of general physiological decompensation, we have little to offer except the basic Hippocratic values of care and comfort. However, for the larger proportion of patients whose physiology is salvageable, we can realistically aim for improved survival and reduced morbidity as a result of integrated multiprofessional care by the many health care workers involved.

References

Anonymous. (1998). "Country Profiles: Economy: Labor Force by occupation. CIA World Factbook." Central Intelligence Agency, Washington, DC. Available: <www.odci.gov/cia/publications/factbook>

Aspray, T. J., Prentice, A., Cole, T. J., Sawo, Y., Reeve, J., and Francis, R. M. (1996). Low bone mineral content is common but osteoporotic fractures are rare in elderly rural Gambian women. *J. Bone Miner. Res.* **11**(7); 1019–1025.

Audit Commission (1995). "United They Stand: Co-ordinating Care for Elderly Patients with Hip Fracture," pp. 11–33. H. M. Stationery Office, London.

Baillie, S. P., Davison, C. E., Johnson, F. J., and Francis, R. M. (1992). Pathogenesis of vertebral crush fractures in men. *Age Ageing* **21**, 139–141.

Barrett-Connor, E. (1995). The economic and human costs of osteoporotic fracture. *Am. J. Med.* **98**(Suppl. 2A); 3S–7S.

Bloom, R. A., and Pogrund, H. (1982). Humeral cortical thickness in female Bantu—its relationship to the incidence of femoral neck fracture. *Skeletal Radiol.* **8**(1), 59–62.

Burger, H., vanDaele, P. L. A., Grashuis, K., Hofman, A., Grobbee, D. E., Schutte, H. E., Birkenhager, J. C., and Pols, H. A. P. (1997). Vertebral deformities and functional impairment in men and women. *J. Bone Miner. Res.* **12**, 152–157.

Carani, C., Qin, K., Simoni, M., Faustini-Fustini, M., Serpente, S., Boyd, J., Korach, K. S., and Simpson, E. R. (1997). Effect of testosterone and estradiol in a man with aromatase deficiency. *N. Engl. J. Med.* **337**, 91–95.

Clemson, L., Cumming, R. G., and Roland, M. (1996). Case control study of hazards in the home and risk of falls and hip fractures. *Age Ageing* **25**, 97–101.

Cooper, C., Wickham, C., and Coggon, D. (1990). Sedentary work in middle life and fracture of the proximal femur. *Br. J. Ind. Med.* **47**, 69–70.

Cooper, C., Campion, G., and Melton, L. J., III (1992a). Hip fractures in the elderly: A worldwide projection. *Osteoporosis Int.* **2**, 285–289.

Cooper, C., Atkinson, E. J., O'Fallon, W. M., and Melton, L. J., III (1992b). The incidence of clinically diagnosed vertebral fracture: A population-based study in Rochester, Minnesota. *J. Bone Miner. Res.* **7**, 221–227.

Cooper, C., O'Neill, T., and Silman, A. J. (1993a). The epidemiology of vertebral fractures. *Bone;* **14,** S89–S97.

Cooper, C., Atkinson, E. J., Jacobsen, S. J., O'Fallon, W. M., and Melton, L. J., III (1993b). Population-based study of survival after osteoporotic fractures. *Am. J. Epidemiol.* **137,** 1001–1005.

Cummings, S. R., Cauley, J. A., Palermo, L., Ross, P. D., Wasnich, R. D., Black, D., and Faulkner, K. G. (1994a). Racial differences in hip axis lengths might explain racial differences in rates of hip fracture. Study of Osteoporotic Fractures Research Group. *Osteoporosis Int.* **4**(4), 226–229.

Cummings, S. R., Xu, L., Chen, X., Zhao, X., Yu, W., and Ge, Q. (1994b). Bone mass, rates of osteoporotic fractures, and prevention of fractures: Are there differences between China and Western countries? *Chin. Med. Sci. J.* **9**(3), 197–200.

Cummings, S. R., Nevitt, M. C., Browner, W. S., Stone, K., Fox, K. M., Ensrud, K. E., Cauley, J., Black, D., and Vogt, T. M. (1995). Risk factors for hip fracture in white women. Study of Osteoporotic Fractures Research Group. *N. Engl. J. Med.* **332,** 767–773.

Daniels, E. D., Pettifor, J. M., Schnitzler, C. M., Russell, S. W., and Patel, D. N. (1995). Ethnic differences in bone density in female South African nurses. *J. Bone Miner. Res.* **10**(3), 359–367.

Dargent-Molina, P., Favier, F., Grandjean, H., Baudoin, C., Schott, A. M., Hausherr, E., Meunier, P. J., and Bréart, G. (1996). for EPIDOS Study Group. Fall-related factors and the risk of hip fracture: The EPIDOS prospective study. *Lancet* **348,** 145–149.

Dennison, E., and Cooper, C. (1996). The epidemiology of osteoporosis. *Br. J. Clin. Pract.* **50,** 33–36.

Diaz, M. N., O'Neill, T. W., and Silman, A. J. (1997). The influence of alcohol consumption on the risk of vertebral deformity. *Osteoporosis Int.* **7,** 65–71.

Dolan, P., and Torgerson, D. J. (1998). The cost of treating osteoporotic fractures in the United Kingdom female population. *In* "Current Research in Osteoporosis and Bone Mineral Measurement" (E. F. J. Ring, D. M. Elvins, and A. K. Bhalla, eds.), Vol. 5, p. 87. British Institute of Radiology, London.

Eastell, R., Cedel, S. L., Wahner, H. W., Riggs, B. L., and Melton, L. J., III (1991). Classification of vertebral fractures. *J. Bone Miner. Res.* **6,** 207–215.

Einhorn, T. A. (1992). Bone strength: The bottom line. *Calcif. Tissue Int.* **51,** 333–339.

Ekman, A., Mallmin, H., Michaelsson, K., and Ljunghall, S. (1997). External hip protectors to prevent osteoporotic hip fractures. *Lancet* **350,** 563–564.

Grisso, J. A., Kelsey, J. L., OBrien, L. A., Miles, C. G., Sidney, S., and Maislin, G. (1997). Risk factors for hip fracture in men. *Am. J. Epidemiol.* **145,** 786–793.

Hayes, W. C., Myers, E. R., Morris, J. N., Gerhart, T. N., Yett, H. S., and Lipsitz, L. A. (1993). Impact near the hip dominates fracture risk in elderly nursing home residents who fall. *Calcif. Tissue Int.* **52,** 192–198.

Horowitz, M., Wishart, J. M., O'Loughlin, P. D., Morris, H. A., Need, A. G., and Nordin, B. E. C. (1992). Osteoporosis and Klinefelter's syndrome. *Clin. Endocrinol.* **36,** 113–118.

Jackson, J. A., and Spiekerman, A. M. (1989). Testosterone deficiency is common in men with hip fracture after simple falls. *Clin. Res.* **37,** 131.

Jacobsen, S. J., Sargent, D. J., Atkinson, E. J., O'Fallon, W. M., and Melton, L. J., III (1995). Population-based study of the contribution of weather to hip fracture seasonality. *Am. J. Epidemiol.* **141,** 79–83.

Jaglal, S. B., Kreiger, N., and Darlington, G. (1993). Past and recent physical activity and risk of hip fracture. *Am. J. Epidemiol.* **138,** 107–118.

Jensen, J. S., and Bagger, J. (1982). Long term social prognosis after hip fractures. *Acta Orthop. Scand.* **53,** 97–101.

Kalache, A. (1996). Ageing worldwide. *In* "Epidemiology in Old Age" (S. Ebrahim and A. Kalache, eds.), pp. 22–31. BMJ Publishing Group, London.

Kanis, J. A., Minne, W. H., Meunier, P. J., Ziegler, R., and Allender, E. (1992). Quality of life and vertebral osteoporosis. *Osteoporosis Int.* **2,** 161–163.

Kannus, P., Parkkari, J., Sievanen, H. *et al.* (1996). Epidemiology of hip-fractures. *Bone* **18** (Suppl. 1), S57–S63.

Karlsson, K. M., Sernbo, I., Obrant, K. J., Redlund-Johnell, I., and Johnell, O. (1996). Femoral neck geometry and radiographic signs of osteoporosis as predictors of hip fracture. *Bone* **18**, 327–330.

Kasperk, C. H., Wakley, G. K., Hierl, T., and Ziegler, R. (1997). Gonadal and adrenal androgens are potent regulators of human bone cell metabolism in vitro. *J. Bone Miner. Res.* **12**, 464–471.

Kiel, D. P., Zhang, Y., Hannan, M. T., Anderson, J. J., Baron, J. A., and Felson, D. T. (1996). The effect of smoking at different life stages on bone mineral density in elderly men and women. *Osteoporosis Int.* **6**, 240–248.

Lau, E. M., and Cooper, C. (1996). The epidemiology of osteoporosis. The oriental perspective in a world context. *Clin. Orthop. Rel. Res.* **323**, 65–74.

Lauritzen, J. B., Petersen, M. M., and Lund, B. (1993). Effect of external hip protectors on hip fractures. *Lancet* **341**, 11–13.

Liu, G., Peacock, M., Eilam, O., Dorulla, G., Braunstein, E., and Johnston, C. C. (1997). Effect of osteoarthritis in the lumbar spine and hip on bone mineral density and diagnosis of osteoporosis in elderly men and women. *Osteoporosis Int.* **7**, 564–569.

Ljunghall, S., Gardsell, P., Johnell, O., Larsson, K., Lindh, E., Obrant, D., and Sernbo, I. (1991). Synthetic human calcitonin in postmenopausal osteoporosis: A placebo-controlled, double-blind study. *Calcif. Tissue Int.* **49**, 17–19.

Maitland, L. A., Myers, E. R., Hipp, J. A., Hayes, W. C., and Greenspan, S. L. (1993). Read my hips: Measuring trochanteric soft tissue thickness. *Calcif. Tissue Int.* **52**, 85–89.

McCloskey, E. V., Spector, T. D., Eyres, K. S., Fern, E. D., O'Rourke, N., Vasikaran, S., and Kanis, J. A. (1993). The assessment of vertebral deformity—a method for use in population studies and clinical trials. *Osteoporosis Int.* **3**, 138–147.

McColl, A., Roderick, P., and Cooper, C. (1998). Hip fracture incidence and mortality in an English region: A study using routine National Health Service data. *J. Public Health Med.* **20**, 196–205.

Melton, L. J., III, Chrischilles, E. A., Cooper, C., Lane, A. W., and Riggs, B. L. (1992). Perspective: How many women have osteoporosis? *J. Bone Mine. Res.* **7**, 1005–1010.

Melton, L. J., III, Lane, A. W., Cooper, C., Eastell, R., O'Fallon, W. M., and Riggs, B. L. (1993). Prevalence and incidence of vertebral deformities. *Osteoporosis Int.* **3**, 113–119.

Melton, L. J., III, Atkinson, E. J., and Madhok, R. (1996). Downturn in hip fracture incidence. *Public Health Rep.* **111**, 146–150.

Melton, L. J., III, Thamer, M., Ray, N. F., Chan, J. K., Chesnut, C. H., Einhorn, T. A., Johnston, C. C., Raisz, L. G., Silverman, S. L., and Siris, E. S. (1997). Fractures attributable to osteoporosis: Report from the National Osteoporosis Foundation. *J. Bone Miner. Res.* **12**, 16–23.

Millar, W. J., and Hill, G. B. (1994). Hip fractures: Mortality, morbidity and surgical treatment. *Health Rep.* **6**(3), 323–337.

Miller, P. D., Bonnick, S. L., Rosen, C. J., Altman, R. D., Avioli, L. V., Dequeker, J. *et al.* (1996). Clinical utility of bone mass measurements in adults: Consensus of an international panel. The Society for Clinical Densitometry. *Semin. Arthritis Rheum.* **25**(6), 361–372.

Morishima, A., Grumbach, M. M., Simpson, E. R., Fisher, C., and Qin, K. (1995). Aromatase deficiency in male and female siblings caused by a novel mutation and the physiological-role of estrogens. *J. Clin. Endocrinol. Metab.* **80**, 3689–3698.

Nelson, D. A., Jacobsen, G., Barondess, D. A., and Parfitt, A. M. (1995). Ethnic differences in regional bone density, hip axis length, and lifestyle variables among healthy black and white men. *J. Bone Mine. Res.* **10**(5), 782–787.

Nguyen, T. V., Eisman, J. A., Kelly, P. J., and Sambrook, P. N. (1996). Risk factors for osteoporotic fractures in elderly men. *Am. J. Epidemiol.* **144**, 255–263.

Nielsen, H. E., Mosekilde, L., Mosekilde, L., Melsen, B., Christensen, P., Olsen, K. J., and Melsen, F. (1980). Relations of bone mineral content, ash weight and bone mass: Implication for correction of bone mineral content for bone size. *Clin. Orthop. Rel. Res.* **153,** 241–247.

Obrant, K. J., Bengner, U., Johnell, O., Nillson, B. E., and Sernbo, I. (1989). Increasing age-adjusted risk of fragility fractures: A sign of increasing osteoporosis in successive generations? *Calcif. Tissue Int.* **44,** 157–167.

O'Neill, T. W., Felsenberg, D., Varlow, J., Cooper, C., Kanis, J. A., and Silman, A. J. (1996). The prevalence of vertebral deformity in European men and women: The European Vertebral Osteoporosis Study. *J. Bone Miner. Res.* **11,** 1010–1018.

Parker, M. J., and Pryor, G. A. (1992). The timing of surgery for proximal femoral fractures. *J. Bone Jt. Surg., Br. Vol.* **74,** 203–205.

Parker, M. J., Twemlow, T. R., and Pryor, G. A. (1996). Environmental hazards and hip fractures. *Age Ageing* **25,** 322–325.

Poor, G., Atkinson, E. J., O'Fallon, W. M., and Melton, L. J., III (1995a). Predictors of hip fractures in elderly men. *J. Bone Miner. Res.* **10,** 1900–1907.

Poor, G., Atkinson, E. J., O'Fallon, W. M., and Melton, L. J., III (1995b). Determinants of reduced survival following hip fractures in men. *Clin. Orthop. Relat. Res.* **319,** 260–265.

Poor, G., Atkinson, E. J., Lewallen, D. G., O'Fallon, W. M., and Melton, L. J. III (1995c). Age-related hip fractures in men: clinical spectrum and short-term outcomes. *Osteoporosis Int.* **5,** 419–426.

Ranstam, J., Elffors, L., and Kanis, J. A. (1996). A mental-functional risk score for prediction of hip fracture. *Age Ageing* **25,** 439–442.

Ravn, P., Rix, M., Andreassen, H., Clemmesen, B., Bidstrup, M., and Gunnes, M. (1997). High bone turnover is associated with low bone mass and spinal fracture in postmenopausal women. *Calcif. Tissue Int.* **60,** 255–260.

Ray, N. F., Chan, J. K., Thamer, M., and Melton, L. J., III (1997). Medical expenditures for the treatment of osteoporotic fractures in the United States in 1995: Report from the national osteoporosis foundation. *J. Bone Miner. Res.* **12,** 24–35.

Riggs, B. L., Melton, L. J., III, and O'Fallon, W. M. (1996). Drug therapy for vertebral fractures in osteoporosis: Evidence that decreases in bone turnover and increases in bone mass both determine antifracture efficacy. *Bone* **18**(3 Suppl.), 197S–201S.

Ross, P. D. (1997). Clinical consequences of vertebral fractures. *Am. J. Med.* **103**(2A), 30S–42S.

Scane, A. C., Sutcliffe, A. M., and Francis, R. M. (1994). The sequelae of vertebral crush fractures in men. *Osteoporosis Int.* **4,** 89–92.

Selby, P. L., Braidman, I. P., Mawer, E. B., and Freemont, A. J. (1996). Differential effects of estrogen and testosterone on the skeleton in male osteoporosis. *J. Bone Miner. Res.* **11**(Suppl. 1), S497–S498.

Sernbo, I., and Johnell, O. (1993). Consequences of a hip fracture: A prospective study over 1 year. *Osteoporosis Int.* **3,** 148–153.

Silman, A. J., O'Neill, T. W., Cooper, C., Kanis, J., and Felsenberg, D. (1997). Influence of physical activity on vertebral deformity in men and women: Results from the European Vertebral Osteoporosis Study. *J. Bone Miner. Res.* **12,** 813–819.

Sixsmith, A. (1986). Independence and home in later life. *In* "Dependency and Interdependency in Old Age" (C. Phillipson, ed.), pp. 338–347. Croom Helm, London.

Smith, E. P., Boyd, J., Frank, G. R., Takahashi, H., Cohen, R. M., Specker, B., Williams, T. C., Lubahn, D. B., and Korach, K. S. (1994). Estrogen resistance caused by a mutation in the estrogen-receptor gene in a man. *N. Engl. J. Med.* **331,** 1056–1061.

Solomon, L. (1979). Bone density in ageing Caucasian and African populations. *Lancet* **2,** 1326–1330.

Soule, S. G., Conway, G., Prelevic, G. M., Prentice, M., Ginsburg, J., and Jacobs, H. S. (1995). Osteopenia as a feature of the androgen insensitivity syndrome. *Clin. Endocrinol.* **43,** 671–676.

Stanley, H. L., Schmitt, B. P., Poses, R. M., and Deiss, W. P. (1991). Does hypogonadism contribute to the occurrence of a minimal trauma hip fracture in elderly men? *J. Am. Geriatr. Soc.* **39,** 766–771.

Štepán, J. J., Lachman, M., Zverina, J., Pacovský, V., and Baylink, D. J. (1989). Castrated men exhibit bone loss: Effect of calcitonin treatment on biochemical indices of bone remodelling. *J. Clin. Endocrinol. Metab.* **69,** 523–527.

Tinetti, M. E., Baker, D. I., McAvay, G., Claus, E. B., Garrett, P., Gottschalk, M., Koch, M. L., Trainor, K., and Horwitz, R. J. (1994). A multifactorial intervention to reduce the risk of falling among elderly people living in the community. *N. Engl. J. Med.* **331,** 821–827.

Villar, M. T. A., Hill, P., Inskip, H., Thompson, P., and Cooper, C. (1998). Will elderly rest home residents wear their hip protectors? *Age Ageing* **27,** 195–198.

Chapter 4

Deborah T. Gold

Departments of Psychiatry and Behavioral Sciences and Sociology
Center for the Study of Aging and Human Development
Duke University Medical Center
Durham, North Carolina

Outcomes and the Personal Impact of Osteoporosis

I. Introduction

Osteoporosis is the most prevalent metabolic bone disease in the United States, with over 28 million Americans either suffering from the disease or from osteopenia (low bone mass), the clinical precursor of osteoporosis (Melton and Chrischilles, 1992; Melton et al., 1997). Age is an important risk factor, with nearly half of all individuals older than 75 affected by this disease (Mazess et al., 1990). Although fractures of the hip threaten quality of life (QOL) more than do other osteoporotic fractures (especially in old age), all fractures cause serious morbidity. In addition, hip fractures result in substantial excess mortality (Poor et al., 1995b). In short, osteoporosis is a major public health problem of particular concern in an aging society (Ross, 1998).

A. Osteoporosis and Men: What We Know

1. Knowledge of Osteoporosis

During the past decade, the understanding of postmenopausal osteoporosis has grown substantially. This growth has occurred both in terms of basic biology as well as outcomes research (e.g., Gold et al., 1993; Roberto, 1988a). However, this improved biological and clinical understanding has a substantial gender bias. The subjects of pharmaceutical and clinical studies of osteoporosis have been almost exclusively postmenopausal women. This age and gender group has been the focus of most research on epidemiology, diagnosis, and management of osteoporosis (Melton and Riggs, 1983).

2. The Epidemiology of Osteoporosis: Do Studies Include Men?

Despite the growing interest in postmenopausal women, another group of individuals with potentially serious bone density loss has escaped the notice of many osteoporosis researchers: men. Health care providers often are surprised to discover that 20% of those people in the United States who develop osteoporosis are male (Wasnich, 1997). One of the better epidemiologic studies was completed by Looker and colleagues (1997). Using the NHANES III data, these investigators estimated the prevalence of osteoporosis in the United States for different age, race, and sex groups of men using bone densitometry. Correcting for the higher bone density of men, they found that 7% of white men, 3% of Hispanic men, and 5% of African-American men met diagnostic criteria for osteoporosis (also see Melton, 1997). The aging of the population is resulting in increased incidence and prevalence of this chronic and debilitating disease in men (Scane et al., 1993, 1994).

Recently, several large epidemiologic studies with sample sizes in the thousands have been completed. Many of them have included no males at all; others have small numbers of male subjects. For example, the Study of Osteoporotic Fractures (SOF) enrolled 9704 women age 65 or older; not a single man was included (Cauley et al., 1995). In addition, the Fracture Intervention Trial (FIT) examined whether alendronate reduced the risk of osteoporotic fracture and had a sample of 2027 women aged 55–81 with low femoral-neck bone mineral density; again, no men were recruited (Ensrud et al., 1997). A third such study occurred in Europe: the *Epidemiologie de l'osteoporose* or EPIDOS. Investigators recruited 7575 French women age 75 and older but no men (Garnero et al., 1996).

However, the epidemiology of male osteoporosis has not been totally neglected. Three recent studies included male subjects: the Dubbo study (a population-based sample of 110 men and 172 women 60 years and older in Australia) (Jones et al., 1996), the EVOS study ($n = 16,047$ with 7454 men and 8593 women in Germany) (Lunt et al., 1997), and the Rotterdam Study (a prospective population-based cohort study with a stratified subsample of

750 men and 750 women ages 55–75+ in the Netherlands) (Burger *et al.*, 1997). All had samples which included men, but only EVOS had over 1000 male subjects (Johnell *et al.*, 1997). Note also that none of these studies occurred in the United States.

3. Men with Osteoporosis: Outcomes Research

a. Vertebral Deformity.   One outcome of male osteoporosis that has been explored by several investigators is vertebral deformity. For example, Mann *et al.* (1992) studied vertebral deformity in a group of male patients recruited from a VA hospital in Portland. Investigators found that vertebral deformity was relatively common among men age 64 years and older and typically occurs in the presence of low bone density. Using a different strategy, Burger *et al.* (1997) compared deformity in males with that in females and found that, even though men had increased moderate deformity (8% versus 7%), the prevalence of serious deformity was higher in women (8% versus 4%). This study also showed that all types of functional impairment occurred more frequently in women than in men except impaired bending. The authors conclude that gender differences might result from men loading their spines differently or more heavily; however, they could not answer that question with data from this study.

Finally, Lau *et al.* (1998) examined three specific health consequences of vertebral deformity in elderly Chinese men and women: back pain, disability, and morale. This study found that the prevalence of back pain was high in men in general. Sixty-eight percent reported back pain in definite cases of osteoporosis, whereas 63% of the controls also reported back pain. In comparison, only 50% of females with definite osteoporosis and 30% of controls reported back pain. The disability findings were somewhat surprising. Men in the definite osteoporosis and control groups reported similar problems with disability (4.9%); women differed slightly across the groups (3.4% disability in the definite group and 2.8% disability in the control group). The gender differences were not significant.

Men showed no differences in morale scores between the definite osteoporosis cases (11%), the mild cases (11.2%), and the controls (10.8) ($p > 0.05$). For women, definite cases scored an average of 10, mild cases scored an average of 8.8, and controls scored 10.2 (a significant difference between mild and controls, $p < 0.01$). These findings show that morale was low in women who had mild fractures but not for those with definite fractures. The authors speculate that those with definite fractures may have already learned to compensate for their fractures, whereas the mild fracture cases are still working out their adaptation.

b. Vertebral Fractures.   Although the prevalence of vertebral deformity seems to have been studied with great interest, the outcomes of vertebral fractures seem to be presented much less frequently in the literature. Scane *et al.* (1994) found the following changes in its sample of 63 men with vertebral fractures (age range, 31–80 years; mean age = 59 years): height loss (49%), kyphosis (54%), unbearable pain (30%), thinking that life was not worth living (11%), analgesic use (52%), and sleeping pill use (24%). Using the Nottingham Health Profile, they compared the subscale scores of their men with vertebral fractures to those of two groups in the literature: same-age nonfracture controls and elderly controls. Their vertebral fracture patients reported worse problems in all six domains (energy, pain, emotion, sleep, social isolation, and physical mobility) [see Hunt *et al.* (1981) for more information about these domains].

    c. Hip Fracture Outcomes. Both the lay public and the medical profession recognize that the osteoporotic fracture that results in the greatest amount of pain and disability is the hip fracture. This is true in both men and women. Poor and colleagues (1995a) identify some of the negative short-term outcomes of hip fractures in men living in Rochester, Minnesota: early mortality (see the following discussion), loss of functioning, need for cane or walker, and discharge to nursing home. In an additional work with the same Rochester data set, Poor *et al.* (1995c) identified important predictors of hip fracture in men. Although men with disorders associated with secondary osteoporosis had a twofold increase in risk of hip fracture, conditions associated with increased risk of falling resulted in a sevenfold risk increase. The authors suggest that reducing the impact of these factors associated with hip fractures in men will also reduce the substantial human and dollar cost associated with these fractures.

    d. Mortality. The issue of excess mortality associated with osteoporotic fractures is one of great importance. As early as 1979, Jensen and Tondevold reported that 1-year mortality associated with hip fracture was 27% in men and women. A year later, Dahl (1980) found that hip fracture mortality had doubled between 1948–1957 to 1961–1970. In addition, Dahl found that mortality was related to the age and sex of the hip-fracture patient. Schroder and Erlandsen (1993) reported similar findings from their study of hip fracture and mortality in Denmark. One of their principal findings was that, although there were more hip fractures in women, men experienced higher excess mortality from hip fractures. Poor and colleagues (1995a) identified three determinants of mortality in men with hip fractures: comorbidity (hazard ratio 3.2), age (hazard ratio 1.4), and mental confusion during hospitalization (hazard ratio 4.2). They stressed that the interaction of hip fracture and serious comorbidity in men is a major threat to survival.

    Even though data exist on mortality and hip fracture in men, the same cannot be said of vertebral fractures and mortality. Cooper *et al.* (1993) used data from Rochester, Minnesota, to estimate survival of individuals with vertebral fractures. They found that, among vertebral fracture patients who received medical care, there was reduced survival; further, they noted that the odds of survival were higher for women than for men. Ismail and colleagues (1998) reported on vertebral fractures and mortality in the EVOS study. Their results were somewhat different from those of Cooper *et al.* (1993). Women had a moderate excess risk of mortality; men, on the other hand, had a smaller relative risk which was nonsignificant. After controlling for other factors such as smoking, alcohol consumption, steroid use, and other variables, the excess risk of mortality was reduced and not significant in both men and women.

B. Osteoporosis: Its Social/Emotional Impact and Quality of Life

In recent years, a major trend in the chronic illness literature has been to identify QOL as a dominant chronic disease outcome. This is especially true in studies of nonterminal, degenerative chronic diseases such as Parkinson's disease, diabetes, or osteoarthritis (Thongprasert, 1998; Tacconelli *et al.*, 1998; Wikby *et al.*, 1998). Not surprisingly, this trend has surfaced in the osteoporosis literature as well. Again we find that empirical research on QOL and osteoporosis is limited exclusively to postmenopausal women. Next, I briefly review this literature in the following order: (1) the psychological, (2) the social, and (3) the overal QOL impact of osteoporosis.

I. Psychological Factors and Osteoporosis

Osteoporosis has been reported to have a substantial impact on the psychological function of patients (Gold, 1996). In an early study on the psychological impact of osteoporosis and fractures, Gold *et al.* (1989) identified specific areas of psychological distress associated with osteoporosis; self-reported anxiety and depression were noted as recurring in many if not all of the subjects they interviewed. The sample for this study included men, but their number was so small that gender-based analyses could not be done. Gold and colleagues (1993) more specifically evaluated the impact of participation in a medical education program for adults with vertebral osteoporosis. Although no mental health component was included in the multidisciplinary program of interest (such as a support group, counseling, or stress reduction), psychological outcomes including stress symptoms and overall psychiatric symptomatology significantly improved in the intervention group and diminished in the control group after the intervention. Again, older men with primary osteoporosis were included in the sample, but the number of men was too small for gender comparisons of responses to this intervention. Finally, Roberto (1988a) also examined the stress of and adaptation to osteoporosis. Although she found substantial evidence of stress emerging from managing this disease, her sample was entirely female.

2. Social Factors and Osteoporosis

In addition to the psychological ramifications of osteoporosis, there appear to be disease influences on both the nature and the content of social relationships as well. For example, Roberto (1988b) showed the importance of social support for women in managing this disease as well as how osteoporosis diminishes the range of individual social roles of its sufferers. These findings were evident in sample members regardless of whether they had a hip or vertebral fracture. Roberto (1988a) also noted that individuals with serious disease cannot continue in their usual patterns of social behavior. One need only glance at the list of tasks that required change to determine that this sample had no males; the tasks included laundry, housekeeping, cooking, gardening, and engaging in strenuous social activities. Finally, Roberto and Gold (1997) examined the impact of osteoporosis on marriage by interviewing a longitudinal sample of osteoporosis patients and their spouses. Again, the sample was entirely female, and men's opinions were solicited only as spouses of women with osteoporosis. Thus, we are beginning to understand the social and psychological dimensions of osteoporosis in women but have made no progress whatsoever toward even identifying potential problems in men.

3. Quality of Life and Osteoporosis

Many, if not most, of the articles written about osteoporosis and QOL have been centered on the development and validation of instruments used to measure life quality, and much work has gone into designing scales that measure osteoporosis-specific QOL. Cook *et al.* (1993) were among the first to explore the measurement issues surrounding QOL in the osteoporotic patient with the scale they call the Osteoporosis Health-Related Quality of Life Scale (OHRQoL). The OHRQoL was constructed to measure the impact of vertebral fractures on women who had extensive chronic pain. Lydick and colleagues (1997) developed the Osteoporosis-Targeted Quality of Life Scale (OPTQoL) which, according to the authors, is unique because, ". . . it attempts to measure the total impact of the disease on QOL within a population at a single point in time" (p. 456). This scale measures the domains of physical difficulty, adaptations to one's daily life, and fears about the future (Chandler *et al.*, 1998). Believing that QOL issues in western Europe differed from those in the United States, the European Foundation for Osteoporosis designed the Quality of Life from the European Foundation for Osteoporosis (Qualeffo) scale (Lips *et al.*, 1997). Qualeffo was designed to be used in clinical trials and has been translated into several European languages for use throughout the continent. A final scale, called the Osteoporosis Assessment Questionnaire or OPAQ, has been created for use with postmenopausal vertebral fracture patients; it measures dimensions of QOL including physical function, emotional status, symptoms (Silverman *et al.*, 1998a). The

OPAQ and Qualeffo investigators compared the effect of osteoporosis on health-related QOL in postmenopausal osteoporotic women in Los Angeles and the Netherlands (Silverman *et al.*, 1998b). Both samples answered both OPAQ and Qualeffo scales. The investigators found no differences between the two cities in physical functioning and social interaction; however, anxiety, health perception, and self-report of pain did differ, suggesting some cultural influences on response to osteoporosis.

As is evident from the number of scales listed earlier, there is no shortage of QOL instruments in osteoporosis. Unfortunately, each of these four scales measures specific content in postmenopausal *women* with osteoporosis. A single-item QOL measure (*Overall, how would you rate the quality of your life?*) could certainly be used with men, but no norms for males have been established. The only other potential QOL measurement strategy in men would be a general QOL assessment tools such as the SF-36 (Ware *et al.*, 1995) or the Sickness Impact Profile (Bergner *et al.*, 1981). Yet those investigators who have used the SF-36 in postmenopausal women with osteoporosis have found that it does not measure some of the domains relevant to QOL and osteoporosis (Lydick *et al.*, 1997).

In a recent supplemental issue of *Bone,* a relevant abstract appeared (Pande *et al.*, 1998). Two aspects of the report are of interest. First is the use of an exclusively male hip-fracture sample, composed of 100 men 50+ years old with hip fractures and 100 matched community controls. Second is the use of the SF-36 as the QOL instrument. Comparing SF-36 scores of the hip-fractured men at the time of admission to nursing and residential care, there were no significant QOL differences between cases living in their homes prior to fracture and those in care. However, the cases as a group reported significantly worse prefracture QOL than did controls in all domains except pain. Why these differences did not continue to be significant after fracture is an enigma.

An assessment of the studies reviewed above raises two important questions. First, given that there are no (or almost no) empirical studies examining the impact of osteoporosis on QOL in men, can we extrapolate from the studies of women and predict what men's problems will be? Second, given limited research resources, what direction should investigators take as they begin to quantify the impact of this prevalent metabolic bone disease on men?

4. Using Women's Data to Infer Osteoporotic Men's Psychosocial Experience

In the broadest terms, role loss and psychological dysfunction—two common consequences of osteoporosis on women—could have similar psychological or social effects on men. However, if we look at more specific components of role behavior, the assumption of gender-neutral role loss no longer holds up. This is true for several reasons. First, men's and women's roles are still distinguished from each other, especially for the cohorts born in 1940 and earlier. Women now begin adult life with *a priori* desires for a career, but older women's lives are for the most part centered on home and family. At the same time, men's lives have been centered around their work. Although this pattern has changed, we cannot forget that today's older adults spent their adolescence and young adulthood playing under different gender rules. Only reluctantly did men express feelings at all, let alone feelings about pain, dysfunction, frustration, and depression. Thus, any research in this area may be stymied by less than accurate reports of the osteoporosis experience by men. It is apparent that we cannot simply apply the findings based on women's lives to men.

II. Men and Osteoporosis: Where Do We Start to Understand Outcomes?

In general, the important first strategy for studying the nonmedical outcomes of osteoporosis in men must start with listening to the experiences of men who have this disease. By listening to patients describe how osteoporosis affects their lives, we will be able to identify the psychological and social stress the disease causes as well as its impact on QOL.

A. Focus Groups

The use of focus groups as a means of eliciting qualitative information from osteoporotic men would permit a more systematic examination of the impact of this chronic disease (Powell and Single, 1996). Focus groups have been used widely to examine other chronic illnesses including cancer (Ashbury *et al.*, 1995) and diabetes (Anderson *et al.*, 1996). Because focus groups concentrate on issues of importance to the subjects rather than the investigators, they often generate speculation about fascinating biopsychosocial phenomena. In osteoporosis, the only recent use of focus groups has been by Lydick *et al.* (1997), in developing OPTQoL. As mentioned earlier, this was completed with a female sample.

Because osteoporosis usually occurs at the time of life when age asserts its most negative pressures on individuals, it can be challenging to manage. Challenges can occur in the physical, functional, and socioemotional domains, and all chronic illnesses of late life may share certain QOL outcomes. Therefore, it would be important to construct focus groups with age homogeneity; this design decision might help provide a common starting point for discussion. It is also possible that the men who experience osteoporosis would feel uneasy about discussing it with those younger than they.

B. Instrumentation

Once focus groups have occurred, relevant dimensions have been identified, and individual comments have been coded on those dimensions, one of the most difficult aspects of the research process must be faced: the design and evaluation of data collection instruments. Although all existing QOL scales are designed for use with women, they may remain useful. A first step is to test those existing instruments to determine whether they do assess a gender difference in reaction to osteoporosis as well as whether minor modifications could render them useful in male samples. The range of assessment and measurement tools is far beyond the scope of this chapter; however, the importance of instrument development cannot be overemphasized. Validation and reliability testing are also critical steps in the instrumentation process. The ultimate test would be a randomized clinical trial in which a particular psychosocial and/or physical intervention was tested. It is only through rigorous and ordered scientific work that this aspect of the osteoporosis world can be uncovered.

III. Commentary

In the last decade, osteoporosis has entered the lexicon of many adults in the United States. From television ads to newspaper stories, osteoporosis is far more in the public eye than ever before. In the process, we have also modified the stereotype of hunchbacked, bent over, and useless older women for whom nothing could be done. The American people now better understand the broad scope of afflicted women and have been exposed to information about the availability of multiple pharmaceutical products to prevent and treat this insidious disease.

One stereotype, however, that certainly has not been discarded relates to the gender specificity of this disease. Osteoporosis is almost inextricably linked to women, perhaps especially so because the recent flood of information and advertisement has focused entirely on postmenopausal females. However, we note that nearly 20% of the people who have diagnosed osteoporosis are male. Our medical views and treatment protocols must change in response to the changing demographics of disease impact.

In some sense, osteoporosis in men today faces the same challenges as did osteoporosis in women a quarter century ago. Although we better understand the natural history of this disease in women than in men, there is much yet to be learned about this disease in both genders. However, we do have some treatment protocols that appear to work effectively with women (Gold *et al.,* 1989), and it will be important to establish similar multidisciplinary treatment protocols for the long-term management of osteoporosis in men.

What of the men who experience substantial decrements in physical performance, appearance, function, self-image, and QOL secondary to osteoporosis? Although little is known about the social and psychological outcomes in male patients, this is also an understudied area in women. Orwoll et al. (1990), Orwoll and Bliziotes (1994), and Mann et al. (1992) have contributed to a substantial nucleus of research focused on men, and some of the more recent studies such as The Rotterdam Study (Burger et al., 1997) have compared men's deformity and functional impairment to those of women. But the existing research has not focused on men and nonphysical consequences of osteoporosis, and it is imperative that researchers extend their QOL and psychosocial research protocols to examine men's outcomes of this disease.

IV. Conclusion

As life expectancy of both men and women continues to increase and more cases of primary osteoporosis in men are diagnosed and treated (Francis, 1998), it will become imperative to include both genders in pharmaceutical trials and outcomes studies. In addition to the primary diagnoses of osteoporosis, the increase in secondary osteoporosis in men associated with organ transplantation (Rodino and Shane, 1998), hypogonadism (Nyquist et al., 1998), steroid use (McEvoy et al., 1998), alcoholism (Anderson, 1998), and other causes compounds the problem. As we increase our empirical evidence about ways in which this disease affects the physiological, psychological, social, and economic dimensions of men's lives, we will also increase the number and effectiveness of treatment protocols for men. Thus, our ultimate goal—to improve the QOL of people with osteoporosis—can surely be reached soon.

Acknowledgments

Support for this project provided in part by NIH Grants AG 11269 (Duke OAIC/Pepper Center) and HD 30442 (Osteoporosis and Disability in Life-Care Community Women) and a research grant from AARP/Andrus Foundation.

References

Anderson, F. H. (1998). Osteoporosis in men. *Int. J. Clin. Pract.* 52, 176–180.
Anderson, R., Barr, P. A., Edwards, G. J., Funnell, M. M., Fitzgerald, J. T., and Wisdom, K. (1996). Using focus groups to identify psychosocial issues of urban black individuals with diabetes. *Diabetes Educator* 22, 28–33.

Ashbury, F. D., Gospodarowicz, M., Kaegi, E., and O'Sullivan, B. (1995). Focus group methodology in the development of a survey to measure physician use of cancer staging systems. *Can. J. Oncol.* **5**, 361–368.

Bergner, M., Bobitt, R. A., Carter, W. B., and Gilson, B. S. (1981).The Sickness Impact Profile: Development and final revision of a health status measure. *Med. Care* **19**, 787–805.

Burger, H., van Daele, P. L. A., Grashuis, K., Hofman, A., Grobbee, D. E., Schutte, H. E., Birkenhager, J. C., and Pols, H. A. P. (1997). Vertebral deformities and functional impairment in men and women. *J. Bone Miner. Res.* **12**, 152–157.

Cauley, J. A., Seeley, D. G., Ensrud, K., Ettinger, B., Black, D., and Cummings, S. R. (1995). Estrogen replacement therapy and fractures in older women. Study of Osteoporotic Fractures Research Group. *Ann. Intern. Med.* **122**, 9–16.

Chandler, J. M., Martin, A. R., Tenehouse, A., Poliquin, S., Hanley, D., Adachi, A., Anastassiades, T., Olszynski, W., and Joyce, C. (1998). The impact of osteoporosis on quality of life of Canadian women: CaMos. *Bone* **23**, S305.

Cook, D. J., Guyatt, G. H., Adachi, J. D., Clifton, J., Griffith, L. E., Epstein, R. S., and Juniper, E. F. (1993). Quality of life issues in women with vertebral fractures due to osteoporosis. *Arthritis Rheum.* **36**, 750–756.

Cooper, C., Atkinson, E. J., Jacobsen, S. J., O'Frallon, W. M., and Melton, L. J., III, (1993). Population-based study of survival after osteoporotic fracture. *Am. J. Epidemiol.* **137**, 1001–1005.

Dahl, E. (1980). Mortality and life expectancy after hip fractures. *Acta Orthop. Scand.* **51**, 163–170.

Ensrud, K. E., Black, D. M., Palermo, L., Bauer, D. C., Barrett-Connor, E., Quandt, S. A., Thompson, D. E., and Karpf, D. B. (1997). Treatment with alendronate prevents fractures in women at highest risk: Results from the Fracture Intervention Trial. *Arch. Intern. Med.* **157**, 2617–2624.

Francis, R. M. (1998). Cyclical etidronate in the management of osteoporosis in men. *Rev. Contemp. Pharm.* **9**, 261–266.

Garnero, P., Hausherr, E., Chapuy, M. C., Marcello, C., Grandjean, H., Muller, C., Cormier, C., Breart, G., Meunier, P. J., and Delmas, P. D. (1996). Markers of bone resorption predict hip fracture in elderly women: The EPIDOS Prospective Study. *J. Bone Miner. Res.* **11**, 1531–1538.

Gold, D. T. (1996). The clinical impact of vertebral fractures: Quality of life in women with osteoporosis. *Bone* **18**, 185S–190S.

Gold, D. T., Bales, C. W., Lyles, K. W., and Drezner, M. K. (1989). Treatment of osteoporosis: The psychological impact of a medical education program on older patients. *J. Am. Geriatr. Soc.* **37**, 417–422.

Gold, D. T., Stegmaier, K., Bales, C. W., Lyles, K. W., Westlund, R. E., and Drezner, M. K. (1993). Psychosocial functioning and osteoporosis in late life: Results of a multidisciplinary intervention. *J. Women's Health* **2**, 149–155.

Hunt, S. M., McKenna, S. P., McEwen, J., Williams, J., and Papp, E. (1981). The Nottingham Health Profile: Subjective health status and medical consultations. *Soc. Sci. Med.* **15**, 221–229.

Ismail, A. A., O'Neill, T. W., Cooper, C., Finn, J. D., Bhalla, A. K., Cannata, J. B., Delmas, P., Falch, J. A., Felsch, B., Hoszowski, K., Johnell, O., Diaz-Lopez, J. B., Lopez Vaz, A., Marchand, F., Raspe, H., Reid, D. M., Todd, C., Weber, K., Woolf, A., Reeve, J., and Silman, A. J. (1998). Mortality associated with vertebral deformity in men and women: Results from the European Prospective Osteoporosis Study (EPOS). *Osteoporos. Int.* **8**(3), 291–297.

Jensen, J. S., and Tondevold, E. (1979). Mortality after hip fractures. *Acta Orthop. Scand.* **50**, 161–167.

Johnell, O., O'Neill, T., Felsenberg, D., Kanis, J., Cooper, C., and Silman, A. J. (1997). Anthropometric measurements and vertebral deformities: European Vertebral Osteoporosis Study (EVOS) Group. *Am. J. Epidemiol.* **146**, 287–293.

Jones, G., White, C., Nguyen, T., Sambrook, P. N., Kelly, P. J., and Eisman, J. A. (1996). Prevalent vertebral deformities: Relationship to bone mineral density and spinal osteophytosis in elderly men and women. *Osteoporosis Int.* **6**, 233–239.

Lau, E. M. C., Woo, J., Chan, H., Chan, M. K. F., Griffith, J., Chan, Y. H., and Leung, P. C. (1998). The health consequences of vertebral deformity in elderly Chinese men and women. *Calcif. Tissue Int.* **63**, 1–4.

Lips, P., Cooper, C., Agnusdei, D., Caulin, F., Egger, P., Johnell, O., Kanis, J. A., Liberman, U., Minne, H., Reeve, J., Reginster, J. Y., de Vernejoul, M. C., and Wiklund, I. (1997). Quality of life as outcome in the treatment of osteoporosis: The development of a questionnaire for quality of life by the European Foundation for Osteoporosis. *Osteoporosis Int.* **7**, 36–38.

Looker, A. C., Orwoll, E. S., Johnston, C. C., Jr., Lindsay, R. L., Wahner, H. W., Dunn, W. L., Calvo, M. S., Harris, T. B., and Heyse, S. P. (1997). Prevalence of low femoral bone density in older U.S. adults from NHANES III. *J. Bone Miner. Res.* **12**, 1761–1768.

Lunt, M., Felsenberg, D., Reeve, J., Benevolenskaya, L., Cannata, J., Dequeker, J., Dodenhof, C., Falch, J. A., Masaryk, P., Pols, H. A., Poor, G., Reid, D. M., Scheidt-Nave, C., Weber, K., Varlow, J., Kanis, J. A., O'Neill, T. W., and Silman, A. J. (1997). Bone density variation and its effects on risk of vertebral deformity in men and women studied in thirteen European centers: The EVOS Study. *J. Bone Miner. Res.* **12**, 1883–1894.

Lydick, E., Zimmerman, S. I., Yawn, B., Love, B., Kleerekoper, M., Ross, P., Martin, A., and Holmes, R. (1997). Development and validation of a discriminative quality of life questionnaire for osteoporosis (the OPTQoL). *J. Bone Miner. Res.* **12**, 456–463.

Mann, T., Oviatt, S. K., Wilson, D., Nelson, D., and Orwoll, E. S. (1992). Vertebral deformity in men. *J. Bone Miner. Res.* **7**, 1259–1265.

Mazess, R. B., Barden, H. S., Drinka, P. J., Bauwens, S. F., Orwoll, E. S., and Bell, N. H. (1990). Influence of age and body weight on spine and femur bone mineral density in U.S. white men. *J. Bone Miner. Res.* **5**, 645–652.

McEvoy, C. E., Ensrud, K. E., Bender, E., Genant, H. K., Yu, W., Griffith, J. M., and Niewoehner, D. E. (1998). Association between corticosteroid use and vertebral fractures in older men with chronic obstructive pulmonary disease. *Am. J. Respir. Crit. Care Med.* **157**, 704–709.

Melton, L. J., III (1997). Editorial: The prevalence of osteoporosis. *J. Bone Miner. Res.* **12**, 1769–1771.

Melton, L. J., III, and Chrischilles, E. A. (1992). Perspective: How many women have osteoporosis? *J. Bone Miner. Res.* **7**, 1001–1010.

Melton, L. J., III, and Riggs, B. L. (1983). Epidemiology of age-related fractures. *In* "The Osteoporotic Syndrome" (L. V. Avioli, ed.), Vol. 45, pp. 45–72. Grune & Stratton, New York.

Melton, L. J., III, Thamer, M., Ray, N. F., Chan, J. K., Chestnut, C. H., III, Einhorn, T. A., Johnston, C. C., Raisz, L. G., Silverman, S. L., and Siris, E. S. (1997). Fractures attributable to osteoporosis: Report from the National Osteoporosis Foundation. *J. Bone Miner. Res.* **12**, 16–23.

Nyquist, F., Gardsell, P., Sernbo, I., Jeppsson, J. O., and Johnell, O. (1998). Assessment of sex hormones and bone mineral density in relation to occurrence of fracture in men—a prospective, population-based study. *Bone* **22**, 147–151.

Orwoll, E. S., and Bliziotes, M. (1994). Heterogeneity in osteoporosis: Men versus women. *Rheum. Dis. Clin. North Am.* **20**, 671–689.

Orwoll, E. S., Oviatt, S. K., McClung, M. R., Deftos, L. J., and Sexton, G. (1990). The rate of bone mineral loss in normal men and the effects of calcium and cholecalciferol supplementation. *Ann. Intern. Med.* **112**, 29–34.

Pande, I., O'Neill, T. W., Scott, D. L., and Woolf, A. D. (1998). Quality of life, residence, comorbidity and outcome following osteoporotic hip fracture in men: Results of the Cornwall Hip Fracture Study. *Bone* **23**, S397.

Poor, G., Atkinson, E.J., Lewallen, D. G., O'Fallon, W. M., and Melton, L. J., III (1995a). Age-related hip fractures in men: Clinical spectrum and short-term outcomes. *Osteoporosis Int.* 5, 419–426.

Poor, G., Atkinson, E. J., O'Fallon, W. M., and Melton, L. J., III (1995b). Determinants of reduced survival following hip fractures in men. *Clin. Orthop.* 319, 260–265.

Poor, G., Atkinson, E. J., O'Fallon, W. M., and Melton, L. J., III (1995c). Predictors of hip fractures in elderly men. *J. Bone Miner. Res.* 10, 1900–1907.

Powell, R., and Single, H. M. (1996). Focus groups. *Int. J. Qual. Health Care* 8, 499–504.

Roberto, K. A. (1988a). Stress and adaptation patterns of older osteoporotic women. *Women Health* 14, 105–119.

Roberto, K. A. (1988b). Women with osteoporosis: The role of the family and service community. *Gerontologist* 28, 224–228.

Roberto, K. A., and Gold, D. T. (1997). Spousal support of older women with osteoporotic pain: Congruity of perceptions. *J. Women Aging* 9, 17–31.

Rodino, M. A., and Shane, E. (1998). Osteoporosis after organ transplantation. *Am. J. Med.* 104, 459–469.

Ross, P. D. (1998). Risk factors for osteoporotic fracture. *Endocrinol. Metab. Clin. North Am.* 27, 289–301.

Scane, A. C., Sutcliffe, A. M., and Francis, R. M. (1993). Osteoporosis in men. *Baillieres Clin. Rheumatol.* 7, 589–601.

Scane, A. C., Sutcliffe, A. M., and Francis, R. M. (1994). The sequelae of vertebral crush fractures in men. *Osteoporosis Int.* 4, 89–92.

Schroder, H. M., and Erlandsen, M. (1993). Age and sex as determinants of mortality after hip fracture: 3,895 patients followed for 2.5–18.5 years. *J. Orthop. Trauma* 7, 525–531.

Silverman, S. L., Minshall, M. E., Shen, W., Harper, K. D., and Xie, S. (1998a). The impact of vertebral fracture(s) on health related quality of life (HRQOL) in established postmenopausal osteoporosis depends on the number and location of the fracture(s). *Bone* 23, S305.

Silverman, S. L., Lips, P., Minshall, M. E., Oleksik, A., and Spritzer, K. (1998b). Does the impact of established postmenopausal osteoporosis on health-related quality of life differ between Amsterdam and Los Angeles? *Bone* 23, S398.

Tacconelli, E., Tumbarello, M., Ventura, G., Leone, F., Cauda, R., and Ortona, L. (1998). Risk factors, nutritional status, and quality of life in HIV-infected patients with enteric salmonellosis. *Ital. J. Gastroenterol. Hepatol.* 30, 167–172.

Thongprasert, S. (1998). Lung cancer and quality of life. *Aust. N. Z. J. Med.* 28, 397–399.

Ware, J. E., Jr., Kosinski, M., Bayliss, M. S., McHorney, C. A., Rogers, W. H., and Raczek, A. (1995). Comparison of methods for the scoring and statistical analysis of SF-36 health profile and summary measures: Summary of results from the Medical Outcomes Study. *Med Care* 33, AS264–AS279.

Wasnich, R. D. (1997). Epidemiology of osteoporosis in the United States of America. *Osteporosis Int.* 7, S68–S72.

Wikby, A., Stenstrom, U., Andersson, P. O., and Hornquist, J. (1998). Metabolic control, quality of life, and negative life events: A longitudinal study of well-controlled and poorly regulated patients with type 1 diabetes after changeover to insulin pen treatment. *Diabetes Educator* 24, 61–66.

Chapter 5

Vicente Gilsanz

Childrens Hospital Los Angeles
Radiology Department
Los Angeles, California

Accumulation of Bone Mass during Childhood and Adolescence

I. Introduction

Osteoporosis is a disease characterized by low bone mass and the development of nontraumatic fractures (Kleerekoper and Avioli, 1993). Although research on osteoporosis has focused mainly on the role of bone loss in the elderly, it is becoming increasingly clear that the amount of bone that is gained during growth is also an important determinant of future resistance to fractures (Johnston *et al.*, 1981; Ott, 1990). Therefore, considerable interest has recently been placed on defining the genetic and environmental factors that contribute to the variations in bone accumulation in healthy children, such as heredity, gender, race, nutrition, body weight, physical activity, and hormonal status (Gilsanz *et al.*, 1988a,b, 1997; Ott, 1990; Krall and Dawson-Hughes, 1993). Such knowledge will provide a means and a more rational way to diagnose, prevent, and treat osteoporosis.

II. Techniques for Bone Measurements in Children _____

The development of precise noninvasive methods for measuring bone mineral content has significantly improved our ability to study the influence of genetic and environmental factors on the attainment of bone. These techniques have not only helped to quantify the loss of bone associated with the various disorders that cause osteopenia in children (Kovanlikaya et al., 1996), but they have also improved our understanding of the childhood antecedents of a condition that happens to manifest in adults—osteoporosis.

Currently, the most commonly used quantitative radiologic method to assess bone mass is dual-energy x-ray absorptiometry (DXA). This technique is readily available and used in the early diagnosis of osteoporosis, the prediction of fracture risk, and the assessment of response to therapy. DXA bone determinations are based on a two-dimensional projection of a three-dimensional structure, and the values are a function of three skeletal parameters: the size of the bone being examined, the volume of the bone, and its mineral density (Carter et al., 1992). These values are frequently expressed as measurements of the bone content per surface area (g/cm^2), as determined by scan radiographs. However, scan radiographs provide only an approximation of the size of the bone, and any correction based on these radiographs is only a very rough estimate of the "density." Attempts to overcome this disadvantage with the use of correction factors [i.e., the squared root of the projected area; the height of the subject, the width of the bone, assuming that the cross-sectional area of the vertebrae is a square, a circle, or an ellipse or that the femur can be modeled as a cylinder, etc. (Katzman et al., 1991; Kröger et al., 1992, 1993; Moro et al., 1996; Plotkin et al., 1996)] are subject to error because there is no closed formula that defines the size of the vertebrae or the femur.

DXA values are also influenced by the unknown composition of soft tissues in the beam path of the region of interest. Because corrections for the soft tissues are based on a homogenous distribution of fat around the bone, changes in DXA measurements are observed if fat is distributed inhomogeneously around the bone measured. It has been determined that inhomogeneous fat distribution in soft tissues, resulting in a difference of 2 cm fat layer between soft tissue area and bone area, will influence DXA measurements by 10% (Hangartner, 1990). Although this is not a limitation when studying subjects whose weight and body size remain constant, DXA bone measurements in growing children reflects a large number of biological parameters.

Quantitative computed tomography (CT) allows for the independent study of the marked alterations that occur in the size and the shape of the skeleton during growth, as well as the concomitant changes in bone volume and bone density, without influence of surrounding soft tissues (Rüegsegger et al., 1976; Cann and Genant, 1980; Hangartner and Overton, 1982; Genant et al., 1996; Hangartner and Gilsanz, 1996). Even though magnetic resonance (MR) imaging is an ideal modality for measuring the volume of any tissue, including bone, the value of this technique in measuring the density of bone is in developmental stages (Fowler *et al.*, 1991; Wehrli *et al.*, 1995; Genant *et al.*, 1996). Ultrasound (US) has also been used as a bone measurement technique (Genant *et al.*, 1996; Glüer *et al.*, 1996). Because, in adults, US can predict fracture risk in patients with osteoporosis, these measurements must be related to some aspects of bone strength (Genant *et al.*, 1996; Glüer *et al.*, 1996). Unfortunately, the values depend on so many structural parameters, yet to be fully defined, that it is difficult to use this information in a meaningful way in children (Genant *et al.*, 1996).

III. Peak Bone Mass

Bone mass increases during growth, reaches peak values in early adult life, and decreases with age both in men and women (Gilsanz *et al.*, 1988b; Mosekilde, 1989; Bonjour *et al.*, 1991). The exact age at which values for bone mass reach their peak has received considerable attention, with varying results. It is likely, however, that the timing of peak values differs between the axial and appendicular skeletons and between men and women.

In the axial skeleton, bone mass achieves peak values by the end of the second decade of life. Studies in women using CT have demonstrated that the density and the size of vertebral bone reach their peak soon after the time of sexual and skeletal maturity (Gilsanz *et al.*, 1988b; Gilsanz *et al.*, 1994a,b), corroborating anatomical data indicating trabecular bone loss as early as the third decade of life, and that there is no change in the cross-sectional area of the vertebral body from 15 to 90 years of age (Weaver and Chalmers, 1966; Merz and Schenk, 1970; Arnold, 1973; Marcus *et al.*, 1983; Mosekilde and Mosekilde, 1990). The data regarding whether vertebral cross-sectional area in men continues to grow after cessation of longitudinal growth are controversial; even though some authors find no change in the cross-sectional dimensions after skeletal maturity, others have suggested that vertebral size increases with age throughout adulthood (Dunnill *et al.*, 1967; Mosekilde and Mosekilde, 1990).

In the appendicular skeleton, the range of ages published in cross-sectional studies for the timing of peak bone mass has varied significantly, from 17–18 years of age to as late as 35 years of age (Halioua and Anderson, 1990; Gordon *et al.*, 1991; Recker *et al.*, 1992; Matkoyic *et al.*, 1994). Longitudinal DXA studies indicate that the rate of increase in skeletal mass slows markedly in late adolescence and that peak values in the femoral neck, like those in the spine, are achieved near the end of puberty in normal females (Bonjour *et al.*, 1991; Theintz *et al.*, 1992; Lu *et al.*, 1994). It should, however, be stressed that, in both men and women, the cross-sectional dimensions of the long bones in the appendicular skeleton continue to grow throughout adulthood and into old age by subperiosteal bone apposition. This increase in bone width occurs in all sample populations studied (Parfitt, 1997).

As bone mass and bone strength decline, the skeleton becomes unable to withstand the loads associated with normal daily activities; consequently, fragility fractures occur. For many years, it was thought that a greater bone loss with aging was responsible for the lower bone mass of patients with fractures when compared with controls. It is now acknowledged that lesser bone gains during growth and a lower peak bone mass are also important determinants of fractures in the elderly (Seeman *et al.*, 1989). Support for this view comes from studies showing a strong resemblance in bone mass values between females with hip and vertebral fractures and values for bone mass in the spine and the femurs of their premenopausal daughters (Seeman *et al.*, 1989). If reduced bone mass was solely the result of excessive age-related bone loss, no reduction in bone mass of the daughters would have been seen. Even though rapid bone loss may contribute to fractures in elderly women, this mechanism is not needed to explain the lower bone mass in these women.

IV. Age-Related Changes in the Axial and Appendicular Skeletons

The human skeleton contains approximately 85% cortical bone and 15% cancellous bone. The appendicular skeleton consists mostly of cortical bone, whereas the vertebral bodies are mainly composed of cancellous bone. Studies have shown that the patterns of gain during growth and the rate of loss with aging differ considerably between cortical and cancellous bone and that these two skeletal compartments may respond differently to hormonal and mechanical stimuli (Gong *et al.*, 1964; Riggs *et al.*, 1981; Rüegsegger *et al.*, 1991; Mora *et al.*, 1994).

The apparent density of cancellous bone is strongly influenced by hormonal and/or metabolic factors associated with sexual development during late adolescence (Gilsanz *et al.*, 1988b). On average, cancellous bone density in the spine increases by 13% during puberty in Caucasian boys and girls. After controlling for puberty, vertebral bone density fails to correlate significantly with age, sex, weight, height, surface area, or body mass index (Gilsanz *et al.*, 1988b). Whether the increase in the apparent density of cancellous bone during the later stages of puberty is a reflection of a greater number of trabeculae, a greater thickness, or a higher degree of mineralization of the trabeculae is not known because of technical limitations (Genant *et al.*, 1996). Due to the relatively small size of the trabeculae, *in vivo* measurements for cancellous bone density reflect not only the amount of mineralized bone and osteoid but also the amount of marrow per pixel (Genant *et al.*, 1996). Similar limitations apply to *in vitro* determinations of the volumetric density of trabecular bone which are obtained by washing the marrow from the pores of a specimen of cancellous bone, weighing it, and dividing the weight by the volume of the specimen, including the pores (Dyson *et al.*, 1970). Both CT and anatomical bone density determinations of cancellous bone are, therefore, directly proportional to the bone volume fraction and inversely proportional to the porosity of the bone.

The factors which account for the increase in cancellous vertebral bone density during late puberty remain to be determined. It is reasonable to suspect that many of the physical changes undergone, such as the accelerated growth spurt and the increases in body and bone mass, are, at least in part, mediated by the actions of sex steroids (Mauras *et al.*, 1994). Some of these effects may be caused by changes in protein and calcium metabolism induced by sex steroids; alternatively, they may be secondary to the cascade of events triggered by the increase in growth hormone and insulin growth factor I production observed after sex steroid exposure (Mauras *et al.*, 1987, 1989). In this regard, both growth hormone deficiency and delayed puberty have been suggested as a cause of a deficient accumulation of bone and low peak bone mass during adolescence (Finkelstein *et al.*, 1992; Hyer *et al.*, 1992; De Boer *et al.*, 1994). Animal models have also been employed to investigate the role of sex steroids as modifiers of bone density during skeletal development. Longitudinal quantitative CT measurements in growing, castrated, rabbits after administration of normal saline, Depo testosterone, or Depo estrogen from six weeks of age until the time of skeletal maturity showed that bone density increased during growth, was highest at the time of epiphyseal closure, and was significantly greater in hormone-treated animals (Gilsanz *et al.*, 1988c).

In the appendicular skeleton, CT values for the material density of cortical bone in children are remarkably similar and constant—2.00 ± 0.065 g/cm^3 (Figure 1) (Rüegsegger *et al.*, 1991; Hangartner and Gilsanz, 1996). Neither puberty, age, gender, race, height, nor weight influence these measurements. These data contradict the common belief that, during the adolescent growth spurt, bone formation transiently outstrips mineral deposition and that there is a temporary decrease in bone density (Kleerekoper *et al.*, 1981). It should be stressed that, because of the thickness and the relative lack of porosity of the femoral cortex, CT values for cortical bone density reflect the true density of the bone—the amount of collagen and mineral in a given amount of bone (Hangartner and Gilsanz, 1996). These values are eight times higher than cancellous bone density values, a finding consistent with histomorphometric studies indicating an equivalent difference in the porosity of these two forms of bone (Gong *et al.*, 1964; Dyson *et al.*, 1970).

Cross-sectional growth of the bones in the axial and the appendicular skeletons results from two different processes which are likely to be regulated by different means (Carter *et al.*, 1996). Bone growth at the midshaft of the femur is achieved by subperiosteal formation of new bone, a process

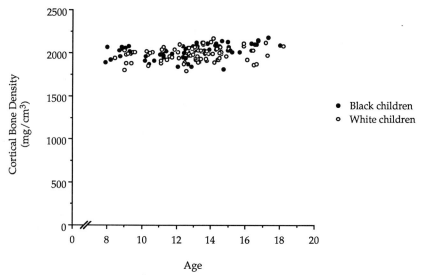

FIGURE I   Female cortical bone density in 80 black and 80 white children from 7 to 20 years of age. Adapted with permission from Gilsanz *et al.* (1998). Differential effect of race on the axial and appendicular skeletons of children. *J. Clin. Endocrinol. Metab.* **68**, 1420–1427. © The Endocrine Society.

that begins before birth and continues throughout life. Simultaneous to the age-specific subperiosteal bone apposition, a complex activity characterized by resorption and apposition occurs at the endosteal surface of the bone. Whereas subperiosteal activity determines the width of the bone, edosteal activity determines the width of the medullary canal. The combination of the relative activities at the two modeling surfaces over a period of time determines the thickness of the cortex. On the other hand, endochondral ossification determines the cross-sectional area of the vertebrae. Endochondral ossification commences in the central area of the cartilage anlage in the vertebrae and, from this region, expands and progresses towards the periphery in all directions. It is generally assumed that normal development and growth of the diaphysis of the femur is mainly dependent upon mechanical loading, whereas endochondral growth and ossification may occur without mechanical stress (Carter *et al.*, 1996).

V. Nutrition

The earliest data suggesting an influence of dietary calcium on peak bone mass comes from a study of two Croatian populations with substantially different calcium intakes (Matkovic *et al.*, 1979). The differences seen in bone mass were present at 30 years of age, suggesting that the effects of dietary calcium probably occurred during growth rather than in adulthood. Subsequent studies on calcium supplementation have, however, proved inconclusive (Johnston *et al.*, 1992; Chan *et al.*, 1995; Lee *et al.*, 1995; Lloyd *et al.*, 1996). This issue was most rigorously addressed by Johnston *et al.* (1992). In their study, the influence of genetic factors on bone mass was controlled by evaluating 45 pairs of identical twins, one of whom was given an oral calcium supplement in the amount sufficient to nearly double the recommended daily intake of calcium. Subjects were followed for three years during the period of rapid skeletal growth when the demand for calcium is high and the beneficial effects of calcium supplementation would be expected to be greatest. The results demonstrated that a twofold increase in calcium intake has little effect on bone mass in the growing skeleton. Calcium supplementation enhanced the radial bone mass in prepubertal children, but this difference did not persist once children entered puberty (Johnston *et al.*, 1992).

Because it is difficult to obtain longitudinal data in normal children throughout the long developmental period of childhood and adolescence, animal models have been employed to determine whether differences in daily calcium intake during skeletal growth influenced peak values for bone. Quantitative CT was used to monitor changes longitudinally in vertebral bone density in rabbits maintained on low, normal, and high calcium diets from birth to skeletal maturity (Gilsanz *et al.*, 1991b). Values for vertebral bone density between rabbits fed high Ca and rabbits fed normal Ca did not differ during growth or at epiphyseal closure in these two groups. However, vertebral bone density was lower throughout the study in rabbits fed low Ca, and peak values at epiphyseal closure remained below those in either normal-Ca or high-Ca groups (Figure 2). Thus, raising dietary calcium intake above normal levels did not increase peak bone mass, but dietary calcium restriction during growth reduced peak bone mass at skeletal maturity in this experimental model (Gilsanz *et al.*, 1991b).

VI. Physical Activity

Physical activity has also been proposed as an intervention for increasing bone mass before it reaches its peak, as well as delaying bone loss during adulthood. Available evidence would indicate that the skeleton is most responsive to exercise during growth and that the benefits obtained from exercise in childhood persist into adulthood (Kannus *et al.*, 1995; Bass *et al.*, 1998). Competitive squash or tennis players who began playing before puberty had 11–24% higher bone mass in their playing than nonplaying arm, two to four times the side-side differences of individuals who began playing the sport after puberty (Jones *et al.*, 1977; Kannus *et al.*, 1995). Because strenuous exercise during puberty may interrupt hormonal cyclicity, delay

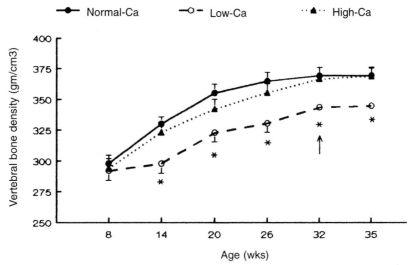

FIGURE 2   Vertebral bone density during growth as measured by quantitative CT in rabbits ingesting diets containing 0.15% (low Ca), 0.45% (normal Ca), or 1.35% (high Ca) calcium; $n = 8$ for each group. Values are means $\pm$ SE; for data points without error bars, symbol size exceeds SE. Vertical arrow denotes confirmation of epiphysial closure. *$P < 0.01$ vs. normal Ca; $^{+}P < 0.05$ vs. high Ca. Reproduced with permission from Gilsanz et al. (1991a).

progression of puberty, and result in attainment of a lower peak bone mass, the prepubertal years are likely to be the most opportune time for exercise to increase bone mass (Drinkwater et al., 1984). Support for this view comes from studies of prepubertal female gymnasts showing that residual benefits in bone mass are maintained into adulthood (Bass et al., 1998).

Nonetheless, prospective clinical trials have not consistently found exercise to be effective in improving bone mass. It has been hypothesized that calcium intake may modify the response of bone to exercise. Specker reviewed 17 published trials and found that physical activity had beneficial effects on bone mass at high calcium intakes, with no effect at calcium intakes less than a mean of 1000 mg/day. This modifying effect of calcium intake on bone mass among exercise groups was more pronounced in the lumbar spine than in the radius and may explain the conflicting results of trials on the effects of physical activity on bone mass (Specker, 1996).

The effect of relative inactivity on the bone has also received considerable attention, most studies finding a significant negative impact on bone mass. Children who limp because weight bearing is painful have considerably lower bone mass in the spine than normally active children of the same age, gender, race, and size (Gilsanz et al., 1989). The deleterious effect of immobilization is, however, greatest on the appendicular skeleton. Fetuses and infants with a variety of neuromuscular disorders characterized by striking hypotonia or flaccidity have marked decreases in periosteal diameter, cortical thickness, and cortical areas of the long bones (Donaldson *et al.,* 1985; Rodriguez *et al.,* 1988). A similar pattern of reduced bone mass with immobilization has been seen at the mid-diaphysis of long bones in young growing Beagles (Uhthoff and Jaworski, 1978), and slow bone growth was found in embryonic chicks after muscle paralysis (Hall and Herring, 1990).

VII. Genetics

A convergence of data from mother-daughter pairs, sib pairs, and twin studies have estimated the heritability of bone mass to account for 60–90% of its variance (Christian *et al.,* 1989; Pocock *et al.,* 1991). Support for this genetic influence comes from investigations reporting a link between several "candidate" genes and bone mass (Ralston, 1997a), and from clinical studies showing reduced bone mass in daughters of osteoporotic women when compared with controls (Seeman *et al.,* 1989), in men and women with first-degree relatives who have osteoporosis (Evans *et al.,* 1988) and in perimenopausal women who have a family history of hip fracture (Torgerson *et al.,* 1995). In addition, recent data shows a familial resemblance for bone mass between premenopausal mothers and their prepubertal daughters (Ferrari *et al.,* 1998).

The obvious application of genetic studies to osteoporosis is the discovery of genetic markers that consistently predict osteoporotic fractures and allow the identification of subjects at risk. Understanding the roles played by genetic factors may also facilitate the prediction of response to treatment. As an example, the response of bone mass to dietary supplementation with vitamin D and calcium is partly dependent on VDR polymorphisms (Dawson-Hughes *et al.,* 1995; Howard *et al.,* 1995; Graafmans *et al.,* 1997), and it is possible that other genes may aid in establishing who would benefit from treatments such as hormone replacement therapy, bisphosphonates, or even exercise.

Two approaches are usually used to determine the genetic contribution to complex diseases, linkage, and association studies (Ralston, 1997a). Linkage studies are expensive, time-consuming, and require sophisticated technology and a detailed understanding of the complex phenotype of osteoporosis. As our knowledge of phenotypes increases and we are able to identify this disease unambiguously before it clinically manifests, linkage studies searching for the genotypes of osteoporosis will become more feasible. Association studies examine specific genomic regions at or near candidate genes and, in osteoporosis research, are facilitated by our knowledge of the factors that regulate bone turnover and the proteins that make up normal bone matrix (Morrison *et al.,* 1994; Cooper and Umbach, 1996; Ralston, 1997a). Given the wide range of factors involved in bone metabolism, there is a seemingly unlimited supply of candidate genes for osteoporosis, even though relatively few have been studied thus far. The first candidate gene to be identified was the vitamin-D receptor (VDR) gene in 1994 (Morrison *et al.*, 1994). Claims that the VDR gene accounted for 80% of the variance in bone mass were exaggerated, and reanalysis of the data indicates a much weaker association (Cooper and Umbach, 1996; Nguyen *et al.*, 1996). Other studies have also found significant associations between bone mass and polymorphisms in the estrogen receptor gene, the interleukin-6 genes, the transforming growth factor β, and the Sp1 binding site of the collagen type I alpha 1 (COLIA1) gene (Grant *et al.*, 1996; Ralston, 1997b).

Because the risk of osteoporosis is greatly determined by peak bone mass, it is foreseen that any gene linked to fractures in the elderly will be found to be associated with low bone mass in children. This association, moreover, is likely to be present even in early childhood, as bone mass, bone density, and bone size measurements can be tracked from childhood to early adulthood and do not change percentiles during growth (Ferrari *et al.*, 1998; V. Gilsanz, personal observation). Indeed, recent studies in prepubertal girls have shown that both the VDR and COLIA1 genes are linked with the density of bone, providing clear evidence that osteoporosis has its antecedents in childhood (Figure 3) (Sainz *et al.*, 1997; Van Tornout *et al.*, 1997).

VIII. Gender

Bone mass is lower in women than in men, and this gender difference is considered to be an important determinant of the greater occurrence of osteoporosis and fractures in women (Cummings *et al.*, 1985). Because most data suggest that this disparity is present early in life, defining the factors that influence bone mass during growth, and whether they regulate the size and/or the density of bone, may help explain why girls are more "at risk" for osteoporosis than boys. Recent observations indicate that, throughout childhood and adulthood, females have smaller vertebral body size but similar cancellous bone density, when compared with males matched for age, degree of sexual development, height, and weight (Gilsanz *et al.*, 1994a,b).

On average, the cross-sectional area of the vertebral bodies is 11% smaller in prepubertal girls than in prepubertal boys matched for age, height, and weight (Gilsanz *et al.*, 1994a, 1997). Although vertebral cross-sectional area increases with weight in all children, the values are substantially greater in boys than in girls. Moreover, this disparity increases with growth and is greatest at skeletal maturity, when the cross-sectional dimensions of the vertebrae are about 25% smaller in women than in men, even after taking into consideration differences in body size (Figure 4) (Gilsanz *et al.*, 1994b).

Because the compressive strength of the vertebrae is determined by cancellous bone density and the cross-sectional area of the vertebral body, a

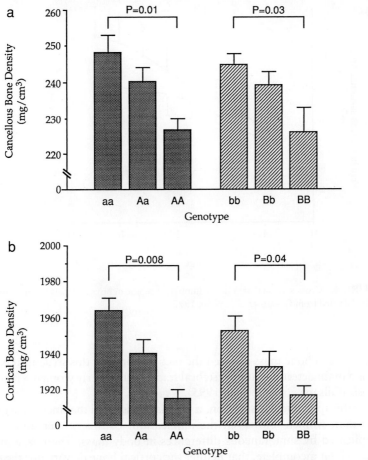

FIGURE 3   (A) Vertebral cancellous bone density and (B) femoral cortical bone density in relation to the VDR gene in 100 prepubertal girls. Values are means ± SE. Reproduced with permission from Sainz *et al.* (1997).

small cross-sectional area is a major mechanical disadvantage and an important determinant of vertebral fractures (Gilsanz *et al.*, 1995). In a case control study, elderly women with reduced bone density and vertebral fractures had smaller vertebral bodies than women with the same bone density, age, and body habitus, who do not experience vertebral fractures. In women with fractures, the cross-sectional area of the unfractured vertebrae was approximately 10% smaller than in women without fractures. The smaller vertebral size in women with fractures resulted in greater mechanical stress for all physical activities and was a major contributor to their vertebral fractures (Gilsanz *et al.*, 1995). Thus, deciphering that bone size accounts for gender

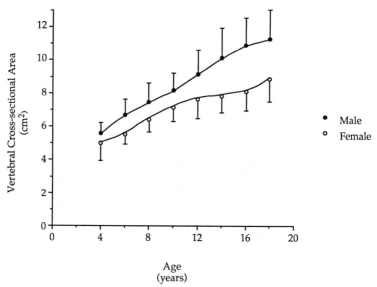

FIGURE 4   Cross-sectional area of the lumbar vertebrae in boys and girls. Values are means ± SD. Adapted from Gilsanz *et al.*, 1988b, 1997.

differences in bone mass allowed the recognition that this structural parameter is a main determinant of vertebral fractures in elderly women with osteoporosis (Gilsanz *et al.*, 1994b, 1995).

In the appendicular skeleton, it is usually assumed that men have greater mass than women. However, the implications of this gender difference is complicated by simultaneous differences in body mass. There is some evidence, albeit incomplete, that neither the cortical bone density nor the cross-sectional dimensions of the femur differ between males and females matched for age, height, and weight. Moro *et al.* (1996) found that with body mass considered multiple regression analysis revealed little gender influence in the determination of appendicular skeletal dimensions in a group of adolescents and young adults (ages 9–26 years). Regardless of gender, body weight was the primary determinant of the cross-sectional and cortical bone areas at the midshaft of the femur, a notion consistent with analytical models proposing that long bone cross-sectional growth is strongly driven by mechanical stimuli associated with increases in body mass during growth (van der Meulen *et al.*, 1993). Gilsanz *et al.* (1997) reported similar findings in a group of preadolescents.

The reasons for the larger cross-sectional dimensions of the bones in the axial but not the appendicular skeleton of boys are unknown. Testosterone, however, has been implied to have a preferential effect on the growth of the axial skeleton. Observations on the treatment of children with hypopituitarism suggest that growth in the upper body segment, indicated by sitting height, is relatively more dependent on testosterone, whereas growth in the lower body segment, indicated by the difference between standing and sitting heights, is primarily under the control of growth hormone (Aynsley-Green *et al.*, 1976; Tanner *et al.*, 1976).

Even though both androgens and estrogens promote accretion and maintenance of bone mass, there are major differences in the effects that these two hormones have on musculoskeletal development (Bachrach and Smith, 1996). Recent studies indicate that, in boys and girls, skeletal maturation is regulated by estrogen and that the lack of estrogens leads to delayed epiphyseal closure, eunochoid habitus, and decreased bone mass (Bachrach and Smith, 1996; Carani *et al.*, 1997). The advanced skeletal age and greater rate of skeletal maturation in girls, when compared to boys, is likely the result of higher estrogen levels (Greulich and Pyle, 1959). Androgens, unlike estrogens, increase protein synthesis in skeletal muscle in prepubertal children, which could account for the differences in muscle mass among sexes (Mauras *et al.*, 1994; Mauras, 1995). In addition, testosterone, either directly or indirectly through its effect on muscle mass, has an effect on the overall size of the bones (Snow-Harter *et al.*, 1990). In men, testosterone deficiency results in smaller bones and blockage of the neonatal secretion of gonadotropins and testosterone in newborn male monkeys results in diminished bone mass and smaller bone size (Mann *et al.*, 1993; Seeman, 1997). Thus, higher testosterone levels in boys during infancy and puberty may account for gender differences in skeletal size.

Regardless of the mechanism by which gender influences skeletal growth, its discrepant effect on the appendicular and axial skeletons may account for the sex difference in the incidence of fractures in elderly subjects with osteoporosis. Theoretically, the smaller vertebral cross-sectional dimensions in women could explain their higher incidence of vertebral fractures when compared to men (Cummings *et al.*, 1985). Likewise, the lack of gender differences in the cross-sectional dimensions of the femur may partially account for the less discrepant incidence of hip fractures between women and men (Melton, 1995).

IX. Race

The prevalence of osteoporosis and the incidence of fractures are substantially lower in black than in white persons, a finding generally attributed to racial differences in adult bone mass (Cummings *et al.*, 1985; Melton and Riggs, 1987). Whether these racial differences are present in childhood has been the subject of considerable interest. Several reports, including those of cadavers (Arnold *et al.*, 1966; Trotter and Peterson, 1970) and those using radiogrammetry (Garn *et al.*, 1972), have suggested a greater skeletal size in black children, and most studies with single photon absorptiometry have indicated radial bone mass to be greater in black subjects (Specker *et al.*, 1987; DePriester *et al.*, 1991). More recent investigations using dual x-ray or photon absorptiometry techniques have yielded conflicting results. Some studies found the bone mass of black children to be greater than that of white children (Li *et al.*, 1989; Bell *et al.*, 1991), whereas others detected no racial differences in bone mass, either in the axial or appendicular skeleton (Southard *et al.*, 1991; Moro *et al.*, 1996).

Studies using CT indicate that, regardless of gender, race has significant and differential effects on the density and the size of the bones in the axial and appendicular skeletons (Gilsanz *et al.*, 1998). In the axial skeleton, the density of cancellous bone in the vertebral bodies is greater in black than in white adolescents, regardless of gender. This difference first becomes apparent during late stages of puberty and persists throughout life. Before puberty, cancellous bone density is similar in black and white children, and, during puberty, it increases in all adolescents. The magnitude of the increase from prepubertal to postpubertal values is, however, substantially greater in black than in white subjects (34% vs. 11%, respectively) (Figure 5) (Gilsanz *et al.*, 1998). The cross-sectional areas of the vertebral bodies, however, do not differ between black and white children (Gilsanz *et al.*, 1998). Thus, theoretically, the structural basis for the lower vertebral bone strength and the greater incidence of fractures in the axial skeleton of white subjects resides in their lower cancellous bone density.

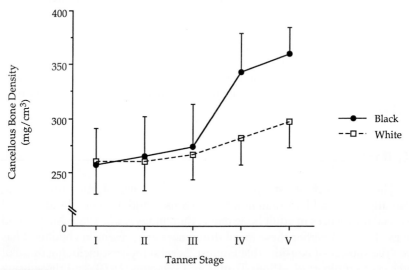

FIGURE 5   Vertebral cancellous bone density in black and white children at each stage of sexual development. Values are means ± SD. Reproduced with permission from Gilsanz *et al.*, 1988b, 1991a.

In contrast, in the appendicular skeleton, race influences the cross-sectional areas of the femurs, but not the cortical bone area nor the material density of cortical bone (Gilsanz *et al.*, 1998). Although values for femoral cross-sectional area increase with height, weight, and other anthropometric parameters in all children, this measurement is substantially greater in black children. On average, the cross-sectional area of the femur at skeletal maturity is 7% and 11% greater in black than in white females and males, respectively (Gilsanz *et al.*, 1998). Because the same amount of cortical bone placed further from the center of the bone results in greater bone strength, the skeletal advantage for blacks in the appendicular skeleton is likely the consequence of the greater cross-sectional size of the bones (van der Meulen *et al.*, 1993).

X. Conclusion

Among the main areas of progress in osteoporosis research during the last decade or so are the general recognition that this condition, which is the cause of so much pain in the elderly, has its antecedents in childhood; the identification of the structural basis accounting for much of the differences in bone strength among humans; and the recent insight into the complex genotypes of this disease. Advances in our understanding of racial and gender differences in bone fragility have come from using techniques that allow three-dimensional comparative analyses of the various parameters of bone mass. Of note are the findings that vertebral fractures may be more common in women than in men because women have smaller vertebrae and that they may be more common in white persons than in black persons because whites have lower spinal bone density. It is anticipated that future studies will show that regardless of race or gender, osteoporosis results, in part, from inherited variations in genes involved in the regulation of the two components of bone mass—bone size and bone density. It is also foreseen that any gene linked to fractures in the elderly will be found to be associated with low bone density and/or small bones in children because the risk of osteoporosis is greatly determined by peak bone mass. Indeed, recent studies in children indicate that the VDR and COLIA1 genes, which have been associated with low bone mass and/or fractures in the elderly, are also related to bone density in prepubertal girls. Thus, it is tempting to think that we will soon be in a position to identify the phenotype(s) and genotype(s) in children at risk for osteoporosis later in life and design appropriate early interventions for this condition.

Acknowledgments

The author thanks Ms. Cara L. Beck for her technical assistance and comments on this manuscript.

This work was supported in part by a grant (R01-AR4-1853-01A1) from the National Institute of Arthritis and Musculoskeletal and Skin Diseases and a grant (1RO1 LM06270-01) from the National Library of Medicine.

References

Arnold, J. S. (1973). Amount and quality of trabecular bone in osteoporotic vertebral fractures. *Clin. Endocrinol. Metab.* **2,** 221–238.

Arnold, J. S., Bartley, M. H., Tont, S. A., and Jenkins, D. P. (1966). Skeletal changes in aging and disease. *Clin. Orthop.* **49,** 17–38.

Aynsley-Green, A., Zachmann, M., and Prader, A. (1976). Interrelation of the therapeutic effects of growth hormone and testosterone on growth in hypopituitarism. *J. Pediatr.* **89,** 992–999.

Bachrach, B. E., and Smith, E. P. (1996). The role of sex steroids in bone growth and development: Evolving new concepts. *Endocrinologist* **6,** 362–368.

Bass, S., Pearce, G., Bradney, M., Hendrich, E., Delmas, P. D., Harding, A., and Seeman, E. (1998). Exercise before puberty may confer residual benefits in bone density in adulthood: Studies in active prepubertal and retired female gymnasts. *J. Bone Miner. Res.* **13,** 500–507.

Bell, N. H., Shary, J., Stevens, J., Garza, M., Gordon, L., and Edwards, J. (1991). Demonstration that bone mass is greater in black than in white children. *J. Bone Miner. Res.* **6,** 719–723.

Bonjour, J. P., Theintz, G., Buchs, B., Slosman, B., and Rizzoli, R. (1991). Critical years and stages of puberty for spinal and femoral bone mass accumulation during adolescence. *J. Clin. Endocrinol. Metab.* **73,** 555–563.

Cann, C. E., and Genant, H. K. (1980). Precise measurement of vertebral mineral content using computed tomography. *J. Comput. Assist. Tomogr.* **4,** 493–500.

Carani, C., Qin, K., Simoni, M., Faustini-Fustini, M., Serpente, S., Boyd, J., Korach, K. S., and Simpson, E. R. (1997). Effect of testosterone and estradiol in a man with aromatase deficiency. *N. Engl. J. Med.* **337,** 91–95.

Carter, D. R., Bouxsein, M. L., and Marcus, R. (1992). New approaches for interpreting projected bone densitometry data. *J. Bone Miner. Res.* **7,** 137–145.

Carter, D. R., van der Meulen, M. C. H., and Beaupre, G. S. (1996). Skeletal development: Mechanical consequences of growth, aging and disease. *In* "Osteoporosis" (R. Marcus, D. Feldman, and J. Kelsey, eds.), pp. 333–350. Academic Press, San Diego, CA.

Chan, G. M., Hoffman, K., and McMurry, M. (1995). Effects of dairy products on bone and body composition in pubertal girls. *J. Pediatr.* **126,** 551–556.

Christian, J. C., Yu, P. L., Slemenda, C. W., and Johnston, C. C. (1989). Heritability of bone mass: A longitudinal study in ageing male twins. *Am. J. Hum. Genet.* **44,** 429–433.

Cooper, G. S., and Umbach, D. M. (1996). Are vitamin D receptor polymorphisms associated with bone mineral density? A meta-analysis. *J. Bone Miner. Res.* **11,** 1841–1849.

Cummings, S. R., Kelsey, J. L., Nevitt, N. C., and O'Dowd, K. J. (1985). Epidemiology of osteoporosis and osteoporotic fractures. *Epidemiol. Rev.* **7,** 178–208.

Dawson-Hughes, B., Harris, S. S., and Finneran, S. (1995). Calcium absorption on high and low calcium intakes in relation to vitamin D receptor genotype. *J. Clin. Endocrinol. Metab.* **80,** 3657–3661.

De Boer, H., Blok, G. J., Van Lingen, A., Teule, G. J., Lips, P., and ven der Veen, E. A. (1994). Consequences of childhood-onset growth hormone deficiency for adult bone mass. *J. Bone Miner. Res.* **9,** 1319–1326.

DePriester, J. A., Cole, T. J., and Bishop, N. H. (1991). Bone growth and mineralization in children aged 4 to 10 years. *Bone Miner.* **12,** 57–65.

Donaldson, J. S., Gilsanz, V., Gonzalez, G., Wittel, R. A., and Gilles, F. (1985). Tall vertebrae at birth: A radiographic finding in flaccid infants. *Am. J. Roentgenol.* **145,** 1293–1295.

Drinkwater, B. L., Nilson, K., Chestnut, C. H., III, Bremner, W. J., Shainholtz, S., and South-worth, M. B. (1984). Bone mineral content of amenorrheic and eumenorrheic athletes. *N. Engl. J. Med.* **311,** 277–281.

Dunnill, M. S., Anderson, J. A., and Whitehead, R. (1967). Quantitative histological studies on age changes in bone. *J. Pathol. Bacteriol.* **94,** 275–291.

Dyson, E. D., Jackson, C. K., and Whitehouse, W. J. (1970). Scanning electron microscope studies of human trabecular bone. *Nature (London)* **225,** 957–959.

Evans, R. A., Marel, G. H., Lancaster, E. K., Kos, S., Evans, M., and Wong, Y. P. (1988). Bone mass is low in relatives of osteoporotic patients. *Ann. Intern. Med.* **109,** 870–873.

Ferrari, S., Rizzoli, R., Slosman, D., and Bonjour, J. P. (1998). Familial resemblance for bone mineral mass is expressed before puberty. *J. Clin. Endocrinol. Metab.* **83,** 358–361.

Finkelstein, J. S., Neer, R. M., Biller, B. M. K., Crawford, J. D., and Klibanski, A. (1992). Osteopenia in men with a history of delayed puberty. *N. Engl. J. Med.* **326,** 600–604.

Fowler, P. A., Fuller, M. F., Glasbey, C. A., Foster, M. A., Cameron, G. G., McNeil, G., and Maughan, R. J. (1991). Total and subcutaneous adipose tissue in women: The measurement of distribution and accurate prediction of quantity using magnetic resonance imaging (MR). *Am. J. Clin. Nutr.* **54,** 18–25.

Garn, S. M., Nagy, J. M., and Sandusky, S. T. (1972). Differential sexual dimorphism in bone diameters of subjects of European and African ancestry. *Am. J. Anthropol.* **37,** 127–130.

Genant, H. K., Engelke, K., Fuerst, T., Gluer, C. C., Grampp, S., Harris, S. T., Jergas, M., Lang, T., Lu, Y., Majumdar, S., Mathur, A., and Takada, M. (1996). Noninvasive assessment of bone mineral and structure: state of the art. *J. Bone Miner. Res.* **11,** 707–730.

Gilsanz, V., Gibbens, D. T., Carlson, M., Boechat, M. I., Cann, C. E., and Schulz, E. E. (1988a). Peak trabecular vertebral density: A comparison of adolescent and adult females. *Calcif. Tissue Int.* **43,** 260–262.

Gilsanz, V., Gibbens, D. T., Roe, T. F., Carlson, M., Senac, M. O., Boechat, M. I., Huang, K. H., Schulz, E. E., Libanati, C. R., and Cann, C. C. (1988b). Vertebral bone density in children: Effect of puberty. *Radiology* **166,** 847–850.

Gilsanz, V., Roe, T. F., Gibbens, D. T., Schulz, E., Carlson, M. E., Gonzalez, O., and Boechat, M. I. (1988c). Effect of sex steroids on peak bone density of growing rabbits. *Am. J. Physiol.* **255,** 416–421.

Gilsanz, V., Gibbens, D. R., Carlson, M., Boechat, M. I., and Tolo, V. T. (1989). The effect of limping on vertebral bone density: A study of children with arsal coalition. *J. Pediatr. Orthop.* **9,** 33–36.

Gilsanz, V., Roe, T. F., Mora, S., Costin, G., and Goodman, W. G. (1991a). Changes in vertebral bone density in black girls and white girls during childhood and puberty. *N. Engl. J. Med.* **325,** 1597–1600.

Gilsanz, V., Roe, T. F., Antunes, J., Carlson, M., Duarte, M. A., and Goodman, W. G. (1991b). Effect of dietary calcium on bone density in growing rabbits. *Am. J. Physiol.* **260,** 471–476.

Gilsanz, V., Boechat, M. I., Roe, T. F., Loro, M. L., Sayre, J. W., and Goodman, W. G. (1994a). Gender differences in vertebral body sizes in children and adolescents. *Radiology* **190,** 673–677.

Gilsanz, V., Boechat, M. I., Gilsanz, R., Loro, M. L., Roe, T. F., and Goodman, W. G. (1994b). Gender differences in vertebral sizes in adults: Biomechanical implications. *Radiology* **190,** 678–682.

Gilsanz, V., Loro, M. L., Roe, T. F., Sayre, J., Gilsanz, R., and Schulz, E. (1995). Vertebral size in elderly women with osteoporosis. Mechanical implications and relationship to fractures. *J. Clin. Invest.* **95,** 2332–2337.

Gilsanz, V., Kovanlikaya, A., Costin, G., Roe, T. F., Sayre, J., and Kaufman, F. (1997). Differential effect of gender on the size of the bones in the axial and appendicular skeletons. *J. Clin. Endocrinol. Metab.* **82,** 1603–1607.

Gilsanz, V., Skaggs, D. L., Kovanlikaya, A., Sayre, J., Loro, M. L., Kaufman, F., and Korenman, S. G. (1998). Differential effect of race on the axial and appendicular skeletons of children. *J. Clin. Endocrinol. Metab.* **68,** 1420–1427.

Glüer, C. C., Cummings, S. R., Bauer, D. C., Stone, K., Pressman, A., Mathur, A., and Genant, H. K. (1996). Osteoporosis: Association of recent fractures with quantitative US findings. *Radiology* **199**, 725–732.

Gong, J. K., Arnold, J. S., and Cohn, S. H. (1964). Composition of trabecular and cortical bone. *Anat. Rec.* **149**, 325–331.

Gordon, C. L., Halton, J. M., Atkinson, S., and Webber, C. E. (1991). The contributions of growth and puberty to peak bone mass. *Growth, Dev. Aging* **55**, 257–262.

Graafmans, W. C., Lips, P., Ooms, M. E., van Leeuwen, J. P. T. M., Pols, H. A. P., and Uitterlinden, A. G. (1997). The effect of vitamin D supplementation on the bone mineral density of the femoral neck is associated with vitamin D receptor genotype. *J. Bone Miner. Res.* **12**, 1241–1245.

Grant, S. F., Reid, D. M., Blake, G., Herd, R., Fogelman, I., and Ralston, S. H. (1996). Reduced bone density and osteoporosis associated with a polymorphic Sp1 binding site in the collagen type I alfa 1 gene. *Nat. Genet.* **14**, 203–205.

Greulich, W. W., and Pyle, S. I. (1959). "Radiographic Atlas of Skeletal Development of the Hand and Wrist." Stanford University Press, Stanford, CA.

Halioua, L., and Anderson, J. J. B. (1990). Age and anthropometric determinants of radial bone mass in premenopausal Caucasian women: A cross-sectional study. *Osteoporosis Int.* **1**, 50–55.

Hall, B. K., and Herring, S. W. (1990). Paralysis and growth of the musculoskeletal system in the embryonic chick. *J. Morphol.* **206**, 45–56.

Hangartner, T. N. (1990). Influence of fat on bone measurements with dual-energy absorptiometry. *Bone Miner.* **9**, 71–78.

Hangartner, T. N., and Gilsanz, V. (1996). Evaluation of cortical bone by computed tomography. *J. Bone Miner. Res.* **11**, 1518–1525.

Hangartner, T. N., and Overton, T. R. (1982). Quantitative measurement of bone density using gamma-ray computed tomography. *J. Comput. Assist. Tomogr.* **6**, 1156–1162.

Howard, G., Nguyen, T., Morrison, N., Watanabe, T., Sambrook, P., Eisman, J., and Kelly, P. J. (1995). Genetic influences on bone density: Physiological correlates of vitamin D receptor gene alleles in premenopausal women. *J. Clin. Endocrinol. Metab.* **80**, 2800–2805.

Hyer, S. L., Rodin, D. A., Robias, J. H., Leiper, A., and Nussey, S. S. (1992). Growth hormone deficiency during puberty reduces adult bone density. *Arch. Dis. Child.* **67**, 1472–1474.

Johnston, C. C., Hui, S. L., and Wiske, P. (1981). Bone mass at maturity and subsequent rates of loss as determinants of osteoporosis. *In* "Osteoporosis: Recent Advances in Pathogenesis and Treatment" (H. F. DeLuca, H. M. Frost, and W. S. S. Jee, eds.), p. 285. University Park Press, Baltimore, MD.

Johnston, C. C., Miller, J. Z., Slemenda, C. W., Reister, T. K., Hui, S., Christian, J. C., and Peacock, M. (1992). Calcium supplementation and increases in bone mineral density in children. *N. Engl. J. Med.* **327**, 82–87.

Jones, H., Priest, J., Hayes, C., Tichenor, C., and Nagel, D. (1977). Humeral hypertrophy in response to exercise. *J. Bone Jt. Surg.* **59**, 204–208.

Kannus, P., Haapasalo, H., Sankelo, M., Sievanen, H., Pasanen, M., Heinonen, A., Oja, P., and Vuori, I. (1995). Effect of starting age of physical activity on bone mass in the dominant arm of tennis and squash players. *Ann. Intern. Med.* **123**, 27–31.

Katzman, D. K., Bachrach, L. K., Carter, D. R., and Marcus, R. (1991). Clinical and anthropometric correlates of bone mineral acquisition in healthy adolescent girls. *J. Clin. Endocrinol. Metab.* **73**, 1332–1339.

Kleerekoper, M., and Avioli, L. V. (1993). Evaluation and treatment of postmenopausal osteoporosis. *In* "Primer on the Metabolic Bone Diseases and Disorders of Mineral Metabolism" (M. J. Favus, ed.), pp. 223–229. Raven Press, New York.

Kleerekoper, M., Tolia, K., and Parfitt, A. M. (1981). Nutritional, endocrine, and demographic aspects of osteoporosis. *Orthop. Clin. North Am.* **12**, 547–558.

Kovanlikaya, A., Loro, M. L., Hangartner, T. N., Reynolds, R. A., Roe, T. F., and Gilsanz, V. (1996). Osteopenia in children: CT assessment. *Radiology* **198**, 781–784.

Krall, E. A., and Dawson-Hughes, B. (1993). Heritable and life-style determinants of bone mineral density. *J. Bone Miner. Res.* **8**, 1–9.

Kröger, H., Kotaniemi, A., Vainio, P., and Alhava, E. (1992). Bone densitometry of the spine and femur in children by dual-energy x-ray absorptiometry. *Bone Miner.* **17**, 75–85.

Kröger, H., Kotaniemi, A., Kröger, L., and Alhava, E. (1993). Development of bone mass and bone density of the spine and femoral neck—a prospective study of 65 children and adolescents. *Bone* **23**, 171–182.

Lee, W. T. K., Leung, S. S. F., Leung, D. M. Y., Tsang, H. S. Y., Lau, J., and Cheng, J. C. Y. (1995). A randomized double-blind controlled calcium supplementation trial, and bone and height acquisition in children. *Br. J. Nutr.* **74**, 125–139.

Li, J. Y., Specker, B. L., Ho, M. L., and Tsang, R. C. (1989). Bone mineral content in black and white children 1 to 6 years of age. Early appearance of race and sex differences. *Am. J. Dis. Child.* **143**, 1346–1349.

Lloyd, T. L., Martel, J. K., Rollings, N., Andon, M. B., Kulin, H., Demers, L. M., Eggli, D. F., Kieselhorst, K., and Chinchilli, V. M. (1996). The effect of calcium supplementation and Tanner stage on bone density, content and area in teenage women. *Osteoporosis Int.* **6**, 276–283.

Lu, P. W., Briody, J. N., Ogle, G. D., Morley, K., Humphries, I. R. J., Allen, J., Howman-Giles, R., Sillence, D., and Cowell, C. T. (1994). Bone mineral density of total body, spine, and femoral neck in children and young adults: A cross-sectional and longitudinal study. *J. Bone Miner. Res.* **9**, 1451–1458.

Mann, D. R., Akingami, M. A., Gould, K. G., Tanner, J. M., and Wallen, K. (1993). Neonatal treatment of male monkeys with a gonadotropin-releasing hormone agonist alters differentiation of central nervous system centers that regulate sexual and skeletal development. *J. Clin. Endocrinol. Metab.* **76**, 1319–1324.

Marcus, R., Kosen, J., Pfefferbaum, A., and Horning, A. (1983). Age-related loss of trabecular bone in premenopausal women: A biopsy study. *Calcif. Tissue Int.* **35**, 406–409.

Matkovic, V., Kostial, K., Simonovic, I., Buzinz, R., Brodarec, A., and Nordin, B. E. (1979). Bone status and fracture rates in two regions of Yugoslavia. *Am. J. Clin. Nutr.* **32**, 540–549.

Matkovic, V., Jelic, T., Wardlaw, G. M., Ilich, J. Z., Goel, P. K., Wright, J. K., Andon, M. B., Smith, K. T., and Heaney, R. P. (1994). Timing of peak bone mass in Caucasian females and its implication for the prevention of osteoporosis. *J. Clin. Invest.* **93**, 799–808.

Mauras, N. (1995). Estrogens do not affect whole-body protein metabolism in the prepubertal female. *J. Clin. Endocrinol. Metab.* **80**, 2842–2845.

Mauras, N., Blizzard, R. M., Link, K., Johnson, M. L., Rogol, A. D., and Veldhuis, J. D. (1987). Augmentation of growth hormone secretion during puberty: Evidence for a pulse amplitude-modulated phenomenon. *J. Clin. Endocrinol. Metabl.* **64**, 596–601.

Mauras, N., Rogol, A. D., and Veldhuis, J. D. (1989). Specific, time-dependent actions of low dose ethinyl estradiol administration on the episodic release of growth hormone, follicle-stimulating hormone and lutenizing hormone in prepubertal girls with Turner's syndrome. *J. Clin. Endocrinol. Metab.* **69**, 1053–1058.

Mauras, N., Haymond, M. W., Darmaun, D., Vieira, N. E., Abrams, S. A., and Yergey, A. (1994). Calcium and protein kinetics in prepubertal boys—positive effects of testosterone. *J. Clin. Invest.* **93**, 1014–1019.

Melton, L. J., III (1995). Epidemiology of fractures. *In* "Osteoporosis" (B. L. Riggs and L. J. Melton, III, eds.), pp. 225–247. Lippincott-Raven, Philadelphia.

Melton, L. J., III, and Riggs, B. L. (1987). Epidemiology of age-related fractures. *In* "The Osteoporotic Syndrome: Detection, Prevention, and Treatment" (L. V. Avioli, ed.), pp. 1–30. Grune & Stratton, Orlando, FL.

Merz, W. A., and Schenk, R. K. (1970). A quantitative histological study on bone formation in human cancellous bone. *Acta Anat* **76**, 1.

Mora, S., Goodman, W. G., Loro, M. L., Roe, T. F., Sayre, J., and Gilsanz, V. (1994). Age-related changes in cortical and cancellous vertebral bone density in girls: Assessment with quantitative CT. *Am. J. Roentgenol.* **162**, 405–409.

Moro, M., van der Meulen, M. C. H., Kiratli, B. J., Marcus, R., Bachrach, L. K., and Carter, D. R. (1996). Body mass is the primary determinant of midfemoral bone acquisition during adolescent growth. *Bone* **19**, 519–526.

Morrison, N. A., Qi, J. C., Tokita, A., Kelly, P. J., Crofts, L. Nguyen, T. V., Sambrook, P. N., and Eisman, J. A. (1994). Prediction of bone density by vitamin D receptor alleles. *Nature (London)* **327**, 284–287.

Mosekilde, Li. (1989). Sex differences in age-related loss of vertebral trabecular bone mass and structure—biomechanical consequences. *Bone* **10**, 425–432.

Mosekilde, Li., and Mosekilde, Le. (1990). Sex differences in age-related changes in vertebral body size, density and biomechanical competence in normal individuals. *Bone* **11**(2), 67–73.

Nguyen, T. V., Morrison, N. A., Sambrook, P. N., Kelly, P. J., and Eisman, J. A. (1996). Vitamin D receptor gene and osteoporosis (letter). *J. Clin. Endocrinol. Metab.* **81**, 1674–1675.

Ott, S. (1990). Editorial: Attainment of peak bone mass. *J. Clin. Endocrinol. Metab.* **71**, 1082A–1082C.

Parfitt, A. M. (1997). Genetic effects on bone mass and turnover-relevance to black/white differences. *J. Am. Coll. Nutr.* **16**, 325–333.

Plotkin, H., Núñez, Alvarez Filgueira, M. L., and Zanchetta, J. R. (1996). Lumbar spine bone density in Argentine children. *Calcif. Tissue Int.* **58**, 144–149.

Pocock, N. A., Eisman, J. A., Hopper, J. L., Yeates, M. G., Sambrook, P. N., and Ebert, S. (1991). Genetic determinants of bone mass in adults: A twin study. *J. Clin. Invest.* **80**, 706–710.

Ralston, S. H. (1997a). Genetic markers of bone metabolism and bone disease. *Scand. J. Clin. Lab.* **227**, 114–121.

Ralston, S. H. (1997b). Osteoporisis. *Br. Med. J.* **315**, 469–472.

Recker, R. R., Davies, K. M., Hinders, S. M., Heaney, R. P., Stegman, M. R., and Kimmel, D. B. (1992). Bone gain in young adult women. *JAMA, J. Am. Med. Assoc.* **268**, 2403–2408.

Riggs, B. L., Wahner, H. W., Dunn, W. L., Mazess, R. B., Offord, K. P., and Mellon, L. J. (1981). Differential changes in bone density of the appendicular skeleton with aging. *J. Clin. Invest.* **67**, 328–335.

Rodriguez, J. I., Palacios, J., Garcia-Aliz, A., Pastor, I., and Paniagua, I. (1988). Effects of immobilization on fetal bone development. A morphometric study in newborns with congenital neuromuscular diseases with intrauterine onset. *Calcif. Tissue Int.* **43**, 335–339.

Rüegsegger, P., Elsasser, U., Anliker, M., Gnehm, H., Kind, H., and Prader, A. (1976). Quantification of bone mineralization using computed tomography. *Radiology* **121**, 93–97.

Rüegsegger, P., Durand, E. P., and Dambacher, M. A. (1991). Differential effects of aging and disease on trabecular and compact bone density of the radius. *Bone* **12**, 99–105.

Sainz, J., van Tournout, J. M., Loro, M. L., Sayre, J., Roe, T. F., and Gilsanz, V. (1997). Vitamin D receptor gene polymorphisms and bone density in prepubertal girls. *N. Engl. J. Med.* **337**, 77–82.

Seeman, E. (1997). Osteoporosis in men. *Adv. Osteoporosis* **4**, 6–7.

Seeman, E., Hopper, J. L., Bach, L. A., Cooper, M. E., Parkinson, E., McKay, J., and Jerums, G. (1989). Reduced bone mass in daughters of women with osteoporosis. *N. Engl. J. Med.* **320**, 554–558.

Snow-Harter, C., Bouxsein, M., Lewis, B., Charette, S., Weinstein, P., and Marcus, R. (1990). Muscle strength as a predictor of bone mineral density. *J. Bone Miner. Res.* **5**, 589–595.

Southard, R. N., Morris, J. D., Mahan, J. D., Hayes, J. R., Tochr, M. A., Sommer, A., and Zipf, W. B. (1991). Bone mass in healthy children: Measurements with quantitative DXA. *Radiology* **179**, 735–738.

Specker, B. L. (1996). Evidence for an interaction between calcium intake and physical activity on changes in bone mineral density. *J. Bone Miner. Res.* **11**, 1539–1544.

Specker, B. L., Brazerol, W., Tsang, R. C., Levin, R., Searcy, J., and Steichen, J. (1987). Bone mineral content in children 1 to 6 years of age: Detectable sex differences after 4 years of age. *Am. J. Dis. Child.* **141**, 343–344.

Tanner, J. M., Whitehouse, R. H., Hughes, P. C. R., and Carter, B. S. (1976). Relative impor-
    tance of growth hormone and sex steroids for the growth at puberty of trunk length, limb
    length, and muscle width in growth hormone-deficient children. *J. Pediatr.* **89,** 1000–1008.
Theintz, G., Buchs, B., Rizzoli, R., Slosman, D., Clavien, H., Sizonenko, P. C., and Bonjour,
    J. P. (1992). Longitudinal monitoring of bone mass accumulation in healthy adolescents:
    Evidence for a marked reduction after 16 years of age at the levels of lumbar spine and
    femoral neck in female subjects. *J. Clin. Endocrinol. Metab.* **75,** 1060–1065.
Torgerson, D. J., Campbell, M. K., and Reid, D. M. (1995). Life-style, environmental and
    medical factors influencing peak bone mass in women. *Br. J. Rheum.* **34,** 620–624.
Trotter, M., and Peterson, R. R. (1970). Weight of the skeleton during postnatal development.
    Am. J. Phys. Anthropol. **33,** 313–324.
Uhthoff, H. K., and Jaworski, Z. F. (1978). Bone loss in response to long-term immobilization.
    J. Bone Jt. Surg. **60,** 420–429.
van der Meulen, M. C. H., Beaupre, G. S., and Carter, D. R. (1993). Mechanobiologic influences
    in long bone cross-sectional growth. *Bone* **14,** 635–642.
Van Tornout, J. M., Sainz, J., and Gilsanz, V. (1997). Towards a multigenetic predictive model
    for bone density in healthy, prepubertal girls. *J. Bone Miner. Res.* **12,** S492
Weaver, J. K., and Chalmers, J. (1966). Cancellous bone: Its strength and changes with aging
    and an evaluation of some methods for measuring its mineral content. I. Age changes in
    cancellous bone. *J. Bone Jt. Surg.* **48,** 289–298.
Wehrli, F. W., Ford, J. C., and Haddad, J. G. (1995). Osteoporosis: Clinical assessment with
    quantitative MR imaging in diagnosis. *Radiology* **196,** 631–641.

Chapter 6

Ego Seeman

Austin & Repatriation Medical Center
The University of Melbourne
Melbourne, Australia

Bone Size, Mass, and Volumetric Density:
The Importance of Structure in Skeletal Health

I. Introduction

The purpose of this review is (i) to describe the changes in skeletal size, mass, and internal architecture that occur during growth and aging in men and women of different racial groups and (ii) to describe the differences in skeletal size, mass, and internal architecture found in men with fractures relative to men without fractures. Because the modeling and remodeling of the periosteal and endosteal (endocortical, intracortical, and trabecular) surfaces during growth and aging determine the external and internal structure of bone, insight into the mechanisms responsible for the development of bone fragility in men and women can be gained by comparing and contrasting the age-, gender-, and race-specific patterns of modeling and remodeling that occur on these bone surfaces.

The growth of the periosteal surface defines the external bone size—an independent determinant of bone strength. The growth of the endocortical surface relative to the periosteal surface determines cortical thickness. The subsequent expansion of the periosteal surface and endocortical remodeling during aging determines the extent of cortical thinning and the distance of the mass of cortical bone relative to the neutral axis of the long bone in old age. The development of trabecular numbers during growth, and the thickening of the trabeculae during pre- and peripubertal growth establishes peak trabecular bone density and the size of surface available for remodeling during aging. The subsequent intensity of remodeling and the remodeling imbalance between bone formation and resorption within each BMU on the trabecular surfaces during aging establish the extent of trabecular bone loss and the degree of trabecular thinning, loss of trabecular connectivity, and so trabecular bone fragility.

II. Comparing Men and Women of Different Races _____

Fractures may occur less commonly in men than in women because bone fragility is less or trauma is less common or less severe. The mechanisms that are more likely to contribute to the lower bone fragility in men than women include the following: (i) attainment of a higher peak bone mass and size at the completion of growth, (ii) less bone loss as a percentage of the (higher) peak bone mass in men, (iii) trabecular bone loss by thinning caused by reduced bone formation in men (Trabecular plate perforation and loss of connectivity is primarily the result of a menopause-related increase in the extent of remodeling and perhaps resorption depth in women.), (iv) less endocortical resorption, (v) greater periosteal expansion during aging, thus increasing bone size and strength, and counteracting cortical bone thinning due to endocortical resorption, and (vi) perhaps less intracortical porosity (Seeman, 1994, 1995).

A. Growth in Size, Mass, and Volumetric Density of the Axial Skeleton

Males have bigger bones than females, and bone size is an independent determinant of bone strength (Ruff and Hayes, 1988). Whether gender and racial differences in bone size are present before birth or shortly thereafter is uncertain. Rupich *et al.* (1996) suggest gender and ethnic differences in total body bone mineral content (BMC) and areal bone mineral density (BMD) are present in infants aged 1 to 18 months. Gilsanz *et al.* (1988), using quantitative computed tomography (QCT) in a study of 196 healthy children aged 4 to 20 years, reported that the cross-sectional area of vertebral bodies was 17% greater in boys at Tanner stage I and higher throughout childhood and adolescence. There were no gender differences in vertebral height. By contrast, blacks matched by height have longer legs and shorter sitting height than whites. Vertebral height was less in black men and women when compared to their white counterparts. Vertebral width was similar in black and white men and in black and white women (Gilsanz *et al.*, 1998). This suggests that there may be race-specific factors regulating vertebral height and gender-specific factors regulating vertebral width.

Areal BMD is greater in the spine in men than women in large part because vertebral width (not height) is greater. The greater amount of bone gained during growth in men than women builds a bigger skeleton, but not necessarily a denser skeleton. For volumetric BMD (the amount of bone contained within *the* bone) to increase during growth, the increase in bone mass (*relative* to the population mean for bone mass) must be greater than the increase in bone size (*relative* to the population mean for bone size). This may occur in predominantly trabecular structures such as the vertebral body by increasing trabecular numbers or thickness or by increasing the true (material) density of the trabeculae themselves (Seeman, 1998).

Volumetric BMD is no different in men and women of the same race (i.e., at peak, trabecular number and thickness are the same in white men and women and in black men and women). Gilsanz *et al.* (1994), reported no differences in cancellous or cortical BMD in 25 women and 18 men aged between 25 and 46 years. Vertebral bodies in women had a lower cross-sectional area (7.9 ± 1.1 versus 10.9 ± 1.3 cm², $P < 0.001$) and volume (22.4 ± 2.4 versus 30.9 ± 2.6 cm³, $P < 0.001$) than men. As a consequence, mechanical stresses within vertebral bodies were predicted to be 30–40% greater in women than in men. Similarly, neither trabecular number nor thickness differ in South African black men and women nor in Japanese men and women (Schnitzler *et al.*, 1990). Fugii *et al.* (1989), using QCT, showed that Japanese men and women have similar trabecular volumetric BMD. By contrast, volumetric BMD is greater in blacks than whites of the corresponding gender because blacks have thicker trabeculae than whites (Han *et al.*, 1996; Parfitt, 1998). Thus, males may have greater peak vertebral bone strength than females of the same race as a result of greater vertebral width, not vertebral BMD. Blacks may have greater peak vertebral bone strength than whites of the corresponding gender because of greater trabecular BMD, despite the smaller vertebral size. (Blacks have a shorter vertebral body containing more bone as a result of thicker trabeculae.)

Before puberty, trabecular volumetric BMD at the spine is similar in boys and girls, blacks and whites, and is independent of age during the prepubertal years. During puberty, trabecular volumetric BMD increases comparably in males and females of a given race but increases more greatly in blacks than whites (Gilsanz *et al.*, 1998) (Figure 1). The increase in trabecular BMD in males and females, as well as the greater increase in trabecular BMD in blacks than whites, is likely to be the result of increased trabecular thickness, not

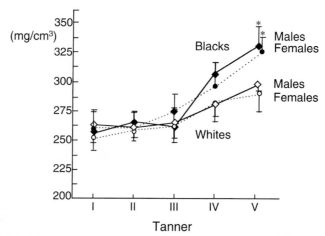

FIGURE I   Vertebral cancellous bone mineral density (mg/cm³) in black and white girls and boys does not differ before puberty, during puberty, increases comparably in girls and boys of the same race but increases more greatly in blacks than whites. Males (full lines), females (broken lines), blacks (full symbols), whites (open symbols). Reproduced from Gilsanz *et al.*, Differential effects of race on the axial and appendicular skeleton of children, *J. Clin. Endocrinol. Metab.* 5, 1420–1427, 1998, © The Edocrine Society.

numbers (Han *et al.*, 1996; Parfitt, 1998). Fugii *et al.* (1989), using QCT, showed that Japanese men and women had lower trabecular BMD than their white gender counterparts. The authors suggest that the differences were greater than can be explained by differences in the methods of measurement used in the two countries. Whether the Japanese have thinner or fewer trabeculae than whites is unknown because no histomorphometric data are available.

Thus, trabecular numbers are independent of race and gender (trabecular numbers are the same in males and females, blacks and whites). Trabecular thickness is independent of gender, being similar before puberty and increasing by a similar amount in males and females at puberty. Trabecular thickness is race-specific, being greater in blacks than whites and probably greater in whites than Japanese. The similarity in thickness in both genders suggests that estrogen may be the common factor regulating trabecular endosteal formation in males and females. Why does trabecular thickness increase more greatly in blacks than whites at puberty (and perhaps more greatly in whites than Japanese at puberty)? Why is vertebral height less and leg length greater in blacks? Why is leg length less in Japanese than whites, whereas trunk length is similar? An increased sensitivity or early exposure to estrogen in blacks may result in earlier fusion of epiphyses, producing shorter vertebra with thicker trabeculae. However, this would produce shorter legs in blacks than whites. Early exposure to estrogen produces smaller bones with higher volumetric BMD in animals (Migliaccio *et al.*, 1996).

B. Growth in Size, Mass, and Volumetric Density of the Appendicular Skeleton

The longer (2 years) prepubertal growth in boys, the more rapid pubertal growth spurt (reaching 10–12 cm/yr in boys and 8–10 cm/yr in girls), and the longer duration of puberty in boys all contribute to size differences. Only 3 cm of the 13-cm difference in height between men and women is attributable to pubertal growth, 10 cm is attributable to prepubertal growth, and most of this difference is in leg length (Cameron *et al.*, 1982; Preece *et al.*, 1992). Thus, on average, men are taller than women because they have longer legs rather than longer trunks. Similarly, black men matched by height with white men have longer legs (Gilsanz *et al.*, 1998). Whether the greater length is present at birth or emerges prior or during puberty is unclear.

Periosteal growth accelerates at puberty in males, enlarging bone diameter. In females, periosteal diameter ceases to expand at puberty, whereas endocortical contraction narrows the medullary cavity. This is illustrated in Figure 2 (Garn, 1970). Any existing gender difference in bone width before puberty increases further at puberty by this mechanism. Thus, bone length is greater in males because of the longer prepubertal and intrapubertal growth, whereas bone width is probably greater because of the androgen-mediated increase in periosteal expansion. Similarly, long bone width is greater in blacks than whites because of greater width at birth and/or greater periosteal expansion before or during puberty. Why blacks have wider and longer femurs than whites of the corresponding gender is uncertain.

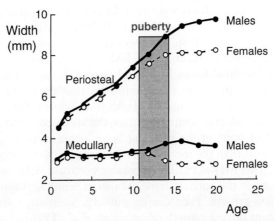

FIGURE 2 Metacarpal periosteal diameter increases in males and females before puberty and increases more greatly in males than females at puberty (gray bar), largely accounting for the gender difference in metacarpal width. Medullary (endocortical) width contracts at puberty in girls and minimally in boys so that final cortical thickness is similar in males and females. Adapted from tables in Garn (1970).

There is little evidence to support the notion that cortical thickness is greater in men than women or greater in blacks than whites. On the contrary, femoral cortical thickness is similar both in young men and women and in blacks and whites. Gilsanz *et al.* (1998) reported that white boys and girls have the same cortical thickness at the midfemur. Similarly, cortical thickness of the midfemur is similar in black males and females and is no different from their white counterparts.

Cortical thickness is the net result of the relative growth of the periosteal and endocortical surfaces. Before puberty, periosteal expansion proceeds rapidly, whereas endocortical (medullary) diameter expands modestly and then contracts, perhaps more in females than in males. Cortical thickness does not differ in males and females because the greater periosteal expansion in males is accompanied by greater endocortical expansion before puberty and less endocortical contraction during puberty. Females achieve the same cortical thickness as males because 25% of final thickness is the result of endocortical contraction during puberty, whereas 75% is the result of periosteal expansion. Cortical thickness in males is largely the result of periosteal expansion.

Similarly, for blacks to have the same cortical thickness as whites (despite the larger bone diameter), either endocortical expansion before and during puberty must be greater or endocortical contraction at puberty must be less in blacks. Garn *et al.* (1972) studied 4379 whites and 1589 blacks. Black men had 7% higher subperiosteal, 30% higher medullary, and 3% higher resultant cortical areas than whites. Black women had 14% higher subperiosteal, 49% higher medullary areas, and 7% higher cortical areas than white women. Whether differences of this magnitude account for the ethnic and gender differences in fracture rates is unknown. By contrast, in a study of 950 South African blacks and 782 whites, Solomon (1979) found that blacks had *lower* cortical area than whites (despite a lower fracture incidence).

Femoral midshaft BMC and areal BMD increase during growth because size increases. Proximal femur BMC and areal BMD are higher in men than women and higher in blacks than whites because the femur is longer and wider in men than women and in blacks than whites. For predominantly cortical structures like the femur or radius, the volumetric BMD will increase if the amount of bone in the growing bone increases more (relative to its population mean) than the increase in external volume (relative to its population mean). This may occur by increasing cortical thickness or increasing the true density of the cortical bone. Midshaft femoral volumetric BMD is constant during growth, even during puberty. Similarly, radial volumetric BMD is constant during growth (Zamberlan *et al.*, 1996). (Note that vertebral trabecular BMD increases at puberty.)

This constancy implies that the increase in size is matched by a commensurate increase in mass within the periosteal envelope of the growing long bone. Although the bones in males and females differ in size, they do not differ by volumetric BMD (Lu *et al.*, 1996). Although vertebral volumetric BMD is greater in blacks than whites, midshaft volumetric BMD was not higher in blacks than whites in the study by Gilsanz *et al.* (1998). This information suggests that any difference in bone fragility in childhood and early adulthood may be a function of the gender and racial differences in bone size rather than "density."

Thus, to summarize, femur length and width is greater in men than women and greater in blacks than whites. Cortical thickness is independent of gender and race. The greater diameter of the midfemur in the male than female and in blacks than whites results in the larger bone having a greater perimeter, and so the greater mass of cortical bone is placed farther from the neutral axis of the long bone conferring greater bone strength in men than women and in blacks than whites. Vertebral size is greater in men than women because vertebral width, not height, is greater. Men and women have the same trabecular number and thickness; at peak, bone strength is greater because bone size is greater. Vertebral size is less in blacks because vertebral height is less; width is similar. Blacks have thicker trabeculae; the vertebrae are smaller in blacks, but trabecular BMD is greater because the trabeculae are thicker.

The surfaces that form these dimensions and structures behave differently because they are regulated differently. Comparative studies within and between genders and races is likely to give insight into the genetic and environmental factors regulating these surfaces. An understanding of the hormonal regulators of periosteal and endocortical growth and remodeling in men and women and blacks and whites may contribute to the development of new drugs that increase periosteal growth (increasing the bending strength of cortical bone), increase endocortical apposition (increasing cortical thickness), or reduce endocortical resorption (preventing cortical thinning).

C. Delayed Puberty

Delayed puberty in males may result in increased femur length because of delayed epiphyseal fusion. Bone width may be reduced because periosteal growth is androgen-dependent. Whether delayed puberty results in reduced volumetric BMD is uncertain. Moore *et al.* (1997) report normal volumetric BMD in adult males with a history of delayed puberty. If volumetric BMD is reduced, this must be the result of reduced cortical width in long bones which may be the result of continued endocortical expansion despite reduced periosteal expansion (due to androgen deficiency) or of failed endocortical contraction (a process that may be dependent on estrogen synthesis from testosterone in males).

Finkelstein *et al.* (1992, 1996) suggest that men with constitutionally delayed puberty may have a low peak areal BMD in adulthood. In the first study, there were two control groups, 21 men 2 years younger and 39 men

2 years older than the cases. Lumbar spine areal BMD in the cases was 1.03 g/cm^2—0.10 g/cm^2 less than the younger controls and 0.05 g/cm^2 less than the 60 controls *combined*. Results for the 39 older controls were not provided but must have been lower than the younger controls to bring the mean from 1.13 g/cm^2 in the younger controls to 1.08 g/cm^2 for all 60 controls; lumbar spine areal BMD should be about 1.03 g/cm^2 in the older controls, which is no different than the cases. In the follow-up study conducted 2 years later in 18 men, radial and spinal areal BMD were reduced. Femoral neck areal BMD was lower than in the controls: 0.88 ± 0.11 versus 0.98 ± 0.14 g/cm^2 ($P < 0.02$). These subjects may have suffered from hypogonadotrophic hypogonadism rather than delayed puberty; they exercised 48 ± 104 miles/week, 35% ran more than 15 miles/week, and 57% were regular weight lifters. Whether the deficits are the result of reduced bone size is also unclear (Seeman, 1997, 1998). If delayed puberty reduces bone width, areal BMD may be reduced because of the smaller size. If bone length is increased (because of delayed epiphyseal closure), BMC or areal BMD may be higher or no different than the controls. For example, Luisetto *et al.* (1995) reported that 42 patients with Klinefelters' syndrome had normal areal BMD (z scores: lumbar spine, 0.5 SD; femoral neck, 0.002 SD; total femur, 0.2 SD). Failure to account for size may have resulted in finding no deficit at the proximal femur (probably a larger bone than in the controls).

III. Changes in Bone Size, Mass, and Volumetric Density during Aging

Bone remodeling occurs on the trabecular surfaces, on the endocortical surfaces, within the cortices of bone, and on the periosteal surfaces. The purpose of remodeling is to maintain bone strength. Remodeling imbalance, the failure to replace the old bone with the same amount of new bone, is the morphological basis of bone loss. Remodeling imbalance (i) on trabecular surfaces results in trabecular thinning, perforation, and loss of connectivity; (ii) on the endocortical surface results in cortical thinning; and (iii) within cortical bone results in increased cortical porosity. Periosteal appositional growth partly offsets the bone loss occurring on the endosteal surfaces.

A. Trabecular and Cortical Bone Loss

The amount of trabecular bone lost in women and men is similar whether assessed by histomorphometry of the iliac crest or quantitative computed tomography of the spine (Kalender *et al.*, 1989; Meunier *et al.*, 1990) (Figure 3). Trabecular bone loss occurs mainly by thinning in men and mainly by loss of connectivity in women (Aaron *et al.*, 1987) (Figure 4). Loss of connectivity may be less in men than in women because there is no

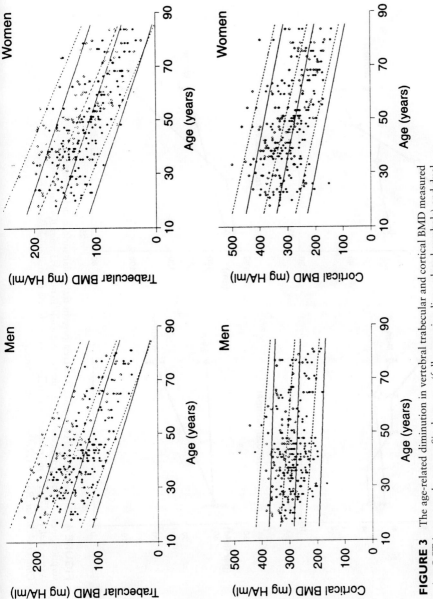

FIGURE 3 The age-related diminution in vertebral trabecular and cortical BMD measured using QCT in men and women. Single energy (full regression lines, closed symbols) and dual energy (full regression lines, closed symbols). Reproduced from *Eur. J. Radiol.* 9, Kalender *et al.*, Reference values for trabecular and cortical vertebral bone density in single and dual energy quantitative computed tomography, pp. 75–80, Copyright 1989, with permission from Elsevier Science.

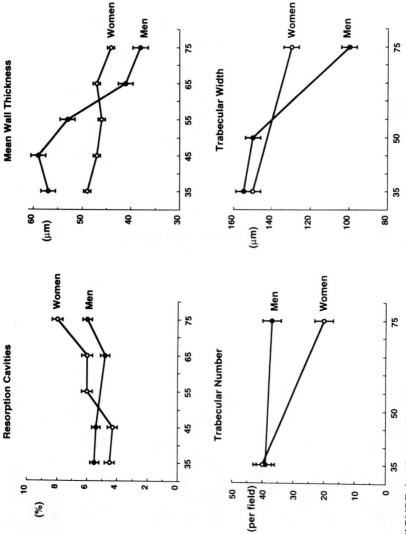

FIGURE 4 The age-related changes in iliac crest percent trabecular surface undergoing resorption, mean wall thickness, trabecular number, and width in men and women. Adapted from Aaron *et al.* (1987), The microanatomy of trabecular bone loss in normal aging men and women. *Clin. Orth. Relat. Res.* **215**, 260–271, with permission.

comparable menopause-related increase in remodeling intensity. In women, loss of trabeculae occurs because of the increased surface extent of remodeling and may produce perforation and complete loss of trabeculae. As trabeculae are lost, there is less trabecular surface available for remodeling, and trabecular bone loss slows. In men, progressive thinning of trabeculae may increase the trabecular surfaces available for remodeling. This may result in continued trabecular bone loss in men. Studies of vertebral trabecular bone loss in elderly men and women using QCT are not available.

Bone loss from the proximal femur is detected soon after attainment of peak areal BMD in cross-sectional studies using densitometry in men and in women. In part, the changes reported in cross-sectional studies may be an artifact of a fall in cellularity and an increase in adipose cells of the marrow in the proximal femur (Kuiper *et al.*, 1996). Studies are needed to clarify when bone loss commences at this site. Trabecular bone may reach its peak earlier than cortical bone and may start to decline while cortical mineral accrual and consolidation is still occurring. The age of attainment of peak areal BMD and commencement of bone loss may vary by race (Looker *et al.*, 1995).

Cortical bone loss is the result of endocortical remodeling imbalance, intracortical remodeling imbalance and periosteal apposition. Thus, the same amount of bone may be lost by fundamentally different mechanisms in males and females, in different races, and in the same individual at different times of life. For example, the 150 g less total bone "loss" in men than women is the net result of less endocortical bone resorption in men than women, greater periosteal apposition in men than in women, and less intracortical porosity in men than women.

The greater periosteal apposition in men than in women results in a bone with a larger cross-sectional area. Ruff and Hayes (1988) studied 99 tibia from 73 individuals and 103 femora from 75 individuals. Changes per decade included the following. (i) Medullary area (reflecting endosteal resorption) increased by 7% in men and 8% in women. (ii) Subperiosteal area (reflecting periosteal deposition) increased by 2.5% in men and 1.1% in women. (iii) Cortical area decreased by 1.6% in men and 7% in women. (iv) The polar second moment of area (bending rigidity), increased by 2.1% in men but declined by 3.3% in women.

Secular trends may obscure a true increase in periosteal diameter. Height and bone width have increased in the last 70 years. In a cross-sectional study, this age-related increase in bone width in (earlier born) current 80 year olds may bring bone width to equal the (later born) current 20 year olds. Femoral width increases more greatly in men than in women across age (Y. Duan and E. Seeman, unpublished data, 1998). However, secular increases in bone width have been reported in women in other studies (Looker *et al.*, 1995). The differing observations in cross-sectional studies may reflect either measurement error or the heterogeneous nature of secular changes in growth. Depending on the community studied, increases are found in one or both genders and in one or both upper and lower body segment lengths (Bakwin, 1964; Meredith, 1978; Cameron *et al.,* 1982; Tanner *et al.,* 1982; Malina and Brown, 1987).

Prospective studies suggest that bone loss accelerates, rather than decelerates, in old age. Ensrud *et al.* (1995) showed that rates of decline in areal BMD at the proximal femur, measured in 5698 community-living white women aged over 61 years, increased fivefold in women 70 to 85 years old. Jones *et al.* (1994) suggest that rates of bone loss at the proximal femur increase with advancing age, based on 241 men and 385 women followed an average of 2.5 years (range 1 to 4 years). More rapid rates of bone loss were not found at the lumbar spine, perhaps because of coexistent osteoarthritis and, in part, because of the loss of trabecular surface. Hannan *et al.* (1994) found similar rates of diminution (percent per year) in 437 men and 698 women 68 to 98 years old: -0.69 ± 0.15 versus -0.68 ± 12 (femoral neck); -0.45 ± 0.17 versus $-0.53 + 0.15$ (trochanter); and -0.88 ± 0.23 versus -0.94 ± 0.12 (Wards triangle).

Secondary hyperparathyroidism is likely to contribute to accelerated cortical bone loss in men and women. Increased endocortical and intracortical remodeling increase the surface available for resorption in cortical bone and may explain the increasing rate cortical bone loss in the elderly. The increased numbers of sites undergoing remodeling on the progressively increasing surface contributes to accelerating bone loss because of the negative bone balance within each remodeling unit. Reduced cortical areal BMD is also the result of increased porosity. Laval-Jeantet *et al.* (1983) report cortical porosity of the humerus increased from ~4% in white men and women aged 40 years to ~10% in over 80 year olds. The fall in apparent density with age correlated with porosity. True mineral density (ash weight per volume unit of bone free of vascular channels) was unchanged.

B. Relative Contributions of Peak Bone Mass and Bone Loss to Bone Mass in Old Age

Men have a net gain of 1200 g calcium to build their skeleton and lose 100 g net (~8%). Women have a net gain of 900 g calcium and lose 250 g (~30%). Thus, bone mass in old age, when fractures occur, is determined more by the amount of bone gained during growth than lost during aging. Compared to women, men gain 300 g more calcium during growth to build a bigger skeleton than women (1200 − 900 g). Because the difference in net loss is 150 g (250 − 100 g), of the 450 g (1100 − 650 g) greater total bone calcium in elderly men than women, 300 g is attributable to the greater net gain, whereas only 150 g is attributable to the lesser net amount of bone lost during aging in men. Of this lesser amount lost, a proportion will be attributable to greater loss in women than men, and the remainder will be attributable to greater bone formation in men.

Because puberty occurs about 2 years later in boys than girls, the prepubertal contribution to total BMC in young adulthood in males is 80%, the pubertal contribution is 20%. In girls, prepubertal and pubertal growth each contribute about 50% of the total BMC in adulthood (Gordan *et al.*, 1991). Thus, a smaller proportion of total BMC at maturity may be sex-hormone-dependent in men than women. If so, then delayed puberty or hypogonadism during growth may be less deleterious in males than in females. If the amount of bone loss caused by hypogonadism is a function of the amount of bone gained during puberty, then hypogonadism during aging in males should be less deleterious than in females.

Comparisons of different racial/ethnic groups suggest that differences in total BMC in old age—when fractures occur—are constituted by different combinations of bone gain and loss (Looker *et al.*, 1995). For example, comparing the total BMC of the proximal femur in old age in whites, blacks, and Mexican-American men, blacks have higher BMC than whites in old age because they gain more and lose similar amounts. Blacks have higher BMC than Mexican-Americans because they gain more but lose more, attenuating the difference in peak BMC. White men gain more than Mexican-Americans but *lose* more, and so Mexican American men have *higher* BMC than whites in old age. The gains and losses are net changes; the relative contributions of the endosteal and periosteal surface modeling and remodeling to *both* peak BMC and net bone loss are unknown.

The changes are region-specific (Perry *et al.*, 1996). Data are available in women, not men. Upper body calcium net losses were 48 g in blacks and 70 g in whites, whereas lower body net losses were 146 g in blacks (14%) and 160 g in whites (16%). Thus, net bone loss is greater in whites than blacks in absolute terms and as a percentage of their (lower) peaks. Net loss relative to peak at the upper body in whites (70 g, 24%) was twice that in blacks (48 g, 14%), but similar net losses occurred in the lower body. The higher BMC in blacks than whites in the postmenopausal years is largely accounted for by the greater net gain in BMC by blacks during growth than by the greater net loss in whites during aging. How much of the greater net loss in whites than blacks is accounted for by more endocortical resorption in whites than blacks and/or more periosteal gain in blacks than whites is unknown.

C. Hip Axis Length

Hip axis length (HAL) is purported to be an independent predictor of hip fracture. These data are based mainly on studies in women. There is little evidence that men with hip fractures have shorter HAL than age-matched controls. Gomez (1994) studied 188 men and 300 women with hip fractures aged 75 ± 7 years. There was no difference in HAL between men or women with hip fractures relative to gender-matched controls. The neck-shaft angle was lower in the fracture cases. Femoral neck cross-sectional area was *higher* in the men with hip fractures (12.1 ± 2.3 cm) than in the controls (9.6 ± 2.1 cm, $P < 0.001$). This is an unusual observation because greater cross-sectional area is associated with greater bone strength. HAL was greater in men than women.

The finding of a shorter HAL in women compared to men is difficult to reconcile with the higher hip fracture rate in women. Racial differences in hip fracture incidence are also attributed to differences in HAL. Blacks have longer legs and shorter trunks than whites. The finding of a shorter HAL in blacks may be a conservative error; HAL may be even shorter if adjustment is made by leg length rather than total height. Asians have similar trunk length but shorter leg length than whites. A shorter HAL reported in Japanese may not be observed after adjustment for total height compared to whites after adjustment for leg length. There are secular trends in upper and/ or lower body segment lengths in whites, blacks, and Asians. Secular increases have been reported in upper and lower body segments in females and males, and secular increases in HAL may parallel the changes in segment lengths (referenced earlier). Whether they are responsible for the increase in hip fracture incidence is uncertain. Whether HAL is an independent predictor of hip fracture will not be resolved until a prospective randomized trial is performed by stratifying HAL and matching the groups for BMD, age, height, weight, and menopausal status.

IV. Comparing Men with and without Fractures ───────────

Areal BMD is reduced at most sites in men with fractures. Men with spine fractures have reduced areal BMD at the spine and proximal femur, whereas men with hip fractures have reduced areal BMD at the proximal femur with more modest deficits at the spine (in part because arthrosis artifactually increases BMD at that site). Because the areal BMD measurement does not entirely correct for differences in bone size, the deficits in areal BMD may be, in part, the result of reduced bone size in men with fractures. The remaining deficit between men with fractures and those without fractures (after accounting for differences in bone size) may be caused by reduced accrual, excessive bone loss, or both.

A. Reduced Bone Size

Reduced vertebral body width, but not femoral neck width, can be found in men with spine fractures (Vega *et al.*, 1998), and reduced femoral neck width, but not spine width, may be present in men with hip fractures (Y. Duan and E. Seeman, unpublished data, 1998). Approximately 16–20% of the deficit in areal BMD at the spine in men with spine fractures and at the proximal femur in men with hip fractures is explained by the smaller bone size. Vertebral body and femoral neck width increase as age advances

(Y. Duan and E. Seeman, unpublished data, 1998). Thus, the smaller bone size may be the result of the attainment of a reduced peak bone size, failure of periosteal apposition during advancing age, or both.

The site selectivity of the deficit in size may be related to reduced regional growth. Before puberty, growth in leg length is more rapid than growth in spine length. During puberty, growth in spine length increases, while leg epiphyses fuse and growth velocity slows. Illness, deficiency in growth hormone or IGF-1, and sex steroid deficiency may have differing effects depending on the age of exposure to the illness or hormone deficiency state. Regions growing more rapidly may be more adversely affected than those that either have not started their growth spurt or have completed it. Illness before puberty may have a greater effect on the growth in size, mass, and volumetric BMD of the legs than on that of the spine; illness during puberty may have greater effects on growth in size, mass, and volumetric BMD of the axial skeleton (Bass et al., 1998). Growth hormone, IGF-1 deficiency, or testosterone deficiency during early growth may result in reduced femoral neck width. Sex steroid deficiency in puberty may result in reduced expansion of the vertebral width. These hypotheses remain untested.

B. Less Bone in the Bone—Reduced Accrual and Excessive Bone Loss

The deficit in areal BMD remaining after accounting for the contribution of reduced bone size reflects the reduced amount of bone in *the* bone— reduced volumetric BMD. Reduced volumetric BMD may be the result of reduced accrual, excessive bone loss, or both. A reduction in the peak volumetric BMD (reduced accrual) in long bones may occur if endocortical expansion is excessive *relative* to periosteal expansion. Alternatively, thinner cortices may result if endocortical contraction during puberty is reduced, perhaps as a result of sex hormone deficiency. A reduced volumetric BMD in trabecular sites may result if growth of primary and secondary spongiosa is disturbed. For instance, testosterone or estrogen deficiency may prevent trabecular thickening during pubertal development and so contribute to reduced trabecular BMD.

Excessive bone loss may also be responsible for the reduced volumetric BMD in patients with fractures. An imbalance between bone resorption and formation at the basic modeling unit (BMU) is the morphological basis for bone loss. Thus, for there to be "excessive bone loss" in patients with fractures, bone balance at the BMU must be more negative than the negative bone balance in controls on one or more of its three endosteal surfaces— endocortical, intracortical, and trabecular. The imbalance will be greater if resorption depth is greater, if formation is lower, or if both are present. Alternatively, if the remodeling rate is higher, bone loss may be greater, even though the negative bone balance is no different. The amount of bone removed from the skeleton as a result of the remodeling imbalance on one or more of these surfaces and the rate of remodeling will be modified according to the extent of subperiosteal bone formation in men with fractures relative to controls.

This potential heterogeneity in the pathogenesis of the deficit in volumetric BMD is poorly characterized. The relative contributions of reduced accrual versus excessive bone loss is unknown and may vary from patient to patient. Whatever the deficit attributable to excessive bone loss, little data are available defining the possible heterogeneous morphological basis of the greater bone loss. Is trabecular bone loss more rapid in men coming to sustain spine fractures? If so, is this caused by an increased depth of resorption within each remodeling site, reduced bone formation within the remodeling site, or increased numbers of remodeling sites?

Do men who sustain hip fractures lose cortical bone more rapidly than the controls? If so, is this the result of increased endocortical resorption, reduced endocortical formation, or both? The greater porosity may be caused by greater numbers and/or larger canals—the former reflecting increased intracortical remodeling and the latter reflecting increased BMU imbalance caused by larger remodeling units (increased resorption or reduced formation).

C. Histomorphometry and Reduced Bone Formation

Histomorphometric studies in men are difficult to interpret because most sample sizes are small, the studies often lack controls, the men with fractures often range in ages by several decades, and men with primary and secondary osteoporosis are often combined. Several studies have been instructive. Mosekilde (1988) reports a reduction in the thickness and loss of horizontal trabeculae in vertebral specimens. There was loss of vertical trabeculae with an increase in intertrabecular space in women, not men. No compensatory thickening of vertical trabeculae was observed. Mellish et al. (1989) report that trabecular thinning occurred with advancing age in 49 men and 47 women. Perforation occurred in both sexes but more so in women. Parfitt et al. (1983) report the age-related decline in iliac crest trabecular bone volume in men and women occurred by a reduction in trabecular density, but not trabecular thinning. In patients with vertebral fractures, trabecular bone volume deficits (of 38% in women and 48% in men relative to age-predicted mean values) occurred by reduction in trabecular density (of about 30% in both sexes). Trabecular thinning contributed to both, although perhaps more so in men (deficits were 18% in men and 7% in women). In patients with hip fractures, the deficits in trabecular bone volume (of 27% in women and 23% in men below age-predicted mean values) occurred by reduction in trabecular thickness (28% in men and 17% in women). The deficit in trabecular density was 11% in women. No deficit in trabecular density occurred in men (relative to age predicted value), but a deficit of 37% relative to the young normals was observed.

Bordier *et al.* (1973) studied 11 cases of osteoporosis in young adult men. Bone formation was reduced when assessed by quantitative histology, by calcium-45 accretion rate, and by serum alkaline phosphatase. Active bone resorption surfaces (the proportion of surface exhibiting osteoclasts within their lacunae) were normal in 8 of 11 subjects and increased in 3. Zerwekh *et al.* (1992) showed that, relative to controls, 16 nonalcoholic eugonadal men with osteoporosis had reduced bone volume (11.4 ± 4% versus 23.2 ± 4.4%), reduced osteoid surfaces (5.6 ± 3.9% versus 12.1 ± 4.6%), osteoblastic surfaces (2.0 ± 2.3% versus 3.9 ± 1.9%), and reduced bone formation rate (0.004 ± 0.001 $mm^3/mm^2/yr$ versus 0.01 ± 0.006 $mm^3/mm^2/yr$). Clarke *et al.* (1996) reported histomorphometric data in 43 healthy men 20 to 80 years old. Cancellous volume of the iliac crest decreased by 40%, as did osteoblast-osteoid interface (19.2%), and double- and single-labeled osteoid (18.6% and 18.0%, respectively). On multiple regression analysis, the log-free androgen index and body weight best predicted the age-related decline in cancellous bone volume ($r^2 = 0.19$, $P = 0.015$). Johansson *et al.* (1997) reported that 11 men with idiopathic osteoporosis aged 43 ± 9 years had reduced wall thickness (48.3 ± 7.2 μm versus 61.7 ± 5.4 μm, $P < 0.001$), *reduced* resorption depth (54.4 ± 3.8 μm versus 60.7 ± 5.3 μm, $P < 0.01$), and a negative balance (-6.04 ± 9.8 μm versus 0.96 ± 3.2 μm, $P < 0.05$), relative to 11 controls aged 31 ± 10 years. Preosteoblastic resorption depth correlated positively with wall thickness in controls ($r = 0.82$, $P < 0.01$) and negatively with wall thickness in patients ($r = -0.56$, $P = 0.07$).

Thus, loss of trabeculae contribute to age-related bone loss and the pathogenesis of fractures in both men and women. Loss of trabeculae is likely to be the main mechanism in vertebral fractures in men and women and in trabecular thinning in hip fractures in men and women. Thus, it is likely that both thinning and loss of trabeculae contribute to bone loss. Bone loss in men is likely to be caused by reduced bone formation rather than increased bone resorption.

D. Cellular Evidence of Reduced Bone Formation

The reduced bone formation may be caused by reduced osteoblastic progenitor cell availability. Bergman *et al.* (1996) reported that cultured marrow stromal mesenchymal stem cells from male mice aged 24 months yielded 41% fewer osteogenic progenitor cell colonies than cells from 4 month old mice. Cultures from older animals had a threefold higher basal proliferative rate, measured by 3H-thymidine uptake, relative to cultures from young mice, but the increase in proliferation in response to serum stimulation was tenfold in cultures from young animals and nonsignificant in cultures from older mice. The age-related decrease in osteoblast number and function may be caused by a reduction in the number and proliferative potential of stem cells.

Jilka *et al.* (1996) used the murine model of accelerated senescence and osteopenia, SAMP6, to determine whether the age-related decrease in bone mass is associated with reduced osteoblastogenesis. Osteoblast progenitor numbers were normal in SAMP6 marrow at one month of age but decreased threefold at 3 to 4 months. This reduction was temporally associated with decreased bone formation (determined using histomorphometry) and decreased BMD. In *ex vivo* bone marrow cultures, osteoclastogenesis was decreased in tissue from SAMP6 mice but was restored by addition of osteoblastic cells from normal mice, suggesting that the osteoclastogenesis defect was secondary to impaired osteoblast formation. Kajkenova *et al.* (1997) suggest that a change in the differentiation program of multipotential mesenchymal progenitors may explain the reduced osteoblastogenesis in SAMP6. *Ex vivo* marrow cultures from SAMP6 mice aged 3 to 5 months had increased numbers of colony-forming unit—adipocytes (14.7-fold in unstimulated cultures) and of fully differentiated marrow adipocytes relative to control SAMR1 mice. The number of colony-forming unit—fibroblasts did not differ. In long-term cultures, the adherent stromal layer capable of supporting hematopoiesis was generated more rapidly, more nonadherent myeloid progenitors were generated, and more IL-6 and colony stimulating activity was produced.

Weinstein *et al.* (1997) report that orchiectomy of SAMR1 mice induced fourfold increases in activation frequency, bone formation rate per bone perimeter and per bone area, increases in osteoclast number, percent osteoclast perimeter, and cancellous osteoclast number, whereas orchiectomized SAMP6 mice showed no such changes. In SAMR1, cancellous bone area decreased by 61%, and trabecular spacing increased by 160%; these parameters changed similarly in SAMP6 but were blunted in magnitude.

Mineralized perimeter in lumbar vertebrae increased in SAMR1, with augmentation in formation rate and appositional rate. No such changes occurred in SAMP6. Global BMD decreased 6.6% in SAMR1 and was unchanged in SAMP6. Orchiectomy increased formation of colonies of fibroblastoid cells (CFU-F) and of colonies producing mineralized bone nodules (CFU-OB) in *ex vivo* bone marrow cultures from SAMR1 but not SAMP6 mice. Thus, cells of osteoblastic lineage are essential mediators of skeletal changes following orchidectomy.

Marie *et al.* (1991) showed that reduced osteoblastic proliferative activity may be responsible for reduced bone formation in men with osteoporosis. Thymidine incorporation into DNA was normal in cells of normal subjects and patients with normal bone formation but was reduced in cells isolated from patients with osteoporosis with reduced bone formation (doubly labeled surfaces, mean wall thickness, osteoblast surface, and mineral apposition rate). Synthetic activity, assessed by osteocalcin responsiveness to vitamin D, was normal. These studies substantiate the importance of reduced bone formation in the pathogenesis of bone loss in men.

V. Summary

Bone fragility in men in old age may be the result of reduced bone size or architectural changes accompanying bone loss such as cortical thinning, trabecular thinning, and loss of connectivity. Men may have fewer spine fractures than women because their peak bone size is greater; greater vertebral width (not height) confers greater breaking strength. Although men have bigger bones, the amount of bone in the (bigger) bone—the peak vertebral volumetric trabecular BMD (trabecular number and thickness)—is the same in men and women. Vertebral body fragility increases less in men than in women during aging because the loss of trabecular bone proceeds primarily by thinning caused by reduced bone formation, whereas increased remodeling in women caused by menopause contributes to trabecular thinning and loss of connectivity.

Men may have fewer hip fractures than women, in part, because proximal femur bone mass and size is greater in men. Femur length and width is greater in men than women because prepubertal growth is two years longer, and pubertal growth velocity is more rapid and ceases later in males. Although femoral neck and shaft cortical thickness is the same in men and women, the cortex is placed farther from the neutral axis in men conferring greater bending strength. The higher proximal femoral BMC and areal BMD in men is the result of greater bone size; volumetric cortical BMD does not differ by gender. Femoral neck axis length is longer in men than in women in absolute terms, an observation difficult to reconcile with lower hip fracture rates in men. Net cortical bone loss during aging is less in men than in women because endocortical resorption is less, and periosteal apposition may be greater; the latter increases bone size, offsetting the bone fragility conferred by cortical thinning.

Bone remodeling in old age increases in men (and remains elevated in women) perhaps because of secondary hyperparathyroidism, calcium malabsorption, and vitamin D deficiency, particularly in house-bound subjects. The increasing cortical porosity and endocortical remodeling "trabecularize" cortical bone, increasing the surface available for remodeling. Cortical bone loss accelerates as a result of the increased remodeling activity and negative bone balance in each remodeling unit, predisposing it to hip fractures.

Men with spine fractures have reduced vertebral width (not height) relative to controls; femoral neck width is normal. Men with hip fractures have reduced femoral neck width; vertebral size is normal. Reduced size accounts for ~16–20% of the deficit in areal BMD. The site specificity of the deficits in bone size may be the result of a regional deficits in bone growth, failed periosteal apposition during aging, or both. The residual deficit in volumetric BMD—the amount of bone in the (smaller) bone in both types of fracture— may be caused by reduced accrual, excessive bone loss, or both. Reduced accrual may be caused by (i) reduced cortical thickness, itself the net result of excessive expansion of endocortical surface *relative* to the periosteal expansion before puberty, failed endocortical contraction during puberty, (ii) reduced development of trabecular numbers in early growth, or (iii) reduced trabecular thickening in puberty.

Studies of racial/ethnic patterns of skeletal growth, aging, and fracture rates in males are scarce. Blacks have fewer fractures than whites. Regional differences in bone mass and HAL are in part, caused by differences in bone size. Blacks have shorter trunks and shorter (not wider) vertebral bodies than whites. (Men have wider, not shorter, vertebrae than women.) Blacks have wider and *longer* femurs with the same cortical width. (Men also have wider and longer femurs with similar cortical width compared to women.) Because the femur is wider, the greater cortical mass is farther from the neutral axis of the long bone in blacks. Asians have similar trunk length as whites but shorter legs. Vertebral trabecular BMD is higher in blacks than whites because of greater trabecular thickness (not numbers) so that blacks have less surface and a lower bone turnover than whites. Because blacks do not appear to lose less bone than whites, bone balance at the BMU may be more negative in blacks. The thicker trabeculae may preserve connectivity during aging.

Periosteal expansion during growth and aging determine external bone size, an independent determinant of bone strength; endosteal (intracortical, endocortical, trabecular) modeling and remodeling establish cortical thickness and porosity, trabecular number, thickness, and connectivity. Understanding the structural basis of bone fragility in men requires the study of the modeling and remodeling of the surfaces of the axial and appendicular skeleton in men and women of different races.

VI. Questions

There are many unresolved questions. One of the most fundamental questions is whether the differences in fracture rates between men and women, between men with fractures and men without fractures, and between races can be explained by the structural differences observed between these groups. If bone size is a critical determinant of its breaking strength, then what genetic and environmental factors contribute to the variance in bone size between men and women of the same race, and between individuals of the same gender but different race? What factors account for the variance in trabecular numbers and their thicknesses? Why do blacks have a greater increase in trabecular thickness at puberty than whites of the corresponding gender? What is the role of estrogens in trabecular and endocortical bone remodeling? What factors regulate periosteal expansion during aging? Do black men lose less bone than white men in absolute terms, or as a percentage of their higher bone mass? Of this putative lesser bone loss, what proportion is caused by less resorption, what proportion is caused by greater bone formation?

References

Aaron, J. E., Makins, N. B., and Sagreiy, K. (1987). The microanatomy of trabecular bone loss in normal aging men and women. *Clin. Orth. Relat. Res.* **215**, 260–271.

Bakwin, H. (1964). Secular increase in height: Is the end in sight? *Lancet* **2**, 1195–1196.

Bass, S., Pearce, G., Bradney, M., Hendrich, E., Delmas, P., Harding, A., and Seeman, E. (1998). Exercise before puberty may confer residual benefits in bone density in adulthood: Studies in active prepubertal and retired female gymnasts. *J. Bone Miner. Res.* **13**, 500–507.

Bergman, R. J., Gazit, D., Kahn, A. J., Gruber, H., McDougall, S., and Hahn, T. J. (1996). Age-related changes in osteogenic stem cells in mice. *J. Bone Miner. Res.* **11**, 568–577.

Bordier, P. J., Miravet, L., and Hioco, D. (1973). Young adult osteoporosis. *Clin. Endocrinol. Metab.* **2**, 277–292.

Cameron, N., Tanner, J. M., and Whitehouse, R. H. (1982). A longitudinal analysis of the growth of limb segments in adolescence. *Ann. Hum. Biol.* **9**, 211–220.

Clarke, B. L., Ebeling, P. R., Jones, J. D., Wahner, H. W., O'Fallon, W. M., Riggs, B. L., and Fitzpatrick, L. A. (1996). Changes in quantitative bone histomorphometry in aging healthy men. *J. Clin. Endocrinol. Metabl.* **81**, 2264–2270.

Ensrud, K. E., Palermo, L., Black, D. M., Cauley, J., Jergas, M., Orwoll, E. S., Nevitt, M. C., Fox, K. M., and Cummings, S. R. (1995). Hip and calcaneal bone loss increase with advancing age: Longitudinal results from the study of osteoporotic fractures. *J. Bone Miner. Res.* **10**, 1778–1787.

Finkelstein, J. S., Neer, R. M., Biller, B. M. K., Crawford, J. D., and Klibanski, A. (1992). Osteopenia in men with a history of delayed puberty. *N. Engl. J. Med.* **326**, 600–604.

Finkelstein, J. S., Klibanski, A., and Neer, R. M. (1996). A longitudinal evaluation of bone mineral density in adult men with histories of delayed puberty. *J. Clin. Endocrinol. Metab.* **81**, 1152–1155.

Fugii, Y., Tsutsumi, M., Tsunenari, T., Fukuase, M., Yoshimoto, Y., Fujita, T., and Genant, H. K. (1989). Quantitative computed tomography of lumbar vertebrae in Japanese patients with osteoporosis. *Bone Miner.* **6**, 87–94.

Garn, S. M. (1970). "The Earlier Gain and Later Loss of Cortical Bone." Thomas, Springfield, IL.

Garn, S. M., Nagy, J. M., and Sandusky, S. T. (1972). Differential sexual dimorphism in bone diameters of subjects of European and Africa Ancestry. *Am. J. Phys. Anthropol.* **37**, 127–130.

Gilsanz, V., Gibbens, D. T., Roe, T. F., Carlson, M., Senac, M. O., Boechat, M. I., Huang, H. K., Schulz, E. E., Libanati, C. R., and Cann, C. C. (1988). Vertebral bone density in children: Effect of puberty. *Radiology* **166**, 847–850.

Gilsanz, V., Boechat, M. I., Gilsanz, R., Loro, M. L., Roe, T. F., and Goodman, W. G. (1994). Gender differences in vertebral size in adults: Biomechanical implications. *Radiology* **190**, 678–694.

Gilsanz, V., Skaggs, D. I., Kovanlikaya, A., Sayre, J., Loro, M. L., Kaufman, F., and Korenman, S. G. (1998). Differential effects of race on the axial and appendicular skeleton of children. *J. Clin. Endocrinol. Metab.* **68**, 1420–1427.

Gomez, C. (1994). Bone mineral density in hip fracture. The Spanish Multi-Centre Study. Abstracts of the Spanish Society for Bone and Mineral Research, Cordoba, Spain, October 20–23, 1993. *Calcif. Tissue Int.* **55**, 440.

Gordan, C. L., Halton, J. M., Atkinson, S. A., and Webber, C. E. (1991). The contributions of growth and puberty to peak bone mass. *Growth, Dev. & Aging* **55**, 257–262.

Han, Z., Palnitkar, S., Rao, S., Nelson, D., and Parfitt, A. (1996). Effect of ethnicity and age or menopause on the structure and geometry of iliac bone. *J. Bone Miner. Res.* **11**, 1967–1975.

Hannan, M. T., Kiel, D. P., Mercier, C. E., Anderson, J. J., and Felson, D. T. (1994). Longitudinal bone mineral density change in elderly men and women: The Framingham Osteoporosis Study. *J. Bone Miner. Res.* **9**(Suppl. 1), S130 (abstr. 37).

Jilka, R. L., Weinstein, R. S., Takahashi, K., Parfitt, A. M., and Manolagas, S. C. (1996). Linkage of decreased bone mass with impaired osteoblastogenesis in a murine model of accelerated senescence. *J. Clin. Invest.* **97**, 1732–1740.

Johansson, A. G., Eriksen, E. F., Lindh, E., Langdahl, B., Blum, W. F., Lindahl, A., Ljunggren, Ö., and Ljunghall, S. (1997). Reduced serum levels of the growth hormone-dependent insulin-like growth factor binding protein and a negative bone balance at the level of individual remodeling units in idiopathic osteoporosis in men. *J. Clin. Endocrinol. Metab.* **82**, 2795–2798.

Jones, G., Nguyen, T., Sambrook, P., Kelly, P. J., and Eisman, J. A. (1994). Progressive loss of bone in the femoral neck in elderly people: Longitudinal findings from the Dubbo osteoporosis epidemiology study. *Br. Med. J.* **309**, 691–695.

Kajkenova, O., Lecka-Czernik, B., Gubrij, I., Hauser, S. P., Takahashi, K., Parfitt, A. M., Jilka, R. L., Manolagas, S. C., and Lipschitz, D. A. (1997). Increased adipogenesis and myelopoiesis in the bone marrow of SAMP6, a murine model of defective osteoblastogenesis and low turnover osteopenia. *J. Bone Miner. Res.* **12**, 1772–1779.

Kalender, W. A., Felsenberg, D., Louis, O., Lopez, O., Lopez, P., Klotz, E., Osteaux, M., and Fraga, J. (1989). Reference values for trabecular and cortical vertebral bone density in single and dual-energy quantitative computed tomography. *Eur. J. Radiol.* **9**, 75–80.

Kuiper, J. W., van Kujik, C., Grashuis, J. L., Ederveen, A. G. H., and Schotte, H. E. (1996). Accuracy and the influence of marrow fat on quantitative CT and dual-energy X-ray absorptiometry measurements of the femoral neck in vitro. *Osteoporosis Int.* **6**, 25–30.

Laval-Jeantet, A.-M., Bergot, C., Carroll, R., and Garcia-Schaefer, F. (1983). Cortical bone senescence and mineral bone density of the humerus. *Calcif. Tissue Int.* **35**, 268–272.

Looker, A. C., Wahner, H. W., Dunn, W. L., Calvo, M. S., Harris, T. B., Heyse, S. P., Johnston, C. C., Jr., and Lindsay, R. L. (1995). Proximal femur bone mineral levels of US adults. *Osteoporosis Int.* **5**, 389–409.

Lu, P. W., Cowell, C. T., Lloyd-Jones, S. A., Brody, J. N., and Howman-Giles, R. (1996). Volumetric bone mineral density in normal subjects aged 5–27 years. *J. Clin. Endocrinol. Metab.* **81**, 1586–1590.

Luisetto, G., Mastrogiacomo, I., Bonanni, G., Pozzan, G., Botteon, S., Tizian, L., and Galuppo, P. (1995). Bone mass and mineral metabolism in Klinefelter's syndrome. *Osteoporosis Int.* **5**, 455–461.

Malina, R. M., and Brown, K. H. (1987). Relative lower extremity length in Mexican American and in American black and white youth. *Am. J. Phys. Anthropol.* **72**, 89–94.

Marie, P. J., De Vernejoul, M. C., Connes, D., and Hott, M. (1991). Decreased DNA synthesis by cultured osteoblastic cells in eugonadal osteoporotic men with defective bone formation. *J. Clin. Invest.* **88**, 1167–1172.

Mellish, R. W. E., Garrahan, N. J., and Compston, J. E. (1989). Age-related changes in trabecular width and spacing in human iliac crest biopsies. *Bone Miner.* **6**, 331–338.

Meredith, H. V. (1978). Secular change in sitting height and lower limb height of children, youths, and young adults of Afro-black, European, and Japanese ancestry. *Growth* **42**, 37–41.

Meunier, P. J., Sellami, S., Briancon, D., and Edouard, C. (1990). Histological heterogeneity of apparently idiopathic osteoporosis. *In* "Osteoporosis: Recent Advances in Pathogenesis and Treatment" (H. F. Deluca, H. M. Frost, W. S. S. Jee, C. C. Johnston, and A.M. Parfitt, eds.), pp. 293–301. University Park Press, MD.

Migliaccio, S., Newbold, R. R., Bullock, B. C., Jefferson, W. J., Sutton, F. G., Jr., McLachlan, J. A., and Korach, K. S. (1996). Alterations of maternal estrogen levels during gestation affect the skeleton of female offspring. *Endocrinology (Baltimore)* **137**, 2118–2125.

Moore, B., Briody, J., Cowell, C. T., and Mobbs, E. (1997). Does maturational delay affect bone mineral density? *Eur. Soc. Paediatr. Endocrinol. 5th J. Meet.*, Stockholm.

Mosekilde, Li. (1988). Age-related changes in vertebral trabecular bone architecture assessed by a new method. *Bone* **9**, 247–250.

Mosekilde, Li, and Mosekilde, Le. (1990). Sex differences in age-related changes in vertebral body size, density and biochemical competence in normal individuals. *Bone* **11**, 67–73.

Parfitt, A. (1997). Genetic effects on bone mass and turnover-relevance to black/white differences. *J. Am. Coll. Nutr.* **16**, 325–333.

Parfitt, A. M. (1998). Perspective: A structural approach to renal bone disease. *J. Bone Miner. Res.* **13**, 1213–1220.

Parfitt, A. M., Mathews, C. H. E., Villanueva, A. R., Kleerkoper, M., Frame, B., and Rao, D. S. (1983). Relationships between surface, volume, and thickness of iliac trabecular bone in aging and in osteoporosis. *J. Clin. Invest.* **72**, 1396–1409.

Perry, H. M., III, Horowitz, M., Morley, J. E., Fleming, S., Jensen, J., Caccione, P., Miller, D. K., Kaiser, F. E., and Sundarum, M. (1996). Aging and bone metabolism in African American and Caucasian women. *J. Clin. Endocrinol. Metab.* **81**, 1108–1117.

Preece, M. A., Pan, H., and Ratcliffe, S. G. (1992). Auxological aspects of male and female puberty. *Acta Paediatr.* **383**, 11–13.

Ruff, C. B., and Hayes, W. C. (1988). Sex differences in age-related remodeling of the femur and tibia. *J. Orthop Res.* **6**, 886–896.

Rupich, R. C., Specker, B. L., Lieuw-A-Fa, M., and Ho, M. (1996). Gender and race differences in bone mass during infancy. *Calcif. Tissue Int.* **58**, 395–397.

Schnitzler, C. M., Pettifor, J. M., Mesquita, J. M., Bird, M. D. T., Schnaid, E., and Smith, A. E. (1990). Histomorphometry of iliac crest bone in 346 normal black and white South African adults. *Bone Min.* **10**, 183–199.

Seeman, E. (1994). Osteoporosis in men. *Am. J. Med.* **95**, 22–28.

Seeman, E. (1995). The dilemma of osteoporosis in men. *Am. J. Med.* **98** (Suppl. 1A), 75S–87S.

Seeman, E. (1997). From density to structure: Growing up and growing old on the surfaces of bone. *J. Bone Miner. Res.* **12**, 1–13.

Seeman, E. (1998). Growth in bone mass and size—are racial and gender differences in bone mineral density more apparent than real? *J. Clin. Endocrinol. Metab.* **68**, 1414–1419.

Solomon, L. (1979). Bone density in ageing caucasian and African populations. *Lancet* **2**, 1327–1329.

Tanner, J. M., Hayashi, T., Preece, M. A., and Cameron, N. (1982). Increase in length of leg relative to trunk in Japanese children and adults from 1957 to 1977: Comparison with British and with Japanese Americans. *Ann. Hum. Biol.* **9**(5), 411–423.

Vega, E., Ghiringhelli, G., Mautalen, C., Valzacchi, G. R., Scaglia, H., and Zylberstein, C. (1998). Bone mineral density and bone size in men with primary osteoporosis and vertebral fractures. *Calcif. Tissue Int.* **62**, 465–469.

Weinstein, R. S., Jilka, R. L., Parfitt, A. M., and Manolagas, S. C. (1997). The effects of androgen deficiency on murine bone remodeling and bone mineral density are mediated via cells of the osteoblastic lineage. *Endocrinology (Baltimore)* **138**, 4013–4021.

Zamberlan, N., Radetti, G., Paganini, C., Gatti, D., Rossini, M., and Braga, V. (1996). Evaluation of cortical thickness and bone density by roentgen microdensitometry in growing males and females. *Eur. J. Pediatr.* **155**, 377–382.

Zerwekh, J. E., Sakhaee, K., Breslau, N. A., Gottschalk, F. G., and Pak, C. Y. C. (1992). Impaired bone formation in male idiopathic osteoporosis: Further reduction in the presence of concomitant hypercalciuria. *Osteoporosis Int.* **2**, 128–134.

Chapter 7

R. Bruce Martin

Orthopaedic Research Laboratories
University of California—Davis Medical Center
Sacramento, California

Aging and Changes in Cortical Mass and Structure

I. Introduction

There are distinct differences between age-related fracture risks in men and women. There are also distinct gender differences in the age-related changes in cortical bone structure. How the structural differences are related to the fracture risks is not entirely clear, but several fundamental principles seem to be important. The elucidation of these is the goal of this chapter.

Generally speaking, cortical bone serves two roles in the skeleton. First, it forms the shafts of long bones, whose lengths provide height and reach to the owner. Whereas long limbs are often desirable, bulky limbs make speed and efficiency of movement difficult. Minimization of the bulk of the limbs requires compact skeletal structure in their cores. Therefore, in most animals the diaphyses of limb bones are primarily composed of compact or cortical bone. The exception to this occurs at the ends of these bones, where more cross-sectional area is desirable to reduce stresses in the cartilage of synovial joints. Because the stress is correspondingly reduced in the metaphyseal and epiphyseal bone, these locations may be filled with lighter, cancellous bone. The integrity of the network of tiny bone struts and marrow in this kind of bone depends, however, on the existence of a surrounding, continuous shell of solid bone. Mechanically, this shell provides a foundation for the trabecular framework so that applied loads do not impinge directly on fragile individual trabeculae. Physiologically, the cortical shell serves to contain the marrow within the interstices of the cancellous bone. These requirements for a cortical shell apply equally to vertebral bodies and flat bones containing cancellous bone, and the general need for a cortical shell around cancellous bone provides the second role for cortical bone in the skeleton. In considering the significance of cortical bone in the pathomechanics of osteoporosis, both of these roles need to be considered.

II. Basic Mechanical Considerations in Diaphyseal Modeling

In the process of giving the skeleton height and reach, long bone diaphyses subject themselves to bending and twisting as well as compressive loads. Whereas resistance to compressive loads depends simply on cross-sectional area, resistance to bending and twisting depends on how that area is distributed about the center of the cross-section. To be specific, it depends on the ratio of a quantity called the *cross-sectional moment of inertia* to the bone's outer diameter (see Figure 1). This ratio, called the *section modulus*, turns out to be proportional to the cube of the bone's radius or diameter. Consequently, if two bones have the same cortical area (and bone mass), but one is larger in diameter (with a correspondingly larger medullary canal), the one with the larger diameter will be stronger and stiffer when bent or twisted. This mechanical principle finds great utility in skeletal biomechanics. As children grow, gain weight, and become more active, the loads on their skeletons increase. To prevent these increased loads from producing increased stresses in the bone tissue, their bones grow in diameter through periosteal modeling. Simultaneously, their hematopoietic capacity must increase, so the diameter of the medullary canal must increase as well, through endosteal modeling. This has the effect of moving the bone mass further from the center of the diaphysis, and that makes the bone material more effective in resisting bending and twisting forces. In fact, the bones' ability to resist bending and twisting loads usually increases disproportionately in comparison to the changes in bone mass (Figure 2). [For a brief introduction to engineering mechanics as it applies to the skeleton, see Turner and Burr (1993).]

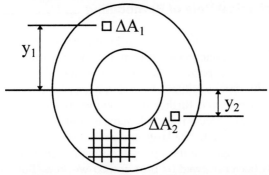

FIGURE I   Cross-sectional moment of inertia (CSMI) and section modulus are defined for a long bone cortex. The circles represent the endosteal and periosteal surfaces. The long horizontal line represents a plane through the bone called the *neutral plane*. When the bone is bent by a force that is perpendicular to this plane, stresses and strains on one side of the neutral plane are tensile, and those on the other side are compressive. The CSMI helps determine these stresses. To see what it is, imagine that the cross-section is divided into many small areas, ΔA, by a grid of lines, a portion of which is sketched in the inferior cortex. Each such element of area is located a distance y from the neutral plane; two examples are shown. Multiply each ΔA by the square of its particular value of y. Then the CSMI is simply the sum of *all* of these products: CSMI $= \Sigma(\Delta Ay^2)$. For a bone of circular cross-section, it turns out that CSMI $= \pi\,(R_p^4 - R_e^4)/4$, where R_p and R_e are the periosteal and endosteal radii, respectively. Finally, the section modulus is just the CSMI divided by the periosteal radius. What is important here is the fact that, because of the y^2 term, bone added to the periosteal surface contributes more to the CSMI and section modulus than bone added to the endosteal surface.

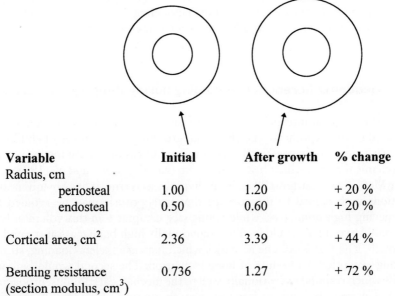

Variable	Initial	After growth	% change
Radius, cm			
periosteal	1.00	1.20	+ 20 %
endosteal	0.50	0.60	+ 20 %
Cortical area, cm^2	2.36	3.39	+ 44 %
Bending resistance (section modulus, cm^3)	0.736	1.27	+ 72 %

FIGURE 2   As a child's long bone grows in diameter, the section modulus grows faster than the cross-sectional area of the diaphyseal cortex.

III. The Mechanical Role of Remodeling ─────────────

A fundamental postulate of skeletal biomechanics is that bone physiology acts to minimize bone mass while maintaining stiffness and strength at levels which enable the species to flourish. As we have seen, the mass of bone required to do this can be reduced by giving bones appropriate shapes. Bone mass can be lowered even further by allowing strains to rise to the point where fatigue damage occurs if such damage is limited by histologic structure and is constantly repaired. The large and growing literature on bone's resistance to fatigue damage and its capacity to repair such damage by remodeling has recently been reviewed by Burr and co-workers (Burr, 1997a,b; Burr *et al.*, 1997). In cortical bone, lamellar organization and osteonal cement lines are thought to be particularly important in controlling the propagation of fatigue "microcracks" so that they are unlikely to develop into catastrophic cracks. Also, it has been established that when loading is sufficient to produce microcracks in cortical bone, remodeling is activated (Burr *et al.*, 1985; Mori and Burr, 1993; Bentolila *et al.*, 1997). Thus, it appears that damage results in a signal activating its repair by remodeling. Even though bone remodeling undoubtedly serves both metabolic and mechanical purposes, it is not unreasonable to postulate that in ordinary, healthy individuals, whose bones are not responding to abnormal metabolic imbalances, the principal stimulus for remodeling is the repair of fatigue damage. This requirement should be particularly high in children, whose growth constantly presses the skeleton to keep up with the demands of steadily increasing body weight, muscle forces, and activity levels. With adulthood this challenge abates, and bone turnover slows, but remodeling continues at a level determined by daily physical activities and metabolic considerations.

IV. Gender Differences in Modeling during Puberty ──────────

The growing interest in the role of mechanical factors in bone biology has led to the hypothesis that the radial growth of the cortices of children's bones is not simply genetically programmed but is driven by the increasing mechanical forces which bear upon them (van der Meulen *et al.*, 1993; van der Meulen and Carter, 1995). If this hypothesis is true, it has obvious implications with regard to the concept that osteoporosis may be avoided by achieving high bone mass while young (see Chapter 6 in this volume). Presumably two things could lead to exceptionally high bone mass at the end of growth. The first would be activities which increase skeletal loading, stimulating exceptional amounts of bone formation. The second would be bone cells which respond exceptionally well to the mechanical stimulus, producing above-average amounts of bone for a given amount of loading. In this scenario, gender differences could arise because of cultural factors leading one sex to pursue activities which place greater loads on their bones, and/or because the bone cells of males and females function in different hormonal environments which affect their responses to mechanical loading. Studies of the first of these possibilities in humans are possible but are confounded by the frequency with which abnormal menstrual cycles occur in female athletes, since menstrual cycle irregularities negatively impact bone mass (Snow-Harter, 1994).

The second possibility was elaborated by Frost (1987), who suggested that estrogen influences the "set point" of the skeleton's control system for adjusting bone strength to the applied loads. Specifically, he proposed that increased estrogen lowers the set point so that less mechancial loading is required to stimulate a given increment of bone mass. A recent paper by Schiessl *et al.* (1998) lends support to this hypothesis. Using data from Zanchetta *et al.* (1995), they plotted DXA-determined whole body bone mineral content vs. lean body mass for groups of boys and girls of increasing age (Figure 3). Assuming that most of the loading on the skeleton is due to muscle forces and that these are proportional to lean body mass, the slopes of the resulting curves should represent the capacity for increasing bone mass when a given amount of loading is present. The curves for boys and girls show two important differences. First, the one for girls has a distinct increase

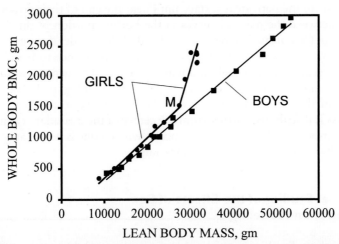

FIGURE 3   Graph of bone mass (whole body bone mineral content) versus muscle mass (lean body mass) for boys and girls. Each data point represents means of these two variables for boys or girls of similar age. Boys show a relatively steady increase in both variables as they grow. In girls, however, there is a change in slope of the graph at 12 years of age; this point is marked with an M because this age corresponds to the mean age of menarche. Reprinted from *Bone* **22**, Schiessl, H., Frost, H. M., and Jee, W. S. S. Estrogen and bone-muscle strength and mass relationships. Pp. 1–6, © 1998 with permission from Elsevier Science.

in slope at the age of menarche, when estrogen levels rise. This strongly supports Frost's hypothesis that estrogen adjusts the skeleton's "mechanostat." The other difference is the abrupt halt in the gains of both bone and muscle mass that occurs at about age 14 in girls but not boys. This is represented by the cluster of points at the end of the girls' curve. The data also suggest the possibility of a slight change in slope of the boys' curve at about age 15, but this possible androgenic effect seems much more tenuous. In any event, several years are required before the boys' muscle mass grows to the point that its forces have stimulated a bone mass surpassing that of the girls. To reiterate: the change in the bone/muscle mass relationship seen at the menarche is hypothesized to be caused by an effect of estrogen on the set point for adaptation of bone mass to strain.

Turner (1991) provided additional insight regarding the effect of menarche on cortical bone using Garn's (1970) data on age changes in the endosteal and periosteal diameters of the second metacarpal bone. As shown in Figure 4, bone formation on the periosteal surface of this bone essentially stops at menarche, but it simultaneously begins on the endosteal surface and continues until about age 20. Thereafter, there is little change in cortical area until menopause, when resorption resumes on the endosteal surface and formation resumes (albeit slowly) on the periosteal surface. Within this particular bone [and it is typical of others, according to Garn (1970)], the postmenarchal addition of bone appears to occur on the endosteal rather than the periosteal surface. Figure 4 shows that males, on the other hand, continue to add bone to the periosteal surface until near the end of their growth. The distance between the pairs of curves in the bottom portion of this figure is the width of the cortex. Between ages 20 and 50 the gender difference in this width is small. This is not true, however, of the resistance to bending and torsion possessed by these male and female cortices. This geometric quantity, the section modulus, is plotted in the upper portion of Figure 4. The section modulus of the male bones is about 60% greater due to the fact that the bone mass is distributed further from the center of the medullary canal. This in turn comes from the gender difference in where bone is added at puberty: periosteally in men and endosteally in women.

V. Animal Studies of the Effects of Sex Hormones on Modeling

Animal studies have confirmed that estrogen inhibits periosteal bone formation and suppresses endosteal resorption. Periosteal bone formation is arrested when prepubescent female rats are given estrogen (Turner *et al.*, 1990a). In this model the existing endosteal resorption is stopped, but endosteal formation is not provoked. Conversely, loss of gonadal hormones also has distinct skeletal effects in male and female rats (Turner *et al.*, 1989,

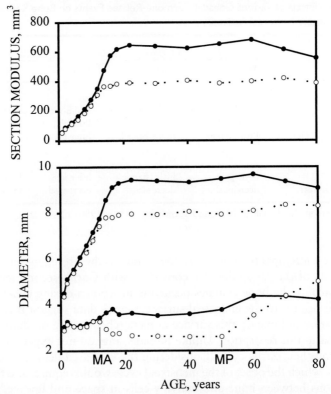

FIGURE 4   Lower graph shows diameters of the periosteal (upper curves) and medullary (lower curves) surfaces in second metacarpal bones of males (filled circles) and females (open circles) of varying age. The upper graph shows male and female section moduli calculated from these diameters. MA and MP, respectively, denote the ages at which menarche and menopause occur. Note that both sexes gain cortical bone mass during the final stages of growth, but in different locations. In men this bone is formed through periosteal apposition, whereas in women it is formed on the endosteal surface. Reprinted from *Bone* **12**, Turner, C. H. Do estrogens increase bone formation? Pp. 305–306, © 1991 with permission from Elsevier Science, using data from Garn (1970).

1990b). In females, bone formation on the periosteal surface is increased by about 25% after ovariectomy, and both the periosteal and endosteal diameters of the tibia increase. In males, periosteal bone formation was reduced a similar amount following orchiectomy. Estrogen or androgen treatment, respectively, reversed these changes. In cancellous bone of the tibial metaphysis, on the other hand, both ovariectomy and orchiectomy decreased bone volume fraction. Thus, the primary gonadal hormones of males and females have distinctly different effects with respect to cortical bone modeling but similar effects (at least in the end result) on trabecular bone remodeling.

TABLE I   Effects of Various Gonadal Hormone-Related Events on Bone Responses at Periosteal and Endosteal Surfaces[a]

	Endosteal surface		Periosteal surface	
Event	Male	Female	Male	Female
Life phase				
Puberty	stop bone loss	add bone	add bone	stop bone gain
Mid-life	slight bone loss	little change	little change	little change
Menopause/Old age	little change	much bone loss	bone loss	bone gain
Gonadectomy				
Bone ±	bone gain	little change	bone loss	little change
Bone form rate	decreased	decreased	decreased	increased

[a]According to studies by Garn (1970) and Turner *et al.* (1989, 1990a,b).

Table I attempts to summarize the results in the preceding paragraphs. The results of the rat studies are consistent with Garn's second metatarsal data regarding the bone changes occurring in women during menarche except with respect to the endosteal surface. Garn's data suggest that women gain substantial bone on this surface at menarche, but the rat data indicate only cessation of resorption. Unlike humans, rats do not experience blood loss during their estrus cycle. Considering the increased demand for hematopoiesis, which the onset of the menstrual cycle would require, and the close connections between bone and marrow cells in space and lineage, it is intriguing to see that the cortical bone surface in contact with marrow is responsible for the increased bone formation when estrogen levels rise in girls. Clearly, Garn's data are inadequate to firmly define the human side of this situation, in terms of men as well as women, and this is an area begging for further study.

VI. Male Hypogonadism

Orwoll and Klein (1994, 1996) have reviewed the effects of hypogonadism on the male skeleton. Early onset hypogonadism seems to be particularly associated with reduced cortical bone mass in the peripheral skeleton. The mechanical implications of this may be of importance when one recalls that the emphasis is on periosteal bone formation during male pubertal skeletal development and endosteal bone formation in girls. The mechanical advantage of periosteally disposed bone, which specifically confers resistance to bending and torsional loads, would presumably be reduced in men who are hypogonadal during puberty, increasing their risk of fracture in the appendicular skeleton. Orwoll and Klein also surmise that vertebral rather than cortical bone is where the greater loss occurs when hypogonadism is post-pubertal. If the addition of cortical bone is primarily associated with modeling drifts in the developing skeleton, postpubertal hypogonadism would not affect this aspect of skeletal mass accumulation. Instead, rat experiments indicate that testosterone deficiency in adults produces trabecular bone loss (Turner *et al.*, 1989).

VII. Remodeling, Fatigue Damage, and Mechanical Properties in the Aging Skeleton

Over one's lifetime the remodeling of cortical bone steadily increases its porosity through the accumulation of secondary Haversian canals (Kerley, 1965). In addition, age-related increases in mineralization, cement lines, and osteon fragments affect the mechancial properties of the bone tissue. These changes are apparently responsible for the age-related diminishment of the stiffness, strength, and other mechanical properties of bone material (Yamada, 1973; Burstein *et al.*, 1976; Evans, 1976; Smith and Smith, 1976). Figure 5 shows typical reductions in the strength properties of femoral bone material between the ages of 20 and 90 years. These reductions are significant but small relative to those in the energy required for fracture, known as "energy-to-failure." This aspect of strength is also called toughness and is

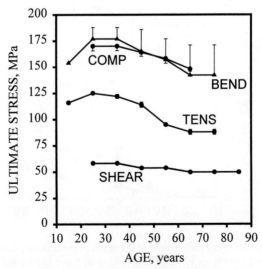

FIGURE 5 Graph showing age changes in the material strength of human femoral cortical bone with age. COMP = compression, BEND = bending, TENS = tension, and SHEAR = shear or torsion. Reprinted from Martin (1993) with permission; data from Yamada (1973).

particularly relevant to fatigue resistance. Working with human femora, Currey and co-workers (1996) have shown that the toughness of cortical bone is inversely related to mineralization. The mineralization of bone is normally tightly controlled and is largely determined by the rate of remodeling because it takes many months for new osteons to mineralize fully. Thus, the ash content of elderly people's bones (65–70%) is slightly more than that of children's bones (60–65%). In Currey's experiments, this modest increase in mineral content, combined with other age-related changes in the cortical tissue, cut toughness in half. It must be emphasized that these declines in cortical material properties seem to occur similarly in men and women.

There is, however, at least one measure of bone's material properties which does not diminish equally with age in men and women. There is growing evidence that fatigue damage and damagability may increase more with age in women that in men, particularly in cortical bone (Burr, 1997b; Schaffler *et al.*, 1995a; Wenzel *et al.*, 1996). Figure 6 shows that the number of microcracks in the cortex of the femur increases exponentially with age in both men and women, but more so in women. Although such damage has been shown to increase with cyclic loading (Burr *et al.*, 1985; Mori and Burr, 1993), it is as yet unclear precisely how such damage affects the mechanical properties of bone, including its fatigue strength. It seems that microcracks

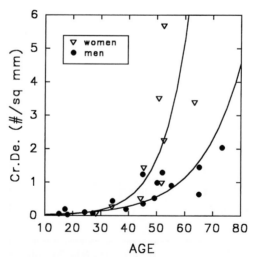

FIGURE 6   Graph of microcrack density in the shafts of the male and female human femur versus age. Reprinted from *Bone* 17, Schaffler, M. B., *et al.* Aging and microdamage accumulation in human compact bone. Pp. 521–525, © 1995 with permission from Elsevier Science. After about age 40 microcracks increase exponentially in number, with a faster rise in women than in men.

and other fatigue damage affect bone's toughness and postyield behavior[1] more than its strength and stiffness (Currey *et al.*, 1996; Martin *et al.*, 1995).

Perhaps microdamage is responsible for the fact that the incidence of fractures is higher in aging women than in aging men. However, one must also consider gender differences in age-related changes in the *structural* properties of cortical bone.

VIII. Compensatory Modeling in the Aging Skeleton ──────────

As the material within the cortex becomes more porous with increasing age, bone may be simultaneously added to or removed from the periosteal and endosteal surfaces. Garn's (1970) radiographic studies of the second metacarpal bone (Figure 4) indicated that the postpubertal periosteal addition of bone was inconsequential, but different results have been seen in other bones. Sedlin *et al.* (1963) found that substantial bone is added to the rib during adulthood, and Smith and Walker (1964) radiographically measured periosteal expansion in one plane of the femurs of aging women. Indeed, they calculated that this addition of bone overcompensated for endosteal loss so that the section modulus of the bone increased past age 75. This conclusion was later reversed when other workers made measurements directly on excised, sectioned femurs and tibias (Martin and Atkinson, 1977; Martin *et al.*, 1980; Ruff and Hayes, 1982, 1988). These studies confirmed that there is radial expansion of both the periosteal and endosteal surfaces of these bones, but there is a gender difference with respect to the resulting section modulus. In men, cross-sectional moment of inertia and section modulus increase throughout adulthood until perhaps age 80. In women, on the other hand, section modulus declines starting at age 35 or earlier. These trends persist when attempts are made to correct the data for possible secular changes due, for example, to the subjects who lived more recently perhaps having had better diets (Ruff and Hayes, 1988). However, studies of archaeological specimens indicate that in some cultures the section modulus has increased or decreased with age similarly in both sexes (Ruff and Hayes, 1982; Martin *et al.*, 1985). Note also the occurrence of periosteal resorption rather than formation in Garn's data for the metacarpals of older men (Table 1 and Figure 4). These studies suggest that diet, habitual activities, and genetics may combine to decide the net results of radial expansion on diaphyseal surfaces.

[1]The term *yield* refers to an event on the way to fracture which is distinguished by a sudden decrease in the stiffness of the bone and marks a damage threshold. A "tough" bone is one which "hangs together" and requires a lot of energy to break after passing the yield point. A brittle bone is one which breaks quickly and absorbs little additional energy once the yield point is exceeded.

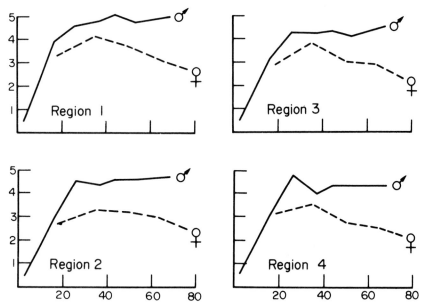

FIGURE 7   Graphs of bending moment at failure for four regions along the shaft of the human femur as functions of age and sex. This measure of whole bone strength is the product of material bending strength, which declines after age 35 in both sexes, and section modulus, which declines after age 35 in women but increases until about age 80 in men. Reprinted from *Journal of Biomechanics* 10, Martin, R. B., and Atkinson, P. J. Age and sex-related changes in the structure and strength of the human femoral shaft. Pp. 223–231, © 1977 with permission of Elsevier Science.

When these structural data are combined with estimates of the decline in material strength occurring equally in aging men and women, the resulting prediction of bone strength in bending or torsion is again very different in men and women (Figure 7). In men, the structural benefit of periosteal expansion fully compensates for intracortical and endosteal loss of bone, and strength is maintained well into old age. In women, on the other hand, declining material and structural components of strength combine to produce decidedly negative regressions with age, essentially throughout adulthood. It is not clear whether this gender difference is due to insufficient periosteal formation or excessive endosteal resorption in women; perhaps it is a combination of both.

Although these diaphyseal results are very interesting and may relate to the generally greater incidence of geriatric fractures in women compared to men, they do not address two obvious issues. First, the most serious, life-threatening fractures in the elderly occur in the hip, not the femoral diaphysis. Does radial expansion occur there, and with what effect in men and women? Second, why does the incidence of fractures in men begin to increase

YOUNG   OLD

MALE

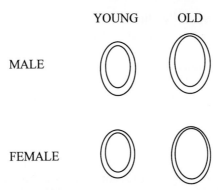

FEMALE

FIGURE 8   Typical age-related changes in the geometry of the neck of male and female femurs as deduced by Beck *et al.* (1992).

well before age 80, when it is not until then that strength compensation by radial expansion seems to deteriorate?

IX. The Neck of the Femur

Ruff and Hayes (1988) found little difference in the male and female radial expansion data for the femoral neck, but other studies have suggested that radial expansion does protect against fracture at this site, at least to some extent. Measuring human subjects noninvasively using x-ray or photon absorptiometry, Beck *et al.*, (1992, 1993) found that femoral neck cross-sectional moment of inertia decreased in postmenopausal women but remained constant in aging men. Both sexes lost cortical bone on the endocortical surface, but in men there was a more decided increase in periosteal diameter. They calculated that, based solely on cortical bone changes, femoral neck stresses ought to increase three times faster with age in women than in men, or 4–12% per decade. Similar studies by Yoshikawa and co-workers (1994) did not find significant age-changes in cross-sectional moment of inertia in either men or women but did conclude that the *strength* of the femoral neck (relative to forces produced in walking or falling) decreased faster with age in women than in men. It should be understood that there is a great deal of variability in these data and considerable overlap of the data for men and women. More recently, on the basis of standardized plane film radiographs, Heaney (1997) reported a slight but statistically significant age-related increase in femoral neck diameter in women.

Both Beck's and Yoshikawa's groups reported another important aspect of the age-related changes in the distribution of cortical bone in the neck of the femur which is more conclusive. As shown in Figure 8, the neck of the normal femur is essentially elliptical, with its major axis oriented in the superior-inferior direction. Furthermore, the cortex is thicker on the inferior side than on the superior (or cranial) side. With age this eccentricity is exaggerated so that the superior cortex becomes even thinner, and more so in women than in men. Thus, the side of the neck which incurs tensile loads when the neck is bent by the hip force becomes critically thin in elderly men and especially women. Generally, the tensile loads at this site are low because, in addition to bending, the hip force applies substantial uniaxial compression to the neck.[2] However, when the femur is in an abducted position, the neck experiences more bending and reduced compression. Because bone is weaker in tension than in compression, situations involving abducted loading (e.g., loss of balance) could be catastrophic for a femur with a thin superior cortex.

The criticality of the situation just described is compounded by observations from another study of aging changes in the cortical bone of the femoral neck. Boyce and Bloebaum (1993) studied the structure of the cortex in the femoral necks of young (26 ± 7 years) and old (63 ± 3 years) men. They confirmed that cortical thinning occurred primarily in the superior aspect of the neck. They also found that the thinning of this region was associated with the development of substantial areas of hypermineralized, dead bone. Cracks which developed in these regions during the preparation of their specimens were assumed to be artifactual, but they nevertheless drove home the point that this tissue was brittle and would be particularly weak in tension and fatigue. Indeed, the same group reported that microdamage per square millimeter increased exponentially with age in the cortex of the femoral neck (Schaffler *et al.*, 1995b). However, this damage was greatest in the inferior cortex and minimal in the superior neck, in both young and old men. An explanation for the lack of association between the microcracks and the hypermineralized region remains to be found, but it is clear that both the superior and inferior portions of the femoral neck are mechanically compromised as men age. Unfortunately, specimens from women were not examined, but the data suggest a plausible explanation for increased numbers of hip fractures in aging men as well as women. Furthermore, as suggested by Smith and Walker (1964), radial expansion of the male femoral diaphysis, while protecting the diaphysis from fracture, may ultimately increase the risk of fracture through the neck. As the cortex is redistributed outward, the femoral shaft should become relatively stiff in bending. This means that shock absorption due to bowing of the femur during gait would diminish and the forces applied to the neck would increase, relatively speaking. Taken together, these events—reduced shock absorption, cortical thinning focussed in the superior neck and exacerbated by embrittlement due to hyperminer-

---

[2]The tensile ($+$) and compressive ($-$) stresses in a bent and compressed structure add algebraically, reducing if not eliminating tensile stress.

alization, and rapidly increasing microdamage in the inferior neck—constitute a credible picture of male hip fracture pathomechanics.

X. Summary and Research Directions ⸻⸻⸻⸻

When osteoporosis is discussed, attention is usually centered on trabecular rather than cortical bone. Nevertheless, cortical bone is important in this context because osteoporotic fractures do occur in long bone cortices as well and because cortical bone surrounds and is integral with all cancellous bone. Perhaps the best case in point is the neck and femur, where osteoporotic fracture is common and often lethal. Indeed, as the preceding discussion makes clear, the virtual disappearance of cortical bone from the superior aspect of the aging femoral neck is likely to be a predisposing factor in femoral neck fracture.

The mechanical significance of cortical bone modeling and remodeling have been surveyed here with particular attention to the changes which occur at puberty and in old age. Obviously, the differences between males and females are largely due to the effects of the principal sex hormones. In skeletal terms, the changes wrought by these hormones at puberty construct the bony frameworks peculiar to men and women and within which postmenopausal and senile osteoporosis may arise. We have seen that there are distinct differences in the effects of estrogen and testosterone on cortical bone surfaces at puberty. On the periosteal surface, testosterone stimulates bone formation and estrogen inhibits it. On the endosteal surface, testosterone has little effect, whereas estrogen inhibits resorption (in rats) or perhaps stimulates formation (in humans). These distinctions are the key to understanding gender differences in skeletal development. Another key concept is the hypothesis that the "set point" for bone's adaptation to mechanical loading is tied to estrogen. This hypothesis provides a new view as to why menarche and menopause are so critical to women's skeletal integrity. (There is apparently no equivalent effect of testosterone.) Finally, it is important to bear in mind that the skeleton is an organ which has evolved in a long line of competing organisms. Survival could arguably have been enhanced by a skeleton that was not only mechanically sufficient but as light as possible. Skeletal weight could be reduced by allowing strains to increase if remodeling was used to repair the resulting fatigue damage. This system has apparently worked well in many vertebrates for millions of years, but it is a dynamic system with, in a sense, many "moving parts" (i.e., biological components) which can get out of adjustment or wear out. Skeletal fragility in old age may occur simply because there is a limit to how long the damage repair system, as it is presently constituted, can work. In addition, a woman's skeleton must cope with demands secondary to the capacity for pregnancy and lactation. These circumstances create specific physiologic requirements which often result in postmenopausal osteoporosis. In men, these particular problems do not occur, but there remains the problem of keeping the system going for far longer than the 40 to 50 years that were necessary from an evolutionary viewpoint. In any event, understanding the basic processes and mechanical principles of cortical bone biology helps clarify the issues which arise in male as well as female osteoporosis.

Several important directions for new research are evident in this chapter. Much of our knowledge concerning the basic science is quite superficial. We need to know a lot more details about the roles of testosterone and estrogen in bone biology, not to mention all the other associated reproductive and calciotrophic hormones. Do boys and girls preferentially form bone on the periosteal and endosteal surfaces, respectively, of all their major long bones during the pubertal years, as suggested by Garn's metacarpal data? Does the menstrual cycle change the effect of estrogen on the endosteal envelope from simply stopping resorption (as seen in rats) to active formation? Is Frost's hypothesis about estrogen and the mechanical set point correct? Do the problems elite women athletes have with irregularities in their menstrual cycle also reflect a physiologic connection between estrogen and bone's system for adapting to mechanical loading? Is postmenopausal bone loss simply a manifestation of resetting the set point at menopause? Was postmenopausal bone loss, so important now, simply inconsequential from an evolutionary viewpoint? Why does radial expansion of the femur seem to compensate for intracortical bone loss in men but not in women? Does microdamage increase more rapidly in women than in men simply because the system controlling their bone strains is reset higher at menopause? Why does hypermineralization of cortical bone in the neck of the femur occur in men? Does it occur in women, too? Does compensatory enlargement of the femoral diaphysis in men really increase strains in the femoral neck? These are just some of the many questions that offer direction to future research on cortical bone's role in male and female osteoporosis.

References

Beck, T. J., Ruff, C. B., Scott, W. W., Plato, C. C., Tobin, J. D., and Quan, C. A. (1992). Sex differences in geometry of the femoral neck with aging: A structural analysis of bone mineral data. *Calcif. Tissue Int.* 50, 24–29.

Beck, T. J., Ruff, C. B., and Bissessur, K. (1993). Age-related changes in female femoral neck geometry: Implications for bone strength. *Calcif. Tissue Int.* 53, S41–S46.

Bentolila, V., Hillam, R. A., Skerry, T. M., Boyce, T. M., Fyhrie, D. P., and Schaffler, M. B. (1997). Activation of intracortical remodeling in adult rat long bones by fatigue loading. *Trans. Orthop. Res. Soc.* 22, 578.

Boyce, T. M., and Bloebaum, R. D. (1993). Cortical aging differences and fracture implications for the femoral neck. *Bone* 14, 769–778.

Burr, D. B. (1997a). Bone, exercise, and stress fractures. *Exercise Sport Sci. Rev.* 25, 171–194.

Burr, D. B. (1997b). Microdamage in bone. *Curr. Opin. Orthop.* **8,** 8–14.

Burr, D. B., Martin, R. B., Schaffler, M. B., and Radin, E. L. (1985). Bone remodeling in response to in vivo fatigue microdamage. *J. Biomech.* **18,** 189–200.

Burr, D. B., Forwood, M. K., Fyhrie, D. P., Martin, R. B., Schaffler, M. S., and Turner, C. H. (1997). Bone microdamage and skeletal fragility in osteoporotic and stress fractures. *J. Bone Miner. Res.* **12,** 6–15.

Burstein, A. H., Reilly, D. T., and Martens, M. (1976). Aging of bone tissue: Mechanical properties. *J. Bone J. Surg., Am. Vol.* **58–A,** 82–86.

Currey, J. D., Brear, K., and Zioupos, P. (1996). The effects of ageing and changes in mineral content in degrading the toughness of human femora. *J. Biomech.* **29,** 257–260.

Evans, F. G. (1976). Age changes in mechanical properties and histology of human compact bone. *Yearb. Phys. Anthropol.* **20,** 57–72.

Frost, H. M. (1987). Bone "mass" and the "mechanostat": A proposal. *Anat. Rec.* **219,** 1–9.

Garn, S. M. (1970). "The Earlier Gain and the Later Loss of Cortical Bone." Thomas, Springfield, IL.

Heaney, R. P. (1997). Bone dimensional change with age: Interactions of genetic, hormonal, and body size variables. *Osteoporosis Int.* **7,** 426–431.

Kerley, E. R. (1965). The microscopic determination of age in human bone. *Am. J. Phys. Anthropol.* **23,** 149–164.

Martin, B. (1993). Aging and strength of bone as a structural material. *Calc. Tissue International* **53** (Suppl.), 534–540.

Martin, R. B., and Atkinson, P. J. (1977). Age and sex-related changes in the structure and strength of the human femoral shaft. *J. Biomech.* **10,** 223–231.

Martin, R. B., Pickett, J. C., and Zinaich, S. (1980). Studies of skeletal remodeling in aging men. *Clin. Orthop. Relat. Res.* **149,** 268–282.

Martin, R. B., Burr, D. B., and Schaffler, M. B. (1985). Effects of age and sex on the amount and distribution of mineral in eskimo tibiae. *Am. J. Phys. Anthropol.* **67,** 371–380.

Martin, R. B., Gibson, V. A., Stover, S. M., Gibeling, J. C., and Griffin, L. V. (1995). Residual strength of equine third metacarpal bone is not reduced by intense fatigue loading: Implications for stress fracture. *J. Biomech.* **30,** 109–114.

Mori, S., and Burr, D. B. (1993). Increased intracortical remodeling following fatigue damage. *Bone* **14,** 103–109.

Orwoll, E. S., and Klein, R. F. (1994). Osteoporosis in men. *In* "Osteoporosis" (R. Marcus, ed.), pp. 146–201. Blackwell Scientific Publications, Boston.

Orwoll, E. S., and Klein, R. F. (1996). Osteoporosis in men. Epidemiology, pathophysiology, and clinical characterization. *In* "Osteoporosis" (R. Marcus, D. Feldman, and J. Kelsey, eds.), pp. 745–784. Academic Press, San Diego, CA.

Ruff, C. B., and Hayes, W. C. (1982). Subperiosteal expansion and cortical remodeling of the human femur and tibia with aging. *Science* **217,** 945–948.

Ruff, C. B., and Hayes, W. C. (1988). Sex differences in age-related remodeling of the femur and tibia. *J. Orthop. Res.* **6,** 886–896.

Schaffler, M. B., Choi, K., and Milgrom, C. (1995a). Aging and microdamage accumulation in human compact bone. *Bone* **17,** 521–525.

Schaffler, M. B., Boyce, T. M., Lundin-Cannon, K. D., Milgrom, C., and Fyhrie, D. P. (1995b). Age-related architectural changes and microdamage accumulation in the femoral neck cortex. *Trans. Orthop. Res. Soc.* **20,** 549.

Schiessl, H., Frost, H. M., and Jee, W. S. S. (1998). Estrogen and bone-muscle strength and mass relationships. *Bone* **22,** 1–6.

Sedlin, E. D., Frost, H. M., and Villanueva, A. R. (1963). The eleventh rib biopsy in the study of metabolic bone disease. *Henry Ford Hosp. Med. Bull.* **11,** 217–219.

Smith, C. B., and Smith, D. A. (1976). Relations between age, mineral density and mechanical properties of human femoral compacta. *Acta Orthop. Scand.* **47,** 496–502.

Smith, R. W., and Walker, R. R. (1964). Femoral expansion in aging women: Implications for osteoporosis and fractures. *Science* **145,** 156–157.

Snow-Harter, C. M. (1994). Bone health and prevention of osteoporosis in active and athletic women. *Clin. Sports Med.* **13**, 389–404.

Turner, C. H. (1991). Editorial: Do estrogens increase bone formation? *Bone* **12**, 305–306.

Turner, C. H., and Burr, D. B. (1993). Basic biomechanical measurements of bone: A tutorial. *Bone* **14**, 595–608.

Turner, R. T., Hannon, K. S., Demers, L. M., Buchanan, J., and Bell, N. H. (1989). Differential effects of gonadal function on bone histomorphometry in male and female rats. *J. Bone Miner. Res.* **4**, 557–563.

Turner, R. T., Colvard, D. S., and Spelsberg, T. C. (1990a). Estrogen inhibition of periosteal bone formation in rat long bones: Down-regulation of gene expression for bone matrix proteins. *Endocrinology (Baltimore)*, **127**, 1346–1351.

Turner, R. T., Wakley, G. K., and Hannon, K. S. (1990b). Differential effects of androgens on cortical bone histomorphometry in gonadectomized male and female rats. *J. Orthop. Res.* **8**, 612–617.

van der Meulen, M. C. H., and Carter, D. R. (1995). Developmental mechanics determine long bone allometry. *J. Theor. Biol.* **172**, 323–327.

van der Meulen, M. C. H., Beaupre, G. S., and Carter, D. R. (1993). Mechanobiological influences in long bone cross-sectional growth. *Bone* **14**, 635–642.

Wenzel, T. E., Schaffler, M. B., and Fyhrie, D. P. (1996). In vivo trabecular microcracks in human vertebral bone. *Bone* **19**, 89–95.

Yamada, H. (1973). "Strength of Biological Materials." Krieger Publ. Co., Huntington, NY.

Yoshikawa, T., Turner, C. H., Peacock, M., Slemenda, C. W., Weaver, C. M., Teegarden, D., Markwardt, P., and Burr, D. B. (1994). Geometric structure of the femoral neck measured using dual-energy x-ray absorptiometry. *J. Bone Miner. Res.* **9**, 1053–1064; errata: *Ibid.* **10**(3), 510 (1995).

Zanchetta, J. R., Plotkin, H., and Filgueira, M. L. A. (1995). Bone mass in children: Normative values for the 2–20–year–old population. *Bone* **16**, 393S–399S.

Chapter 8

Belinda Beck
Robert Marcus

Geriatrics Research, Education, and Clinical Center
Veterans Affairs Medical Center
Palo Alto, California;
and Department of Medicine
Stanford University
Stanford, California

Skeletal Effects of Exercise in Men

I. Introduction

It is generally accepted that bone adapts to changes in habitual mechanical loading in order to best withstand future loads of the same nature. This phenomenon, loosely referred to as Wolff's Law, honors the 19th century scientist who attempted a mathematical description of the process. Evidence of Wolff's Law emerges in the findings of both animal and human studies. In the human realm, a much larger body of evidence exists for the skeletal effects of exercise loading on females than on males. Consequently, no systematic discussion of the relationship of exercise to bone mass specific to men has been presented.

To initiate such a discussion, this chapter will address: characteristic features of male bone health, fundamental aspects of the response of bone to loading, and findings of cross-sectional and intervention trials investigating the effect of exercise on the skeleton of male subjects. Specifically, the relationships of body mass, exercise type, intensity and history, site specificity, and muscle strength to male bone density and geometry will be examined.

The influence of age on the response of bone to loading as well as the impact of exercise on male hormone status will be considered. Finally, we will briefly address the comparative effects of exercise on the bones of men and women.

II. Definitions

A number of terms are commonly employed to describe bone mass and density. Even though actual bone mass is a difficult element to quantify, it is a relatively simple process to measure the amount of mineral in bone. Bone mass and mineral are highly correlated quantities (given normal matrix mineralization); thus, bone mineral can be used to estimate reliably the mass of normal skeletal tissue. **Bone mineral content** (BMC) is a measure of the amount of mineral in a defined region of bone (in grams). To account for differences in bone size among individuals, bone is commonly evaluated in terms of tissue density or porosity. Areal **bone mineral density** (BMD) is derived by dividing BMC by the area of bone measured and is expressed in grams per square centimeter. **Bone mineral apparent density** (BMAD) is an approximation of volumetric BMD (Katzman *et al.*, 1991; Carter *et al.*, 1992) introduced to minimize the effect of bone size on two-dimensional scans by considering the dimension of bone depth. It is calculated from densitometry-derived bone area and other skeletal length dimensions and is expressed in grams per cubic centimeter.

III. The Male Skeleton—Why Care about It?

A. Bone Density: Gender Comparison

A clear gender difference exists between the mass of male and female skeletons. Men attain greater values of BMC and BMD than women (Hannan *et al.*, 1992), primarily by virtue of having larger bones. Peak BMD in men compared with women is approximately 1.033 versus 0.942 gm/cm^2 at the hip, 1.115 versus 1.079 gm/cm^2 at the spine (L2–L4), and 0.687 versus 0.579 gm/cm^2 at the forearm (radius). When bone size is fully taken into account, however, these differences essentially disappear; that is, volumetric bone density is approximately equal between men and women.

B. Fracture Risk

Attainment of greater peak bone mass in men is associated with superior bone integrity throughout life and a lower ultimate risk of osteoporotic fracture than for women. In 1990, male hip fractures accounted for 30% of the 1.7 million hip fractures which occurred worldwide (Cooper *et al.*, 1992).

Even though a comparison between genders clearly indicates a problem of greater magnitude for the female population, a closer look at real numbers lends perspective to the situation. Thirty percent of 1.7 million amounts to a total of 510,000 male hip fractures, clearly a non-trivial figure. Perhaps even more noteworthy is the fact that men over 75 years of age have been observed to suffer a 21% mortality rate following hip fracture compared to 8% in women (Poor *et al.*, 1995). With current trends of increasing life expectancy, the prevalence of men who suffer from osteoporosis and related fractures in the future is also likely to rise. Thus, efforts to determine methods of preserving bone in the male population are required.

C. Acquisition and Loss of Bone

Because a comprehensive discussion of this topic appears elsewhere in this volume (Chapters 5, 7, 15, 16, 24), only a brief summation will be presented here. In adults, the amount of bone in the skeleton at any time represents that which was formed during growth, minus that which has been subsequently lost. Although considerable information is now available regarding the trajectory of bone acquisition in girls, understanding is less complete for boys. In both sexes, greatest bone acquisition occurs during pubertal growth (Boot *et al.*, 1997). The rate of BMD gain in 11-year-old boys may be 2.5 times that of younger children (Gunnes and Lehmann, 1996), whereas rates of gain increase fourfold to sixfold in the 4 years encompassing ages 13–17 (Theintz *et al.*, 1992; Bonjour *et al.*, 1994). During this period, changes in long bone diaphyses are less marked than in the spine and hip and largely reflect increases in cortical width. Following puberty, the rate of gain in males declines but remains significant at the spine and mid-femoral shaft between the ages of 17 and 20 (Theintz *et al.*, 1992). In females, by contrast, the rate of BMC and BMD increment is greatest between 11 and 14 years, falling dramatically after the age of 16 (Theintz *et al.*, 1992). The rate of change in cortical BMD is thought to peak around 16 ± 0.3 years in boys and 14 ± 0.3 years in girls (Gunnes and Lehmann, 1996).

Thus, even though it has commonly been accepted that both sexes attain peak bone mass during the mid thirties, 95% of peak bone mass is actually attained by age 20. Peak bone mass in both sexes is characterized by substantial interindividual variation (Theintz *et al.*, 1992). The standard deviation of BMD values in the population varies from one skeletal region to the next but is generally about 10–12% of the mean value. Thus, variation in peak bone mass greatly exceeds the variation associated with rates of bone loss later in life. Childhood and adolescence therefore represent crucial periods during which diet, physical activity, and other factors may exert long-term influence on skeletal integrity.

After the acquisition of peak bone mass, men and women experience similar rates of decline in bone mass across most of the lifespan, the obvious exception being the first 5 to 8 years after menopause, when women lose bone at an accelerated rate.

A study of adult human cadavera revealed the following age-related changes in male long bones (femur and humerus): cortical areas increase until approximately 60 to 75 years of age and then decline, cortical porosity increases throughout life, the number of Haversian canals increases until approximately 80 years of age and then declines, and osteon areas decrease gradually with age (Martin *et al.*, 1980). The contribution of bone size and shape to bone strength, and the effect of aging on this relationship, is addressed in Section IVC.

IV. The Response of Bone to Loading— Fundamental Aspects

Repeated observations of relatively high bone mass in athletes have led many to conclude that physical exercise is beneficial to bone. To understand why this is so, it is necessary to achieve a better understanding of the fundamental mechanisms by which bone responds to mechanical stimulation. The skeleton is routinely exposed to the forces of gravity and muscle contraction. To optimize strength without unduly increasing weight, bones accommodate the loads that are imposed upon them by undergoing alterations in mass, external geometry, and internal microarchitecture. In recent years, considerable energy has been directed toward elucidating mechanical load parameters which optimally stimulate a response from bone.

A. Characteristics of Effective Mechanical Loading

Mechanical loads may be characterized by several independent parameters, including type of load, load magnitude, number of load cycles, and rate at which strain is induced. Bone loads are generally expressed in terms of stress and strain. **Stress** is the force applied to an object, expressed per unit area. Stress in a bone is calculated by dividing the load on the bone by its cross-sectional area. **Strain** is a measure of bone deformation in response to the application of stress (i.e., loading) and can be calculated by dividing the change in bone length by its original length.

1. Dynamic versus Static Loading

To be an effective initiator of remodeling, mechanical stimulation must be dynamic. Hert and colleagues (1971) and Lanyon and Rubin (1984) found that simple application of a static load produced no adaptive bone remodeling nor did it protect bone from atrophy. Application of the same load in a cyclical manner, however, induced bone deposition and increased diaphyseal cross-sectional area.

2. Load Intensity versus Cycle Number

From a model comparing the relative effects of load intensity and cycle number on bone mass, Whalen *et al.* (1988) concluded that load intensity is a more important contributor than cycle number. This conclusion is substantiated by indications from clinical literature, in which highest bone density values have been observed in athletes whose activities include lifting of heavy loads and application of high-impact forces (Block *et al.*, 1989; Heinonen *et al.*, 1995; Robinson *et al.*, 1995). It is also consonant with animal data indicating that the number of load cycles necessary to maintain bone mass is relatively small (Rubin and Lanyon, 1984); that although modest running activity is associated with higher bone mass in rats, running 3 or 18 km per day has the same effect on bone mineral content (Newhall *et al.*, 1991); and that increasing the magnitude of loads with weighted backpacks is a more effective stimulus to increase bone mass than increasing the duration of treadmill running (van der Wiel *et al.*, 1995).

3. Rate of Strain

Peak load magnitude per se does not describe the intensity of loading nor does it determine skeletal response. **Rate of strain** is a term used to describe the time over which strain develops after load application and is roughly comparable to the term *impact*. In several experimental models, rate of strain has been shown to be of critical importance to skeletal response, a principle that applies even at large peak strains (O'Connor *et al.*, 1982; Turner *et al.*, 1995a). Turner and associates (1995a) applied loads of 54 N[1] at 2 cycles per second for 18 seconds each day to rat tibiae and measured the effect of varying the rate of strain on bone formation and mineral apposition. Results showed a marked linear elevation in both variables as rate of strain increased.

B. The Curvilinear Nature of Skeletal Response

Complete immobilization, as seen with high-level spinal cord injury, leads rapidly to devastating bone loss. By contrast, imposition of even substantial training regimens on normally ambulatory people or animals increases bone mass by only a few percent over a similar period. This phenomenon is illustrated in Figure 1, where the effect of walking on bone mass is schematized. As an individual goes from immobility to full ambulation, duration of time spent walking becomes a progressively less efficient stimulus for increasing bone mass. A person who habitually walks 6 hours each day might require another 4–6 hours just to add a few more percent BMD. On the other hand, adding a more rigorous stimulus, such as high-impact loading, for even a few cycles would increase the response slope.

[1]N = Newtons. One Newton is the force necessary to accelerate 1 kg of mass 1 m/sec^2.

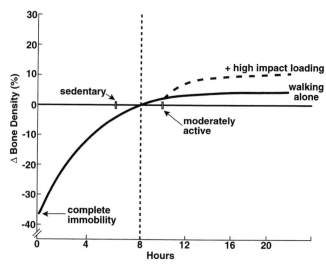

FIGURE I   The curvilinear nature of skeletal response. From Marcus (1996).

C. The Role of Bone Geometry

In addition to bone density, geometric features make a substantial contribution to bone strength. Such features include overall size, shape, and distribution of mass, as well as internal microscopic architecture, such as trabecular connectivity. Exercise loading is known to exert an influence on bone geometry.

I. Bone Deformation with Loading

Because long bones are curved, compressive loads applied at joint surfaces rarely act through the center of the bone; hence, bending occurs. In 1964, Frost proposed a Flexural Neutralization Theory of bone remodeling, by which he suggested that bone seeks the shape, size, and location that equalizes and minimizes the amount of tissue deformation incurred by normal usage. Although more recent evidence suggests that in reality this condition is neither achieved nor desirable (Rubin, 1984), it is indeed likely that bone models and remodels to maintain functional stiffness with optimal resistance to injurious bending (Schaffler, 1985). Diaphyseal width contributes significantly to the ability of bone to resist bending loads. Martin and Burr (1989) stated that "If 100 mm² is removed from the inner cortex of . . . bone . . . bending strength can be maintained by putting only approximately 30 mm² back onto the outside surface" (p. 231). **Cross-sectional moment of inertia (CSMI)** is a measure of bone geometry which determines the resistance of bone to bending at a particular site. It is a function of cross-sectional area and the distribution of bone in that area relative to the point about which the bone bends (axis of rotation). The further the bone is distributed from the axis of rotation, the wider the bone and the more resistance it will have to bending.

2. Age-Related Geometric Adaptation

The diameters of long bone diaphyses tend to expand with age. Expansion is achieved via the concomitant effects of periosteal bone deposition and increased endosteal resorption, such that net thickness of the bone cortex is reduced. The effect is seen in both weight-bearing (Ruff and Hayes, 1988) and non-weight-bearing (Burr and Martin, 1983) bone. Increased diaphyseal width acts to maintain the CSMI of long bones and, correspondingly, to maintain bone strength in the face of cortical thinning and increased porosity. Remains of pre-industrial bones indicate no gender-specific differences in adaptive ability in this respect (Ruff and Hayes, 1983); however, in modern times, males appear to have maintained the ability to expand diaphyseal widths to a greater extent than females (Martin and Atkinson, 1977; Burr and Martin, 1983; Ruff and Hayes, 1988). Although forearm bones in older women do reflect increased cross-sectional moments of inertia, the magnitude of change may not be enough to compensate for excessive endosteal loss of bone (Bouxsein *et al.*, 1994). Cultural and behavioral changes, particularly in physical activity type and intensity, between pre- and post-industrial times likely contribute to gender differences in age-related geometric adaptation today. It is also likely that the superior resistance to osteoporosis in men is at least partly attributable to this more effective geometric compensation for the weakening effect of age-related increases in porosity and cortical thinning.

V. Translating Theory into Practice—Exercise and Bone _____

A. Limitations of the Literature

I. Implications of Study Design

It is routinely recommended that regular lifelong physical exercise is important for the prevention of osteoporosis (Jackson and Kleerekoper, 1990; Seeman, 1997); however, very few exercise trials that actually confirm or clarify this presumed relationship have been reported. The recommendation to exercise has been based primarily on data from cross-sectional studies comparing BMD between already-exercising and nonexercising groups. Unfortunately, cross-sectional studies contain inherent limitations of selection bias and, as such, may not accurately represent the general population. It is conceivable that individuals who choose to exercise have certain predisposing skeletal characteristics which influence their choice and ability to initiate and maintain regular physical activity. For example, Bennell and associates

(1997) reported greater BMD in power athletes than controls, but they also found that the athletes had engaged in more physical activity during childhood than had the controls. As discussed presently, childhood activity is likely to exert a strong influence on bone mass across the lifespan.

2. Methodological Concerns

Exercise-loading bone research is rife with methodological problems which complicate data interpretation. Important examples include reliance on questionnaires and recall for accounts of previous activity, under-representation of ethnic minorities, inability to control for the effects of anabolic steroid use in athletes, variations in bone mineral measurement tools among studies, variations in the precision error of similar measurement tools, and use of "inactive" control groups which actually participate in nontrivial amounts of physical activity. In addition, many early studies utilized BMC to estimate bone mass, a value which, by failing to account for bone size, is less valid for the purposes of comparison between individuals than BMD or BMAD.

Perhaps the most worrisome methodological concern is the fact that instruments used to assess physical activity vary widely, and few data exist to establish their validity or reliability. Many instruments currently in use, designed originally to assess aerobic work or energy expenditure, may simply fail to reflect the loads actually experienced by the skeleton. Even devices that quantify the number of steps taken in a 24-hour period generally do not distinguish the intensity of impact and, therefore, do not fully describe skeletal loading.

A review of cross-sectional exercise studies is further complicated by the variety of subject groupings utilized: exercise versus sedentary, low-intensity activity versus high-intensity activity, sport versus sport, dominant-side limb versus non-dominant-side limb, and sport versus retired from sport. Given an awareness of these inherent limitations, a review of the literature can be presented for interpretation with appropriate circumspection. In spite of methodological shortcomings in many studies, the relative uniformity of findings suggests that some generalizations about the effect of exercise on bone in men can nevertheless be made with confidence.

B. Relationship of Body Mass to BMD

Many report a strong positive relationship of body mass with bone mineral density or content (Hamdy et al., 1994; Suominen and Rahkila, 1991; Snow-Harter et al., 1992; Smith and Rutherford, 1993; Welten et al., 1994; Karlsson et al., 1995; Glynn et al., 1995; Sone et al., 1996; Boot et al., 1997), although a minority of investigators have found otherwise (Nilsson and Westlin, 1971; Bevier et al., 1989). This relationship is in keeping with the tenets of Wolff's Law in that increased body mass effectively increases the magnitude of daily gravitational load on the skeleton. Of course, a similar gene may influence both lean body mass and bone mass, a feature which would naturally establish a fundamental relationship between them. In addition, the BMD measurement is itself influenced by bone size (positive correlation) so that genes determining body size can further influence bone density measures.

C. Relationship of Muscle Strength to BMD

The positive effects of exercise on BMD are likely to be due in part to the beneficial effects of exercise on muscle strength. That exercisers have greater muscle strength in most muscle groups than nonexercisers has been repeatedly shown (Snow-Harter *et al.*, 1992). It is also known that muscle mass is highly correlated with muscle strength and that lean body mass is positively correlated with bone mass and cross-sectional properties (Moro *et al.*, 1996; Doyle *et al.*, 1970). In addition to the influence of common genetic determinants, increased muscle mass may exert an effect on bone mass in two ways: (1) by increasing total body mass and the consequent magnitude of gravitational load on the skeleton and (2) by enhancing local bone strains by virtue of an enhanced ability to apply contractile forces at sites of origin and insertion. The observation that power athletes have greater BMD than endurance athletes or controls (Bennell *et al.*, 1997) somewhat illustrates this relationship.

Back, biceps, quadriceps, and grip strength have all been positively correlated with hip, spine, whole body, and tibial BMD. Back extensor muscle mass and strength in particular have been found to be the strongest, most robust predictors of BMD at many sites, particular the spine and hip (Bevier *et al.*, 1989; Snow-Harter *et al.*, 1992). Grip and biceps strength correlate positively with forearm BMC (Myburgh *et al.*, 1993; Bevier *et al.*, 1989), quadriceps strength is a positive determinant of hip BMD (Glynn *et al.*, 1995), and leg strength is similarly positively correlated with hip BMD (Block *et al.*, 1989), illustrating a site specificity of bone response to loading.

Some authors, however, have reported that quadriceps strength is not an independent predictor of BMD (Duppe *et al.*, 1997) and is not related to distal femoral BMD (Nilsson and Westlin, 1971). In order to elucidate the nature of the BMD-muscle strength relationship fully and account for the influence of genetic commonality between the two factors, intervention trials designed to primarily address this issue must be completed.

D. Exercise Effects—Cross-Sectional Study Findings

Animal studies have indicated that the skeletal response to mechanical loading may be tempered with age (Rubin *et al.*, 1992; Turner *et al.*, 1995b). Adequacy of skeletal response reflects bone cell numbers and vigor as well as hormonal and cytokine milieu. Cell populations, circulating growth factors, and production of bone matrix proteins all decline with age (Benedict *et al.*, 1994; Termine, 1990) and may all contribute to an age-related deficit in skeletal response to loading. To account for this effect, subsequent discussion will be grouped according to the age of subjects. Data for children and adolescents (<20 years) will be discussed initially, followed by those for adult (20–65 years) and finally, older men (>65 years).

1. Young Males

Investigations of exercise effects on bone have not typically targeted the pediatric population. As a consequence, only a small amount of data is available for analysis.

a. Current Activity   Even in very young children, exercise appears to promote the acquisition of bone. In a study of premature infants, Moyer-Mileur and associates (1995) found that five repetitions of range of motion, gentle compression, flexion, and extension exercises five times a week resulted in greater acquisition of BMD at 4 weeks in exercised babies than in controls.

Slemenda and associates (1994) studied factors influencing the rate of skeletal mineralization in male and female children and adolescents. Even though a combined-gender analysis limits male-specific inferences which can be drawn from their report, the authors noted that physical activity was a significant predictor of BMD at the radius, spine, and hip in prepubertal but not peripubertal children. These findings suggest that exercise exerts an influence on BMD before puberty, but during puberty other factors become more influential on bone acquisition.

Researchers have repeatedly found significant associations between physical activity and forearm, total body, and spine BMD in adolescent boys of various races (Duppe *et al.*, 1997; Boot *et al.*, 1997; Welten *et al.*, 1994; Gunnes and Lehmann, 1996; Tsai *et al.*, 1996). VandenBergh and associates (1995), however, found that after adjustments for body weight, height, skeletal age, and chronological age were made, no correlation between physical fitness (measured by VO_{2max}) and middle-phalanx BMC existed in 7- to 11-year-old boys. Upon closer analysis, greater BMC was actually found in boys categorized as highly fit versus low-fit boys older than 10, but not younger. The latter study illustrates the methodological limitations inherent in the search for a relationship between exercise per se and bone density. Maximal oxygen consumption is not an adequate surrogate for more specific measures of skeletal loading. The finding of greater BMC in highly fit boys compared to low-fit boys is likely to reflect the increased chance that more active boys will participate in activities that beneficially load the skeleton than less-active boys, but it cannot be confirmed.

b. Site Specificity   Considerable evidence suggests that the adaptive bone response is site-specific; that is, only bones or regions of bone that are loaded undergo significant load-related change. Nordstrom and associates (1996) compared tibial tuberosity BMD between highly active and less-active teenage boys (average age 15). They observed significantly greater tuberosity BMD in the more active group (when Osgood Schlatters[2] sufferers were excluded from the analysis) and found that the difference was related to quadricep strength. As the quadricep muscles insert at the tibial tuberosity, these findings support a localized muscle-loading effect on bone.

Adolescent Chinese athletes were found to exhibit sport-specific differences in BMD. Judo athletes had greater spine BMD than baseball, swimming, and track athletes, whereas baseball players had greater hip BMD than swimmers, judo, and track athletes (Tsai *et al.,* 1996). Variations in BMD response to different sports reflect the different loading patterns of each sport.

2. Adult Males

a. Current Activity   In adult men (approximately 20 to 65 years old), individuals exercising at relatively high loads have consistently greater BMD than nonexercisers or those exercising at low loads. These differences have been found in the whole body (Snow-Harter *et al.,* 1992; Karlsson *et al.,* 1996; Bennell *et al.,* 1997), spine, and/or proximal femur (Block *et al.,* 1986, 1989; Colletti *et al.,* 1989; Snow-Harter *et al.,* 1992; Karlsson *et al.,* 1993, 1996; Need *et al.,* 1995; Sone *et al.,* 1996; Duppe *et al.,* 1997), distal femur (Nilsson and Westlin, 1971), tibia (Leichter *et al.,* 1989; MacDougall *et al.,* 1992; Snow-Harter *et al.,* 1992; Karlsson *et al.,* 1993), calcaneus (Hutchinson *et al.,* 1995), and distal forearm (Karlsson *et al.,* 1993). An example of bone mineral density differences observed between exercising and nonexercising men is shown in Figure 2 (Snow-Harter *et al.,* 1992).

Even though such differences are easily shown between athletes and controls, differences between athletes participating in different sports (e.g., water polo and weight training; Block *et al.,* 1989) or at different intensities of the same sport (MacDougall *et al.,* 1992) may not be as evident. This observation is predictable from the previously described curvilinear nature of the skeletal response to loading.

Moderate exercise may not apply a sufficient stimulus to the skeleton to precipitate an adaptive response. Myburgh and associates (1993) observed no differences in ulna BMC between moderately active subjects and controls, whereas differences between highly active versus moderately active subjects and controls were significant.

Some have stated that individuals who participate in reduced-weight-bearing activities such as swimming and bicycling have BMD similar to nonexercisers (Nilsson and Westlin, 1971; Taaffe *et al.,* 1995). Discrepancies

---

[2]Osgood Schlatters Disease is a condition of inflammation of the tibial tuberosity at the growth apophysis, generally resulting from excessive, repetitive, forceful knee extension (e.g., kicking and jumping) during the growth spurt.

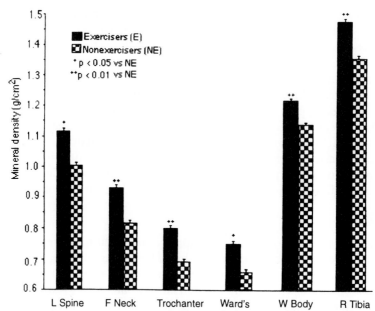

FIGURE 2 Bone mineral density differences in exercising ($n = 27$) versus nonexercising ($n = 18$) men. L Spine, lumbar spine; F Neck, femoral neck; W Body, whole body; R Tibia, right tibia. Reproduced from Snow-Harter *et al.* (1992) *J. Bone Miner. Res.* 7, Fig. 3, p. 1291–1296, with permission.

exist, however, concerning the effect of non-weight-bearing activity on bone density because some have found that male swimmers have greater radial and spine BMD than controls (Orwoll *et al.*, 1989). Given the location of the BMD increment in the swimmers in Orwoll's study, disparities may be based in the site specificity of bone response to loading. During swimming, contraction of muscles acting on the upper extremity may place substantial loads on the spine (latissimus dorsi) and radius (biceps brachii, brachioradialis). Alternatively, degree of swimming participation may strongly influence the effect of the activity on bone density. Elite swimmers who train intensively effectively *unload* their skeletons by spending extended periods of time in a reduced-gravity environment. Exercise loads placed on the skeleton during swimming may be of insufficient magnitude to overcome the negative impact of substantially reduced daily weight bearing.

High-intensity impact activities such as running, jumping, and power lifting are thought to be more effective bone stimulators than low-intensity or non-weight-bearing activities. Need and colleagues (1995) found that spine and hip BMD are positively correlated with activity levels in men 20 to 83 years old and that femoral neck BMD was significantly greater in joggers than sedentary subjects. Dalen and Olsson (1974) found that 50- to 59-year-old men with 25 years running experience had significantly greater BMC at the distal forearm, humeral head, femoral shaft, and calcaneus than controls. Bennell and associates (1997) reported baseline cross-sectional data on power and endurance athletes versus controls (19 to 20 years olds) and again after 12 months in order to observe longitudinal sport-specific BMD changes. They found that total body and femoral BMD increased in all groups, a generalized effect attributed to continued growth of the study subjects; however, power athletes gained more BMD than endurance athletes or controls.

Interestingly, some have observed lower skull (Karlsson *et al.*, 1996) and rib (Smith and Rutherford, 1993) BMD in athletes than controls, raising the question of whether nonloaded bone actually suffers at the expense of BMD enhancement in loaded bone.

b. Previous Activity   A previous history of substantial sports participation is likely to be beneficial to bone, although study findings are often confounded by continued activity participation. Sone and associates (1996) found men who had exercised "often" or "sometimes" in the past had greater spine and femoral neck BMD than those who had exercised "not at all." (Those who exercised "often" in the present also had greater spine BMD than nonexercisers.)

Karlsson and associates (1996) noted that ex-weight lifters who had retired from their sport 25 ± 13 years previously maintained a significant difference in total body and hip BMD from controls. (Because 72% of ex-lifters continued to exercise for 5 ± 3 hours per week after retirement, the contributions of historical versus current levels of exercise are difficult to discern.) Ex-weight lifters in the age range of 50–65 were observed to maintain significantly higher total body (Karlsson *et al.*, 1996) and spine BMD (Karlsson *et al.*, 1995) than controls, but not after age 65 (Karlsson *et al.*, 1996). Significant positive correlations were also found between current exercise frequency, exercise intensity, and BMD.

c. Site Specificity   As with children and adolescents, the effects of exercise loading on BMD of adult men are likely to be site-specific. BMD differences in athletes are often observed only at certain skeletal locations. Hamdy and associates (1994) found BMD differences between weight lifters, runners, cross trainers, and recreational sport participants to be present only in the upper limbs. Weight lifters had greater upper limb BMD than runners and recreational athletes, and cross-trained athletes also exhibited greater upper limb BMD than runners. Because weight lifting typically loads the upper limbs to a much greater extent than running, these findings make intuitive sense. In an illustration of the vagaries of cross-sectional data, however, other studies have shown power and weight lifters to have greater spine and hip but not upper or lower limb BMD than endurance athletes or controls (Bennell *et al.*, 1997; Colletti *et al.*, 1989). Aloia and associates (1978) found that even though total body calcium in marathon runners exceeds that of nonrunners, no such difference was observed in radial BMC and width. Such a finding is likely to reflect the fact that the radius is not substantially loaded during running and is thus unlikely to undergo running-related adaptation. Although not specifically measured, the increments in total body calcium are likely to have resided in the weight-bearing limbs.

Limb domination ("handedness" or "footedness") provides an elegant model of the site specificity of skeletal adaptation. Commonly, the dominant arm exhibits greater total and cortical bone mass than the nondominant arm (Rico et al., 1994). Even greater differences between right and left side limb bone masses become evident when the dominant limb is chronically overloaded. Up to a 40% difference between the playing and nonplaying arm humeral BMD of professional tennis players has been observed, compared to a 3% difference between right and left arms of non-tennis-playing controls (Haapasalo et al., 1996; Dalen et al., 1985). Dominant leg BMD has also been observed to be greater than nondominant leg BMD in players of a variety of weight-bearing sports (Nilsson and Westlin, 1971). Rowers and triathletes appear to have no such BMD sidedness (Smith and Rutherford, 1993), an observation which is predictable given that rowing, running, swimming and biking load bilateral limbs essentially equally.

d. Does an "Exercise Intensity Benefit Ceiling" Exist?   A number of investigations have reported seemingly anachronistic results describing the effect of exercise on BMD. MacDougall and associates (1992) observed a generalized increase in BMD with running mileage up to 15–20 miles per week; thereafter, the trend reversed, suggesting a possible detrimental effect of overtraining. The reduction in bone density, however, was accompanied by an increase in bone area which was significantly different between controls and runners covering 40–50 miles per week. Bilanin and associates (1989) found 9% less vertebral BMD in runners who ran an average of 92 km per week for several years than in controls. Similarly, Hetland and colleagues (1993) reported a negative correlation between weekly running distance and BMC at the spine, total body, hip, and forearm. Even though the use of BMC limits the utility of these results, other findings support a negative effect of ever-increasing exercise loads. These findings suggest the existence of an "exercise intensity ceiling" beyond which bone mass declines. However, no direct evidence for such a ceiling has ever been presented, and it is equally plausible that low BMD in successful ultra-distance runners reflects a self-selection effect based on pretraining characteristics or other effects such as low body mass or nutritional inadequacy.

3. Older Males

a. Current Activity   Studies of older men (>65 years) report responses of bone to exercise loading which are similar to those of younger men. Endurance and speed athletes aged 70–81 were found to have greater calcaneal BMD than controls (Suominen and Rahkila, 1991). In a study of men aged 50 to 72, Michel and associates (1989) found a positive association between weight-bearing exercise and lumbar spine BMD but no significant correlation between BMD and non-weight-bearing exercise.

By contrast, Need and associates (1995) found significant relationships of activity to BMD in younger men to dissipate after the age of 50. It is likely that the lack of relationship of BMD to current level of activity in their study reflected the low intensity of activities pursued. Pollock and associates (1997) measured whole body, spine, and hip BMD of current and exathlete men aged 60 to 90+ who continued to participate in low-, moderate-, and high-intensity forms of exercise. Even though investigators did not stratify BMD data by exercise intensity, they found that bone density was generally maintained in all men observed. This finding argues against a critical role of exercise intensity for bone density maintenance in older men.

b. Previous Activity   Glynn and associates (1995) found that historical physical activity was a positive determinant of hip BMD in men aged 50 to 88, but that current leisure or occupational activities were not influential. Greendale and colleagues (1995) also reported a significant linear trend in older men between both lifetime and current exercise and hip BMD, although no significant relationship was found at other sites. Neither was there a relationship between osteoporotic fracture rate and exercise profile, a reminder that maintenance of bone mass is arguably not a primary clinical or functional goal in and of itself. In fact, BMD maintenance is largely a method of achieving the more practical goal of minimizing risk of fracture.

4. Exercise-Related Geometric Adaptation

Expanded diaphyseal diameters are frequently seen in dominant side limbs of athletes who preferentially load them. Krahl and colleagues (1994) observed significant differences in diameter and length of playing arm ulnae of tennis players compared to their contralateral arms. The second metacarpals of playing hands were also wider and longer than in contralateral hands. No differences were observed between limbs of controls. Dalen and associates (1985) observed a 27% difference in cortical cross-sectional area between left and right humeri of tennis players compared to a nonsignificant 5% difference in controls. Significant differences between playing and nonplaying arm humeral cortical wall thickness, length, width, and cross-sectional moment of inertia were likewise observed by Haapasalo and associates (1996).

E. Exercise Effects—Intervention Trial Findings

Prospective studies designed to expose randomly selected, previously untrained subjects to exercise are a more rigorous and valid method of observing the effect of exercise on BMD than cross-sectional designs. The inherent difficulties of subject recruitment and compliance associated with exercise intervention trials are, however, reflected in the substantially reduced volume of reports in the literature.

I. Adult Men

One prospective trial concluded that there were no significant differences between calcaneal BMC of consistent runners, inconsistent runners, and nonexercising controls after 9 months of marathon training (Williams *et al.*, 1984). A closer analysis of the data, however, revealed that consistent runners indeed increased calcaneal BMC and that the amount of change in BMC was significantly different from controls. The correlation between average distance run and percent change in BMC also indicated a strong positive relationship.

Army recruits completing 14 weeks of intensive physical training have been observed to increase right and left leg BMC by 8.3 and 12.4%, respectively (Margulies *et al.*, 1986). In a similar trial, a 7.5% increase in tibial bone density was observed in Army recruits after 14 weeks of basic training (Leichter *et al.*, 1989). Recruits who began the training period with the lowest bone density gained the greatest amount. Those who temporarily ceased training due to stress fracture also gained bone density, but to a lesser degree (5%). It is an interesting question to consider whether reduced bone density contributed to the incidence of stress fracture in the injured group, or if the cessation of training reduced the opportunity to accrue a similar amount of bone as those who completed training. Also notable is the fact that 10% of recruits actually lost bone density. This effect was likely to stem from resorption-related remodeling porosity which had not yet been matched by replacement formation owing to the short time frame of the study. The discrepancy in results across recruits highlights the phenomenon of substantial individual variation in bone adaptation response to exercise loading.

The effects of 4 months of high-intensity resistance training three times per week on the bone metabolism of 23- to 31-year-old Asian males were investigated by Fujimura and associates (1997). They found that indicators of bone formation (serum osteocalcin concentration and serum bone-specific alkaline phosphatase activity) were increased within a month of initiating training and remained elevated throughout the training period. Markers of bone resorption (plasma procollagen type I and urinary deoxypyridinoline) were never significantly elevated. Although the findings led the authors to conclude that resistance training stimulated bone formation but not bone resorption, no significant changes in BMD were evident following training to confirm the assertion.

The influence of training intensity on bone response becomes apparent when the results of army trials are compared with those of Dalen and Olsson (1974). In the latter trial, subjects aged 25 to 52 failed to gain bone mass at the forearm, spine, humerus, femur, or calcaneus after 3 months of either walking (3 km, 5 days a week), or running (5 km, 3 days a week). In comparison, the bone mineral gains observed in the aforementioned army recruits reflect the considerably more intense nature of exercise loading during basic army training.

2. Older Men

Results from exercise intervention trials with older men are conflicting, with some suggestion that exercise does not strongly stimulate bone accretion in this population. McCartney and associates (1996) reported that 42 weeks of weight training in 60 to 80 year olds increased muscle strength and functional ability but caused no changes in whole body and spine BMD. Conversely, Welsh and Rutherford (1996) found that trochanteric BMD increased significantly in 50- to 73-year-old men performing step and jumping exercises. The effect is likely to be related to the enhancement of the strength of hip extensor muscles inserting at that site. Although gluteal muscle strength was not measured, quadriceps strength was increased after 12 months of exercise.

Sixteen weeks of progressive resistance training of 64- to 75-year-old men, with or without growth hormone supplementation, had no significant effect on BMD of either growth hormone treated or placebo groups. (A minor BMD increase only at Ward's triangle in the placebo group, and minor decreases in whole body and femoral neck BMD in the growth hormone treatment group are of questionable significance) (Yarasheski et al., 1997). Similarly, 24 weeks of exercise intervention, with or without growth hormone, increased muscle strength (independent of growth hormone) but effected no change in BMD of older men (Taaffe et al., 1994, 1996, personal communication, 1998).

VI. Unloading Bone—In Brief

Although a thorough review of the subject is beyond the scope of the present chapter, it is appropriate to mention the effects of skeletal unloading— the opposite extreme of the loading continuum to chronic exercise. In keeping with Wolff's Law, unloading bone provokes the converse reaction to that of loading it. A substantial body of evidence exists to support this claim, particularly regarding the effects of spinal cord injury, prolonged bed rest, and limb immobilization on BMD. Paraplegic and quadriplegic patients may lose more than 2% of lower extremity bone mass for the first 4–6 months after injury, thereafter losing approximately 1% a month for the remainder of the first year (Kiratli, 1996). Krølner and Toft (1983) observed patients who were hospitalized at bed rest for an average of 27 days. The average decrease in BMD during bed rest was 3.6%, equivalent to about 0.9% bone loss per week. After an average of 15 weeks of reambulation, an average gain of 4.4% BMD was observed. Even more dramatic descriptions of bone loss have been reported in astronauts exposed to microgravity.

VII. Hormonal Factors

A. Acute Exercise Response

Acute hormonal perturbation has been observed in individuals under exercise stress. Significant increases in serum concentrations of testosterone, lutenizing hormone (LH), dehydroepiandrosterone (DHEA), follicle stimulating hormone (FSH), cortisol, prolactin and androstenedione have been observed during maximum endurance exercise (Cumming et al., 1986; MacConnie et al., 1986).

Markers of bone turnover and parathyroid hormone (PTH) are also acutely stimulated by exercise (Brahm et al., 1997). Rong and associates (1997) found that strength exercise increased acute levels of PTH and that both strength and prolonged endurance exercise caused a pronounced decrease in type I collagen telopeptide (marker of bone resorption).

B. Chronic Exercise Response

The ability of chronic exercise to substantially modify hormone balance has not been shown. Investigators have found that male athletes exercising at a range of intensities appear to have serum concentrations of testosterone which lie within the normal range (MacConnie et al., 1986; Suominen and Rahkila, 1991; MacDougall et al., 1992; Hetland et al., 1993; Smith and Rutherford, 1993), including adolescents (Rowland et al., 1987). Others factors, such as LH, FSH, prolactin, cortisol, and estradiol (Rogol et al., 1984; Wheeler et al., 1984; MacConnie et al., 1986; Hackney et al., 1988) have also been found to circulate at normal levels in male athletes.

Increased concentrations of parathyroid hormone have been observed in response to a maximal exercise test before and after 6 weeks of endurance training (Zerath et al., 1997). Before training, the exercise test effected increased circulating osteocalcin (a marker of bone formation) but not after. In fact, osteocalcin concentrations decreased significantly after training. This finding may further illustrate the characteristic of diminishing returns in terms of exercising for bone mass. That is, greatest changes are seen in bone which has not previously undergone load-related bone adaptation. These responses clearly require further investigation, however, because Rong and associates (1997) found that prolonged endurance exercise increased osteocalcin levels. Long-term exercise has not been shown to preserve the decline in activity of the growth hormone-IGF-I axis (Cooper *et al.*, 1998).

These generalizations notwithstanding, a degree of subtle hormonal perturbation may be evident in some athletes. Smith and Rutherford (1993) found that, while in the normal range, serum total testosterone was significantly lower in triathletes than controls, but not rowers. Further, Wheeler and associates (1984) found that total serum testosterone, non-sex hormone binding globulin (SHBG)-bound testosterone, and "free" testosterone concentrations in men running more than 64 km per week to be 83, 69.5, and 68.1% that of controls, respectively. Prolactin concentrations were also significantly lower in runners than controls. In contrast, Suominen and Rahkila (1991) found that endurance athletes had significantly greater levels of SHBG than strength athletes and controls, and Cooper and associates (1998) showed substantially increased circulating SHBG in elderly long-term runners than in age-matched nonexercising men. Hackney and associates (1988) also found resting and free testosterone concentrations of trained athletes to be 68.8 and 72.6% that of controls and LH to be slightly higher in athletes than controls.

The implications of exercise-related hormonal perturbation to bone mass is somewhat unclear. Suominen and Rahkila (1991) detected a negative correlation between BMD and SHBG in endurance athletes but no relationship of BMD with testosterone. Interestingly, Fiore and associates (1991) found that intense body-building training and self-administered anabolic steroids (testosterone: 193.75 ± 147.82 mg/week) did not stimulate greater osteoblastic activity or bone formation than exercise alone. Given sparse data from long-term intervention trials, a connection between exercise, hormone status, and bone metabolism remains difficult to make.

VIII. Sex Comparison of Exercise Effect on Bone ─────────

Once again, there is only a modicum of data comparing male and female responses to exercise intervention, and information regarding an interaction of age with these responses is essentially nonexistent. Welsh and Rutherford (1996) observed the effect of 12 months of high-impact aerobics two to three times a week on hip, spine, and total body BMD of elderly men and women. They found that both men and women increased BMD a similar amount (men, approximately 1.2%; women, approximately 1.3%) at all sites, whereas controls lost BMD.

Even though evidence suggests that exercise training improves BMD in women of all ages, and it is likely that these results are indicative of the male response to exercise, the known influence of hormones on bone mass precludes premature inferences from gender-specific findings.

IX. Maintaining Bone Mass—Exercise Prescription _____

The common prescription of walking three to four times per week for bone health has not altered over the past 20 years (Sidney *et al.*, 1977; Katz and Sherman, 1998). Even though a recommendation to walk is certainly appropriate for the purposes of general health maintenance, available data specific to bone gain or maintenance do not necessarily support this belief (Dalen and Olsson, 1974; Hutchinson *et al.*, 1995). Low-impact activities may, in fact, be relatively ineffective for the purposes of increasing or maintaining bone mass in any age group, with the exception of the very young. While Michel and associates (1989) reported that up to 300 minutes of weight-bearing exercise, including walking, was linearly related to BMD in older men, a causal relationship was not established. The only other evidence for walking as a bone stimulus comes from research involving postmenopausal women, where walking more than 7.5 miles per week was associated with higher whole body, leg, and trunk BMD than walking less than 1 mile per week (Krall and Dawson-Hughes, 1994).

High-intensity resistance training or relatively high-impact weight-bearing exercise appears to impose the greatest stimulus on bone. It is something of a conundrum to design an exercise program which sufficiently loads the skeleton without placing it at risk of impact-related fracture, particularly in an osteoporotic population. In addition, running and other higher-impact activities may increase the risk of falls and possible fracture. Such injury is to be avoided at all costs, given the negative repercussions of prolonged immobilization and/or bed rest on BMD and health in general. Because exercise is known to enhance balance and neuromuscular function, activities of higher impact than walking should be given at least passing consideration as a viable option for some individuals. Examples of the controlled circumstances under which a running regimen may be effectively implemented include: establishing an adequately graduated program of increasing intensity (beginning with walking in most cases), wearing appropriate footwear and exercise clothing, obtaining clearance for other medical conditions for which high-intensity exercise is contraindicated, and monitoring exercise bouts by family members or friends. Running and other high-impact activities are not recommended for those suffering from grossly compromised skeletal components such as advanced vertebral osteoporosis.

Resistance training is also a viable option for bone health maintenance. The benefit of weight lifting resides primarily in the opportunity to load non-weight-bearing bones in a controlled exercise environment that offers minimal risk for falling. It could also be argued that, even in the absence of bone gain with resistance training, the benefits of muscle strength gains for the purposes of reducing fracture risk are sufficient in and of themselves to warrant such a recommendation. It has been recommended that resistance-training loads be chosen for their ability to induce muscle fatigue after 10 to 15 repetitions and should be increased gradually. A resistance workout should be performed approximately every 3 days to allow time for muscle recovery. Rowing machines should be avoided by individuals suffering from osteoporosis owing to the risk of vertebral fracture from deep forward bending. Resistance exercise is not optimally recommended for individuals suffering from hypertension as transient increases in blood pressure associated with forceful large muscle group contractions may be hazardous.

There is no such thing as a "one-size-fits-all" exercise prescription for the purposes of bone gain or, indeed, any other physiological function. It is, however, safe to say that individuals who currently exist in primarily sedentary lifestyles have much to gain by increasing their levels of activity by any degree. For those who fit such a description, moderate-intensity walking of increasing frequency and duration to approximately 30 to 60 minutes, four times per week, in combination with a generalized increase in incidental activity (for example, leaf raking instead of blowing), is likely to confer substantial benefits on bone health. An emphasis on activities which improve general muscle strength, flexibility, and coordination is highly recommended, given the attendant reduced risk of falling associated with these attributes.

For those who are already somewhat active, higher-intensity, impact exercises such as running up and down hills and stairs, aerobics, and jump rope are "bone-friendly" activities. Graduated increments in exercise training intensity are recommended to allow adequate time for bone remodeling and avoid bone stress injury. Resistance training of muscle groups in all regions of the body (triceps surae, quadriceps, hamstrings, gluteals, iliopsoas, erector spinae, abdominals, chest and upper back, biceps brachii/brachialis, triceps, etc.) is also recommended. Novel incidental or recreational exercises (e.g., carrying shopping bags, yard work, arm wrestling, tug-of-war) which load bones in an unusual manner or target non-weight-bearing portions of the skeleton may additionally assist in the maintenance of skeletal mass in moderately active individuals. The essential factor in the prescription of exercise for bone mass maintenance is the recommendation that it be pursued throughout the lifespan and that long periods of immobilization or inactivity are avoided.

X. Conclusions

We have reviewed the conceptual basis for understanding the relationship between mechanical loading and skeletal adaptation, along with the specific effect of exercise on bone mass in men. Complete understanding of the relationship of exercise to bone mass in humans must await development and validation of accurate, quantitative estimates of mechanical loading history. Although this has not yet been accomplished, sufficient information is available to permit general conclusions, as well as speculation about the kinds of exercises that are likely to prove most osteogenic.

Cross-sectional studies, in general, provide support for the notion that habitual athletic endeavor promotes superior bone density in men compared with that of a sedentary life-style. The magnitude of this difference is likely to depend on the nature of the activity, the age at which it was initiated, and the number of years spent in training. Physical activity may enhance peak bone mass attained if initiated before the age of 20. Muscle mass and strength is likely to contribute positively to BMD at this age, as well as during later years. Bone displays a clear site specificity for mechanical load-induced adaptation at all ages.

Exercise intensity may be an important factor in the stimulation of bone adaptation. Moderate- to high-impact weight-bearing activities such as running, jumping, and power lifting appear to be the most bone stimulatory. Walking and long-duration swimming are less effective, with the exception that swimming may have a positive impact on bones not normally loaded during weight bearing.

Although there are inadequate data upon which to make decisive conclusions, the ability of exercise to stimulate significant gains in bone mass in older males appears to be reduced. The strong positive effect of exercise on muscle strength at all ages, however, suggests that exercise indirectly benefits bone, even in older males, as a function of improved or maintained balance, coordination, and related reduction in the risk of falling.

The response of bone to exercise loading is curvilinear in nature. The greatest increments in bone mass are generally observed in individuals with the lowest initial values. It is undoubtedly true that unloading the skeleton for extended periods is detrimental to bone. The addition of even modest activity to an immobilized subject will increase BMD to a much greater extent than will a substantial increase in training for a highly active person. Therefore, one might best consider physical activity to be an effective prevention against bone *loss*, rather than a means to achieving major increases in bone mass.

References

Aloia, J. F., Cohn, S. H., Babu, T., Abesamis, C., Kalici, N., and Ellis, K. (1978). Skeletal mass and body composition in marathon runners. *Metab. Clin. Exp.* **27**, 1793–1796.

Benedict, M. R., Adiyaman, S., Ayers, D. C., Thomas, F. D., Calore, J. D., Dhar, V., and Richman, R. A. (1994). Dissociation of bone mineral density from age-related decreases in insulin-like growth factor-1 and its binding proteins in the male rat. *J. Gerontol.* **49**, B224–B230.

Bennell, K. L., Malcolm, S. A., Khan, K. M., Thomas, S. A., Reid, S. J., Brukner, P. D., Eberling, P. R., and Wark, J. D. (1997). Bone mass and bone turnover in power athletes, endurance athletes, and controls: A 12-month longitudinal study. *Bone* **20**, 477–484.

Bevier, W. C., Wiswell, R. A., Pyka, G., Kozak, K. C., Newhall, K. M., and Marcus, R. (1989). Relationship of body composition, muscle strength, and aerobic capacity to bone mineral density in older men and women. *J. Bone Miner. Res.* **4**, 421–432.

Bilanin, J. E., Blanchard, M. S., and Russek-Cohen, E. (1989). Lower vertebral bone density in male long distance runners. *Med. Sci. Sports Exercise* **21**, 66–70.

Block, J. E., Genant, H. K., and Black, D. (1986). Greater vertebral bone mineral mass in exercising young men. *West. J. Med.* **145**, 39–42.

Block, J. E., Friedlander, A. L., Brooks, G. A., Steiger, P., Stubbs, H. A., and Genant, H. K. (1989). Determinants of bone density among athletes engaged in weight-bearing and non-weight-bearing activity. *J. Appl. Physiol.* **67**, 1100–1105.

Bonjour, J. P., Theintz, G., Law, F., Slosman, D., and Rizzoli, R. (1994). Peak bone mass. *Osteoporosis Int.* **4**,(Suppl. 1), 7–13.

Boot, A. M., de Ridder, M. A. J., Pols, H. A. P., Krenning, E. P., and de Muinck Keizer-Schrama, S. M. P. F. (1997). Bone mineral density in children and adolescents: Relation to puberty, calcium intake, and physical activity. *J. Clin. Endocrinol. Metab.* **82**, 57–62.

Bouxsein, M. L., Myburgh, K. H., van der Meulen, M. C. H., Lindenberger, E., and Marcus, R. (1994). Age-related differences in cross-sectional geometry of the forearm bones in healthy women. *Calcif. Tissue Int.* **54**, 113–118.

Brahm, H., Piehl-Aulin, K., Saltin, B., and Ljunghall, S. (1997). Net fluxes over working thigh of hormones, growth factors and biomarkers of bone metabolism during short lasting dynamic exercise. *Calcif. Tissue Int.* **60**, 175–180.

Burr, D. B., and Martin, R. B. (1983). The effects of composition, structure and age on the torsional properties of the human radius. *J. Biomech.* **16**, 603–608.

Carter, D. R., Bouxsein, M. L., and Marcus, R. (1992). New approaches for interpreting projected bone densitometry. *J. Bone Miner. Res.* **7**, 137–145.

Clarke, B. L., Ebeling, P. R., Jones, J. D., Wahner, H. W., O'Fallon, W. M., Riggs, B. L., and Fitzpatrick, L. A. (1996). Changes in quantitative bone histomorphometry in aging healthy men. *J. Clin. Endocrinol. Metab.* **81**, 2264–2270.

Colletti, L. A., Edwards, J., Gordon, L., Shary, J., and Bell, N. H. (1989). The effects of muscle-building exercise on bone mineral density of the radius, spine, and hip in young men. *Calcif. Tissue Int.* **45**, 12–14.

Cooper, C., Campion, G., and Melton, L. J. (1992). Hip fractures in the elderly: A world-wide projection. *Osteoporosis Int.* **2**, 285–289.

Cooper, C., Taaffe, D. R., Guido, D., Packer, E., Holloway, L., and Marcus, R. (1998). Relationship of chronic endurance exercise to the somatotropic and sex hormone status of older men. *Eur. J. Endocrinol.* **138**, 517–523.

Cumming, D. C., Brunsting, L. A., Strich, G., Ries, A. L., and Rebar, R. W. (1986). Reproductive hormone increases in response to acute exercise in men. *Med. Sci. Sports Exercise* **18**, 369–373.

Dalen, N., and Olsson, K. E. (1974). Bone mineral content and physical activity. *Acta Orthop. Scand.* **45**, 170–174.

Dalen, N., Laftman, P., Ohlsen, H., and Stromberg, L. (1985). The effect of athletic activity on the bone mass in human diaphyseal bone. *Orthopaedics* **8**, 1139–1141.

Doyle, F., Brown, J., and Lachance, C. (1970). Relation between bone mass and muscle weight. *Lancet* **1**, 391–393.

Duppe, H., Gardsell, P., Johnell, O., Nilsson, B. E., and Ringsberg, K. (1997). Bone mineral density, muscle strength and physical activity. A population-based study of 332 subjects aged 15–42 years. *Acta Orthop. Scand.* **68**, 97–103.

Fiore, C. E., Cottini, E., Fargetta, C., di Salvio, G., Foti, R., and Raspagliesi, M. (1991). The effects of muscle-building exercise on forearm bone mineral content and osteoblast activity in drug-free and anabolic steroids self-administering young men. *Bone Miner.* **13**, 77–83.

Frost, H. M. (1964). "The Laws of Bone Structure." Thomas, Springfield, IL.

Fujimura, R., Ashizawa, N., Watanabe, M., Mukai, N., Amagai, H., Fukubayashi, T., Hayashi, K., Tokuyama, K., and Suzuki, M. (1997). Effect of resistance exercise training on bone formation and resorption in young male subjects assessed by biomarkers of bone metabolism. *J. Bone Miner. Res.* **12,** 656–662.

Glynn, N. W., Meilahn, E. N., Charron, M., Anderson, S. J., Kuller, L. H., and Cauley, J. A. (1995). Determinants of bone mineral density in older men. *J. Bone Miner. Res.* **10,** 1769–1777.

Greendale, G. A., Barrett-Connor, E., Edelstein, S., Ingles, S., and Haile, R. (1995). Lifetime leisure exercise and osteoporosis. The Rancho Bernardo Study. *Am. J. Epidemiol.* **141,** 951–959.

Gunnes, M., and Lehmann, E. H. (1996). Physical activity and dietary constituents as predictors of forearm cortical and trabecular bone gain in healthy children and adolescents: A prospective study. *Acta Paediatr.* **85,** 19–25.

Haapasalo, H., Sievanen, H., Kannus, P., Heinenon, A., Oja, P., and Vuori, I. (1996). Dimensions and estimated mechanical characteristics of the humerus after long-term tennis loading. *J. Bone Miner. Res.* **11,** 864–872.

Hackney, A. C., Sinning, W. E., and Bruot, B. C. (1988). Reproductive hormonal profiles of endurance-trained and untrained males. *Med. Sci. Sports Exercise* **20,** 60–65.

Hamdy, R. C., Anderson, J. S., Whalen, K. E., and Harvill, L. M. (1994). Regional differences in bone density of young men involved in different exercises. *Med. Sci. Sports Exercise* **26,** 884–888.

Hannan, M. T., Felson, D. T., and Anderson, J. J. (1992). Bone mineral density in elderly men and women: Results from the Framingham Osteoporosis Study. *J. Bone Miner. Res.* **7,** 547–553.

Heinonen, A., Oja, P., Kannus, P., Sievanen, H., Haapasalo, H., Manittari, A., and Vuori, I. (1995). Bone mineral density in female athletes representing sports with different loading characteristics of the skeleton. *Bone* **17,** 197–203.

Hert, J., Liskova, M., and Landa, J. (1971). Reaction of bone to mechanical stimuli. Part 1. Continuous and intermittent loading of tibia in rabbit. *Folia Morphol.* **19,** 290–317.

Hetland, M. L., Haarbo, J., and Christiansen, C. (1993). Low bone mass and high bone turnover in male long distance runners. *J. Clin. Endocrinol. Metab.* **77,** 770–775.

Hutchinson, T. M., Whalen, R. T., Cleet, T. M., Vogel, J. M., and Arnaud, S. B. (1995). Factors in daily physical activity related to calcaneal mineral density in men. *Med. Sci. Sports Exercise* **27,** 745–750.

Jackson, J. A., and Kleerekoper, M. (1990). Osteoporosis in men: Diagnosis, pathophysiology, and prevention. *Medicine (Baltimore)* **69,** 137–152.

Karlsson, M. K., Johnell, O., and Obrant, K. J. (1993). Bone mineral density in weight lifters. *Calcif. Tissue Int.* **52,** 212–215.

Karlsson, M. K., Johnell, O., and Obrant, K. J. (1995). Is bone mineral density advantage maintained long-term in previous weight lifters? *Calcif. Tissue Int.* **57,** 325–328.

Karlsson, M. K., Hasserius, R., and Obrant, K. J. (1996). Bone mineral density in athletes during and after career: A comparison between loaded and unloaded skeletal regions. *Calcif. Tissue Int.* **59,** 245–248.

Katz, W. A., and Sherman, C. (1998). Osteoporosis. The role of exercise in optimal management. *Phys. Sports Med.* **26,** 33–43.

Katzman, D. K., Bachrach, L. K., Carter, D. R., and Marcus, R. (1991). Clinical and anthropometric correlates of bone mineral acquisition in healthy adolescent girls. *J. Clin. Endocrinol. Metab.* **73,** 1332–1339.

Kiratli, B. J. (1996). Immobilization osteopenia. *In* "Osteoporosis" (R. Marcus, D. Feldman, and J. Kelsey, eds.), 1st ed., pp. 833–853. Academic Press, San Diego, CA.

Krahl, H., Michaelis, U., Pieper, H.-G., Quack, G., and Montag, M. (1994). Stimulation of bone growth through sports. A radiologic investigation of the upper extremities in professional tennis players. *Am. J. Sports Med.* **22,** 751–757.

Krall, E. A., and Dawson-Hughes, B. (1994). Walking is related to bone density and rates of bone loss. *Am. J. Med.* **96**, 20–26.

Krølner, B., and Toft, B. (1983). Vertebral bone loss: An unheeded side effect of therapeutic bed rest. *Clin. Sci.* **64**, 537–540.

Lanyon, L. E., and Rubin, C. T. (1984). Static vs dynamic loads as an influence on bone remodeling. *J. Biomech.* **17**, 897–905.

Leichter, I., Simkin, A., Margulies, J. Y., Bevas, A., Steinberg, R., Giladi, M., and Milgrom, C. (1989). Gain in mass density of bone following strenuous physical activity. *J. Orthop. Res.* **7**, 86–90.

MacConnie, S. E., Barkan, A., Lampman, R. M., Schork, M. A., and Beitins, I. Z. (1986). Decreased hypothalmic gonadotrophin-releasing hormone secretion in male marathon runners. *N. Engl. J. Med.* **315**, 411–417.

MacDougall, J. D., Webber, C. E., Martin, J., Ormerod, S., Chesley, A., Younglai, E. V., Gordon, C. L., and Blimkie, C. J. R. (1992). Relationship among running mileage, bone density, and serum testosterone in male runners. *J. Appl. Physiol.* **73**, 1165–1170.

Marcus, R. (1996). Mechanisms of exercise effects on bone. *In* "Principles of Bone Biology" (J. P. Bilezikian, L. G. Raisz, and G. Rodan, eds.), pp. 1135–1146. Academic Press, San Diego, CA.

Margulies, J. Y., Simkin, A., Leichter, I., Bivas, A., Steinberg, R., Giladi, M., Stein, M., Kashtan, H., and Milgrom, C. (1986). Effect of intense physical activity on the bone-mineral content in the lower limbs of young adults. *J. Bone J. Surg.* **68**, 1090–1093.

Martin, R. B., and Atkinson, P. J. (1977). Age and sex-related changes in the structure and strength of the human femoral shaft. *J. Biomech.* **20**, 223–231.

Martin, R. B., and Burr, D. B. (1989). "Structure, Function, and Adaptation of Compact Bone." Raven Press, New York.

Martin, R. B., Pickett, J. C., and Zinaich, S. (1980). Studies of skeletal remodeling in aging men. *Clin. Orthop.* **149**, 268–282.

McCartney, N., Hicks, A. L., Martin, J., and Webber, C. E. (1996). A longitudinal trial of weight training in the elderly: Continued improvements in year 2. *J. Gerontol. A Biol. Sci. Med. Sci.* **51**, B425–B433.

Michel, B. A., Bloch, D. A., and Fries, J. F. (1989). Weight-bearing exercise, overexercise, and lumbar bone density over age 50 years. *Arch. Intern. Med.* **149**, 2325–2329.

Moro, M., van der Meulen, M. C. H., Kiratli, B. J., Marcus, R., Bachrach, L. K., and Carter, D. R. (1996). Body mass is the primary determinant of midfemoral bone acquisition during adolescent growth. *Bone* **19**, 519–526.

Moyer-Mileur, L., Luetkemeier, M., Boomer, L., and Chan, G. M. (1995). Effect of physical activity on bone mineralization in premature infants. *J. Pediatr.* **127**, 620–625.

Myburgh, K. H., Charette, S., Zhou, L., Steele, C. R., Arnaud, S., and Marcus, R. (1993). Influence of recreational activity and muscle strength on ulnar bending stiffness in men. *Med. Sci. Sports Exercise* **25**, 592–596.

Need, A. G., Wishard, J. M., Scopacasa, F., Horowitz, M., Morris, H. A., and Nordin, B. E. (1995). Effect of physical activity on femoral bone density on men. *Br. Med. J.* **310**, 1501–1502.

Newhall, K. M., Rodnick, K. J., Van Der Meulen, M. C., Carter, D. R., and Marcus, R. (1991). Effects of voluntary exercise on bone mineral content in rats. *J. Bone Miner. Res.* **6**, 289–296.

Nilsson, B. E., and Westlin, N. E. (1971). Bone density in athletes. *Clin. Orthop.* **77**, 179–182.

Nordstrom, P., Nordstrom, G., Thorsen, K., and Lorentzon, R. (1996). Local bone mineral density, muscle strength, and exercise in adolescent boys: A comparative study of two groups with different muscle strength and exercise levels. *Calcif. Tissue Int.* **58**, 402–408.

O'Connor, J. A., Lanyon, L. E., and MacFie, H. (1982). The influence of strain rate on adaptive bone remodelling. *J. Biomech.* **15**, 767–781.

Orwoll, E. S., Ferar, J., Ovaitt, S. K., McClung, M. R., and Huntington, K. (1989). The relationship of swimming exercise to bone mass in men and women. *Arch. Intern. Med.* **149**, 2197–2200.

Pollock, M. L., Mengelkoch, L. J., Graves, J. E., Lowenthal, D. T., Limacher, M. C., Foster, C., and Wilmore, J. H. (1997). Twenty-year follow-up of aerobic power and body composition of older track athletes. *J. Appl. Physiol.* **82**, 1508–1516.

Poor, G., Atkinson, E. J., Lewallen, D. G., O'Fallon, W. M., and Melton, L. J., III (1995). Age-related hip fractures in men: Clinical spectrum and short-term outcomes. *Osteoporosis Int.* **5**, 419–426.

Rico, H., Gonzalez-Riola, J., Revilla, M., Villa, L. F., Gomez-Castresana, F., and Escribano, J. (1994). Cortical versus trabecular bone mass: Influence of activity on both bone compartments. *Calcif. Tissue Int.* **54**, 470–472.

Robinson, T. L., Snow-Harter, C., Taaffe, D. R., Gillis, D., Shaw, J., and Marcus, R. (1995). Gymnasts exhibit higher bone mass than runners despite similar prevalence of amenorrhea. *J. Bone Miner. Res.* **10**, 26–35.

Rogol, A. D., Veldhuis, J. D., Williams, F. A., and Johnson, M. L. (1984). Pulsatile secretion of gonadotrophins and prolactin in male marathon runners. *J. Androl.* **5**, 21–27.

Rong, H., Berg, U., Torring, O., Sundberg, C. J., Granberg, B., and Bucht, E. (1997). Effect of acute endurance and strength exercise on circulating calcium-regulating hormones and bone markers in healthy young males. *Scand. J. Med. Sci. Sports* **7**, 152–159.

Rowland, T. W., Morris, A. H., Kelleher, J. F., Haag, B. L., and Reiter, E. O. (1987). Serum testosterone response to training in adolescent runners. *Am. J. Dis. Child.* **141**, 881–883.

Rubin, C. T. (1984). Skeletal strain and the functional significance of bone architecture. *Calcif. Tissue Int.* **36**, S11–S18.

Rubin, C. T., and Lanyon, L. E. (1984). Regulation of bone formation by applied dynamic loads. *J. Bone J. Surg.* **66**, 397–402.

Rubin, C. T., Bain, S. D., and McLeod, K. J. (1992). Suppression of the osteogenic response in the aging skeleton. *Calcif. Tissue Int.* **50**, 306–313.

Ruff, C. B., and Hayes, W. C. (1983). Cross-sectional geometry of Pecos pueblo femora and tibiae—a biomechanical inverstigation: II. Sex, age, and side differences. *Am. J. Phys. Anthropol.* **60**, 383–400.

Ruff, C. B., and Hayes, W. C. (1988). Sex differences in age-related remodeling of the femur and tibia. *J. Orthop. Res.* **6**, 886–896.

Schaffler, M. B. (1985). Stiffness and fatigue of compact bone at physiological strains and strain rates. Ph.D. Dissertation West Virginia University, Morgantown.

Seeman, E. (1997). Osteoporosis in men. *Bailliere's Clin. Rheumatol.* **11**, 613–629.

Sidney, K. H., Shepard, R. J., and Harrison, J. E. (1977). Endurance training and body composition of elderly. *Am. J. Clin. Nutr.* **30**, 326–333.

Slemenda, C. W., Reister, T. K., Hui, S. L., Miller, J. Z., Christian, J. C., and Johnston, C. C., Jr. (1994). Influences on skeletal mineralization in children and adolescents: Evidence for varying effects of sexual maturation and physical activity. *J. Pediatr.* **125**, 201–207.

Smith, R., and Rutherford, O. M. (1993). Spine and total body bone mineral density and serum testosterone levels in male athletes. *Eur. J. Appl. Physiol.* **67**, 330–334.

Snow-Harter, C., Whalen, R., Myburgh, K., Arnaud, S., and Marcus, R. (1992). Bone mineral density, muscle strength, and recreational exercise in men. *J. Bone Miner. Res.* **7**, 1291–1296.

Sone, T., Miyake, M., Takeda, N., Tomomitsu, T., Otsuka, N., and Fukunaga, M. (1996). Influence of exercise and degenerative vertebral changes on BMD: A cross-sectional study in Japanese men. *Gerontology* **42**, 57–66.

Suominen, H. (1993). Bone mineral density in long term exercise. An overview of cross-sectional athlete studies. *Sports Med.* **16**, 316–330.

Suominen, H., and Rahkila, P. (1991). Bone mineral density of the calcaneus in 70- to 80-yr-old male athletes and a population sample. *Med. Sci. Sports Exercise* **23**, 1227–1233.

Taaffe, D. R., Pruitt, L., Riem, J., Hintz, R. L., Butterfield, G., Hoffmen, A. R., and Marcus, R. (1994). Effect of recombinant human growth hormone on the muscle strength response to resistance exercise in elderly men. *J. Clin. Endocrinol. Metab.* **79**, 1361–1366.

Taaffe, D. R., Snow-Harter, C., Connolly, D. A., Robinson, T. L., Brown, M. D., and Marcus, R. (1995). Differential effects of swimming versus weight-bearing activity on bone mineral status on eumenorrheic athletes. *J. Bone Miner. Res.* **10**, 586–593.

Taaffe, D. R., Jin, I. H., Vu, T. H., Hoffman, A. R., and Marcus, R. (1996). Lack of effect of recombinant growth hormone (GH) on muscle morphology and GH-insulin-like growth factor expression in resistance-trained elderly men. *J. Clin. Endocrinol. Metabl.* **81**, 421–425.

Termine, J. D. (1990). Cellular activity, matrix proteins, and aging bone. *Exp. Gerontol.* **25**, 217–221.

Theintz, G., Buchs, B., Rizzoli, R., Slosman, D., Clavien, H., Sizonenko, P. C., and Bonjour, J. P. (1992). Longitudinal monitoring of bone mass accumulation in healthy adolescents: Evidence for a marked reduction after 16 years of age at the levels of lumbar spine and femoral neck in female subjects. *Clin. Endocrinol. Metab.* **75**, 1060–1065.

Tsai, S. C., Kao, C. H., and Wang, S. J. (1996). Comparison of bone mineral density between athletic and non-athletic Chinese male adolescents. *Kaohsiung J. Med. Sci.* **12**, 573–580.

Turner, C. H., Owan, I., and Takano, Y. (1995a). Mechanotransduction in bone: Role of strain rate. *Am. J. Physiol.* **269**, E438–E442.

Turner, C. H., Takano, Y., and Owan, I. (1995b). Aging changes mechanical loading thresholds for bone formation in rats. *J. Bone Miner. Res.* **10**, 1544–1549.

VandenBergh, M. F. Q., DeMan, S. A., Witteman, J. C. M., Hofman, A., Trouerbach, W. T., and Grobbee, D. E. (1995). Physical activity, calcium intake, and bone mineral content in children in the Netherlands. *J. Epidemiol. Commun. Health* **49**, 299–304.

van der Wiel, H. E., Lips, P., Graafmans, W. C., Danielsen, C. C., Nauta, J., van Lingen, A., and Mosekilde, L. (1995). Additional weight-bearing during exercise is more important than duration of exercise for anabolic stimulus of bone: A study of running exercise in female rats. *Bone* **16**, 73–80.

Welsh, L., and Rutherford, O. M. (1996). Hip bone mineral density is improved by high-impact aerobic exercise in postmenopausal women and men over 50 years. *Eur. J. Appl. Physiol. Occup. Physiol.* **74**, 511–517.

Welten, D. C., Kemper, H. C. G., Post, G. B., Van Mechelen, W., Twisk, J., Lips, P., and Teule, G. J. (1994). Weight-bearing activity during youth is a more important factor for peak bone mass than calcium intake. *J. Bone Miner. Res.* **9**, 1089–1096.

Whalen, R. T., Carter, D. R., and Steele, C. R. (1988). Influence of physical activity on the regulation of bone density. *J. Biomech.* **21**, 825–837.

Wheeler, G. D., Wall, S. R., Belcastro, A. N., and Cumming, D. C. (1984). Reduced serum testosterone and prolactin levels in male distance runners. *J. Am. Med. Assoc.* **252**, 514–516.

Williams, J. A., Wagner, J., Wasnich, R., and Heilbrun, L. (1984). The effect of long-distance running upon appendicular bone mineral content. *Med. Sci. Sports Exercise* **16**, 223–227.

Yarasheski, K. E., Campbell, J. A., and Kohrt, W. M. (1997). Effect of resistance exercise and growth hormone on bone density in older men. *Clin. Endocrinol.* **47**, 223–229.

Zerath, E., Holy, X., Douce, P., Guezennec, C. Y., and Chatard, J. C. (1997). Effect of endurance training on postexercise parathyroid hormone levels in elderly men. *Med. Sci. Sports Exercise* **29**, 1139–1145.

Chapter 9

Clifford J. Rosen

St. Joseph Hospital
Maine Center for Osteoporosis Research and Education
Bangor, Maine

Insulin-like Growth Factors and Bone:
Implications for the Pathogenesis and Treatment of Osteoporosis

I. Introduction

The skeleton has an abundant supply of latent growth factors essential for linear growth and maintenance of adult bone mass (Mohan and Baylink, 1990). Bone is also bathed by circulating peptides and cytokines from the circulation (Rosen, 1994). One of the most abundant growth factors in bone and in the circulation is insulin-like growth factor I (IGF-I), a ubiquitous polypeptide with multiple functions. In the skeleton, IGF-I is essential for differentiated osteoblast function, as well as for chondrocyte proliferation (Hayden *et al.*, 1995). IGF-II supports collagen synthesis, stimulates osteoblast differentiation, and inhibits collagenase activity (Canalis *et al.*, 1991). Despite a relatively greater proportion of IGF-II than IGF-I in human bone and in serum, much more is known about IGF-I as an anabolic factor for the skeleton. In part, this relates to the ease of measuring IGF-I by RIA, its high concentration in serum, and its critical role as a somatomedin, modulating growth hormone activity at the cartilagenous growth plate. Indeed, serum IGF-I is often considered a surrogate end point for the biologic activity of endogenous growth hormone. This chapter will focus almost exclusively on IGF-I and its relationship to acquisition and maintenance of bone mass. A more generic discussion about the role of IGF-II in the skeleton is also undertaken.

There have been major advances in our understanding of the IGFs over the last decade. Several components of the IGF regulatory system have been defined, the function of two IGF receptors have been described, and the subcellular signaling cascades for the IGFs have been delineated. With the advent of recombinant peptide technology, clinical investigations using rhIGF-I in several chronic diseases including diabetes mellitus, renal failure, and osteoporosis have been undertaken. This chapter will focus on the skeletal and circulatory IGF regulatory system, how it is regulated, and what importance these systems might hold with respect to the maintenance of bone mass in both men and women. In fact, gender differences in tissue and circulating IGF-I, even absent excess or deficiency states, may provide key pieces of evidence which will define the relationship of skeletal growth factors to osteoporosis.

II. Physiology of the IGFs

A. IGF-I and IGF-II Structure and Function

1. IGFs and IGFBPs

The IGFs are 7 kilodalton polypeptides which share structural homology with pro-insulin (Canalis *et al.*, 1991). These proteins were initially called somatomedins because of their growth-promoting properties in numerous tissues and the initial inability to suppress their activity with anti-insulin antibodies. Both growth factors are found in high concentration in serum, and nearly every mammalian cell type can synthesize and export IGF-I and IGF-II. The IGF regulatory system in each organ is tissue-specific, but all share certain components. The IGFs circulate in a molar ratio of 2 : 1 (IGF-II : IGF-I) (Jones and Clemmons, 1995). However, neither is free, but rather each is bound to a series of high-affinity IGF-specific binding proteins (IGFBPs) of which six have been fully characterized (Jones and Clemmons, 1995). These binding proteins share about 50% sequence homology and contain highly conserved cysteine residues (Jones and Clemmons, 1995). In serum, their concentrations range from 100 to 5000 ng/ml and, except for IGFBP-3, are relatively unsaturated (Jones and Clemmons, 1995). Recently, a family of IGF-specific, low-affinity IGFBP-like proteins have been identified (IGFBP 7–10) (Oh, 1997). Their precise physiologic role has not been defined, although they possess the capacity to act on target cells independent of the IGFs.

Serum IGFBPs hold IGFs within the circulation and in extracellular tissue as inactive peptides. IGFBP-3 and IGFBP-5 have extracellular matrix binding sites which provide alternative storage sites for both IGFs (Jones and Clemmons, 1995). In bone for example, IGFBP-5 has very strong affinity for the hydroxyapatite crystal and is the principle binding protein which holds IGF-I and IGF-II within the matrix (Jones *et al.*, 1993). All but one of the IGFBPs, IGFBP-3, are small enough to translocate from the circulation into tissue shuttling IGFs to or from cells. The IGFBPs clearly serve as a reservoir for the IGFs but also can enhance or inhibit IGF activity, depending on tissue-specific factors.

Although both IGFs are mitogens, IGF-II is much more active during prenatal life than IGF-I. On the other hand, IGF-I is the principle regulator of linear growth. There is a wealth of information about IGF-I's role in skeletal homeostasis, whereas much less is known about IGF-II despite its relative abundance. Both IGFs act as skeletal mitogens, and each can be activated by a series of cytokines, calcium analogs, or other growth factors.

2. IGF-IR and IGFBP Proteases

IGF receptors and IGFBP proteases comprise two other essential components of all tissue IGF regulatory systems. There are two extra-membrane IGF receptors. The Type I IGF receptor (IGF-IR) is expressed ubiquitously and shares significant sequence homology with the insulin receptor (LeRoith *et al.*, 1995). It can bind insulin, IGF-I or IGF-II. The presence of the Type I receptor may confer special properties on the cell for several reasons. First, receptor binding to ligand can prevent programmed cell death or apoptosis (LeRoith *et al.*, 1997). Also, the presence of IGF-IR on the surface of some neoplastic cells may signify a more proliferative cell type. Third, interference with the Type I IGF-IR can result in tumor cell death (LeRoith *et al.*, 1997).

There are three different properties mediated by the IGF-IR. These include mitogenicity, transforming activity, and anti-apoptotic activity (LeRoith *et al.*, 1997; Baserga *et al.*, 1997). The Type II IGF-II receptor (IGF-IIR) is structurally very different from the Type I receptor and contains a mannose 6-phosphate binding site (LeRoith *et al.*, 1997). It does not bind insulin and preferentially binds IGF-II over IGF-I. Its precise role in cell growth is unclear, although it is a target for disposal of intracellular proteins (LeRoith *et al.*, 1997). Signaling from both IGF receptors occurs after ligand binding; this is followed by autophosphorylation of the receptor (LeRoith *et al.*, 1997; Baserga *et al.*, 1997; Myers *et al.*, 1993). Two major substrates of the receptor, IRS-I and IRS-2, are phosphorylated and then interact with a number of src homology 2(SH2) domain containing proteins (LeRoith *et al.*, 1997; Baserga *et al.*, 1997; Myers *et al.*, 1993). These interactions eventually lead to activation of downstream signaling proteins and kinases.

The other unique component of the IGF regulatory system are the IGFBP-specific proteases which cleave intact IGFBPs, thereby altering binding of the IGFs to IGFBPs (Campbell *et al.*, 1992). These proteases, some of which act only on certain tissues, are under the control of autocrine, paracrine, and hormonal influences. In particular, IGFBP tissue-specific proteases can act as co-mitogens by cleaving intact binding proteins into lower molecular weight fragments that bind the IGFs less avidly (Kanzaki *et al.*, 1994). In addition, the lower molecular weight IGFBP fragments may actually act as agonists to enhance IGF bioactivity (Fowlkes *et al.*, 1994). Finally, some of these proteases act on extracellular components thereby permitting cells to penetrate organic matrices (Thraillkill *et al.*, 1995). All these activities add to the layer of complexity surrounding a particular IGF regulatory system whether it be in bone or in the circulation. Recently, much progress has been made in defining constituents of the skeletal IGF system and its regulation.

B. The Skeletal IGF Regulatory System

1. IGF-I

The IGFs are the most abundant growth factors in bone (Mohan, 1993). As in the circulation, IGF-II is present in much higher concentrations than IGF-I. Both decline with age in cortical and trabecular sites while the relative ratio of IGF-II : I is preserved. In rodent bone and serum, IGF-I is the more abundant growth factor (Mohan, 1993). Both IGFs are stored in the skeletal matrix bound to IGFBP-5 and hydroxyapatite. Acid hydrolysis during bone resorption may be the mechanism whereby inert growth factors are activated (Fig. 1). But active growth factors are also synthesized in the skeleton and are regulated by three major hormones: growth hormone, PTH and 1,25 dihydroxyvitamin D (Mohan, 1993). Estradiol also can be a potent inhibitor of IGF-I synthesis. Recently, McCarthy and colleagues identified a cyclic AMP promoter element within the IGF-I gene of rat osteoblasts which is down regulated by 17-βestradiol (McCarthy *et al.*, 1997). This may have major significance in terms of gender responsiveness to anabolic factors which work through IGF-I and in understanding how estrogen may dampen stimuli that increase bone formation.

IGF-II, the predominant IGF produced by human osteoblasts, is regulated by systemic hormones (e.g., progesterone and glucocorticoids) and local factors (e.g., electromechanical stimuli and BMP-7) (McCarthy *et al.*, 1989a). IGF-I expression has also been noted in osteoclasts, and both IGFs have been premature osteoclasts to bone surfaces (Mahuzuki *et al.*, 1991). Undifferentiated osteoclasts possess the IGF-IR, although it is not clear whether there is an active autocrine IGF loop in differentiated osteoclasts. Based on these studies, there is strong evidence that IGF-I is a major coupling factor which permits bone remodeling to be balanced between resorption and formation.

2. Skeletal IGFBPs and IGFBP Proteases

All six IGFBPs are expressed by bone cells. IGFBP-1, -2, -4, and -6 are inhibitory to skeletal cells under most circumstances, whereas IGFBP-3 and -5

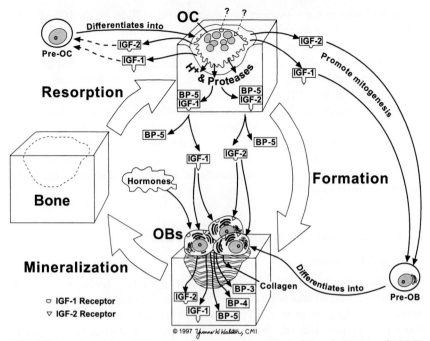

FIGURE I   The skeletal IGF regulatory system is composed of ligands (IGF-I and IGF-II), IGFBPs, IGFBP-specific proteases, and IGF receptors. At the onset of remodeling, osteoblasts are activated to secrete IGFs. With bone resorption, IGFs are released from the skeletal matrix and together with osteoblast-synthesized IGFs recruit new osteoblasts for bone formation.

are stimulatory (Jones and Clemmons, 1995; Mohan, 1993; Mohan and Baylink, 1997). IGFBP-5 is the first binding protein shown to have agonistic effects on osteoblasts independent of the IGFs (Andress *et al.*, 1992). Growth hormone enhances IGFBP-3 and -5 activity, whereas 1,25 dihydroxyvitamin D and PTH stimulate IGFBP-4 synthesis (Andress *et al.*, 1992; Rosen *et al.*, 1992). Insulin can cause suppression of IGFBP-1 production in bone cells, whereas glucocorticoids stimulate IGFBP-1 synthesis (Conover, 1996). The IGFs can also regulate their own bioactivity. For example, IGF-1 increases IGFBP-3 and IGFBP-5 tissue expression in bone, while it simultaneously decreases IGFBP-4 production (Mohan, 1993). Within the skeleton, IGFBP-specific proteases are produced as well as other proteases such as matrix metalloprotease, cathepsin D, and plasmin (Fowlkes *et al.*, 1994; Kudo *et al.*, 1996). These enzymes are capable of breaking down different proteins as well as the IGFBPs. Complete characterization of IGFBP-specific proteases in bone have not been successful to date.

In addition to the transport and modulation of IGFs by the IGFBPs, it is now apparent that some IGFBPs can have IGF independent activity. For example, IGFBP-3 can be activated by the tumor suppressor protein, p53, which in turn can inhibit mitogenesis (Buckbinder *et al.*, 1996). IGFBP-3 can also suppress breast cancer growth irrespective of IGF-I (Buckbinder *et al.*, 1996). Similarly, IGFrBP-1, a member of the new low-affinity IGFBP family (which may number 4), has also been shown to have IGF-independent effects on breast cancer cells (Oh, 1997; Nun *et al.*, 1997). These properties suggest that this unique superfamily of IGFBPs exhibit other properties which could be tailored for certain therapeutic paradigms. For example, in the skeleton, agents that affect the IGFBPs are already being tested and enhance the bone-forming properties of IGF-I.

C. Regulation of Serum and Skeletal IGFs

1. Growth Hormone

There is a dynamic equilibrium between circulating levels of IGF-I and tissue production of this peptide. However, caution must be exercised when interpreting changes in serum IGF-I as a reflection of alterations in local tissue production. Indeed, there can be tremendous divergence in specific regulatory factors which affect hepatic synthesis versus those which control tissue production. But certain hormones are common determinants of IGF-I expression in most tissues. Since its discovery as a sulfation factor more than 40 years ago, IGF-I has been considered a mediator of growth hormone activity in bone (Daughaday *et al.*, 1972). In the skeleton, growth hormone stimulates osteoblast and chondrocyte production of IGF-I (Canalis *et al.*, 1988). Osteoblasts also make IGFBP-3 in response to growth hormone (GH), and there is some *in vitro* evidence that IGFBP-4 production is enhanced by GH (Mohan, 1993; Mohan and Baylink, 1997). Serum levels of IGF-I reflect growth hormone secretion to a certain degree and therefore have been used clinically as a surrogate indicator of GH status. Indeed, low-serum IGF-I is found in growth hormone deficiency states of children and adults, whereas high levels of IGF-I are found in acromegaly (Blum *et al.*, 1993). In these disease states, serum levels are bound to reflect skeletal content and activity, although there are no studies in humans with growth hormone deficiency or excess to prove that thesis. In rats and mice, alterations in serum IGF-I are also reflected in cortical bone content of IGF-I.

2. Nutrition

Although GH represents the principle hormonal regulator of circulating IGF-I, other determinants can affect IGF-I concentrations both in serum and at the tissue level. The nutrient status of an individual can profoundly affect serum IGF-I concentrations (Rosen and Conover, 1997). For example, protein-calorie malnutrition severely limits IGF-I synthesis in the liver and leads to a 50% reduction in circulating concentrations even among healthy volunteers (Estivarez and Ziegler, 1997). Starvation is also associated with reduced bone formation and increased bone resorption. These changes are due to declining skeletal IGF-I concentrations as well as alterations in post-receptor GH action, a decreased number of GH receptors, and alterations in several IGFBPs (Grinspoon et al., 1995). Yet these effects occur despite a marked increase in GH production. Thus during protein calorie malnutrition, there is peripheral resistance to GH leading to dissociation between GH and IGF-I.

As noted earlier, not only do serum levels of IGF-I decline dramatically, but the bioactivity of IGF-I is also markedly reduced by malnutrition. In part, this may be related to a marked increase in IGFBP-1. Nutrient intake and insulin status both determine serum IGFBP-1 concentrations and the extent of phosphorylation of IGFBP-1 which in turn determines IGF binding affinity (Rajaram et al., 1997). With starvation, IGFBP-1 increases and binds IGF-1 more avidly. This occurs because of a decline in substrate availability and suppressed insulin levels. Because IGFBP-1 is also synthesized by osteoblasts, it is conceivable that this IGFBP might contribute to the marked impairment in bone formation noted with starvation. Similarly, during chronic insulin deficiency, serum IGFBP-1 levels are high, and this could lead to growth retardation in poorly controlled Type I insulin-dependent diabetes (Chan and Spencer, 1997). Moreover, osteopenia and reduced bone formation have been noted in IDDM, and this might be a function of high skeletal production of IGFBP-1.

Another inhibitory IGFBP which is increased in some chronic diseases and could impact bone formation is IGFBP-4. This binding protein is principally regulated by PTH (Mohan et al., 1995). However, in one study, the highest levels of IGFBP-4 were found in elders who sustained a hip fracture and had undergone significant weight loss prior to their injury (Cook et al., 1996). This would imply that there may be other regulatory factors associated with poor nutrition (e.g., cytokines) which could trigger local production of inhibitory IGFBPs. A marked change in the bioactivity of IGF-I due to IGFBP perturbations may be responsible for growth retardation in malnourished children. In addition to IGFBP changes, there is also evidence that zinc deficiency, a common accompaniment of protein-calorie malnutrition, can inhibit IGF-I synthesis in liver and bone (Estivarez and Ziegler, 1997). Zinc repletion in experimental animals leads to increased hepatic IGF-I expression, although longitudinal studies in adults have not shown a direct rise in serum IGF-I due to zinc supplementation alone (Estivarez and Ziegler, 1997).

3. Age

Other factors regulate circulating concentrations of IGF-I, and these can have an impact on the skeleton. Advanced age is associated with a progressive decrease in serum IGF-I as GH secretion declines approximately 14% per decade of life (Rosen and Conover, 1997; Borst *et al.*, 1994; Veldhuis *et al.*, 1997; Toogood *et al.*, 1996). Thus over a lifetime, GH production is reduced nearly 30-fold. This decrement is due to increased somatostatinergic tone and a generalized reduction in the pulses of GH-releasing hormones and GH-releasing peptides (Hoffman *et al.*, 1997). Declining sex steroid production may also have a negative impact on the GH/IGF-I axis (Ho *et al.*, 1987). Alterations in body composition, and specifically increases in visceral body fat, can feedback negatively on the hypothalamic GH-GHRH axis, possibly via leptin (Ahren *et al.*, 1997). The sum of altered GH secretion in the elderly includes low levels of serum IGF-I and IGFBP-3.

Aging also affects circulating IGFBPs in both men and women. Serum IGFBP-4, an inhibitory binding protein, increases dramatically with advancing age in both men and women (Mohan and Baylink, 1997; Rosen *et al.*, 1992; Mohan *et al.*, 1995). On the other hand, IGFBP-3 and IGFBP-5 are much lower in older individuals than younger ones (Gelato and Frost, 1997). There is evidence that serum IGFBP-1 concentrations are higher in the elderly than in younger people (Clemmons *et al.*, 1986). These changes in stimulatory and inhibitory IGFBPs are consistent with *in vitro* evidence that senescent cells have impaired cellular responsiveness to the IGFs (Davis *et al.*, 1997). In particular, a recent study demonstrated that osteoblasts from older patients are resistant to IGF-I stimulation (Davis *et al.*, 1997). Although these age-associated changes in IGFs could lead to osteoporosis, there is still much debate about the role IGFs and IGFBPs play with respect to determining overall bone density and fracture risk.

4. Sex Steroids

One consistent finding in serum IGF-I, whether it is measured during puberty or advanced age, is a gender difference. Males exhibit a 10–15% higher serum IGF-I concentration than females across all ages after puberty (Grogean *et al.*, 1997). The cause for this difference is not clear, but several attempts have been made to link high or low serum levels of IGF-I to the pathogenesis of several chronic diseases including osteoporosis, breast cancer, prostate cancer, and Alzheimer's disease. One cause for an age-associated decline in serum IGF-I is reduced sex steroid production (Veldhuis *et al.*, 1995). However, the picture is complex in part because both estrogen and testosterone can affect pituitary GH release as well as tissue IGF-I expression. There is strong evidence that total and free testosterone concentrations in serum correlate with GH secretory bursts in pubertal boys (Martha *et al.*, 1992). Also, administration of testosterone to younger men with hypogonadism and to boys with isolated GnRH deficiency increases serum levels of IGF-I (Hobbs *et al.*, 1993). But the precise mechanism and site of action in the hypothalamus or pituitary are not defined, in part because androgens are converted to estrogen via aromatization, and this may positively affect GH secretion. This mechanism may be extremely important with respect to the aging skeleton since new cross-sectional and longitudinal data demonstrate that total estradiol levels may be a better predictor of bone mineral density in the elderly male than serum testosterone (Andersen et al., 1998). Furthermore, osteoblasts possess the capacity to aromatize androgens to estrogens, thereby providing a local site for regulation (Burich et al., 1992). And, in several case reports of males with osteoporosis and deficient aromatase activity, exogenous estrogens, not androgens, partially restored bone mass (Smith et al., 1994; Carani et al., 1997).

Several lines of evidence suggest that there may be a strong causal relationship between endogenous estrogens and serum IGF-I in women as well. First, cross-sectional studies have demonstrated that serum estradiol levels correlate with IGF-I in both men and women (Greendale et al., 1997). Second, both cross-sectional and now longitudinal data have demonstrated that serum IGF-I declines during the early menopausal years (Poehlman et al., 1997; Ravn et al., 1995). Third, several preliminary studies suggest that low-serum IGF-I levels in women are related more closely to years since menopause than to chronological age (LeBoff et al., 1995). Finally, in contrast to oral conjugated estrogens and tamoxifen, percutaneous estrogen administration to postmenopausal women results in an increase in serum IGF-I (Shewmon et al., 1995).

Adrenal androgens may also affect circulating IGF-I. For example, DHEA-S levels decline with age, and absolute levels in postmenopausal women corelate with serum IGF-I (DePugola et al., 1993). Similarly, in premenopausal women with adrenal androgen excess and insulin resistance, serum IGF-I are relatively high (DePugola et al., 1993). Also, in a randomized placebo-controlled trial of DHEA, serum IGF-I levels rose in both elderly men and women (Morales et al., 1994). Finally, there is some preliminary evidence that in a subset of adolescent women with eating disorders, DHEA-S increases serum IGF-I (Leboff, personal communication; Labrie et al., 1997). Hence, some evidence supports the thesis that weak adrenal androgens may have a positive impact on serum and possibly skeletal IGF-I. There are no data on adrenal androgen action on the IGFBPs. Further randomized trials will have to determine if these compounds prevent bone resorption, stimulate bone formation, or both.

Gonadal steroids regulate several IGFBPs as well as IGF-I. Estrogen stimulates production of IGFBP-4 while it inhibits osteoblastic IGFBP-3 synthesis (Mohan and Baylink, 1997; Rosen et al., 1997a). On the other hand, testosterone stimulates IGFBP-3 synthesis and activates a critical IGFBP-3 protease, prostate-specific antigen (Koperak et al., 1990). Progesterone, PTH, dexamethasone, and 1,25 dihydroxyvitamin D also stimulate IGFBP-4 production in bone cells, although it is unclear precisely how these hormones have an impact on skeletal activity of IGF-I (Tremollières *et al.,* 1992). However, it is certain that there are multiple layers of IGF regulation which could be affected by alterations in gonadal steroids.

5. Genetic Control of Serum IGF-I

There is tremendous heterogeneity in serum IGF-I concentrations among healthy adults. Normal levels can range from 100 to 300 ng/ml, and although GH remains the major regulatory factor controlling serum levels, it is clear that there must be other determinants (Donahue *et al.,* 1990). Indeed, it is likely that the IGF-I phenotype is a continuous variable representing a complex polygenic trait. Hence, there should be some element of heritability for IGF-I expression which may or may not be controlled at the pituitary level. Recently, Comuzzie *et al.* (1996) demonstrated, among Mexican-Americans, strong heritability for serum IGF-I. In a preliminary cross-sectional mother-daughter pair study, serum IGF-I was found to correlate very closely despite a 30 year age difference (Kurland *et al.,* 1998). Moreover, in recombinant inbred strains of mice, serum IGF-I and bone density correlate very closely, and IGF-I co-segregates with BMD across two generations, suggesting strong heritability for IGF-I (Rosen *et al.,* 1997b). And, in a very recent study, it has been reported that a polymorphism in a noncoding region upstream of the transcription start site of the IGF-I gene is associated with significantly lower levels of serum IGF-I in both men and women (Rosen *et al.,* 1998). These new lines of evidence suggest that there may be important genetic regulation of serum and possibly skeletal IGF-I expression.

6. Other Regulatory Factors for IGF-I

The major control over IGF-I synthesis in the liver is growth hormone. Nutritional determinants, possibly including zinc, regulate IGF-I message expression in the liver. Heritable factors may also be important. Deficient gonadal steroids can affect serum IGF-I at the level of hepatic transcription or at the pituitary/hypothalamic level. Estrogen also enhances IGF-I production in the uterus. But, in addition to those factors, adequate insulin is a prerequisite for IGF-I expression in the liver (Rosen *et al.,* 1994; Milne *et al.,* 1998). Thyroxine has recently been shown to upregulate IGF-I expression in rat femorae, and this may explain how hyperthyroidism stimulates bone turnover (Milne *et al.,* 1998). PTH is a major stimulator of skeletal IGF-I expression in rat, mouse, and human bone cells (Linkhart and Mohan, 1989). This effect is most pronounced when it is administered intermittently. Anti-IGF-I antibodies block collagen biosynthesis and other anabolic properties induced by PTH (Canalis *et al.,* 1989). Studies of the IGF-I gene in rat osteoblast have demonstrated that there is a cyclic AMP promoter region in exon 1 which undoubtedly is the site of PTH regulation of IGF-I expression (McCarthy *et al.,* 1989b). Interestingly enough, there is also an estrogen response element in that region which down-regulates IGF-I expression, possibly explaining estrogen's direct suppressive effect on IGF-I expression *in vitro* (McCarthy *et al.*, 1997). Whether there is a gender difference in skeletal PTH responsiveness remains to be determined, although several preliminary studies suggest that male inbred strains of mice, as well as male growth-hormone-deficient mice, have a more vigorous bone density response to PTH than females (I. R. Donahue, personal communication). In humans, there are no side-by-side gender studies with PTH to determine if this effect also occurs. However, it should be noted that the most vigorous skeletal response to PTH has been reported in men (Slowik *et al.*, 1986).

In conclusion, IGF-I is a major coupling factor in bone remodeling. Its regulation is tissue-specific and multifaceted. Changes in serum IGF-I may sometimes reflect tissue activity, but often there is disparity between the two. Many of the studies which have demonstrated a relationship between IGF-I and bone mineral density or fracture risk have used serum IGF-I as a surogate. As noted earlier, this must be viewed with some caution.

III. IGFs and Their Role in Acquisition and Maintenance of Adult Bone Mass

A. Acquisition of Peak Bone Mass—Role of the IGFs

Peak bone mass is acquired by the end of the second decade and remains one of the most important factors in determining adult bone density (BMD) at any point in an individual's life. Longitudinal studies with DXA suggest that the most rapid acquisition phase for bone is between the ages of 12 and 16 years, a time when linear bone growth is just beginning to de-accelerate (Marcus, 1997). Coincident with several hormonal surges (e.g., estrogens and androgens) at that time, GH pulses are more frequent and of greater magnitude (Inzuchki and Robbins, 1994; Slootwigh, 1998). Serum IGF-I levels are also at their highest point in life at this time (Isakson *et al.*, 1987). Hence, ascertaining the role of IGF-I in acquisition of peak bone mass had become a major thrust for investigators.

Several lines of evidence support the importance of IGF-I in the process of peak bone mass acquisition. First, growth-hormone-deficient (but otherwise healthy) mice (*lit/lit*) have reduced volumetric bone mineral density throughout life as a result of markedly reduced serum IGF-I concentrations (Donahue and Beamer, 1993). Similarly, male and female adolescents with acquired GH deficiency have lower peak bone mass than age-matched normals (Bing-you *et al.*, 1993). Second, normal inbred strains of mice have differences in bone density which correspond to similar differences in serum and skeletal IGF-I (Beamer *et al.*, 1996). Inbred strains acquire peak bone mass by 16 weeks of age, a time when large interstrain differences in serum IGF-I are first noted (Beamer *et al.*, 1996). Also, osteoblasts from high-density mice express more IGF-I than do cells from low-density mice. Third, the acquisition of bone mineral density in adolescence corresponds to a similar rise in serum IGF-I (Tanner *et al.*, 1976). Fourth, in a longitudinal trial with young girls (ages 11 to 12), milk supplementation increased bone density more than placebo, and the rise in BMD corresponded to a greater increase in serum IGF-I than in the nontreated group (Cadogan *et al.*, 1997). Finally, surges in sex steroids (both androgens and estrogens) promote peak bone mass acquisition and also enhance GH release from the pituitary, thereby increasing serum IGF-I (Bouillon, 1991). Although these studies indirectly suggest that IGF-I and peak BMD are closely related, it does not establish cause and effect. Furthermore, the mechanism whereby peak bone mass is enhanced by IGF-I has not been fully elucidated. For example, the highest bone mass in mice is noted in strains with reduced bone resorption (D. J. Baylink, personal communication). Similarly, African-American males and females have higher bone density than Caucasians, but this may be a function of slower bone turnover rather than an increase in bone formation.

Peak bone mass in adolescence is associated with a marked increase in the size of the skeleton, as well as incremental changes in mineralization. There is a strong gender effect on size, and this could affect measurement of peak bone mass and future fracture risk. Using volumetric bone density measurements rather than two-dimensional area determinations, investigators have noted that much of the male-female difference in apparent BMD disappears, except in the vertebrae where males continue to have greater true volumetric density (Carter *et al.*, 1992). Since IGF-I promotes periosteal growth, and boys have higher serum IGF-I levels than girls, it is conceivable that IGF-I could affect size, which in turn could affect fracture risk. However, in studies of adult patients with Laron dwarfism (i.e., growth hormone resistance syndrome), area BMD measurements were much lower than age and sex-matched controls, but volumetric determinations failed to reveal differences between the two groups (Rosenfeld, personal communication). These findings would suggest that IGF-I is not the only factor responsible for peak bone mass acquisition. Clearly, further studies will be needed to define how IGF-I affects peak bone mass.

B. IGF-I and Maintenance of Bone Density

1. Cross-Sectional and Cohort Studies

There are several cross-sectional studies which have demonstrated a correlation between serum IGF-I and bone density across a wide age range in men and women (Romagnoli *et al.*, 1994; Boonen *et al.*, 1996; Fall *et al.*, 1998). In one study, serum and skeletal IGF-I levels showed a dramatic age-related decline which could be superimposed on an age-related drop in bone density (Boonen *et al.*, 1996). In addition to the IGF changes, there are data to suggest that IGFBP-3 may affect bone mass in healthy and osteoporotic males (Wuster *et al.*, 1993; Sugimoto *et al.*, 1997; Johansson *et al.*, 1993). However, despite their strengths, all these studies suffer from the absence of longitudinal data relating bone density, bone loss or fracture risk to IGF-I. As noted previously, numerous factors affect serum IGF-I, and some of these are the same determinants of age-related bone loss. For example, declining estrogen production in men and women has been linked directly to low bone mass in males and females, as well as to a decline in serum IGF-I. The nutrient status of individuals can have a profound effect on serum IGF-I, and malnourished elders are more likely to fall, to have low serum vitamin D levels, and to have suffered recent weight loss, other independent predictors of fracture risk. Prospective data on fracture risk and the IGFs are even less convincing, although a pattern has recently emerged.

Three large cohorts have been analyzed for the relationship of IGF-I to bone density. In the Study of Osteoporotic Fractures (SOF), a cohort of more than 9000 women, the lowest quartile of IGF-I has been associated with a significant and independent risk for hip fracture [$RR = 1.7\ (1.1–2.2)$] (D. Bauer, personal communication). This finding might be considered intuitive based on the realization that serum IGF-I integrates several coincidental processes which produce a catabolic state (e.g., acute illness, starvation, immobility, age), as well as predicting risk for fracture and frailty. Since SOF is a prospective observational study, it adds more strength to the thesis that IGF-I may be related to osteoporosis. In another longitudinal observational study, the Framingham Heart Study, it was recently noted that the lowest quartile of IGF-I was associated with the lowest BMD at multiple skeletal sites, even when adjusted for covariables such as body weight and protein intake (D. P. Kiel, personal communication). However the relationship of IGF-I to bone mass held only for women, not for men. In the Rancho Bernardo cohort, serum levels of IGF-I were also higher in men than women, and bone density was also greater at all sites in males than females (Greendale *et al.*, 1997). However, as noted previously, these studies cannot prove cause and effect.

A unique subset of osteoporotic patients who have recently undergone careful reexamination is men with the syndrome of idiopathic osteoporosis. These individuals are middle aged but have very low bone mineral density and suffer from debilitating spinal fractures. A small percentage of these men have hypercalcuria, but the majority have no identifiable cause for their disease. In 1992, Johansson *et al.* reported that these men had low-serum IGF-I concentrations (Ljunghall *et al.*, 1992). Subsequently, Reed *et al.* (1995) also noted low-serum IGF-I and hypercalcuria in males with this syndrome. On bone biopsy, these men were found to have low bone turnover. More recently, Kurland *et al.* (1997) reported on 25 males with idiopathic osteoporosis who had low-serum IGF-I levels and reduced bone formation on bone biopsy. Subsequent studies in this cohort revealed that growth hormone dynamics were normal (Kurland *et al.*, 1996). Ebeling *et al.* in a preliminary study of men with a similar phenotype noted that first-degree male relatives of those subjects had low spine bone mineral density and increased body fat (Ristevski *et al.*, 1997). These findings suggest that IGF-I may play a pathogenic role in maintenance of adult bone density or acquisition of peak bone mass. That thesis was recently reinforced by a study of men with idiopathic osteoporosis in which a homozygous polymorphism in a noncoding region of the IGF-I gene was twice as common in affected men as those in the general population (Rosen *et al.*, 1998). This genotype, labeled 192/192, is also associated with 15–20% lower serum IGF-I levels than any other combination of alleles. Thus, there are several lines of evidence, some direct, some indirect, that serum IGF-I may be related to bone mineral density. Whether serum IGF-I can be used as a diagnostic tool in males presenting with osteoporosis remains to be determined.

2. Intervention Trials with rhGH and rhIGF-I in Osteoporosis

Low bone mineral density as a result of chronic growth hormone deficiency (GHD) in adulthood can lead to osteoporotic fractures (Rosen *et al.*, 1993). Recently, the U.S. FDA approved the use of recombinant human GH (rhGH) for GHD in adults. In part, this indication was based on compelling data from the United States and Europe that rhGH treatment for GHD increases BMD at several skeletal sites after 2 years of treatment (Rosen *et al.*, 1993; Beshyah *et al.*, 1995). These effects are more pronounced in males than females, although this may be related to hormonal replacement with estrogens, which could dampen both the IGF-I response to GH and skeletal activation of remodeling.

There are no trials which have shown that rhGH can increase bone mass in the elderly to the extent noted in GHD, even though both skeletal and serum IGF-I levels are low initially and are increased by exogenous administration (Marcus, 1997). The reasons for the disparate response between young and old skeletons to rhGH or rhIGF-I are not entirely clear, although recent studies suggest that low levels of IGF-I may not be the only pathogenic mechanism in age-related osteoporosis.

Originally, Rudman *et al.* (1990) reported a 1.6% increase in lumbar BMD after 6 months of rhGH treatment in elderly males with low-serum IGF-I. These men were not randomized to treatment or placebo but were selected for very low levels of IGF-I. Subsequent follow-up of that cohort failed to show a significant effect of rhGH on the spine, hip, or total body BMD (Rudman *et al.*, 1991). Other short-term studies have also been unable to show a strong positive effect from rhGH treatment on bone mineral density, even though markers of bone turnover rise (Papadakis *et al.*, 1996; Thompson *et al.*, 1995; Ghiron *et al.*, 1995; Holloway *et al.*, 1997). Similarly, Holloway *et al.* (1997) could not establish a benefit from rhGH treatment alone that was greater than treatment with the antiresorptive medication, calcitonin. Furthermore, McLean *et al.* (1995) recently reported that total body BMD decreased after 1 year of low-dose rhGH in elderly men and women who were classified as frail by indices of physical performance. Moreover, there was no correlation between serum IGF-I and measures of physical performance in that same cohort either at baseline or after treatment (Kiel, personal communication). It is even more notable that the results of these studies were negative despite consistent and significant increases of serum IGF-I into the young normal range. Taken together, these data would suggest that IGF-I deficiency was not the pathogenic factor in age-related osteoporosis, or that other factors, including the IGFBPS, limit the bioactivity of IGF-I in the skeleton of older individuals. However, it should be noted that long-term studies with rhGH or rhIGF-I in elderly indidivuals have not gone beyond 24 months. Based on previous GH trials, it might take several years to see a beneficial effect from growth factor treatment, especially with respect to the aging skeleton (Rosen et al., 1993; Beshyah et al., 1995). In addition, it will be critical to assess the effects of gender on skeletal responsiveness in elderly individuals.

The absence of an anabolic skeletal effect in the elderly has not deterred investigations with rhIGF-I and IGF-I/IGFBP-3 as antiosteoporotic treatments. Ebeling et al. (1993) investigated several doses of rhIGF-I in younger postmenopausal women and found that bone turnover was stimulated and the lowest dose of rhIGF-I could increase bone formation more than resorption. Few side effects were noted with rhIGF-I at doses of 30 and 60 µg/kg/day (Andersen et al., 1998). More recently, Ghiron et al. (1995) administered low-dose IGF-I (15 µg/kg/day b.i.d.) to elderly women and found a selective increase in bone formation without changes in bone resorption. These data suggest that rhIGF-I in low doses may have an effect on bone turnover, and potentially (although not measured in the Ghiron study) BMD. The findings by Ghiron et al. are also consistent with short-term studies by Grinspoon and colleagues (1995) in young fasting women. In those studies, much higher doses of rhIGF-I were well tolerated and produced an increase in bone formation which exceeded bone resorption. These effects were pronounced considering those women exhibited a decline in serum IGF-I and a rise in IGFBP-1, another inhibitory IGF binding protein (Grinspoon et al., 1995).

Serum levels of IGFBP-3 are reduced in some osteoporotic patients, and because of the concern about hypoglycemia during rhIGF-I treatment, an alternative approach for using rhIGF-I in age-related osteoporosis has emerged. IGF-I complexed to IGFBP-3 and administered daily as a soluble complex subcutaneously has been shown to increase serum IGF-I concentrations markedly in the young and elderly without serious adverse effects. Based on earlier animal studies, IGF-I/IGFBP-3 complex can strongly enhance bone formation and bone mass (Bagi et al., 1994). Dose ranging studies using IGF-I/IGFBP-3 complex (0.3–6.0 mg/kg) in young volunteers and healthy elderly adults has shown that this agent is safe and well tolerated (D. Rosen, personal communication). No episodes of hypoglycemia were noted even at high doses of complex. Similarly, in a phase I trial, 7 consecutive days of rhIGF-I/IGFBP-3 at doses of 0.5–2.0 mg/kg/day by continuous subcutaneous infusion via minipump, produced no serious side effects to healthy elders. Furthermore, procollagen peptide (a marker of bone formation) increased 50% over the 7-day period and remained elevated for an addition 7 days after discontinuation of treatment (D. Rosen, personal communication). Despite a concomitant rise in deoxypyridinoline with complex administration, this rise did not persist post-treatment. Thus, this form of IGF-I administration could have utility in patients with osteoporosis.

In conclusion, the evidence is overwhelming that rhGH treatment, which restores IGF-I levels to young normal ranges in growth-hormone deficient adults, leads to a substantial increase in bone mineral density in those patients. This effect seems even more pronounced in males than females, although the reason for this is at present not clear. On the other hand, elders treated with rhGH or rhIGF-I do not demonstrate an increase in bone mass after one year of therapy. This suggests that, although IGF-I may be important in the acquisition of peak bone mass, age-related osteoporosis is not solely a function of reduced GH secretion or deficient serum or skeletal IGF-I.

IV. Summary

There is now very strong evidence that insulin-like growth factors are essential for maintaining homeostatic balance in the skeleton over the lifetime in both men and women. IGFs are one of several coupling factors which link bone resorption to bone formation, thereby maintaining adult bone mass. IGF-I also mediates linear growth and acts in an endocrine manner to modulate growth hormone activity in adolescence. More importantly, data are emerging which suggest that IGF-I expression is heritable, that it cosegregates with bone density, and that disorders in the serum or skeletal IGF-I regulatory system can affect peak bone mass and ultimately fracture risk. Despite these positive findings and several cross-sectional studies which suggest that there is a relatively strong correlation between IGF-I and bone mineral density in both men and women, there is still a paucity of longitudinal data to confirm a causal relationship. However, recent cohort studies support the hypothesis that there is a link between circulating IGF-I and fracture risk. Pedigree and association studies will determine if specific candidate genes such as IGF-I play a major role in determining peak bone mass. Similarly, the rate of decline in serum IGF-I may be a limiting factor in accelerating bone formation rates in response to greater bone resorption in the elderly. Research directions for the future will have to include more gender-based studies to assess differential skeletal responsiveness to anabolic factors such as IGF-I and growth hormone.

On balance, there can be little debate that the IGFs are essential growth factors for the proper function of the skeleton. However, more longitudinal studies will be needed to confirm a causal relationship between changes in circulating IGF-I and bone mineral density in men. Moreover, the lack of a positive effect on bone mineral density when treating elders with recombinant rhGH or rhIGF-I suggests that there must be other factors, possibly the IGFBPs, which will have to be manipulated before a strong skeletal anabolic effect will occur.

References

Ahren, B., Larsson, H., Wilhemsson, C., Nasman, B., and Olsson, T. (1997). Regulation of circulating leptin in humans. *Endocrine* 7–8.

Andersen, G. H., Francis, R. M., Silly, P. L., and Cooper, C. C. (1998). Sex hormones and osteopenia in men. *Calcif. Tissue Int.* **62**, 185–188.

Andress, D. L., and Brinbaum, R. S. (1992). Human osteoblast-derived IGF binding protein-5 stimulates osteoblast mitogenesis and potentiates IGF action. *J. Biol. Chem.* **267,**22467–22472.

Bagi, C. M., Brommage, R., DeLeon, L., Adams, S., Rosen, D., and Sommer, A. (1994). Benefit of systemically administered rhIGF-I/IGFBP-3 on cancellous bone in ovariectomized rats. *J. Bone Miner. Res.* **9**, 1301–1305.

Baserga, R., Resnicoff, M., and Dews, M. (1997). The IGF-I receptor and cancer. *Endocrine* 7, 99–103.

Beamer, W. G., Donahue, L. R., Rosen, C. J., and Baylink, D. J. (1996). Genetic variability in adult bone density among inbred strains of mice. *Bone* 21217–21223.

Beshyah, S. A., Kyd, P., Thomas, E., Fairny, A., and Johnston, D. G. (1995). The effects of prolonged GH replacement on bone turnover and bone mineral density in hypopituitary adults. *Clin. Endocrinol.* **42**, 249–254.

Bing-you, R. G., Denis, M. G., and Rosen, C. J. (1993). Low bone mineral density in adults with previous hypothalamic pituitary tumors. *Calcif. Tissue Int.* **52**, 183–187.

Blum, W. F., Albertson, K., Roseberg, S., and Rnake, M. B. (1993). Serum levels of IGF-I and IGFBP-3 reflect spontaneous GH secretion. *J. Clin. Endocrinol. Metab.* **76**, 1610–1630.

Boonen, S., Lesaffre, E., Dequeker, J., Aerssens, J., Nijs, J., Pelemans, W., and Bouillon, R. (1996). Relationship between baseline IGF-I and femoral neck bone density in women aged over 70 years. *J. Am. Geriatr. Soc.* **44**, 1301–1306.

Borst, S. E., Millard, R. D., and Lowenthal, D. T. (1994). GH exercise and aging. *J. Am. Geriatr. Soc.* **42**, 528–535.

Bouillon, R. (1991). Growth hormone and bone. *Horm. Res.* **36**, 49–55.

Buckbinder, C., Talbetti, R., Velasceo-Wegree, S. (1996). Induction of the growth inhibitor BP-3 by p53. *Nature (London)* 377, 646–650.

Burich, H. B., Wolf, L., Budde, R. *et al.* (1992). Androstenedione metabolism in cultured human osteoblast like cells. *J. Clin. Endocrinol. Metab.* 75, 101–105.

Cadogan, J., Eastell, R., Janes, N., and Bailer, M. (1997). Milk intake and bone mineral acquisition in adolescent girls. *Br. Med. J.* 315, 1255–1261.

Campbell, P. G., Novak, T. F., Yanoscik, T. B., and McMaster, J. H. (1992). Involvement of the plasmin system in dissociation of IGFBP complex. *Endocrinology (Baltimore)* 130, 1401–1402.

Canalis, E., McCarthy, T. L., and Centrella, M. (1988). Growth factors and bone remodeling. *J. Clin. Invest.* 81, 277–281.

Canalis, E., Centrella, M., Bach, W., and McCarthy, T. L. (1989). IGF-I mediates selective anabolic effects of PTH in bone cell cultures. *J. Clin. Invest.* **63**, 60–65.

Canalis, E., Centrella, M., and McCarthy, T. L. (1991). Regulation of IGF-II production in bone cultures. *Endocrinology (Baltimore)* **129**, 2457–2461.

Carani, C., Qin, K., Simoni, M., Faustini-Fustini, M., Serpente, S., Boyd, J., Korach, K. S., and Simpson, B. R. (1997). Effect of testosterone and estradiol in a male with aromatasedeficiency. *N. Engl. J. Med.* **337**, 91–95.

Carter, D. R., Bouxsein, M. L., and Marcus, R. (1992). New approaches for interpreting projectional bone densitometry data. *J. Bone Miner. Res.* **7**, 137–145.

Chan, K., and Spencer, E. M. (1997). General aspects of the IGFBPs. *Endocrine* **1**, 95–97.

Clemmons, D. R., Elgin, R. G., Han, V. K. M., Casella, S. J., D'Ercole, A. J., and Van Wyk, J. J. (1986). Cultured fibroblast monolayers secrete a protein that alters the cellular binding of somatomedin C/IGF-I. *J. Clin. Invest.* **77**, 1548–1556.

Comuzzie, G., Blangero, J., Mahaney, M. C., Henner, A. M. *et al.* (1996). Genetic and environmental correlates among hormone levels and means of body fat accumulation and topography. *J. Clin. Endocrinol. Metab.* **81**, 597–600.

Conover, C. A. (1996). The role of IGFs and IGFBPs in bone cell biology. *In* "Principles of Bone Biology" (J. P. Bilezikian, L. R. Raisz, and G. Rodan, eds.), pp. 607–618. Academic Press, San Diego, CA.

Cook, F., Rosen, C. J., Vereault, D., Steffens, C., Kessenich, C. R., Greenspan, S., Ziegler, T. R., Watts, N. B., Mohan, S., and Baylink, D. J. (1996). Major changes in the circulatory IGF regulatory system after hip fracture surgery. *J. Bone Miner. Res.* **11**, S327.

Daughaday, W. H., Hall, K., Rahn, S., Salmon, W. D., and Van Wyck, J. J. (1972). Somatomedin; a proposed designation for sulfation factor. *Nature (London)* **235**, 107–110.

Davis, P. Y., Frazier, C. R., Shapiro, J. R., and Fedarko, N. S. (1997). Age-related changes in effects of IGF-I on human osteoblast like cells. *Biochem. J.* **324**, 753–760.

DePugola, G., Lespite, L., Grizzulli, V. A. *et al.* (1993). IGF-I and DHEA-S in obese females. *Int. J. Obesity Relat. Metab. Dis.* **11**, 481–483.

Donahue, L. R., and Beamer, W. G. (1993). GH deficiency in little mice. *J. Endocrinol.* **136**, 104–110.

Donahue, L. R., Hunter, S. J., Sherblom, A. P., and Rosen, C. J. (1990). Age-related changes in serum IGFBPs in women. *J. Clin. Endocrinol Metab.* **71**, 575–579.

Ebeling, P., Jones, J., O'Fallon, W., Janess, C., and Riggs, B. L. (1993). Short term effects of recombinant IGF-I on bone turnover in normal women. *J. Clin. Endocrinol. Metab.* **77**, 1384–1387.

Estivarez, C. E., and Ziegler, T. R. (1997). Nutrition and the IGF system. *Endocrine* **7**, 65–71.

Fall, C., Hindmarsh, P., Dennison, E., Kellingray, S., Barker, D., and Cooper, C. (1998). Programming of growth hormone secretion and bone mineral density in elderly men: A hypothesis. *J. Clin. Endocrinol. Metab.* **83**, 135–139.

Fowlkes, J., Enghild, J., Suzuki, K., and Nagase, H. (1994). Matrix metalloproeinases degrade IGFBP-3 in dermal fibroblast cultures. *J. Biol. Chem.* **269**, 25742–25746.

Gelato, M. C., and Frost, R. A. (1997). IGFBP-3 Functional and structural implications in aging and wasting syndrome. *Endocrine* **7**, 81–85.

Ghiron, L., Thompson, J., Halloway, L., Hintz, R. L., Butterfield, G., Hoffman, A., and Marcus, R. (1995). Effects of rhIGF-I and GH on bone turnover in elderly women. *J. Bone Miner. Res.* **10**, 1844–1877.

Greendale, G. A., Delstein, S., and Barrett Connor, E. (1997). Endogenous sex steroids and bone mineral density in older men and women. *J. Bone Miner. Res.* **12**, 1833–1843.

Grinspoon, S. K., Baum, H. B. A., Peterson, S., and Klibanski, A. (1995). Effects of rhIGF-I administration on bone turnover during short-term fasting. *J. Clin. Invest.* **96**, 900–905.

Grogean, T., Vereault, D., Millard, P. S., and Rosen, C. J. (1997). A comparative analysis of methods to measure IGF-I in human serum. *Endocrinol. Metab.* **4**, 109–114.

Hayden, J., Mohan, S., and Baylink, D. J. (1995). The IGF system and the coupling of formation to resorption. *Bone* **17**, 93S–98S.

Ho, K. Y., Evans, W. S., Blizzard, R., Velhuis, J. D., Merriam, G. R., Samojlik, E., Furlanetto, R., Rogol, A. D., Kaiser, D. L., and Thorner, M. O. (1987). Effects of sex and age on twenty four hour profiles of GH secretion in men. *J. Clin. Endocrinol. Metab.* **64**, 51–58.

Hobbs, C. J., Plymate, S. R., Rosen, C. J., and Adler, R. A. (1993). Testosterone administration increases IGF-I in normal men. *J. Clin. Endocrinol. Metab.* **77**, 776–780.

Hoffman, A. R., Lieberman, S. A., Butterfield, G., Thompson, J., Hintz, R. R. L., Ceda, G. P., and Marcus, R. (1997). Functional consequences of th Somatopause and its treatment. *Endocrine* **7**, 73–76.

Holloway, L., Kohlmeier, L., Kent, K., and Marcus, R. (1997). Skeletal effects of cyclic recombinant human GH and salmon calcitonin in osteopenic postmenopausal women. *J. Clin. Endocrinol.* **82**, 1111–1117.

Inzuchki, S. E., and Robbins, R. J. (1994). Effect of GH on human bone biology. *J. Clin. Endocrinol. Metab.* **79**, 691–694.

Isakson, O. G. P., Lendahl, A., Nelson, A. *et al.* (1987). Mechanisms of stimulating effect of GH on long bone growth. *Endocr. Rev.* **8**, 426–438.

Johansson, A., Forslund, A., Hambraeus, L., Blum, W., and Ljunghall, S. (1993). Growth hormone dependent IGFBP-3 is a major determinant of bone mineral density in healthy men. *J. Bone Miner. Res.* **9**, 915–921.

Jones, J., and Clemmons, D. R. (1995). IGFs and their binding proteins. *Endocr. Rev.* **16**, 3–32.

Jones, J., Gockerman, A., Busby, J. W. *et al.* (1993). Extracellular matrix contains IGFBP-5: Potentiation of the effects of IGF-I. *J. Cell Biol.* **121**, 679–687.

Kanzaki, S., Hilliker, S., Baylink, D. J., and Mohan, S. (1994). Evidence that human bone cells in culture produce IGFBP-4 and IGFBP-5 proteases. *Endocrinology (Baltimore)* **134**, 383–392.

Koperak, C., Fittsimmons, R., Stein, D., Mohan, S. *et al.* (1990). Studies of the mechanisms by which androgens enhance mitogenesis and differentiation of bone cells. *J. Clin. Endocrinol. Metab.* **71**, 329–337.

Kudo, Y., Iwashita, M., Itatsu, S., Iguchi, and Takeda, Y. (1996). Regulation of IGFBP-4 protease activity by estrogen and PTH in SaOS-2 cells: Implications for the pathogenesis of postmenopausal osteoporosis. *J. Endocrinol.* **150**, 223–229.

Kurland, E. S., Rackoff, P. J., Adler, R. A., Bilezikian, J. P., Rogers, J., and Rosen, C. J. (1998). Heritability of serum IGF-I and its relationship to bone density. *Endocr. Soc. Meeting*, p. 99.

Kurland, E. S., Chan, F., Vereault, D., Rosen, C. J., and Bilezikian, J. P. (1996). R Growth hormone IGF-I axis in men with idiopathic osteoporosis and reduced circulating levels of IGF-I. *J. Bone Miner. Res.* **11**(S1), 323.

Kurland, E. S., Rosen, C. J., Cosman, E., McMahon, D., Chan, F., Shane, E., Lindsay, R., Dempster, D., and Bilezikian, J. P. (1997). IGF-I in men with idiopathic osteoporosis. *J. Clin. Endocrinol. Metab.* **82**, 2799–2805.

Labrie, F., Bélanger, A., Cusan, L., and Candan, B. (1997). Physiological changes in DHEA are not reflected by serum levels of active androgens and estrogens but their metabolites. *J. Clin. Endocrinol. Metab.* **82**, 2403–2409.

LeBoff, M. S., Rosen, C. J., and Glowacki, J. (1995). Changes in growth factors and cytokines in postmenopausal women. *J. Bone Miner. Res.* **10**, 241.

LeRoith, D., Werner, H., Butner-Johnson, D., and Roberts, C. T. (1995). Molecular and cellular aspects of the IGF-I receptor. *Endocr. Rev.* **16**, 143–153.

LeRoith, D., Parrizas, M., and Blakesley, V. A. (1997). IGF-I receptor and apoptosis. *Endocrine* **7**, 103–105.

Linkhart, T. A., and Mohan, S. (1989). PTH stimulates release of IGF-I and IGF-II from neonatal mouse calvariae. *Endocrinology (Baltimore)* **125**, 1484–1491.

Ljunghall, S., Johansson, G., Burman, K., Kampe, O., and Lindh, E. (1992). Low plasma levels of IGF-I in male patients with idiopathic osteoporosis. *J. Intern. Med.* **232**, 59–64.

Mahuzuki, H., Hakeda, Y., Wakatasuki, N., Useii, N. *et al.* (1991). IGF-I supports formation and activation of osteoclasts. *Endocrinology (Baltimore)* **131**, 1075–1078.

Marcus, R. (1997). Skeletal effects of GH and IGF-I in adults. *Horm. Res.* **48**, 60–67.

Martha, P. M., Gooman, K. M., Blizzard, R. M. *et al.* (1992). Endogenous GH secretion and clearance in normal boys as determined by deconvolution analysis. *J. Clin. Endocrinol. Metab.* **74**, 336–344.

McCarthy, T. L., Centrella, M., and Canalis, E. (1989a). Regulatory effects of IGF-I and IGF-II on bone collagen synthesis in rat calvarial cells. *Endocrinology (Baltimore)* **124**, 301–308.

McCarthy, T. L., Centrella, M., and Canalis, E. (1989b). PTH enhances the transcript and polypeptide levels of IGF-I in osteoblast enriched cultures from fetal rate calvariae. *Endocrinology (Baltimore)* **124**, 1247–1253.

McCarthy, T. L., Ji, C., Slu, H., Langhorne, S., Coates, K., Rowein, P., and Centrella, M. (1997). 17 Beta estradiol suppresses cyclic AMP induced IGF-I gene transcription in primary rat osteoblast cultures. *J. Biol. Chem.* **272**, 18132–18139.

McLean, D., Kiel, D. P., and Rosen, C. J. (1995). Low dose rhGH for frail elders stimulates bone turnover in a dose dependent manner. *J. Bone Miner. Res.* **10** (S1), 458.

Milne, M., Kang, M., Wuail, J. M., and Baran, D. M. (1998). Thyroid hormone excess increases IGF-I transcripts in bone marrow cell cultures: Divergent effects on vertebral and femoral cell cultures. *Endocrinology (Baltimore)* **139** (in press).

Mohan, S. (1993). IGF binding proteins in bone cell regulation. *Growth Regul.* **3**, 65–68.

Mohan, S., and Baylink, D. J. (1990). Autocrine and paracrine aspects of bone metabolism. *Growth Genet. Horm.* **6**, 1–9.

Mohan, S., and Baylink, D. J. (1997). Serum IGFBP-4 and IGFBP-5 in aging and age-associated diseases. *Endocrine* **7**, 87–91.

Mohan, S., Farley, J. R., and Baylink, D. J. (1995). Age-related changes in IGFBP-4 and IGFBP-5 in human serum and bone: Implications for bone loss with aging. *Prog. Growth Factor Res.* **6**, 465–473.

Morales, A. J., Nolan, J. J., Lukes, C. C., and Yen, S. S. C. (1994). Effects of replacement doses of DHEA in men and women. *J. Clin. Endocrinol. Metab.* **78**, 1360–1361.

Myers, M. G., Sur, X. J., Christian, B., Jadreau, B. R., Barker, J. M., White, M. F. (1993). IRS-1 is a common element in insulin and IGF-I signaling to PI-3'kinase. *Endocrinology (Baltimore)* **132**, 1421–1427.

Nuerberg, M., Buckbinder, L., Sizinger, B., and Kley, N. (1997). The p53 IGF-I receptor axis in the regulation of programmed cell death. *Endocrine* **7**, 107–109.

Nun, S. E., Gibson, T. B., Rayak, R., and Cohen, P. (1997). Regulation of prostate cell growth by IGFBPs and proteases. *Endocrine* **7**, 115–118.

Oh, Y. (1997). IGFBPs and neoplastic models: New concepts for roles of IGFBPs in regulation of cancer cell growth. *Endocrine* **7**, 115–117.

Papadakis, M. A., Grady, D., Black, D., Tremey, M. J., Goding, G. A. W., and Grunfeld, C. (1996). GH replacement in healthy older men improves body composition but not functional activity. *Ann. Intern. Med.* **124**, 708–716.

Poehlman, E. T., Toth, M. J., Ades, P. A., and Rosen, C. J. (1997). Menopause associated changes in plasma lipids insulin-like growth factor-I and blood pressure: A longitudinal study. *Eur. J. Clin. Invest.* **27**, 322–326.

Rajaram, S., Baylink, D. J., and Mohan, S. (1997). IGFBPs in serum and other biological fluids. *Endocr. Rev.* **18**, 801–831.

Ravn, P., Overgaard, K., Spencer, E. M., and Christiansen, C. (1995). IGF-I and IGF-II in healthy females. *Eur. J. Endocrinol.* **132**, 313–319.

Reed, B. Y., Zerwick, J. E., Sakhee, K., Binder, N. *et al.* (1995). Serum IGF-I is low and correlated with osteoblast surfaces in IOM. *J. Bone Miner. Res.* **10**, 1218–1225.

Ristevski, S., Yeung, S., Pon, C., Wark, J. W., and Ebeling, J. W. (1997). Osteopenia is common in young first degree male relatives of men with osteoporosis. *Aust. N. Z. Bone Soc.* Abst. No. 60, p. 65.

Romagnoli, E., Minisola, S., Carnevale, V., Rosso, R., Pacitti, M. T., Scarda, A., Scarnecchia, L., and Mazzuoli, G. (1994). Circulating levels of IGFBP-3 and IGF-I in perimenopausal women. *Osteoporosis Int.* **4**, 305–308.

Rosen, C. J. (1994). Growth hormone, IGFs and the senescent skeleton. *J. Cell Biochem.* **58**, 346–348.

Rosen, C. J., and Conover, C. (1997). Growth insulin like growth factor-I axis in aging: A summary of an NIA sponsored synposium. *J. Clin. Endocrinol. Metab.* **82**, 3919–3922.

Rosen, C. J., Donahue, L. R., Hunter, S. J. *et al.* (1992). The 24/25 kDa serum IGFBP is increased in elderly women with hip and spine fractures. *J. Clin. Endocrinol. Metab.* **74**, 24–27.

Rosen, T., Hannsson, H., Granhed, H., Szucs, J., and Bengtsson, B. A. (1993). Reduced bone mineral content in adults with GHD. *Acta Endocrinol. (Copenhagen)* **129**, 201–206.

Rosen, C. J., Donahue, L. R., and Hunter, S. J. (1994). IGFs and bone: The osteoporosis connection. *Proc. Soc. Exp. Biol. Med.* **206**, 83–102.

Rosen, C. J., Vereault, D., Steffens, C., Chilutte, D., and Glowacki, J. (1997a). Effect of age and estrogen status on the skeletal IGF regulatory system. *Endocrine* **7**, 77–80.

Rosen, C. J., Dimai, H. P., Vereault, D., Donahue, L. R., Beamer, W. G., Farley, J., Linkhart, S., Linkhart, T., Mohan, S., and Baylink, D. J. (1997b). Circulating and skeletal IGF-I concentrations in two inbred strains of mice with different bone mineral densities. *Bone* **21**, 217–223.

Rosen, C. J., Kurland, E. S., Vereault, D., Adler, R. A., Rackoff, P. J., Craig, W. Y., Witte, S., Rogers, J., and Bilezikian, J. P. (1998). An assocaition between serum IGF-I and a simple sequence repeat in the IGF-I gene. Implication for genetic studies of bone mineral density. *J. Clin. Endicronol. Metab.* **83**, 2286–2290.

Rudman, D., Feller, A. G., and Nelgrag, H. S. (1990). Effect of human GH in men over age 60. *N. Engl. J. Med.* **323**, 52–60.

Rudman, D., Feller, A. G., and Cohn, L. (1991). Effect of rhGH on body composition in elderly men. *Horm. Res.* **36**, 73–81.

Shewmon, D. A., Stock, J. L, Rosen, C. J. *et al.* (1995). Effects of estrogen and tamoxifen on Lp(a) and IGF-I in healthy postmenopausal women. *Arterioscler. Thromb.* **14**, 1586–1591.

Slootwigh, M. C. (1992). Growth hormone and bone. *Horm. Metab. Res.* **25**, 335–345.

Slowik, D. M., Rosenthal, D. I., Doppelt, S. H. *et al.* (1986). Restoration of spinal bone mass in osteoporotic males by treatment with human PTH and 1,25 dihydroxyvitamin D. *J. Bone Miner. Res.* **1**, 377–381.

Smith, E. P., Boyd, J., Frank, G. R., Takahashi, H., Cohen, R. M., Speeker, B., Williams, T. C., Lubahn, D. B., and Korach, K. S. (1994). Estrogen resistance caused by a mutation in the ER gene in a man. *N. Engl. J. Med.* **33**, 1056–1061.

Sugimoto, T., Nishiyama, K., Kuribayashi, F., and Chihara, K. (1997). Serum levels of IGF-I, IGFBP-2, and IGFBP-3 in osteoporotic patients with and without spine fractures. *J. Bone Miner. Res.* **12**, 1272–1279.

Tanner, J. M., Whitehouse, R. H., Hughes, P. C. R., and Carter, B. S. (1976). Relative importance of GH and sex steroids at puberty of thigh length, limb length and muscle width in GHD children. *J. Pediatr.* **89**, 1000–1008.

Thompson, J. L., Butterfield, G. E., and Marcus, R. (1995). The effects of recombinant rhIGF-I and GH on body composition in elderly women. *J. Clin. Endocrinol. Metab.* **80**, 1845–1852.

Thraillkill, K., Quarles, L. D., Nagase, H., Suzuki, K., Serra, D., and Fowlkes, J. (1995). Characterization of IGFBP-5 degrading proteases produced throughout murine osteoblast differentiation. *Endocrinology (Baltimore)* **136**, 3527–3533.

Toogood, A. A., O'Neil, P. A., and Shalet, S. A. (1996). Beyond the somatopause: GHD in adults over age 60. *J. Clin. Endocrinol. Metab.* **81**, 460–465.

Tremollières, F. A., Strong, D. D., Baylin, D., and Mohan, S. (1992). Progesterone and promogesterone stimulates human bone cell proliferation and IGF-II production. *Acta Endocrinol.* **126,** 329–337.

Veldhuis, J. D., Kerr, T. Y., South, J., Weltman, A., Weltman, J. *et al.* (1995). Differential impact of age, sex steroids and obesity on basal vs pulsatile GH secretion. *J. Clin. Endocrinol. Metab.* **82,** 3209–3222.

Veldhuis, J. D., Iranmanesh, A., and Weltman, A. (1997). Elements in the pathophysiology of diminished GH secretion in aging humans. *Endocrine* **7,** 41–48.

Wuster, C., Blum, W., Sclemilch, S., Ranke, M., and Ziegler, R. (1993). Decreased serum IGFs and IGFBP3 in osteoporosis. *J. Intern. Med.* **234,** 249–255.

Zapf, J., and Froesch, E. (1986). IGFs/somatomedins: Structure, secretion, biological actions and physiological roles. *Horm. Res.* **24,** 121–130.

Zapf, J., Schmid, C., and Froesche, E. R. (1984). Biological and Immunological properties of IGF-I and IGF-II. *Clin. Endocrinol. Metab.* **13,** 7–12.

Chapter 10

Bernard P. Halloran
Daniel D. Bikle

Department of Medicine
University of California
San Francisco, California
Divisions of Endocrinology and Geriatrics
Veterans Affairs Medical Center
San Francisco, California

Age-Related Changes in Mineral Metabolism

I. Introduction

Mineral metabolism is regulated primarily by parathyroid hormone (PTH) and vitamin D but with significant ancillary roles played by the sex steroids, growth hormone (GH), and the insulin-like growth factors (IGF-I, -II). Through the actions of these hormones on the intestine, kidney, and bone, a delicate balance is maintained between Ca and P absorption in the intestine, storage in the bone, and excretion from the kidney. With advancing age, mineral balance gradually becomes negative, excretion exceeds absorption, and skeletal mass diminishes. Osteopenia develops as a consequence of an imbalance in mineral metabolism. To appreciate the pathogenesis of osteoporosis in the male, it is important to understand the process of aging and its effects on cell metabolism and tissue function. In this chapter we will first review the regulation of mineral metabolism, then discuss the fundamentals of human aging, and finally focus on the humoral and tissue changes associated with aging that influence mineral metabolism.

II. Regulation of Mineral Metabolism

The serum concentrations of calcium (Ca) and phosphorus (P) are regulated primarily by parathyroid hormone and vitamin D (Feldman *et al.*, 1997; Bilezikian *et al.*, 1994). Small changes in blood ionized Ca (Ca^{++}) modulate PTH secretion through a membrane-found Ca-receptor (CaR). When Ca^{++} is low, PTH secretion increases, and parathyroid cell proliferation is stimulated. Parathyroid hormone increases renal reabsorption of Ca, stimulates bone turnover, and promotes the release of Ca and P into the serum pool. Through its phosphaturic effect, PTH balances the release of P from bone by increasing its urinary excretion.

Vitamin D is produced in the skin or absorbed from the diet and is converted to 25-hydroxyvitamin D (25-OH-D) in the liver. Conversion of vitamin D to 25-OH-D is poorly regulated, and thus the serum concentration of 25-OH-D provides a good index of vitamin D status. 25-Hydroxyvitamin D undergoes renal metabolism to 1,25-dihydroxyvitamin D ($1,25(OH)_2D$), the active hormonal form of the vitamin. PTH stimulates conversion of 25-OH-D to $1,25(OH)_2D$ through the 25-hydroxyvitamin D-1a-hydroxylase, an enzyme whose activity is inhibited by high extracellular Ca^{++} and P and modulated by the sex steroids, GH, and IGF. 1,25-Dihydroxyvitamin D, acting through the vitamin D receptor (VDR) and, perhaps, nongenomic mechanisms, stimulates Ca and P absorption from the intestine and modulates mineral release from bone. In feedback fashion, $1,25(OH)_2D$ inhibits PTH secretion, parathyroid cell proliferation, and renal 1-hydroxylase activity. Mineral homeostasis depends on the coordinate functioning of each element in this delicately balanced network.

III. Human Aging

A. Aging and Disease

Aging, in the context of this chapter, will refer to postmaturational aging to differentiate growth and development from the gradual degenerative processes that occur after puberty and result in the progressive loss of physiological function. Aging stems from a time-dependent change in somatic cell function. It is both programmed and a consequence of an inability to repair molecular damage. Disease is a confounding factor and complicates how we age. Because tissues age at different rates and because disease burden can vary enormously between individuals, we become increasingly different from one another as we age. This increases the heterogeneity within the elderly population and explains in part the many discrepancies observed among aging studies. In this chapter we will focus on healthy aging. We will examine the effects of aging on mineral metabolism in the absence of overt disease. For a discussion of the effects of disease, Chapters 17 and 20–23 should be consulted.

B. The Basis of Aging: Cell Senescence

Aging begins at the level of the cell (Dice, 1993). Cells age or senesce both in culture and in the whole organism. Cell aging is manifest by changes in both replicative potential and metabolic function. Normal replicating cells are limited in their number of division cycles (Hayflick, 1975). Proliferative capacity is inversely proportional to donor age. Although this limits the ability of tissues to restore themselves, it is generally agreed that aging is not solely a consequence of loss of proliferative potential.

Cell function also changes with aging. Chromosomal abnormalities increase (Crowely and Curtis, 1963), DNA mutations and oxidative damage increase (Garcia de la Asuncion *et al.*, 1996), protein synthetic and degradative rates change (Dice, 1989), and responsiveness to hormones and growth factors are altered (Harley *et al.*, 1981; Carlin *et al.*, 1983; McCormick and Campisi, 1991). These changes impair the ability of organ systems to meet their physiological demands. The changes in organ function alter the metabolism of other tissues, creating a cascade of altered function. The collective effects on organ function induced directly by cell senescence and indirectly by alterations in other tissues result in a gradual degeneration of physiological function.

IV. Aging and Mineral Metabolism

A. Age-Related Endocrine Changes

1. Parathyroid Hormone and Calcitonin

The serum concentration of PTH increases with advancing age (Marcus *et al.*, 1984; Orwoll and Meier, 1986; Sherman *et al.*, 1990; Halloran *et al.*, 1990; Eastell *et al.*, 1991; Minisola *et al.*, 1993; Ledger *et al.*, 1994; Khosla *et al.*, 1997) (Figure 1). Levels of intact hormone in healthy men and women are 35–80% higher at age 70 than at age 30. The increase in serum PTH begins around midlife, reflects increased levels of biologically active hormone (Forero *et al.*, 1987) and, despite a near constant glandular weight between ages 30 and 90 years (Grimelius *et al.*, 1981) is associated with a two- to threefold increase in the minimum and maximum secretory rates (Ledger *et al.*, 1994; Portale *et al.*, 1997).

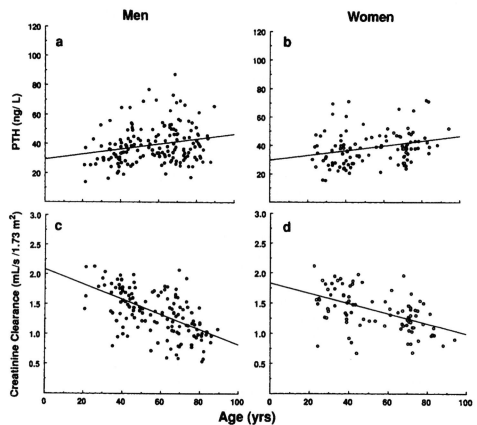

FIGURE I The relationship between the serum concentration of intact PTH(1-84) and age (upper panels) and creatinine clearance and age (lower panels) in men (a and c) and women (b and d). Reprinted from Sherman, S., Hollis, B., and Tobin, J. (1990). Vitamin D status and related parameters in a healthy population: The effects of age, sex and season. *J. Clin. Endocrinol. Metab.* 71(2), 405–413, © The Endocrine Society, with permission.

The mechanisms responsible for the increase in PTH secretion are not clear. Portale *et al.* (1997) have shown under metabolic conditions that morning fasting and mean 24-hr whole blood Ca^{++} concentrations are not different in healthy young and elderly men (Table I). Thus hypocalcemia is not required to sustain the age-related elevation in serum PTH. Periodic bouts of mild hypocalcemia, induced by inadequate dietary Ca (Chapter 11), decreased intestinal Ca absorption, or impaired renal conservation of Ca, may occur, and these could result in increased PTH secretory activity (Akerstrom *et al.*, 1986). McKane *et al.* (1996) report that Ca supplementation in elderly women can decrease serum PTH and maximum secretory capacity by 25 and 35%, respectively.

TABLE I Morning Fasting and 24-Hour Mean Whole Blood Ca^{++} Concentrations in Healthy Young and Elderly Men after 9 Days on a Constant Metabolic Diet

	Young (n = 13)	Elderly (n = 9)
Age (yr)	39 ± 1	74 ± 2
Whole blood Ca^{++} (gm/dl)		
Morning fasting	4.84 ± 0.03	4.84 ± 0.04
24-hour mean[a]	4.77 ± 0.04	4.80 ± 0.04

From Portale et al. (1997).
Values are mean ± SE.
[a]Measurements were taken hourly for 24 hours.

Secondary hyperparathyroidism induced by renal insufficiency may also contribute to increased PTH secretory capacity in the elderly. Although the age-related rise in serum PTH occurs in all men and women including those with normal or near normal glomerular filtration rates (Portale et al., 1997), as GFR falls below 70 ml/min the contribution of renal insufficiency to the age-related rise in serum PTH becomes increasingly important.

Vitamin D deficiency may further augment the rise in serum PTH with age. The normal serum concentrations of 1,25(OH)$_2$D and 25-OH-D provide tonic inhibition of parathyroid cell proliferation and PTH secretion (Russell et al., 1986; Szabo et al., 1989). Mild to moderate vitamin D deficiency is common among the elderly, and an inverse relationship between serum PTH and 25-OH-D is often observed in both elderly men and women (Krall et al., 1989; Gloth et al., 1995). Metabolic changes within the aging parathyroid secretory cell may further contribute to abnormalities in gland function (see Section IV.B.1).

Bone health may be jeopardized by the gradual age-related increase in serum PTH. Parathyroid hormone increases bone turnover, and increased levels of the markers of bone resorption reportedly predict hip fracture in at least some populations of women (Garnero et al., 1996). Resolution of age-related hyperparathyroidism by treatment of elderly men and women with calcium and vitamin D can reduce the rate of bone loss and hip fracture (Chapuy et al., 1996; Dawson-Hughes et al., 1997b).

The serum concentration of calcitonin (CT) is higher in men than in women and is reported to either decrease (Deftos et al., 1980; Reginster et al., 1989; Boucher et al., 1989) or remain unchanged (Tiegs et al., 1986) with advancing age. Calcium challenge elicits a greater increase in serum CT in young than in elderly women (Boucher et al., 1989), but studies in men are lacking. Estrogen administration in postmenopausal women can restore, at least in part, CT responsiveness to Ca (Gennari and Agnusdei, 1990).

2. Vitamin D

Cutaneous production of vitamin D decreases with advancing age (MacLaughlin and Holick, 1985; Webb *et al.*, 1988). Beginning in the third decade of life, epidermal thinning occurs (Lavker, 1979), keratinocyte number and turnover rate decrease (Grove and Kligman, 1983), cholesterol content diminishes (Ghadially *et al.*, 1995), and skin blood flow falls (Tsuchida, 1993). Production of 7-dehydrocholesterol, the precursor to vitamin D, is reduced in the epidermis, and the response in serum vitamin D after one minimal erythemal dose of ultraviolet B radiation is reduced nearly fourfold in elderly subjects (Holick *et al.*, 1989). The ability to produce vitamin D in the elderly is aggravated by sunscreen use and avoidance of sun exposure.

Although dietary intake of vitamin D decreases only slightly or remains the same with advancing age (Chapter 11), and intestinal absorption of vitamin D does not appear to change (Fleming and Barrows, 1982; Clemens *et al.*, 1986), the decrease in cutaneous production results in a decrease in serum vitamin D levels. Because synthesis of 25-OH-D is normal in elderly people as long as liver function is preserved (Matsuoka *et al.*, 1988), circulating levels of 25-OH-D also decrease (Omdahl *et al.*, 1982; Aksnes *et al.*, 1988; McKenna, 1992; Quesada *et al.*, 1992; Need *et al.*, 1993; Van der Wielen *et al.*, 1995; Gloth *et al.*, 1995; Chapuy *et al.*, 1996).

Gender has no effect on cutaneous production of vitamin D (M. Holick, personal communication), but gender differences have been observed in the serum concentration of 25-OH-D. Dawson-Hughes *et al.* (1997a) report that serum 25-OH-D concentrations are higher in elderly ($>$ 65 yr) men than in women (82 versus 69 nM, $p <$ .001).

The serum concentration of $1,25(OH)_2D$ in men has been reported to either decrease (Manolagas *et al.*, 1983; Epstein *et al.*, 1986) or remain the same (Orwoll and Meier, 1986; Halloran *et al.*, 1990; Sherman *et al.*, 1990) with advancing age. Similar results have been found in women and mixed populations (Gallagher *et al.*, 1979; Tsai *et al.*, 1984; Sherman *et al.*, 1990; Prince *et al.*, 1990; Kinyamu *et al.*, 1997). The discrepancies between these reports can be accounted for, at least in part, by differences in the elderly populations studied. Elderly in poor health or confined to rest homes tend to have low (Manolagas *et al.*, 1983) whereas healthy elderly tend to have normal (Halloran *et al.*, 1990; Sherman *et al.*, 1990) serum concentrations of $1,25(OH)_2D$. The production rate and metabolic clearance rate of $1,25(OH)_2D$ are also normal in healthy elderly men (Table II) (Halloran *et al.*, 1990).

Despite the finding that serum $1,25(OH)_2D$ is normal in healthy elderly subjects, the sensitivity of the renal 1-hydroxylase to trophic factors may be reduced. In elderly patients with osteoporosis (Slovik *et al.*, 1981) and in postmenopausal women with mild to moderate renal insufficiency (Tsai *et al.*, 1984), $1,25(OH)_2D$ responsiveness to PTH is impaired. Kinyamu *et al.*

TABLE II   Serum Concentration, Metabolic Clearance Rate, and Production Rate of 1,25(OH)$_2$D in Healthy Young and Elderly Men after 9 Days on a Constant Metabolic Diet

	Young (n = 9)	Elderly (n = 9)
Age (yr)	34 ± 2	72 ± 2
Serum concentration (pg/ml)	37 ± 3	35 ± 3
Metabolic clearance rate (ml/min)	34 ± 2	37 ± 2
Production rate (ng/min)	1.30 ± 0.10	1.27 ± 0.10

From Halloran *et al.* (1990).
Values are mean ± SE.

(1996) studied 199 women between ages 25 and 38 years. Serum creatinine and basal serum PTH increased predictably with age, whereas serum 1,25(OH)$_2$D did not change. Responsiveness to PTH decreased with age, but significant reductions were not noted until after age 70.

In healthy elderly men (70 ± 1 yr) (GFR > 70 ml/min/1.73 m^2), the response of the serum concentration of 1,25(OH)$_2$D to PTH is delayed, but the final magnitude of the change in concentration is similar to that in young men (Halloran *et al.*, 1996) (Table III). The response of nephrogenous cAMP (NcAMP) and P transport to PTH are normal. In these same men, basal serum PTH (+148%), NcAMP (+56%), and fractional excretion of P (+44%) were higher than in young men. That NcAMP and fractional excretion of P are elevated is consistent with the basal elevation in serum PTH. That basal serum 1,25(OH)$_2$D is not elevated may be a consequence of the small reduction in functional renal mass (GFR was 30% lower in the elderly) or a selective loss of 1-hydroxylase enzyme (see Section IV.B.2).

Calcium and phosphorus also directly regulate 1,25(OH)$_2$D synthesis (Hulter *et al.*, 1985). Serum Ca has been reported to be either decreased (Sherman *et al.*, 1990; Quesada *et al.*, 1992), increased (Endres *et al.*, 1987),

TABLE III   Response of Serum 1,25(OH)$_2$D to Exogenous Infusion of hPTH(1-34) for 24 Hours in Healthy Young and Elderly Men

	Young (n = 9)	Elderly (n = 8)
Age (yr)	39 ± 1	70 ± 1
Serum concentration (pg/ml)		
Basal	31 ± 3	32 ± 4
After 24-hour infusion of PTH	47 ± 4	44 ± 5

From Halloran *et al.* (1996).
Values are mean ± SE.

or normal (Epstein *et al.*, 1986; Minisola *et al.*, 1993) in elderly men and women. These discrepancies probably reflect differences in the health status or life-style of the elderly populations studied or in study design. In healthy young and elderly men, studied under metabolic conditions, the morning fasting and mean 24-hr whole blood Ca^{++} concentrations are not significantly different (Table I) (Portale *et al.*, 1997). Serum P concentrations have been observed uniformly to decrease in men but remain unchanged in women with advancing age (Sherman *et al.*, 1990).

Studies to examine the effect of age on the responsiveness of the renal 1-hydroxylase to Ca and P are limited. Attempts to manipulate serum Ca selectively through dietary maneuvers are accompanied by changes in serum PTH which confound assessment of the effect of Ca alone. On the other hand, changes in dietary P can and have been used to manipulate serum P levels selectively without influencing either serum PTH or Ca. We have used this approach to study the effect of aging on the relationship between the serum concentrations of P and $1,25(OH)_2D$ in men (Portale *et al.*, 1996). The results show that the serum concentrations of $1,25(OH)_2D$ in young and elderly men in whom the serum concentration of 25-OH-D is normal and not different respond equally to changes in dietary P. However, at each dietary intake of P, fasting and 24-hr mean serum concentrations of P are lower in elderly men (Table IV). The relationship between serum P and $1,25(OH)_2D$ is altered with aging. Serum $1,25(OH)_2D$ is inappropriately low for the serum concentration of P.

Thus, the predicted trophic effects of both basally elevated serum PTH and low serum P on $1,25(OH)_2D$ production appear to be diminished by aging in men. Serum $1,25(OH)_2D$ may be normal in healthy elderly men, but maintenance of a normal synthetic rate appears to require tonic stimulation by increased serum PTH and decreased serum P. The normal balance between the serum concentrations of P, PTH, and $1,25(OH)_2D$ found in young men is disrupted in elderly men. The reason for these alterations is not clear.

TABLE IV   Response of Serum P to Changes in Dietary P in Healthy Young and Elderly Men

	Young (n = 9)	Elderly (n = 7)
Age (yr)	29 ± 2	71 ± 1
Serum concentration of P (mg/dl)		
Dietary P (mg/d) = 625	3.7 ± 0.1	3.2 ± 0.2[a]
1500	4.2 ± 0.1	3.7 ± 0.2[a]
2300	4.3 ± 0.1	3.8 ± 0.2[a]

From Portale *et al.* (1996).
Values are mean ± SE.
[a] $p < 0.01$, mean differs from young men.

Gradual loss of functional renal mass, alterations in other trophic factors important for 1-hydroxylase activity (e.g., GH), or functional changes in cell metabolism induced by cell aging may be at fault.

3. Testosterone and Estrogen

Serum total and free testosterone concentrations decrease with advancing age in men (Lamberts *et al.*, 1997). Like estrogen replacement in postmenopausal women, testosterone replacement in hypogonadal men can increase serum 1,25(OH)$_2$D levels (Hagenfeldt *et al.*, 1992). Whether the normal age-related fall in circulating testosterone influences either 25-OH-D or 1,25(OH)$_2$D metabolism, however, is not clear.

Estrogen deficiency in postmenopausal women has been linked to oversecretion of PTH. Khosla *et al.* (1997) report that the age-related increase in serum PTH is eliminated in postmenopausal women receiving long-term estrogen therapy. Morley *et al.* (1993), however, treated elderly hypogonadal men with testosterone and found no effect on serum PTH.

Estrogen can increase the serum concentration of the vitamin D binding protein (DBP) and thereby reduce the fraction of free 1,25(OH)$_2$D (Cooke and Haddad, 1997). Estrogen administration to postmenopausal women, however, increases both total and free 1,25(OH)$_2$D, despite a decrease in free fraction (Bikle *et al.*, 1992). Whether testosterone has similar effects and whether the fall in estrogen and testosterone with age influence the circulating levels of DBP and free 1,25(OH)$_2$D is not clear. In men, DBP levels do not appear to change with age (Fujisawa *et al.*, 1984). In women, DBP levels have been reported to be decreased (Fujisawa *et al.*, 1984; Bikle *et al.*, 1992; Dick *et al.*, 1995), normal (Aksnes *et al.*, 1988; Quesada *et al.*, 1992), or increased (Prince *et al.*, 1990) in elderly subjects.

4. Growth Hormone and Insulin-like Growth Factor

Growth hormone (GH) and insulin-like growth factor I (IGF-I) treatment *in vivo* stimulate renal P reabsorption, and IGF-I treatment *in vitro* stimulates P uptake by renal cells (Caverzasio and Bonjour, 1989; Hammerman *et al.*, 1980). Growth hormone and IGF-I treatment *in vivo* also stimulate 1,25(OH)$_2$D production. The action of GH appears to be mediated through IGF-I because IGF-I administration *in vitro* enhances 1,25(OH)$_2$D synthesis, but GH does not (Condamine *et al.*, 1994). Insulin-like growth factor-I sensitizes the renal 1-hydroxylase to changes in serum P (Halloran and Spencer, 1988). In the absence of IGF-I, the stimulatory effect of hypophosphatemia on 1,25(OH)$_2$D synthesis is dramatically reduced.

The serum concentrations of both GH and IGF-I decrease with advancing age in men and women (Florini *et al.*, 1985; Corpas *et al.*, 1993; Martin *et al.*, 1997). Treatment of elderly subjects with GH can increase the serum concentration of 1,25(OH)$_2$D (Marcus *et al.*, 1990; Lieberman *et al.*, 1994), suggesting that the age-related decrease in serum GH and IGF-I may decrease tonic stimulation of the 1-hydroxylase and diminish responsiveness to changes in serum P. Indeed, this may explain the altered relationship between the serum concentrations of P and 1,25(OH)$_2$D observed in healthy elderly men.

B. Age-Related Changes in Tissue Function

I. Parathyroid Gland

The age-related increase in serum PTH is associated with an increase in the concentration of Ca^{++} required to half-maximally suppress PTH release (Ca set point) (Portale *et al.*, 1997). The set point increases from 4.54 ± 0.03 mg/dl in young men (39 ± 1 yr) to 4.71 ± 0.04 mg/dl ($p < .005$) in old men (74 ± 4 yr). In women, the set point for PTH release does not appear to change with age. Ledger *et al.* (1994) report set-point values in young and elderly women receiving no supplemental vitamin D, calcium, or estrogen of 4.76 ± 0.04 and 4.72 ± .04 mg/dl, respectively.

The increase in calcium set point for PTH release in men suggests that parathyroid cell responsiveness to Ca^{++} may decrease with age. Expression of mRNA and protein in the parathyroid gland for the Ca-receptor increases with age in rats (Autry *et al.*, 1997). That PTH secretion is increased despite increased receptor concentration suggests that aging may impair calcium binding or coupling between the Ca-receptor and down-stream effector elements in the pathway regulating PTH release. Alterations in transmembrane signaling have been reported to occur with advancing age for various receptor-mediated functions (Hanai *et al.*, 1989; Miyamoto and Ohshika, 1994). A decrease in signal transduction could result in the cellular perception that Ca^{++} is limited. That receptor expression is increased may reflect upregulation of a feedback loop responsible for maintaining normal cellular responsiveness to Ca. Interestingly, expression of the Ca receptor in the thyroid gland increases in parallel with that in the parathyroid gland with aging in rats (Autry *et al.*, 1997).

2. Kidney

The decreases in renal mass and GFR that occur with advancing age (Figure 1) decrease functional renal capacity (Lindeman *et al.*, 1985). When measured under constant dietary conditions on a metabolic ward, daily urinary excretion of Ca in healthy elderly men decreases with age (Portale *et al.*, 1996). When normalized to GFR, however, fasting urinary Ca excretion (Mol/L GFR) and fractional excretion of Ca are identical in young and old men (Halloran *et al.*, 1996). There is no evidence of an age-induced renal Ca leak in healthy elderly men. However, the relationship between serum PTH and fractional excretion of Ca has not been carefully examined.

Daily urinary excretion of P, fractional excretion of P, and NcAMP in healthy elderly men increase with age (Halloran *et al.*, 1996; Portale *et al.*,

1996). The changes appear to reflect the age-related increase in serum PTH. There is no evidence that processing of P in response to PTH is impaired in healthy elderly men. Animal studies, however, suggest that receptor desensitization in response to rising serum hormone concentrations may blunt at least some PTH-induced functions including $1,25(OH)_2D$ synthesis (Hanai et al., 1989). Production of $1,25(OH)_2D$ may also be impaired because of decreased mitochondrial number and function (Ishida et al., 1987; Ozawa, 1997).

3. Intestine

Crypt cell proliferation increases (Holt and Yeh, 1989), absorptive surface area decreases (Chen et al., 1990), and nutrient transport is impaired (Ferraris and Vinnakota, 1993) in the intestine with advancing age. Intestinal absorption of vitamin D does not change (Clemens et al., 1986). Absorption of Ca is reported either to decrease (Avioli et al., 1965; Heaney et al., 1989; Kinyamu et al., 1997) or to remain the same (Ebeling et al., 1992, 1994) with aging. Decrements in Ca absorption of 10–30% are commonly observed in elderly women. In some cases, these reach significance (Kinyamu et al., 1997), and in others they do not (Ebeling et al., 1992, 1994). Responsiveness to endogenous changes in serum $1,25(OH)_2D$ induced by restriction of dietary Ca is the same in young and old women (Ebeling et al., 1994). Intestinal vitamin D receptor concentrations in elderly women are reported to be slightly decreased (-20%) (Ebeling et al., 1992) or normal (Kinyamu et al., 1997). Parallel studies in men are lacking.

Animal studies support these observations. In the rat, Ca uptake into brush border membrane vesicles and whole duodenal cells is decreased in aged animals (Liang et al., 1991). Vitamin D receptor mRNA and protein are reported to decrease (-25%) or remain unchanged with postmaturational aging (Liang et al., 1994; Johnson et al., 1995).

4. Bone

The skeletal response to exogenous infusion of PTH is blunted in elderly men (Halloran et al., 1996). The increment in whole blood Ca^{++} after a 24-hour infusion of PTH (1-34) is reduced by 40% in elderly when compared to young men. Osteoblast responsiveness to PTH, GH, and platelet-derived growth factor correlates negatively with donor age (Pfeilschifter et al., 1993). Studies in male rats corroborate these findings (Fox and Mathew, 1991). In women, the response of serum Ca and urinary hydroxyproline excretion to PTH increases after the menopause (Joborn et al., 1991). Estrogen repletion can restore the calcemic and hydroxyproline responses to near normal, suggesting that estrogen inhibits the resorptive effects of PTH. Whether estrogen exerts similar effects in men, or whether the age-related fall in circulating testosterone also influences bone sensitivity to PTH have not been examined.

TABLE V Age-Related Changes[a] in Mineral Metabolism in Men and Women

	Men	Women
Dietary Ca and P	↓	↓
Vitamin D synthesis in skin	↓	↓
Serum 25-OH-D	↓	↓
Serum 1,25(OH)$_2$D	NC, ↓	NC, ↓
Serum PTH	↑	↑
Serum Ca	NC, ↓	NC, ↓
Serum P	↓	NC
Intestinal Ca absorption	NC, ↓	NC, ↓
Creatinine clearance	↓	↓

[a] The changes in mineral metabolism that occur with advancing age are strongly influenced by health status and life-style. The changes indicated repesent those generally observed in free-living elderly men and women.

V. Conclusion

Aging stems from a time-dependent change in somatic cell function. Proliferative potential diminishes, and cell metabolic activity is altered. As a consequence, mineral metabolism is similarly altered in men and women (Table V). Changes in parathyroid gland responsiveness to Ca and diminished bioavailability of Ca brought about by reduced dietary intake and impaired intestinal absorption stimulate PTH secretion. Diminished vitamin D production in the skin reduces substrate (25-OH-D) availability to the renal 1-hydroxylase and limits analogue effects of 25-OH-D on PTH secretion and intestinal Ca absorption. Progressive loss of the tonic stimulatory effects of GH, IGF-I, and sex steroids on renal 1-hydroxylase activity are offset by a gradual rise in circulating PTH so that 1,25(OH)$_2$D production and serum concentration, at least in healthy elderly, are normal. The accompanying mild hyperparathyroidism increases urinary P excretion and the lability of the bone Ca pool. The alteration in the relationship between PTH and 1,25(OH)$_2$D, as well as senescent changes in bone cells shift the source of Ca from intestinal absorption to bone demineralization. Osteopenia and osteoporosis predictably ensue.

References

Akerstrom, G., Rudberg, C., and Grimelius, L. (1986). Histological parathyroid abnormalities in an autopsy series. *Hum. Pathol.* **17**, 520–527.

Aksnes, L., Rodland, O., and Aarskog, D. (1988). Serum levels of vitamin D_3 and 25-hydroxy-vitamin D_3 in elderly and young adults. *Bone Miner.* **3**, 351–3537.

Autry, C. P., Kifor, O., Brown, E. M., Fuller, F. H., Rogers, K. V., and Halloran, B. P. (1997). Ca^{2+} receptor mRNA and protein increase in the rat parathyroid gland with advancing age. *J. Endocrinol.* **153**, 437–444.

Avioli, L., McDonald, J., and Lee, S. (1965). Influence of age on intestinal absorption of Ca in women. *J. Clin. Invest.* **44**, 1960–1967.

Bikle, D. D., Halloran, B. P., Harris, S. T., and Portale, A. A. (1992). Progestin antagonism of estrogen stimulated 1,25-dihydroxyvitamin D levels. *J. Clin. Endocrinol. Metab.* **72**, 519–523.

Bilezikian, J. P., Marcus, R., and Levine, M. A., eds. (1994). "The Parathyroids: Basic and Clinical Concepts." Raven Press, New York.

Boucher, A., D'Amour, P., Hamel, L., Fugere, P., Gascon-Barre, M., Lepage, R., and Ste-Marie, L. G. (1989). Estrogen replacement decreases the set point of parathyroid hormone stimulation by calcium in normal postmenopausal women. *J. Clin. Endocrinol. Metab.* **68**, 831–836.

Carlin, C., Phillips, P., Knowles, B., and Cristofalo, V. (1983). Diminished in vitro tyrosine kinase activity of the EGF receptor of senescent human fibroblasts. *Nature (London)* **306**, 617–620.

Caverzasio, J., and Bonjour, J.-P. (1989). IGF-I stimulates Na-dependent P transport in cultured kidney cells. *Am. J. Physiol.* **257**, F712–F717.

Chapuy, M. C., Schott, A. M., Garnero, P., Hans, D., Delmas, P. D., and Meunier, P. J. (1996). Healthy elderly french women living at home have secondary hyperparathyroidism and high bone turnover in winter. *J. Clin. Endocrinol. Metab.* **81**, 1129–1133.

Chen, T. S., Currier, G. J., and Wabner, C. L. (1990). Intestinal transport during the life span of a mouse. *J. Gerontol.* **45**, B129–B133.

Clemens, T. L., Zhou, X. Y., Myles, M., Endres, D., and Lindsay, R. (1986). Serum vitamin D_3 and vitamin D_2 concentrations and absorption of vitamin D_2 in elderly subjects. *J. Clin. Endocrinol. Metab.* **63**, 656–660.

Condamine, L., Vztovsnik, F., and Garabedian, M. (1994). Local action of phosphate depletion and IGF-I on in vitro production of $1,25(OH)_2D$ by kidney cells. *J. Clin. Invest.* **94**, 1673–1679.

Cooke, N. E., and Haddad, J. G. (1997). Vitamin D binding protein. *In* "Vitamin D" D. Feldman, F. H. Glorieux, J. W. Pike (eds.), pp. 87–101. Academic Press, San Diego, CA.

Corpas, E., Harman, M., and Blackman, M. R. (1993). Human growth hormone and human aging. *Endocrinol. Rev.* **14**, 20–39.

Crowley, K., and Curtis, H. J. (1963). The development of somatic mutations in mice with age. *Proc. Natl. Acad. Sci. U.S.A.* **49**, 626–628.

Dawson-Hughes, B., Harris, S. S., and Dallal, G. E. (1997a). Plasma calcidiol, season, and serum parathyroid hormone concentration in healthy elderly men and women. *Am. J. Clin. Nutr.* **65**, 67–71.

Dawson-Hughes, B., Harris, S. S., Krall, E. A., and Dallal, G. E. (1997b). Effect of calcium and vitamin D supplementation on bone density in men and women 65 years of age or older. *N. Engl. J. Med.* **337**, 670–676.

Deftos, L. J., Weisman, M. H., and Williams, G. W. (1980). The influence of age and sex on plasma calcitonon in human beings. *N. Engl. J. Med.* **302**, 1351–1353.

Dice, J. F. (1989). Altered protein degradation in aging: A possible cause of proliferative arrest. *Exp. Gerontol.* **24**, 451–459.

Dice, F. J. (1993). Cellular and molecular mechanisms of aging. *Physiol. Rev.* **73**, 149–159.

Dick, I. M., Prince, R. L., Kelly, J. J., and Ho, K. K. (1995). Estrogen effects on calcitrol levels in postmenopausal women: A comparison of oral verses transdermal administration. *Clin. Endocrinol.* **43**, 219–224.

Eastell, R., Yergey, A. L., Vierira, N. E., Cedel, S. E., Kumar, R., and Riggs, B. L. (1991). Interrelationship among vitamin D metabolism, true calcium absorption, parathyroid function and age in women: Evidence of age-related intestinal resistance to 1,25(OH)$_2$D. *J. Bone Miner. Res.* **6**, 125–132.

Ebeling, P. R., Sandgren, M. E., DiMagno, E. P., Lane, A. W., DeLuca, H. F., and Riggs, B. L. (1992). Evidence of an age-related decrease in intestinal responsiveness to vitamin D: Relationship between serum 1,25-dihydroxyvitamin D$_3$ and intestinal vitamin D receptor concentrations in normal women. *J. Clin. Endocrinol. Metab.* **75**, 176–182.

Ebeling, P. R., Yergey, A. L., Vieira, N. E., Burritt, M. F., O'Fallon, W. M., Kumar, R., and Riggs, B. L. (1994). Influence of age on effects of endogenous 1,25-Dihydroxyvitamin D on calcium absorption in normal women. *Calcif. Tissue Int.* **55**, 330–334.

Endres, D. B., Morgan, C. H., Garry, P. J., and Omdahl, J. L. (1987). Age-related changes in serum immunoreactive parathyroid hormone and its biological action in healthy men and women. *J. Clin. Endocrinol. Metab.* **65**, 724–731.

Epstein, S., Bryce, G., and Hinman, J. W. (1986). The influence of age on bone mineral regulating hormones. *Bone* **7**, 421–425.

Feldman, D., Glorieux, F. H., and Pike, J. W., eds. (1997). "Vitamin D." Academic Press, San Diego, CA.

Ferraris, R. P., and Vinnakota, R. R. (1993). Regulation of intestinal nutrient transport is impaired in aged mice. *J. Nutr.* **123**, 502–511.

Fleming, B. B., and Barrows, C. H. (1982). The influence of aging on intestinal absorption of vitamins A and D by the rat. *Exp. Gerontol.* **17**, 115–120.

Florini, J. R., Prinz, P. N., Vitiello, M. V., and Hintz, R. L. (1985). Somatomedin C levels in healthy young and old men: Relationship to peak and 24-hour integrated levels of growth hormone. *J. Gerontol.* **40**, 2–7.

Forero, M. S., Klein, R. F., Nissenson, R. A., Nelson, K., Heath, H., III, Arnaud, C. D., and Riggs, B. L. (1987). Effect of age on circulating immuno-reactive and bioactive parathyroid hormone levels in women. *J. Bone Miner. Res.* **2**, 363–366.

Fox, J., and Mathew, M. (1991). Heterogeneous response to PTH in aging rats. *Am. J. Physiol.* **260**, E933–E937.

Fujisawa, Y., Kida, K., and Matsuda, H. (1984). Role of change in vitamin D metabolism with age on calcium and phosphorus metabolism in normal human subjects. *J. Clin. Endocrinol. Metab.* **59**, 719–726.

Gallagher, C., Riggs, B. L., Eisman, J. A., Hamstra, A., Arnaud, S. B., and DeLuca, H. F. (1979). Intestinal calcium absorption and vitamin D metabolites in normal subjects and osteoporotic patients. *J. Clin. Invest.* **64**, 729–736.

Garcia de la Asuncion, J., Millan, A., Pla, R., Bruseghini, A. E., Pallardo, F. V., Sastre, J., and Vina, J. (1996). Mitochondrial oxidation correlates with age-associated oxidative damage to mitochondrial DNA. *FASEB J.* **10**, 333–338.

Garnero, P., Hausherr, E., Chapuy, M.-C., Marcelli, C., Grandjean, H., and Delmas, P. D. (1996). Markers of bone resorption predict hip fracture in elderly women: The EPIDOS Prospective Study. *J. Bone Miner. Res.* **11**, 1531–1538.

Gennari, C., and Agnusdei, D. (1990). Calcitonin, esrogens and the bone. *J. Steroid Biochem. Mol. Biol.* **37**, 451–455.

Ghadially, R., Brown, B. E., Sequeira-Martin, S. M., Feingold, K. R., and Elias, P. M. (1995). The aged epidermal permeability barrier. *J. Clin. Invest.* **95**, 2281–2290.

Gloth, F. M., Gundberg, C. M., Hollis, B. W., Haddad, J. G., and Tobin, J. D. (1995). Vitamin D deficiency in homebound elderly persons. *J. Am. Med. Assoc.* **274**, 1683–1686.

Grimelius, L., Akerstrom, G., and Bergstrom, R. (1981). Anatomy of human parathyroid glands. *Pathol. Ann.* **16**, 1–20.

Grove, G. L., and Kligman, A. M. (1983). Age-associated changes in human epidermal cell renewal. *J. Gerontol.* **38**, 137–142.

Hagenfeldt, Y., Linde, K., Sjoberg, H. E., and Arver, S. (1992). Testosterone increases serum 1,25(OH)$_2$D and IGF in hypogonadal men. *Int. J. Androl.* **15**, 93–102.

Halloran, B. P., and Spencer, E. M. (1988). Dietary phosphorus and 1,25-Dihidroxyvitamin D metabolism: Influence of insulin-like growth factor. *J. Endocrinol.* **123**, 1225–1229.

Halloran, B. P., Portale, A. A., Lonergan, E. T., and Morris, R. C. (1990). Production and metabolic clearance of 1,25(OH)$_2$D in men: Effect of advancing age. *J. Clin. Endocrinol. Metab.* **70**, 318–323.

Halloran, B. P., Lonergan, E. T., and Portale, A. A. (1996). Aging and renal responsiveness to PTH in healthy men. *J. Clin. Endocrinol. Metab.* **81**, 2192–2197.

Hammerman, M. R., Karl, I. E., and Kruska, K. A. (1980). Regulation of canine renal vesicle P transport by growth hormone and PTH. *Bochim. Biophys. Acta* **603**, 322–335.

Hanai, H., Liang, c., Cheng, L., and Sacktor, B. (1989). Desensitization to PTH in renal cells in aged rats is associated with alterations in G-protein activity. *J. Clin. Invest.* **83**, 268–277.

Harley, C. B., Goldstein, S., and Posner, B. (1981). Decreased sensitivity of old and progeric human fibroblasts to a preparation of factors with insulin-like activities. *J. Clin. Invest.* **68**, 988–994.

Hayflick, L. (1975). Current theories of aging. *Fed. Proc.* **34**, 9–13

Heaney, R., Recker, R., Stegman, M., and Moy, A. (1989). Calcium absorption in women. *J. Bone Miner. Res.* **4**, 469–475.

Holick, M. F., Matsuoka, L. Y., and Wortsman, J. (1989). Age, vitamin D and solar ultraviolet. *Lancet* **2**, 1104–1105.

Holt, P., and Yeh, K. (1989). Intestinal crypt cell proliferation are increased in senescent rats. *J. Gerontol.* **44**, B9–B14.

Hulter, H. N., Halloran, B. P., Toto, R. D., and Peterson, J. C. (1985). Long term control of calcitriol concentration in dog and man: The dominant role of plasma calcium concentration in experimental hyperparathyroidism. *J. Clin. Invest.* **76**, 695–702.

Ishida, M., Bulos, B., Takamoto, S., and Sacktor, B. (1987). Hydroxylation of 25-Hydroxyvitamin D3 by renal mitochondria from rats of different ages. *Endocrinology* **121**, 443–448.

Joborn, C., Ljunghall, S., Larsson, K., and Rastad, J. (1991). Skeletal responsiveness to PTH. *Clin. Endocrinol.* **34**, 335–339.

Johnson, J., Beckman, M., Christokos, S., Horst, R., and Reinhardt, T. (1995). Age and gender effects of 1,25(OH)$_2$D-regulated gene expression. *Exp. Gerontol.* **30**, 631–643.

Khosla, S., Atkinson, E., Melton, J., and Riggs, B. L. (1997). Effects of age and estrogen status on serum PTH and biochemical markers of bone turnover in women. *J. Clin. Endocrinol. Metab.* **82**, 1522–1527.

Kinyamu, H. K., Gallagher, J. C., Petranick, K. M., and Ryschon, K. L. (1996). Effect of parathyroid hormone (hPTH[1-34]) infusion on serum 1,25-Dihydroxyvitamin D and parathyroid hormone in normal women. *J. Bone Miner. Res.* **11**, 1400–1405.

Kinyamu, H. K., Gallagher, J. C., Prahl, J. M., Deluca, H. F., Petranick, K. M., and Lanspa, S. J. (1997). Association between intestinal vitamin D receptor, calcium absorption, and serum 1,25 Dihydroxyvitamin D in normal young and elderly women. *J. Bone Miner. Res.* **12**, 922–928.

Krall, E., Sahyoun, N., Dallal, G., and Dawson-Hughes, B. (1989). Effect of vitamin D intake on seasonal variations in PTH secretion in postmenopausal women. *N. Engl. J Med.* **321**, 1777–1783.

Lamberts, S., van den Beld, A., and van der Levy, A. (1997). The endocrinology of aging. *Science* **278**, 419–424.

Lavker, R. M. (1979). Structural alterations in exposed and unexposed aged skin. *J. Invest. Dermatol.* **73**, 59–66.

Ledger, G. A., Burritt, M. F., Kao, P. C., O'Fallon, W. M., Riggs, B. L., and Khosla, S. (1994). Abnormalities of PTH secretion in elderly women that are reversible by short term therapy with 1,25(OH)$_2$D. *J. Clin. Endocrinol. Metab.* **79**, 211–216.

Liang, C. T., Barnes, J., Sacktor, B., and Takamoto, S. (1991). Alterations of duodenal vitamin D-dependent calcium-binding protein content and calcium uptake in brush border membrane vesicles in aged Wistar rats: Role of 1,25-dihydroxyvitamin D$_3$. *Endocrinology* **128**, 1780–1784.

Liang, C. T., Barnes, J., Imanaka, S., and DeLuca, H. F. (1994). Alterations in mRNA expression of duodenal 1,25-dihydroxyvitamin D_3 receptor and vitamin D-dependent calcium binding protein in aged rats. *Exp. Gerontol.* **29**, 179–186.

Lieberman, S. A., Holloway, L., Marcus, R., and Hoffman, A. R. (1994). Interactions of growth hormone and parathyroid hormone in renal phosphate, calcium and calcitrol metabolism and bone remodeling in postmenopausal women. *J. Bone Miner. Res.* **9**, 1723–1728.

Lindeman, R. D., Tobin, J., and Shock, N. W. (1985). Longitudinal studies on the rate of decline or renal function with age. *J. Am. Geriatr. Soc.* **33**, 278–285.

MacLaughlin, J., and Holick, M. F. (1985). Aging decreases the capacity of human skin to produce vitamin D. *J. Clin. Invest.* **76**, 1536–1538.

Manolagas, S., Culler, F. L., Howard, J. E., Brickman, A. S., and Deftos, L. J. (1983). The cytoreceptor assay for $1,25(OH)_2D$ and its application to clinical studies. *J. Clin. Endocrinol. Metab.* **56**, 751–760.

Marcus, R., Madvig, P., and Young, G. (1984). Age related changes in PTH and PTH action in normal humans. *J. Clin. Endocrinol. Metab.* **58**, 233–230.

Marcus, R., Butterfield, G., Holloway, L., Gilland, L., Baylink, D., Hintz, R., and Sherman, B. (1990). Effects of short term administration of recombinant human growth hormone to elderly people. *J. Clin. Endocrinol. Metab.* **70**, 519–523.

Martin, F. C., Ai-Lyn, Y., and Sonksen, P. H. (1997). Growth hormone secretion in the elderly: Ageing and the somatopause. *Bailliere's Clin. Endocrinol. Metab.* **11**, 223–250.

Matsuoka, L. Y., Wortsman, J., Hanifin, and Holick, M. F. (1988). Chronic sunscreen use decreases circulating concentrations of 25-hydroxyvitamin D. *Arch. Dermatol.* **124**, 1802–1804.

McCormick, A., and Campisi, J. (1991). Cellular aging and senescence. *Curr. Opin. Cell Biol.* **3**, 230–234.

McKane, W. R., Khosla, S., Egan, K. S., Robins, S. P., Burritt, M., and Riggs, B. L. (1996). Role of calcium intake in modulating age-related increases in parathyroid function and bone resorption. *J. Clin. Endocrinol. Metab.* **81**, 1699–1703.

McKenna, M. J. (1992). Differences in vitamin D status between countries in young adults and the elderly. *Am. J. Med.* **93**, 69–77.

Minisola, S., Pacitti, M., and Scarda, A. (1993). Serum ionized calcium, parathyroid hormone and related variables: Effect of age and sex. *J. Bone Miner.* **23**, 183–193.

Miyamoto, A., and Ohshika, H. (1994). Expression of Gs alpha mRNA in rat ventricular myocardium with aging. *Eur. J. Pharmacol.* **266**, 147–154.

Morley, J. E., Perry, H. M., Kaiser, F. E., and Perry, H. M., Jr. (1993). Effects of testosterone replacement therapy in old hypogonadal males. *J. Am. Geriatr. Soc.* **41**, 149–152.

Need, A. G., Morris, H. A., Horowitz, M., and Nordin, C. (1993). Effects of skin thickness, age, body fat and sunlight on serum 25-OH-D. *Am. J. Clin. Nutr.* **58**, 882–885.

Omdahl, J. L., Garry, P. J., Hunsaker, L. A., Hunt, W. C., and Goodwin, J. S. (1982). Nutritional status in a healthy elderly population: Vitamin D. *Am. J. Clin. Nutr.* **36**, 1225–1233.

Orwoll, E. S., and Meier, D. (1986). Alterations in calcium, vitamin D and PTH physiology in normal men with aging. *J. Clin. Endocrinol. Metab.* **63**, 1262–1269.

Ozawa, T. (1997). Genetic and functional changes in mitochondria associated with aging. *Physiol. Rev.* **77**, 425–464.

Pfeilschifter, J., Diel, I., Pilz, U., and Zeigler, R. (1993). Mitogenic responsiveness of human bone cells in vitro to hormones and growth factors decreases with age. *J. Bone Miner. Res.* **8**, 707–717.

Portale, A., Halloran, B., Morris, R., and Longergan, E. T. (1996). Effect of aging on the metabolism of P and $1,25(OH)_2D$ in men. *Am. J. Physiol.* **270**, E483–E490.

Portale, A. A., Lonergan, E. T., Tanney, D. M., and Halloran, B. P. (1997). Aging alters calcium regulation of serum concentration of parathyroid hormone in healthy men. *Am. J. Physiol.* **272** (Part 1), E139, E146.

Prince, R. L., Dick, I., Garcia, W. P., and Retallack, R. W. (1990). The effects of the menopause on calcitriol and PTH: Responses to a low dietary calcium stress test. *J. Clin. Endocrinol. Metab.* **70,** 1119–1123.

Quesada, J. M., Coopmans, W., Ruiz, B., Aljama, P., Jans, I., and Bouillon, R. (1992). Influence of vitamin D on parathyroid function in the elderly. *J. Clin. Endocrinol. Metab.* **75,** 494–501.

Reginster, J. Y., Deroisy, R., Albert, A., Denis, D., Lacart, M. P., Collette, J., and Franchimont, P. (1989). Relationship between whole plasma calcitonon levels, calcitonon secretory capacity, and plasma levels of estrone in healthy women and postmenopausal osteoporotics. *J. Clin. Invest.* **83,** 1073–1077.

Russell, J., Littieri, D., and Sherwood, L. (1986). Suppression by 1,25(OH)$_2$D of transcription of the pre-parathyroid hormone gene. *Endocrinology* **119,** 2864–2870.

Sherman, S. S., Hollis, B. W., and Tobin, J. D. (1990). Vitamin D status and related parameters in a healthy population: The effects of age, sex, and season. *J. Clin. Endocrinol. Metab.* **71,** 405–413.

Slovik, S. M., Adams, J. S., Neer, R. M., Holick, M. F., and Potts, J. T. (1981). Deficient production of 1,25(OH)$_2$D in elderly patients. *N. Engl. J. Med.* **305,** 372–374.

Szabo, A., Merke, J., Beier, E., and Ritz, E. (1989). 1,25(OH)$_2$D inhibits parathyroid cell proliferation in uremia. *Kidney Int.* **35,** 1049–1056.

Tiegs, R. D., Body, J. J., and Barta, J. M. (1986). Secretion and metabolism of monomeric human calcitonin: Effects of age, sex and thyroid damage. *J. Bone Miner. Res.* **1,** 339.

Tsai, K. S., Health, H., Kumar, R., and Riggs, B. L. (1984). Impaired vitamin D metabolism with aging in women. *J. Clin. Invest.* **73,** 1668–1672.

Tsuchida, Y. (1993). The effect of aging and arteriosclerosis on human skin and blood flow. *J. Dermatol. Sci.* **5,** 175–181.

Van der Wielen, R. P., Lowik, M. R., van den Berg, H., de Groot, L. C., Haller, J., Moreiras, O., and van Staveren, W. A. (1995). Serum vitamin D concentrations among elderly people in Europe. *Lancet* **346,** 207–210.

Webb, A. R., Kline, L., and Holick, M. F. (1988). Influence of season and latitude on cutaneous synthesis of vitamin D$_3$. *J. Clin. Endocrinol. Metab.* **67,** 373–378.

Chapter 11

Bess Dawson-Hughes

Jean Mayer USDA Human Nutrition Research Center on Aging
at Tufts University
Boston, Massachusetts

Calcium and Vitamin D Nutrition[1]

I. Introduction

The relationship between calcium and vitamin D intakes and bone health in adults has been examined in some detail in the last few years. Although most of the studies have been conducted in women, some data are now emerging in men. This chapter will review the effects of calcium and vitamin D intake on calcium-regulating hormone levels, on rates of bone turnover, and on rates of change in bone mineral density (BMD) in men. Findings in men will be compared with women.

[1]The contents of this publication do not necessarily reflect the views or policies of U.S. Department of Agriculture, nor does mention of trade names, commercial products, or organizations imply endorsement by the U.S. government.

II. Calcium and Vitamin D Metabolism

Calcium and vitamin D influence the skeleton both directly and indirectly, by inducing changes in calcium-regulating hormone levels. As illustrated in Figure 1, an inadequate intake of either calcium or vitamin D results in a reduced amount of absorbed calcium and a slightly lower blood concentration of ionized calcium. In response to this, the blood parathyroid hormone (PTH) concentration increases. PTH stimulates bone turnover, and a higher bone turnover rate increases risk of fragility fractures by reducing BMD (Cummings *et al.*, 1993) and by other mechanisms that are not well understood (Garnero *et al.*, 1996b). Much of the evidence supporting this sequence has been accrued in women. More recently, comparative data are becoming available in men.

Several studies have compared 25-hydroxyvitamin D (25(OH)D) levels in men and women. In reports from Europe (Stamp and Round, 1974), Japan (Kobayashi *et al.*, 1983), and the United States (Omdahl *et al.*, 1982; Sherman *et al.*, 1990), 25(OH)D levels were higher in men than in women. The one report of higher 25(OH)D levels in women was in a small group of vitamin D-deficient subjects in Montreal, Canada (Delvin *et al.*, 1988). Several of these studies compared 25(OH)D levels in men and women in different seasons. Kobayashi *et al.* (1983) found men to have relatively higher 25(OH)D levels in summer, whereas Omdahl *et al.* (1982) and Sherman *et al.* (1990) found disproportionately higher 25(OH)D levels in men throughout the year. In men and women over age 65 who enrolled in the National Institute on Aging STOP/IT trial in Boston (latitude 42°N), plasma 25(OH)D levels were higher in men than in women during the time of year when sun exposure promotes vitamin D synthesis but similar in the two groups in the winter and spring when the diet is the major source of vitamin D (Table I;

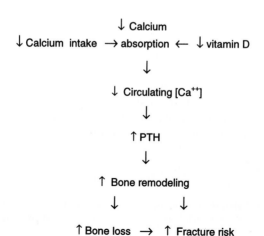

FIGURE 1   Interface of calcium and vitamin D intakes and the skeleton.

TABLE I.   Mean Plasma 25-Hydroxyvitamin D Concentrations by
Season and Travel History in Men and Women[a]

Measurement periods	Plasma 25-hydroxyvitamin D, nmol/L	
	Men	Women
February–May		
Nontravelers	56.9 ± 19.4 [47]	55.6 ± 22.4 [73]
Travelers[b]	82.9 ± 30.7 [5]	73.6 ± 25.4 [10]
June–September		
Nontravelers	104.9 ± 35.0 [50]	82.3 ± 34.8 [64]
Travelers	94.8 ± 16.9 [5]	83.2 ± 23.6 [3]
October–January		
Nontravelers	83.5 ± 36.0 [71]	69.2 ± 35.3 [57]
Travelers	65.5 ± 11.2 [4]	67.4 ± 10.6 [2]

[a]Mean ± SD; n in brackets.
[b]The average number of days spent at latitudes ≤ 35°N was, for men and
women, respectively: February–May, 11 ± 4 and 11 ± 8; June–September,
8 ± 3 and 9 ± 2; October–January 8 ± 5 and 13 ± 8.
Reprinted with permission from Dawson-Hughes *et al.* (1997a), © *Am. J.
Clin. Nutr.* American Society for Clinical Nutrition.

Dawson-Hughes *et al.*, 1997a). In both men and women, mean 25(OH)D levels
varied by season and were lowest in the winter and early spring. Time spent
outdoors and vitamin D intake were positively associated with 25(OH)D
levels, and weight and age were negatively associated with 25(OH)D levels
in these men and women. Notably, short-term travel in the wintertime to
locations below 35°N, where sun exposure promotes vitamin D production
in the skin throughout the year (Webb *et al.*, 1988), was sufficient to raise
25(OH)D concentrations to levels attained during the summer.

Serum PTH and 25(OH)D levels are usually found to be inversely associated, as indicated in Figure 1. An important consideration is whether PTH
levels at different concentrations of 25(OH)D are similar in men and women.
The Boston STOP/IT cohort is suitable for this analysis because the men and
women had similar mean calcium intakes (Dawson-Hughes *et al.*, 1997a).
As expected, serum PTH concentrations were significantly higher at lower
levels of 25(OH)D in the men (ANOVA, $P = 0.032$) and the women ($P =
0.002$, Table II). In each category of 25(OH)D concentration, mean PTH
levels were similar in the men and women. This suggests that the regulation
of PTH by vitamin D, although indirect, is similar in older men and women.

III. PTH Response to Calcium and Vitamin D _____

Another way to compare calcium regulating the hormonal axis in men
and women is to compare changes in serum PTH concentration after supple-

TABLE II.   Mean Parathyroid Hormone Concentrations by Category of Plasma 25-Hydroxyvitamin D Concentration[a]

Plasma 25-hydroxyvitamin D, nmol/L	Serum parathyroid hormone, pmol/L[b]	
	Men	Women
0–50	4.29 ± 1.81 [36]	4.68 ± 1.92 [65]
51–75	4.19 ± 2.17 [52]	3.86 ± 1.51 [80]
76–100	3.44 ± 1.32 [48]	3.73 ± 1.38 [35]
101–125	3.42 ± 1.75 [27]	3.27 ± 1.42 [15]
> 125	3.24 ± 0.88 [19]	3.56 ± 1.17 [14]

[a]Mean ± SD; n in brackets.
[b]Serum parathyroid hormone concentrations changed significantly with changes in concentrations in men, $P = 0.032$ and women, $P = 0.002$, (ANOVA).
Reprinted with permission from Dawson-Hughes *et al.* (1997a), © *Am. J. Clin. Nutr.* American Society for Clinical Nutrition.

mentation with calcium and vitamin D. This was done in STOP/IT subjects (146 men, 147 women) who adhered to treatment with placebo or calcium plus vitamin D (500 mg and 700 IU, respectively) daily for 3 years (Dawson-Hughes *et al.*, 1997b). The men and women were similar in age (mean 71 years) and had similar dietary intakes of vitamin D as well as calcium. With supplementation, urinary calcium excretion rose dramatically, reflecting increased amounts of absorbed calcium. Serum PTH levels, initially similar in the men and women, rose gradually over 3 years in subjects taking placebo and declined in those taking the supplements. At the end of 3 years, the mean PTH level in the supplemented group was 23% lower than that in placebo among the men, and 33% lower among the women. This indicates that the long-term PTH response to calcium and vitamin D supplementation is similar in healthy, older men and women. Responses of younger men and women have not been systematically compared.

IV. Calcium, Vitamin D, and Bone Turnover

One intermediary endpoint for assessing the effect of calcium and vitamin D on the skeleton is change in the bone turnover rate. Serum osteocalcin is a common indicator of bone formation and, because of coupling, also bone turnover. Urine pyridinoline crosslinks reflect bone resorption and turnover. Men appear to have lower turnover rates than women, throughout the age range of 30 to 90 years, as measured by serum osteocalcin (Epstein *et al.*, 1984) and urinary pyridinoline levels (Delmas *et al.*, 1993). The sex difference becomes more exaggerated after age 50, reflecting the increase in turnover in women after menopause (Ebeling *et al.*, 1996).

A higher remodeling rate has been associated with lower bone mass. This association, initially identified in women (Garnero *et al.*, 1996a), has also been seen in a cross-sectional study of 1087 healthy older men and women (Krall *et al.*, 1997). Although mean osteocalcin and N-teleopeptide levels were lower and BMD values were higher in the men, these biochemical markers of bone turnover were as effective in predicting BMD in men as they were in women. Although biochemical markers of bone turnover appear to predict fracture risk independent of BMD (Garnero *et al.*, 1996b), evidence for this is limited to studies in women.

The effects of supplemental calcium (Chevalley *et al.*, 1994; Elders *et al.*, 1994; Riis *et al.*, 1987) and vitamin D (Dawson-Hughes *et al.*, 1995; Ooms *et al.*, 1995) alone and combined (Chapuy *et al.*, 1992) on changes in bone turnover have been examined in several randomized, placebo-controlled studies in women. In these studies, supplementation induced a modest, and often not statistically significant, decrement in serum osteocalcin, averaging about 10%. Prince *et al.* (1995) reported an even more modest decrease in urinary deoxypyridinoline concentration of 4% as a result of calcium supplementation. In another study, 500 mg of supplemental calcium per day induced no change in the urinary N-telopeptide : creatinine ratio in postmenopausal women (Chesnut *et al.*, 1997).

We recently compared the long-term effect of combined calcium and vitamin D supplementation on rates of bone turnover in men and women in the Boston STOP/IT study (Dawson-Hughes *et al.*, 1997b). Supplementation with 500 mg of calcium and 700 IU of vitamin D produced significant and sustained reductions in serum osteocalcin levels in the men and women (Table III). Treatment group differences after 3 years were similar in the

TABLE III.   Initial and Final Laboratory Values in Adherent Subjects[a]

	Men (n = 146)			Women (n = 167)		
	Initial	*Final*	P^b	*Initial*	*Final*	P^b
Serum osteocalcin, nmol/L						
Placebo	0.98 ± 0.32	1.02 ± 0.32[c]	0.24	1.21 ± 0.42	1.21 ± 0.43[c]	0.90
Ca + vit D	0.91 ± 0.23	0.83 ± 0.28	0.003	1.19 ± 0.42	1.03 ± 0.33	<0.001
24-hr N-telopeptide: Cr, nmol/mmol						
Placebo	31.6 ± 15.9	32.2 ± 16.2[d]	0.60	47.6 ± 29.6	45.8 ± 23.4	0.59
Ca + vit D	28.7 ± 9.2	26.6 ± 11.5	0.16	44.8 ± 16.7	42.4 ± 21.6	0.22

[a]Mean ± SD.
[b]These P values are for comparisons of initial with final values, within each treatment group.
[c]Placebo differs from calcium and vitamin D at $P < 0.005$.
[d]Placebo differs from calcium and vitamin D at $P < 0.05$.
Reprinted with permission from Dawson-Hughes *et al.* (1997a), © *Am. J. Clin. Nutr.* American Society for Clinical Nutrition.

men and women (0.19 and 0.18 nmol/L, respectively), representing decrements of 19% and 15%, respectively. After 3 years, the mean 24-hr urinary N-telopeptide : creatinine ratio was significantly lower in men receiving the supplements than in those on placebo (17%). The decrease in women was more modest (7%) and not statistically significant. These data indicate that older men with calcium and vitamin D intakes similar to the 1989 Recommended Dietary Allowances of 800 mg and 200 IU, respectively, can lower their bone turnover rates over the long term by increasing their intakes of calcium and vitamin D. Having considered the effects of calcium and vitamin D on bone turnover, we will now turn to the evidence that calcium and vitamin D intake regulate bone mass in men.

V. Calcium, Vitamin D, and the Skeleton

Because calcium is the major mineral component of bone, it follows that calcium substrate deficiency will result in lower bone calcium content. But calcium and vitamin D have other actions on bone as evidenced by their effects on bone turnover as described earlier. In subjects with an inadequate intake of calcium and vitamin D, increasing intake of these nutrients increases skeletal calcium content; however, further increases in intake, beyond need, will not confer additional benefit to the skeleton. Several approaches have been taken to identify the plateau intake, defined as the intake associated with maximal skeletal retention of calcium.

A. Calcium Balance Studies

Historically, the calcium balance approach was used to identify the calcium requirement. Although short-term in nature, balance studies are valuable because they can provide data on a wide range of intakes. The intake associated with zero calcium balance was frequently used as an endpoint in balance studies, but this choice is limiting in several respects. First, one component of the calcium balance equation, sweat calcium losses, is rarely measured, and this source of error is usually ignored. Second, zero calcium balance is rarely maintained by groups of individuals at risk for osteoporosis, such as the elderly. It is estimated that older postmenopausal women lose bone mass at a rate of about 1% per year and that men loss at about half this rate. In older individuals, a small but discrete amount of calcium is lost from the skeleton with each remodeling cycle. Losses are compounded by many factors that are unrelated to calcium or vitamin D intake, such as lack of physical exercise, loss of estrogen at menopause, and smoking. A useful balance study endpoint is to identify the calcium intake that promotes maximal calcium retention, or the plateau intake. This application of balance data has several advantages. Estimation of the plateau intake does not require quantification of sweat calcium losses, nor does it depend upon the absolute amount of calcium lost or gained at any given intake. In order to identify the plateau intake, a balance study must include a large number of subjects, and the subjects must have a wide range and fairly even distribution of usual calcium intakes. One such balance study has been reported in men. Spencer *et al.* (1984) reported 181 balance measurements in men, age 34 through 71 years. The men were studied on six different calcium intake levels, ranging from 234 to 2320 mg per day. Milk or calcium gluconate supplements were used to reach the higher intake levels. Adaptation periods on the diets were adequate and ranged from 29 to 38 days. Results of these balance studies are shown in Table IV. Calcium balance became significantly more positive as intake increased from 234 to 804 mg per day and from 804 to 1230 mg per day. However, calcium balance did not increase significantly with dietary increases from 1230 to 1431 mg or higher. This places the plateau intake at about 1200 mg of calcium per day. This study also indicates that retention of calcium from milk and from the supplement calcium gluconate is similar. Malm (1958) also conducted a large balance study in men. In his study, men maintained calcium intakes of 460 and 940 mg per day. Balance was more positive at 940 mg intake than at 460 mg intake. Because both intakes studied are below 1200 mg per day, however, Malm's study is not useful in challenging or confirming the plateau intake identified by Spencer.

TABLE IV. Comparative Calcium Balances at Different Calcium Intakes

Calcium intake (mg/day)	No. of studies	Ca balance (mg/day)	Significance[a]
Calcium gluconate studies			
234[b]	22	−95	—
804	67	+22	0.005
1230	7	+106	0.001
1431	13	+104	NS
2021	12	+147	NS
2320	14	+139	NS
Milk studies			
810	22	+10	—
1248	15	+106	< 0.001
1467	9	+147	NS

[a]Significance in comparing calcium balance with the balance at previous calcium intake.
[b]Low calcium intake without the addition of calcium gluconate. All higher calcium intakes were achieved by adding calcium gluconate tablets to the constant low-calcium diet.
From Spencer *et al.* (1984), with permission.

Despite the fact that many elegant balance studies have been conducted in women, comparison of plateau intakes in men and women is difficult because very few balance studies have been conducted in women who were consuming more than 1000 mg of calcium per day. Two such studies have been reported in women with osteoporosis, but none are available in women drawn from the general population. Hasling et al. (1990) found a positive correlation between calcium intake and balance in 85 osteoporotic women with a mean calcium intake of 1225 mg per day. Selby (1994) studied 18 women and 7 men with a mean intake of 1214 mg per day. Again there was a positive correlation between intake and balance. Although the sample size was too small to allow firm conclusions, these older men and women appeared to fit on the same regression line. Balance studies in healthy women studied on a wider range of calcium intakes are needed in order to determine whether the plateau intake of 1200 mg per day identified in men is similar in postmenopausal women.

B. Bone Mineral Density

BMD is a valid intermediary endpoint for assessing the calcium and vitamin D requirements in adults because of the strong inverse association between BMD and fracture incidence. A one standard deviation decrease in hip BMD is associated with a 2.5-fold increased risk of hip fracture in women (Cummings et al., 1993). Presumably the same association applies to men. Intermediary endpoints are needed in studies of men because studies with fracture endpoints would require inordinately large sample sizes and/or duration.

Two randomized, controlled trials testing the effect of calcium plus vitamin D on rates of bone loss in men have been reported. Orwoll et al. (1990) treated 86 men, mean age 58 years (range 30 through 87 years) with either placebo or 1000 mg of elemental calcium and 800 IU of vitamin D daily for 3 years. The men had a relatively high usual mean calcium intake of 1159 mg per day, an intake near the plateau identified by Spencer et al. (1984). BMD was measured at the proximal and distal radius by single-photon absorptiometry and at the spine by dual-energy quantitative computed tomography. Over the 3 years, rates of loss in the two treatment groups were similar at each skeletal site. The main finding of this study, that bone loss cannot be attenuated in men consuming about 1200 mg per day of calcium by increasing intake of calcium and vitamin D, supports the plateau intake of 1200 mg identified by Spencer. The second reported trial in men tested placebo versus 500 mg of calcium plus 700 IU of vitamin D in 176 men age 65 and older (Dawson-Hughes et al., 1997b) participating in the Boston STOP/IT study. These men consumed about 700 mg of calcium and 200 IU of vitamin D per day in their diets. In contrast to the findings of Orwoll et al. (1990), supplementation significantly reduced bone loss from the spine, femoral neck, and total body. Results of this study are also consistent with the balance-based plateau intake of 1200 mg, in that increasing calcium intake from 700 to 1200 mg per day and taking a vitamin D supplement had a significant positive effect on net calcium retention in bone. Studies of the independent effects of calcium and vitamin D on BMD in men are not currently available.

VI. Recommended and Usual Intakes

A. Institute of Medicine Recommendations

After reviewing available evidence, the Institute of Medicine (IOM) (1997) of the National Academy of Sciences recently increased the recommended intakes of calcium and vitamin D for adult men and women (Table V). The calcium recommendations were based on the intakes needed by specific age groups to achieve the desired calcium balance. For adult men, the IOM defined this intake as that resulting in a calcium retention (or balance) of zero, which assumes no net gain or loss of bone mineral density. Supporting evidence was derived from calcium intervention trials with changes in BMD and fracture incidence as outcomes. There was insufficient evidence in the oldest age group (71 and over) to justify recommendations different from those for men and women aged 51 through 70 years. The 1997 calcium intake recommendations for adults represent the first increases since the Academy's initial recommendation of 800 mg in 1941.

The vitamin D intake recommendations were based on the intake needed to maintain the desired circulating level of 25-hydroxyvitamin D to prevent increases in the blood PTH level and to minimize bone loss. The recommendations assume that no vitamin D is available from sun-mediated skin synthesis. The vitamin D intake recommendation of 600 IU per day for the elderly represents a substantial increase above the 1989 value of 200 IU per day (National Research Council, 1989).

TABLE V.   Institute of Medicine Recommendations for Men and Women—1989 and 1997

	Calcium, mg		Vitamin D, IU	
Age	1989	1997	1989	1997
Intakes				
31–50	800	1000	200	200
51–70	800	1200	200	400
71+	800	1200	200	600
Upper limit				
All adults	—	2500	—	2000

B. Tolerable Upper Limits

For the first time, the IOM recommendations included a tolerable upper limit, defined as the maximal intake that can safely be consumed by normal subjects (Table V). For calcium, three potential adverse events were considered: nephrolithiasis, hypercalcemia with renal insufficiency (or milk alkali syndrome, MAS), and the interference of calcium with the absorption of other essential nutrients. High intakes of dietary calcium have been associated with a lower incidence of kidney stones in men and women (Curhan *et al.,* 1993, 1997). In contrast, high intakes of supplemental calcium increased the relative risk for kidney stones by 20% in women (Curhan *et al.,* 1997). A similar trend was noted in men (Curhan *et al.,* 1993). Since the 1982 review by Orwoll (1982), 26 cases of MAS have been reported. Of the three potential adverse effects, data adequate for identification of a dose-response relationship were available only for the MAS. Based on MAS data, the critical intake was defined as 5 g per day. Application of a safety factor of 2 resulted in a tolerable upper limit of 2500 mg per day for calcium.

For vitamin D, the tolerable upper limit was considered the highest intake known not to cause hypercalcemia. Based on the 3-month intervention study of Narang *et al.* (1984) and supporting evidence from other studies (Johnson *et al.,* 1980; Honkanen *et al.,* 1990), the critical intake was 2400 IU per day. At this intake level, serum calcium rose significantly, but the mean level remained in the normal range (Narang *et al.,* 1984). In contrast, an intake of 3800 IU per day increased the mean serum calcium to above 11 mg/dl. Application of a safety factor of 1.2 to the critical intake of 2400 IU resulted in a tolerable upper limit of 2000 IU of vitamin D per day for adults.

C. Usual Intakes in the United States

Based on the 1994 U.S. Department of Agriculture Continuing Survey of Food Intake of Individuals, men in the United States have median calcium intakes of 857 mg per day at ages 31 through 51, 708 mg at ages 51 through 70, and 702 mg at ages 71 and older. The medians have been adjusted for day-to-day variation by the method of Nusser *et al.* (1996). The median intakes for men in each age category are 30–40% below the recommended intake of 1200 mg per day. Comparable national intake data are not available for vitamin D, but several estimates place the mean intake at around 200 IU per day. This intake is inadequate for many over age 50.

VII. Conclusions _____

Many aspects of calcium and bone metabolism in men and women are similar. When their 25(OH)D levels and calcium intakes are similar, men and women have similar mean PTH levels. Although the bone turnover rate is lower in men than in women, the decrease induced by treatment with supplemental calcium and vitamin D is similar in the two groups. Evidence from calcium balance studies and from randomized, controlled calcium and vitamin D intervention trials indicates that a calcium intake of 1200 mg per day is needed to minimize bone loss in adult and older men. Men with a usual mean intake of 1200 mg per day did not benefit demonstrably from increasing their calcium intakes. These findings provided the basis for the recent increase in the recommended calcium intake from 800 to 1200 mg per day (IOM, 1997). Because the hormonal, bone turnover, and BMD responses of older men and women to changes in calcium and vitamin D intake are similar, it is reasonable to expect that men, like women, can reduce their risk of fracture by raising calcium and vitamin D intakes to recommended levels. However, direct evidence for this is needed.

References

Chapuy, M. C., Arlot, M. E., Doboeuf, F., Brun, J., Crouzet, B., Arnaud, S., Delmas, P. D., and Meunier, P. J. (1992). Vitamin D_3 and calcium to prevent hip fractures in elderly women. *N. Engl. J. Med.* **327**, 1637–1642.

Chesnut, C. H., III, Bell, N. H., Clark, G. S., Drinkwater, B. L., English, S. C., Johnston, C. C., Jr., Notelovitz, M., Rosen, C., Cain, D. F., Flessland, K. A., and Mallinak, N. J. S. (1997). Hormone replacement therapy in postmenopausal women: Urinary N-telopeptide of type I collagen monitors therapeutic effect and predicts response of bone mineral density. *Am. J. Med.* **102**, 29–37.

Chevalley, T., Rizzoli, R., Nydegger, V., Slosman, D., Rapin, C.-H., Michel, J.-P., Vasey, H., and Bonjour, J. P. (1994). Effects of calcium supplements on femoral bone mineral density and vertebral fracture rate in vitamin-D-replete elderly patients. *Osteoporosis Int.* **4**, 245–252.

Cummings, S. R., Black, D. M., Nevitt, M. C., Browner, W., Cauley, J., Ensrud, K., Genant, H. K., Palermo, L., Scott, J., and Vogt, T. M. (1993). Bone density at various sites for prediction of hip fractures. *Lancet* **341**, 72–75.

Curhan, G. C., Willett, W. C., Rimm, E. B., and Stampher, M. J. (1993). A prospective study of dietary calcium and other nutrients and the risk of symptomatic kidney stones. *N. Engl. J. Med.* **328**, 833–838.

Curhan, G. C., Willett, W. C., Speizer, F. E., Spiegelman, D., and Stampher, M. J. (1997). Comparison of dietary calcium with supplemental calcium and other nutrients as factors affecting the risk of kidney stones in women. *Ann. Intern. Med.* **126**, 497–504.

Dawson-Hughes, B., Harris, S. S., Krall, E. A., Dallal, G. E., Falconer, G., and Green, C. L. (1995). Rates of bone loss in postmenopausal women randomized to two dosages of vitamin D. *Am. J. Clin. Nutr.* **61**, 1140–1145.

Dawson-Hughes, B., Harris, S. S., and Dallal, G. E. (1997a). Plasma calcidiol, season, and serum parathyroid hormone concentrations in healthy elderly men and women. *Am. J. Clin. Nutr.* **65**, 67–71.

Dawson-Hughes, B., Harris, S. S., Krall, E. A., and Dallal, G. E. (1997b). Effect of calcium and vitamin D supplementation on bone density in men and women 65 years of age or older. *N. Engl. J. Med.* **337**, 670–676.

Delmas, P. D., Gineyts, E., Bertholin, A., Garnero, P., and Marchand, F. (1993). Immunoassay of pyridinoline crosslink excretion in normal adults and in Paget's disease. *J. Bone Miner. Res.* **8**, 643–648.

Delvin, E. E., Imbach A., and Copti, M. (1988). Vitamin D nutritional status and related biochemical indices in an autonomous elderly population. *Am. J. Clin. Nutr.* **48**, 373–378.

Ebeling, P. R., Atley, L. M., Guthrie, J. R., Burger, H. G., Dennerstein, L., Hopper, J. L., and Wark, J. D. (1996). Bone turnover markers and bone density across the menopausal transition. *J. Clin. Endocrinol. Metab.* **81**, 3369–3371.

Elders, P. J. M., Lips, P., Netelenbos, J. C., van Ginkel, F. C., Khoe, E., van der Vijgh, W. J. F., and van der Stelt, P. F. (1994). Long-term effect of calcium supplementation on bone loss in perimenopausal women. *J. Bone Miner. Res.* **9**, 963–970.

Epstein, S., Posner, J., McClintock, R., Johnston, C. C., Jr., Bryce, G., and Hui, S. (1984). Differences in serum bone gla-protein with age and sex. *Lancet* **2**, 307–310.

Garnero, P., Sornay-Rendu, E., Chapuy, M. C., and Delmas, P. D. (1996a). Increased bone turnover is a major determinant of osteoporosis in elderly women. *J. Bone Miner. Res.* **3**, 337–349.

Garnero, P., Hausherr, E., Chapuy, M.-C., Marcelli C., Grandjean, H., Muller, C., Cormier, C., Breart, G., Meunier, P. J., and Delmas, P. D. (1996b). Markers of bone resorption predict hip fracture in elderly women: The EPIDOS Prospective Study. *J. Bone Miner. Res.* **11**, 1531–1538.

Hasling, C., Charles, P., Jensen, F., and Mosekilde, L. (1990). Calcium metabolism in postmenopausal osteoporosis: The influence of dietary calcium and net absorbed calcium. *J. Bone Miner. Res.* **5**, 939–946.

Honkanen, R., Alhava, E., Parviainen, M., Talasniemi, S., and Monkkonen, R. (1990). The necessity and safety of calcium and vitamin D in the elderly. *J. Am. Geriatr. Soc.* **38**, 862–866.

Institute of Medicine (IOM) (1997). "Dietary Reference Intakes: Calcium, Phosphorus, Magnesium, Vitamin D, and Fluoride." National Academy Press, Washington, DC.

Johnson, K. R., Jobber, J., and Stonawski, B. J. (1980). Prophalactic vitamin D in the elderly. *Age Ageing* **9**, 121–127.

Kobayashi, T., Okano, T., Shida, S., Okada, K., Suginohara, T., Nakao, H., Kuroda, E., Kodama, S., and Matsuo, T. (1983). Variation of 25-hydroxyvitamin D_3 and 25-hydroxyvitamin D_2 levels in human plasma obtained from 758 Japanese healthy subjects. *J. Nutr. Sci. Vitaminol.* **29**, 271–281.

Krall, E. A., Dawson-Hughes, B., Hirst, K., Gallagher, J. C., and Dalsky, G. (1997). Bone mineral density and serum osteocalcin levels in healthy elderly men and women. *J. Gerontol.* **52A**, M61–M67.

Malm, O. J. (1958). Calcium requirement and adaptation in adult men. *Scand. J. Clin. Lab. Invest.* **10**(Suppl. 36), 1–280.

Narang, N. K., Gupta, R. C., and Jain, M. K. (1984). Role of vitamin D in pulmonary tuberculosis. *J. Assoc. Physicians India* **32**, 185–188.

National Research Council (1989). "Recommended Dietary Allowances: Subcommittee on the Tenth Edition of the RDA's Food and Nutrition Board, Commission on Life Sciences, National Research Council," 10th rev. ed. National Academy Press, Washington, DC.

Nusser, S. M., Carriquiry, A. L., Dodd, K. W., and Fuller, W. A. (1996). A semiparametric transformation approach to estimating usual daily intake distributions. *J. Am. Stat. Assoc.* **91**, 1140–1449.

Omdahl, J. L., Garry, P. J., Hunsaker, L. A., Hunt, W. C., and Goodwin, J. S. (1982). Nutritional status in a healthy elderly population: Vitamin D. *Am. J. Clin. Nutr.* **36**, 1225–1233.

Ooms, M. E., Roos, J. C., Bezemer, P. D., Van Der Vijgh, W. J. F., Bouter, L. M., and Lips, P. (1995). Prevention of bone loss by vitamin D supplementation in elderly women: A randomized double-blind trial. *J. Clin. Endocrinol. Metab.* **80**, 1052–1058.

Orwoll, E. S. (1982). The milk-alkali syndrome: Current concepts. *Ann. Intern. Med.* **97**, 242–248.

Orwoll, E. S., Oviatt, S. K., McClung, M. R., Deftos, L. J., and Sexton, G. (1990). The rate of bone mineral loss in normal men and the effects of calcium and cholecalciferol supplementation. *Ann. Intern. Med.* **112**, 29–34.

Prince, R., Devine, A., Dick, I., Criddle, A., Kerr, D., Kent, N., Price, R., and Randell, A. (1995). The effects of calcium supplementation (milk powder or tablets) and exercise on bone density in postmenopausal women. *J. Bone Miner. Res.* **10**, 1068–1075.

Riis, B., Thomsen, K., and Christiansen, C. (1987). Does calcium supplementation prevent postmenopausal bone loss? *N. Engl. J. Med.* **316**, 173–177.

Selby, P. (1994). Calcium requirement—a reappraisal of the methods used in it's determination and their application to patients with osteoporosis. *Am. J. Clin. Nutr.* **60**, 944–948.

Sherman, S. S., Hollis, B. W., and Tobin, J. D. (1990). Vitamin D status and related parameters in a healthy population: The effects of age, sex, and season. *J. Clin. Endrocrinol. Metab.* **7**, 405–413.

Spencer, H., Kramer, L., Lesniak, M., DeBartolo, M., Norris, C., and Osis, D. (1984). Calcium requirements in humans. Report of original data and a review. *Clin. Orthop. Relat. Res.* **184**, 270–280.

Stamp, T. C. B., and Round, J. M. (1974). Seasonal changes in human plasma levels of 25-hydroxyvitamin D. *Nature (London)* **274**, 563–565.

Webb, A. R., Kline, L., and Holick, M. F. (1988). Influence of season and latitude on the cutaneous synthesis of vitamin D_3: Exposure to winter sunlight in Boston and Edmonton will not promote vitamin D_3 synthesis in human skin. *J. Clin. Endocrinol. Metab.* **67**, 373–378.

Chapter 12

Kristine M. Wiren
Eric S. Orwoll

Bone and Mineral Unit
Oregon Health Sciences University
and the Portland VA Medical Center
Portland, Oregon

Androgens and Bone:
Basic Aspects

I. Introduction

The obvious importance of the menopause in skeletal biology has focused most research in gonadal steroid action on the effects of estrogen.
However, androgens also have important effects on both skeletal development and the maintenance of bone mass, and the mechanisms by which
androgens affect skeletal homeostasis have become increasingly clear. Androgen receptors are expressed in osteoblasts and direct actions of androgen
in the regulation of both osteoblast proliferation and expression has been
documented *in vitro*. In castrate animals, replacement with nonaromatizable
androgens (e.g., dihydrotestosterone) yields beneficial effects that are notably different than those of estrogen (Turner *et al.*, 1989, 1990b). Furthermore, blockade of the androgen receptor results in osteopenia in intact
females (Goulding and Gold, 1993), and recent data suggest that combination therapy with both estrogen and androgenic steroids is more effective

Osteoporosis in Men
211

than estrogen replacement alone (Raisz *et al.*, 1996; Rosenberg *et al.*, 1997). Thus, in men and women it is probable that androgens and estrogens each have important, and interacting, functions during bone development and in the subsequent maintenance of skeletal homeostasis. An awakening awareness of the importance of the effects of androgen on bone, and the potential to make use of this information for the treatment of bone disorders, has fueled an increase in research.

II. Mechanisms of Androgen Action in Bone: The Androgen Receptor

The cloning of the androgen receptor cDNA (Chang *et al.*, 1988; Lubahn *et al.*, 1988) has allowed a direct characterization of androgen receptor expression in a variety of tissues, including bone. Colvard *et al.* (1989b) first reported the presence of androgen receptor mRNA and specific androgen binding sites in normal human osteoblastic cells. The abundance of androgen and estrogen receptor proteins was similar, suggesting that androgens and estrogens each play important roles in skeletal physiology (Figure 1). Subse-

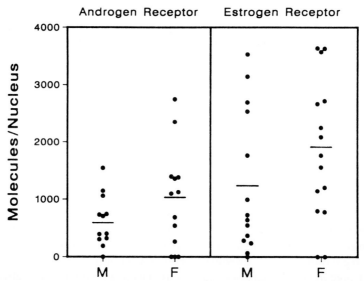

FIGURE I   Nuclear androgen and estrogen receptor binding in normal human osteoblast-like cells. Dots represent the mean calculated number of molecules per cell nucleus for each cell strain. (Left) Specific nuclear binding of [³H]R1881 (methyltrienolone, an androgen analog) in 12 strains from normal men and 13 strains from normal women. (Right) Specific nuclear [³H]estradiol binding in 15 strains from men and 15 strains from women. The horizontal lines indicate the mean receptor concentrations (Colvard *et al.*, 1989b).

quent reports have confirmed androgen receptor mRNA expression and/or the presence of androgen binding sites in both normal and clonal transformed osteoblastic cells derived from a variety of species (Benz *et al.*, 1991; Orwoll *et al.*, 1991; Zhaung *et al.*, 1992; Liesegang *et al.*, 1994; Nakano *et al.*, 1994; Takeuchi *et al.*, 1994). The size of the androgen receptor mRNA transcript in osteoblasts (about 10 kb) is similar to that described in prostate and other tissues (Chang *et al.*, 1988), as is the size of the androgen receptor protein analyzed by Western blotting (~110 kDa) (Nakano *et al.*, 1994). There is a report of two isoforms of androgen receptor protein in human osteoblast-like cells (~110 and ~97 kDa) (Kasperk *et al.*, 1997b) similar to that observed in human prostatic cells (Wilson and McPhaul, 1994). Furthermore, the binding affinity of the androgen receptor found in osteoblastic cells ($K_d = 0.5$–2×10^{-9}) is typical of that found in other tissues. The number of specific androgen binding sites in osteoblasts varies, depending on methodology, from 1,000 to 14,000 sites/cell (Masuyama *et al.*, 1992; Liesegang *et al.*, 1994; Nakano *et al.*, 1994; Kasperk *et al.*, 1997a) but is in a range seen in other androgen target tissues. Androgen binding is specific, without significant competition by estrogen, progesterone, or dexamethasone (Colvard *et al.*, 1989a; Nakano *et al.*, 1994; Kasperk *et al.*, 1997a). Finally, testosterone and dihydrotestosterone (DHT) appear to have similar binding affinities (Benz *et al.*, 1991; Nakano *et al.*, 1994). All these data are consistent with the notion that the direct biologic effects of androgenic steroids in osteoblasts are mediated at least in part via classic mechanisms associated with the steroid hormone receptor superfamily, principally through changes in gene expression.

The distribution of androgen receptors in the bone microenvironment is becoming better characterized. Abu *et al.* (1997) have localized androgen receptor in intact human bone by immunocytochemical analysis. In developing bone, androgen receptors were predominantly expressed in osteoblasts at sites of bone formation, as well as in osteocytes (Figure 2). Androgen receptor was also observed within the bone marrow in mononuclear cells and endothelial cells of blood vessels, and the pattern of expression was similar in males and females. Expression of the androgen receptor has also been characterized in cultured osteoblastic cell populations isolated from bone biopsy specimens, determined at both the mRNA level and by binding analysis (Kasperk *et al.*, 1997a). Expression varied according to the skeletal site of origin and age of the donor of the cultured osteoblastic cells, being higher in osteoblastic cells derived from cortical and mandibular sites and lower in cells derived from trabecular and iliac crest-derived cells. That distribution correlated with androgen responsiveness. In addition, androgen receptor expression was highest in early adulthood osteoblastic cultures and somewhat lower in samples from prepubertal and senescent bone. Again, no differences were found between male and female samples, suggesting that differences in receptor number per se do not underlie development of a sex-

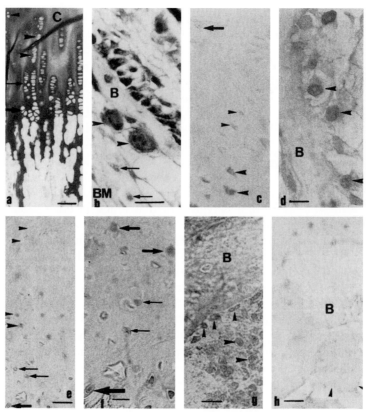

FIGURE 2   The localization of AR in normal tibial growth plate and adult osteophytic human bone. (a) Morphologically, sections of the growth plate consist of areas of endochondral ossification with undifferentiated (small arrowhead), proliferating (large arrowheads), mature (small arrow), and hypertrophic (large arrow) chondrocytes. Bar = 80 μm. An inset of an area of the primary spongiosa is shown in b. (b) Numerous osteoblasts (small arrowheads) and multinucleated osteoclasts (large arrowheads) on the bone surface. Mononuclear cells within the bone marrow are also present (arrows). Bar = 60 μm (c) In the growth plate, AR is predominantly expressed by hypertrophic chondrocytes (large arrowheads). Minimal expression is observed in the mature chondrocytes (small arrowheads). The receptors are rarely observed in the proliferating chondrocytes (arrow). (d) In the primary spongiosa, the AR is predominantly and highly expressed by osteoblasts at modeling sites (arrowheads). Bar = 20 μm. (e) In the osteophytes, AR is also observed at sites of endochondral ossification in undifferentiated (small arrowheads), proliferating (large arrowheads), mature (small arrows), and hypertrophic-like (large arrow) chondrocytes. Bar = 80 μm. (f) A higher magnification of e showing proliferating, mature, and hypertrophic-like chondrocytes (large arrows, small arrows, and very large arrows, respectively) Bar = 40 μm. (g) At sites of bone remodeling, the receptors are highly expressed in the osteoblasts (small arrowheads) and also in mononuclear cells in the bone marrow (large arrowheads). Bar = 40 μm. (h) AR is not detected in osteoclasts (small arrowheads). Bar = 40 μm. B, bone; C, cartilage; BM, bone marrow. Reproduced from Abu, E. O., *et al.* (1997). The localization of androgen receptors in human bone. *J. Clin. Endocrinol. Metab.* **82,** 3493–3497, © The Endocrine Society, with permission.

ually dimorphic skeleton. Androgen and estrogen receptors have also been shown in bone-marrow-derived stromal cells (Bellido *et al.*, 1995), which are responsive to sex steroids during the regulation of osteoclastogenesis. Because androgens are so important in bone development at the time of puberty, it is not surprising that androgen receptors are also present in epiphyseal chondrocytes (Carracosa *et al.*, 1990; Abu *et al.*, 1997). The expression of androgen receptors in such a wide variety of cell types known to be important for bone modeling and remodeling provides evidence for a direct action of androgens in bone and cartilage tissue, and further suggests a complexity of androgen effects.

Estrogen receptors have been reported to be present in osteoclasts (Oursler *et al.*, 1991), suggesting that osteoclasts may be a target for sex steroid regulation, but a direct effect of androgens on osteoclast function has not been demonstrated. Mizuno *et al.* described the presence of androgen receptor immunoreactivity in mouse osteoclast-like multinuclear cells (Mizuno *et al.*, 1994), but expression was not detected in osteoclasts in human bone slices (Abu *et al.*, 1997). Furthermore, the biologic relevance of androgen receptor expression in osteoclasts is unclear, especially because the major effects of androgens on skeletal remodeling and on the maintenance of bone mineral density seem to be mediated by cells of the osteoblast lineage (Weinstein *et al.*, 1997).

Regulation of androgen receptor expression in osteoblasts is incompletely characterized. Autologous regulation by androgen has been described that is tissue-specific; up-regulation by androgen exposure is seen in osteoblasts (Zhuang *et al.*, 1992; Takeuchi *et al.*, 1994; Wiren *et al.*, 1997), whereas down-regulation of androgen receptor occurs after androgen exposure in prostatic tissue. At least in part, this androgen-mediated up-regulation in osteoblasts occurs through changes in androgen receptor gene expression (Figure 3). Increased androgen receptor protein stability may also play a part. No effect, or inhibition, of androgen receptor mRNA by androgen exposure in osteoblastic cells has been described (Hofbauer *et al.*, 1997; Kasperk *et al.*, 1997a). The mechanism(s) underlying the tissue specificity in autologous androgen receptor regulation and the possible biological significance of distinct autologous regulation of androgen receptor is not yet understood. Receptor up-regulation by androgen in bone could indicate an enhancement of androgen responsiveness at times when androgen levels are rising or elevated. Androgen receptor expression in osteoblasts may also be up-regulated by glucocorticoids (Kasperk *et al.*, 1997b), but regulation during osteoblast differentiation, or by other hormones, growth factors, or agents has not yet been described in bone. Furthermore, whether the androgen receptor undergoes post-translational processing (stabilization, phosphorylation, etc.) in osteoblasts as described in other tissues (Kemppainen *et al.*, 1992) is also unknown.

In addition to the classical androgen receptor present in bone cells, several other signaling pathways have been described. Androgens may be spe-

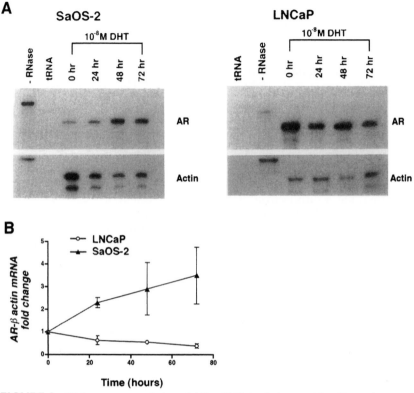

FIGURE 3   Dichotomous regulation of AR mRNA levels in osteoblast-like and prostatic carcinoma cell lines after exposure to androgen. (A) Time course of changes in AR mRNA abundance after DHT exposure in human SaOS-2 osteoblastic cells and human LNCaP prostatic carcinoma cells. To determine the effect of androgen exposure on hAR mRNA abundance, confluent cultures of either osteoblast-like cells (SaOS-2) or prostatic carcinoma cells (LNCaP) were treated with 10^{-8} M DHT for 0, 24, 48, or 72 hr. Total RNA was then isolated and subjected to RNase protection analysis with 50 μg total cellular RNA from SaOS-2 osteoblastic cells and 10 μg total RNA from LNCaP cultures. (B) Densitometric analysis of AR mRNA steady-state levels. The AR mRNA to β-actin ratio is expressed as the mean ± SEM compared to the control value from three to five independent assessments. Reproduced from Wiren *et al.*, 1997, with permission.

cifically bound in osteoblastic cells by a recently described 63-kDa cytosolic protein (Wrogemann *et al.*, 1991) or may regulate osteoblast activity via rapid nongenomic mechanisms through unconventional receptors at the cell surface (Lieberherr and Grosse, 1994), as has been shown for estrogen (Lieberherr *et al.*, 1993). A recent description of specific binding sites for weaker androgens (dehydroepiandrosterone, DHEA) (Meikle *et al.*, 1992) raises the possibility that DHEA or similar androgenic compounds may also have direct effects in bone. In fact, Bodine *et al.* (1995) recently showed that DHEA caused a rapid reduction of c-*fos* expression in human osteoblastic cells that was more robust than that seen with the classical androgens (dihydrotestosterone (DHT); testosterone; androstenedione). Nevertheless, all androgenic compounds significantly increased TGFβ activity in osteoblastic cells. The role of these nonclassical signaling pathways in androgen-mediated responses is still relatively unexplored.

III. Effects of Androgens on the Proliferation and Differentiation of Osteoblastic Cells

Androgens have direct effects on osteoblast proliferation and expression *in vitro.* The effect of androgen exposure on osteoblast proliferation is unclear at this point; both stimulation and inhibition of osteoblast proliferation have been reported. Benz *et al.* (1991) have shown that prolonged androgen exposure in the presence of serum-inhibited proliferation (cell counts) by 15–25% in a transformed human osteoblastic line (TE-85). Testosterone and DHT were nearly equally effective regulators. Kasperk *et al.* (1997b) showed that prolonged DHT treatment inhibited normal human osteoblastic cell proliferation (cell counts) in cultures pretreated with DHT. On the other hand, the same group (Kasperk *et al.,* 1989, 1990) also demonstrated in osteoblast-like cells in primary culture (murine, passaged human) that a variety of androgen in serum-free medium increase DNA synthesis ([³H]thymidine incorporation) up to nearly 300% (Table I) and cell counts by 200%. Again, testosterone and nonaromatizable androgens (DHT and fluoxymesterone) were nearly equally effective regulators. Consistent with increased proliferation, testosterone and DHT have also been reported to cause an increase in creatine kinase activity and [³H]thymidine incorporation into DNA in rat diaphyseal bone (Sömjen *et al.,* 1989). The differences observed with androgen-mediated changes in osteoblastic cell proliferation may be due to the different model systems employed (transformed osteoblastic cells versus

TABLE I   Effect of Androgens (1 nM) on [³H]Thymidine Uptake into DNA of Mouse Bone Cells

	CPM	% control	P
Control	235 ± 14	100 ± 6	
DHT	479 ± 23	204 ± 9	<0.001
Testosterone	429 ± 47	182 ± 20	<0.01
Fluoxymesterone	423 ± 44	180 ± 18	<0.01
Methenolone	633 ± 55	269 ± 23	<0.001

Reprinted from Kasperk *et al.,* 1989, with permission.

second to fourth passage normal human cells) and/or may reflect differences in the culture conditions (e.g., state of differentiation, receptor number, times of treatment, phenol red-containing versus phenol red-free, or serum containing versus serum-free). These differences also suggest an underlying complexity for androgen regulation of osteoblast proliferation.

Increased matrix production has also been shown to result from androgen exposure. Androgen treatment in both normal osteoblasts and transformed clonal human osteoblastic cells (TE-89) appears to increase the proportion of cells expressing alkaline phosphatase activity, possibly representing a shift toward a more differentiated phenotype (Figure 4) (Kasperk *et al.*, 1989, 1997b). There are also reports of increased type Iα-1 collagen protein and mRNA levels (Benz *et al.*, 1991; Gray *et al.*, 1992) and increased osteocalcin secretion (Kasperk *et al.*, 1997b). Consistent with increased collagen production, androgen treatment has been shown to stimulate mineral accumulation (Kapur and Reddi, 1989; Takeuchi *et al.*, 1994; Kasperk *et al.*, 1997b). These results suggest that androgens enhance osteoblast differentiation and may thus play an important role in the regulation of bone matrix production and/or organization, consistent with an overall stimulation of bone formation.

IV. Interaction with Other Factors to Modulate Bone Formation and Resorption

The actions of androgens on the osteoblast certainly must also be considered in the context of the very complex endocrine, paracrine, and autocrine

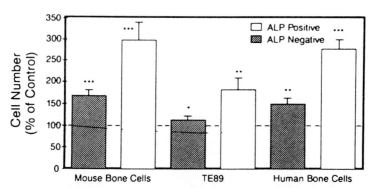

FIGURE 4   Effect of DHT on ALP positive (ALP$^+$) and ALP negative (ALP$^-$) cells in normal mouse, normal human osteoblast-line, and human osteosarcoma (TE89) monolayer cell culture (*** = $P < 0.001$; ** = $P < 0.01$; * = $P < 0.1$). Control values in cells per square millimeter for mouse bone cells: 90 $\pm$ 5; TE89 cells: 75 $\pm$ 7; human bone cells: 83 $\pm$ 14. Reprinted from Kasperk *et al.*, 1989, with permission.

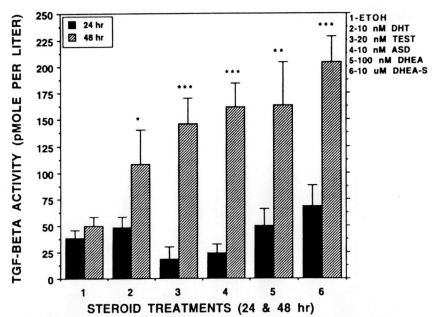

FIGURE 5   Induction of total TGFβ activity by gonadal and adrenal androgens in human osteoblast (hOB) cell conditioned-media. The cells were treated for 24–48 hr with vehicle or steroids. After treatment, the conditioned-media was saved and processed for the TGF-β bioassay. The results are presented as the mean ± SEM of three to four experiments; *$P < 0.05$; **$P < 0.02$; ***$P < 0.0005$ (Behren's-Fisher t-test) compared to the 48-hr ethanol control. ETOH, ethanol; TEST, testosterone; DHT, dihydrotestosterone; ASD, androstenedione; DHEA, dehydroepiandrosterone; DHEA-S, DHEA-sulfate. Reprinted from *J. Steroid Biochem. Molec. Biol.* 52, Bodine, P. V. N., Riggs, B. L., and Spelsberg, T. C. Regulation of c-fos expression and TGF-B production by gonadal and adrenal androgens in normal human osteoblastic cells, pp. 149–158, copyright 1995, with permission from Elsevier Science.

environment where systemic/local factors act in concert to influence bone cell function. In fact, androgens have been shown to regulate other well-known modulators of osteoblast proliferation or function. The most extensively characterized growth factor influenced by androgen exposure is TGFβ. TGFβ activity is increased by androgen treatment in human osteoblast primary cultures (Figure 5). The expression of some TGFβ mRNA transcripts (apparently TGFβ2) is increased, but there was no effect on TGFβ1 mRNA abundance (Kasperk *et al.*, 1990; Bodine *et al.*, 1995). At the protein level, specific immunoprecipitation analysis reveals DHT-mediated increases in TGFβ activity to be predominantly TGFβ2 (Bodine *et al.*, 1995; Kasperk *et al.*, 1997b). On the other hand, TGFβ1 mRNA levels are increased by androgen treatment in human clonal osteoblastic cells (TE-89), under conditions where osteoblast proliferation is slowed (Benz *et al.*, 1991). At the level of bone, orchiectomy drastically reduces bone content of TGFβ and

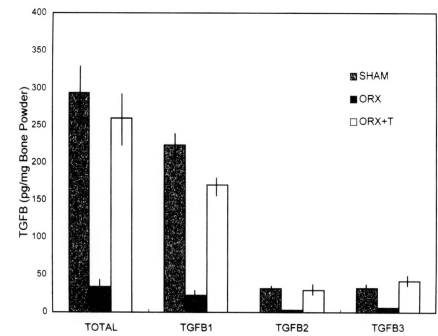

FIGURE 6   Effects of orchiectomy and T replacement on isoforms of TGFβ in long bones. Results are mean ± SE of four to six animals. Rats underwent sham operation or orchiectomy and 1 week later were given either placebo or 100 mg of testosterone in 60-day slow release pellets. Specimens were obtained 6 weeks after surgery. All forms of TGFβ were reduced by orchiectomy (at least $P < 0.0002$), whereas there was no change in those with testosterone replacement. Reprinted from Gill *et al.* (1998), Orchiectomy markedly reduced the concentration of the three isoforms of transforming growth factor β in rat bone, and reduction is prevented by testosterone. *Endocrinologist (Baltimore)* **139**, 546–550, with permission.

testosterone replacement prevents the effect (Gill *et al.*, 1998) (Figure 6). These data support the findings that androgens influence cellular expression of TGFβ and suggest that the bone loss associated with castration is related to a reduction in growth factor abundance induced by androgen deficiency.

Other growth factor systems may also be influenced by androgens. Conditioned media from DHT-treated normal osteoblast cultures are mitogenic, and DHT pretreatment increases the mitogenic response to fibroblast growth factor and to insulin-like growth factor II (IGF-II) (Kasperk *et al.*, 1990). In part, this may be due to slight increases in IGF-II binding in DHT-treated cells (Kasperk *et al.*, 1990), as IGF-I and IGF-II levels in osteoblast-conditioned media are not affected by androgen treatment (Kasperk *et al.*, 1990; Canalis *et al.*, 1991). Androgens may also modulate expression of components of the AP-1 transcription factor, as has been shown with inhibition of c-*fos* expression in proliferating normal osteoblast cultures (Bodine *et al.*, 1995).

Thus, androgens may accelerate osteoblast differentiation via a mechanism whereby growth factors or other mediators of differentiation are regulated by androgen exposure.

Finally, androgens may modulate responses to other important osteotropic hormones/regulators. Testosterone and DHT specifically inhibit the cAMP response elicited by parathyroid hormone or parathyroid hormone-related protein in the human clonal osteoblast-like cell line SaOS-2, whereas the inactive or weakly active androgen 17α-epitestosterone had no effect (Figure 7). This inhibition may be mediated via an effect on the parathyroid hormone receptor-G_S-adenylyl cyclase complex (Fukayama and Tashjian, 1989; Gray *et al.*, 1991; Vermeulen, 1991). The production of prostaglandin E_2 (PGE_2), another important regulator of bone metabolism, is also affected by androgens. Pilbeam and Raisz showed that androgens (both DHT and testosterone) were potent inhibitors of both parathyroid hormone (Figure 8), and interleukin-1 stimulated prostaglandin E2 production in cultured neonatal mouse calvaria (Pilbeam and Raisz, 1990). The effects of androgens on parathyroid hormone action and PGE_2 production suggest that androgens could act to modulate (reduce) bone turnover in response to these agents.

In stromal cells of the bone marrow, androgens have been shown to have potent inhibitory effects on the production of interleukin-6 (Table II) and the

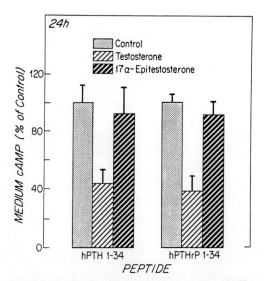

FIGURE 7 Actions of testosterone and 17α-epitestosterone on cAMP accumulation stimulated by hPTH[1-34] (5.0 nM) or hPTHrP[1-34] (5.0 nM) in human SaOS-2 cells. Cells were pretreated without or with the steroid hormones (10^{-9} M) for 24 hr. Each bar gives the mean value, and the brackets give the SE for four to five dishes. Reprinted from Fukayama and Tashjian, 1989, with permission.

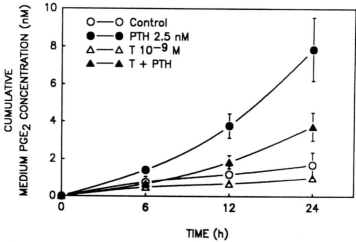

FIGURE 8   Effect of T on PTH-stimulated PGE[2] production in cultured neonatal calvariae as a function of time. Each bone was precultured for 24 hr in 1 ml medium with or without 10^{-9} M T and then transferred to a similar medium with 2.5 nM PTH. Media were sampled (0.1 ml) at the indicated times. Data were corrected for the media removed. Each point represents the mean ± SEM for six bones in one experiment. The effect of T on PTH-stimulated PGE[2] production was significant ($P < 0.05$) at 6, 12, and 24 hr. Reproduced from Pilbeam and Raisz, *J. Bone Miner. Res.* 1990; 5:1183–1188 with permission of the American Society for Bone and Mineral Research.

subsequent stimulation of osteoclastogenesis by marrow osteoclast precursors (Bellido *et al.*, 1995). Interestingly, adrenal androgens (androstenediol, androstenedione, dehydroepiandrosterone) have similar inhibitory activities on interleukin-6 gene expression and protein production by stroma (Bellido *et al.*, 1995). The loss of inhibition of interleukin-6 production by androgen may contribute to the marked increase in bone remodeling and resorption that follows orchidectomy. Moreover, androgens inhibit the expression of the genes encoding the two subunits of the IL-6 receptor (gp80 and gp130) in the murine bone marrow, another mechanism which may blunt the effects of this osteoclastogenic cytokine in intact animals (Lin *et al.*, 1997). In these respects, the effects of androgens seem to be very similar to those of estrogen, which also inhibit osteoclastogenesis via mechanisms that involve interleukin-6 inhibition.

V. Direct Effects of Androgens on Other Cell Types in Bone *in Vitro*

Similar to the effects noted in osteoblastic populations, androgens regulate chondrocyte proliferation and expression. Androgen exposure promotes

TABLE II Effect of Androgens on Cytokine-Induced IL-6 Production by Murine Bone Marrow Stromal Cells

Treatment	IL-6
IL-1 + TNF	4.27 ± 1.43
IL-1 + TNF+ testosterone (10^{-12} M)	3.87 ± 0.33
IL-1 + TNF+ testosterone (10^{-11} M)	2.90 ± 0.42
IL-1 + TNF+ testosterone (10^{-10} M)	2.09 ± 0.33
IL-1 + TNF+ testosterone (10^{-9} M)	1.12 ± 0.49
IL-1 + TNF+ testosterone (10^{-8} M)	1.03 ± 0.04
IL-1 + TNF+ testosterone (10^{-7} M)	1.01 ± 0.48
IL-1 + TNF+ dihydrotestosterone (10^{-12} M)	4.05 ± 0.19
IL-1 + TNF+ dihydrotestosterone (10^{-11} M)	2.97 ± 0.48
IL-1 + TNF+ dihydrotestosterone (10^{-10} M)	2.31 ± 0.86
IL-1 + TNF+ dihydrotestosterone (10^{-9} M)	1.72 ± 0.43
IL-1 + TNF+ dihydrotestosterone (10^{-8} M)	0.65 ± 0.21
IL-1 + TNF+ dihydrotestosterone (10^{-7} M)	1.41 ± 0.82

Murine stromal cells (+/+ LDA11 cells) were cultured for 20 hr in the absence or the presence of different concentrations of either testosterone or dihydrotestosterone. Then IL-1 (500 U/ml) and TNF (500 U/ml) were added, and cells were maintained for another 24 hr. in culture. Values indicate means (±SD) of triplicate cultures from one experiment. Data were analyzed by one-way ANOVA. *$P < 0.05$, versus cells not treated with steroids as determined by Dunnet's test. Neither testosterone nor dihydrotestosterone had an effect on cell number. Reproduced from The Journal of Clinical Investigation, 1995, vol. 95, pp. 2886–2895 by copyright permission of The American Society for Clinical Investigation.

chondrogenesis as shown with increased creatine kinase and DNA synthesis after androgen exposure in cultured epiphyseal chondrocytes (Carracosa *et al.*, 1990; Sömjen *et al.*, 1991). Increased [^{35}S]sulfate incorporation into newly synthesized proteoglycan (Corvol *et al.*, 1987) and increased alkaline phosphatase activity (Schwartz *et al.*, 1994) are androgen-mediated. Regulation of these effects are obviously complex because they were dependent on the age of the animals and the site from which chondrocytes were derived. Thus, in addition to effects on osteoblasts, multiple cell types in the skeletal milieu are regulated by androgen exposure.

VI. Metabolism of Androgens in Bone—Aromatase and 5α-Reductase Activities

There is abundant evidence in a variety of tissues that the eventual cellular effects of androgens may be the result not only of direct action but also of the effects of sex steroid metabolites formed as the result of local enzyme activities. The most important of these metabolites are estradiol (formed by the aromatization of testosterone) and 5α-DHT (the result of 5α reduction of testosterone). Conversion of androstenedione and testosterone into 5α-reduced androgens or into estrogens is both irreversible and mutually exclusive (Mahendroo et al., 1997). There is evidence that both aromatase and 5α-reductase are present in bone tissue, at least to some extent, but the biologic relevance is still controversial.

5α-Reductase activity was first described in crushed rat mandibular bone by Vittek et al. (1974), and Schweikert et al. (1980) reported similar findings in crushed human spongiosa. Two different 5α-reductase genes encode type 1 and type 2 isozymes in many mammalian species (Russell and Wilson, 1994), but the isozyme present in human bone has not been characterized. In osteoblast-like cultures derived from orthopedic surgical waste, androstenedione (the most abundant circulating androgen in women) can be reversibly converted to testosterone via 17β-hydroxysteroid dehydrogenase activity, and to 5α-androstanedione via 5α-reductase activity, whereas testosterone is converted to DHT via 5α-reductase activity (Bruch et al., 1992). The principal metabolite of androstenedione is α-androstanedione in the 5α-reductase pathway and testosterone in the 17β-hydroxysteroid dehydrogenase pathway. Essentially the same results were reported in experiments with human epiphyseal cartilage and chondrocytes (Audi et al., 1984). In general, the K_m values for bone 5α-reductase activity are similar to those in other androgen responsive tissues (Schweikert et al., 1980; Nakano et al., 1994).

The cellular populations in these studies were mixed, and hence the specific cell type responsible for the activity is unknown. Interestingly, Turner et al. found that periosteal cells do not have detectable 5α-reductase activity (Turner et al., 1990a), raising the possibilities that the enzyme may be functional in only selected skeletal compartments and that testosterone may be the active metabolite at this clinically important site.

From a clinical perspective, the general importance of this enzymatic pathway is suggested by the presence of skeletal abnormalities in patients with 5α-reductase type 2 deficiency (Fisher et al., 1978). However, Bruch et al. (1992) found no significant correlation between enzyme activities and bone volume. In mutant null mice lacking 5α-reductase type 1 (mice express very little type 2 isozyme), the effect on the skeleton cannot be analyzed due to midgestational fetal death (Mahendroo et al., 1997). Treatment of male animals with finasteride (an inhibitor of type 1 5α-reductase activity) does not recapitulate the effects of castration (Rosen et al., 1995), indicating that reduction of testosterone to DHT by the type 1 isozyme is not a major element in the effects of gonadal hormones on bone. Even though the available data point to a possible role for 5α-reduction in the mechanism of action for androgen in bone, the clinical impact of this enzyme, which isozyme may be involved, whether it is uniformly present in all cells involved in bone modeling/remodeling, or whether local activity is important all remain certain.

The biosynthesis of estrogens from androgen precursors is catalyzed by the microsomal enzyme aromatase cytochrome P450 (P450$_{arom}$, the product of the CYP19 gene). It is an enzyme well known to be both expressed and regulated in a very pronounced tissue-specific manner (Simpson *et al.*, 1994). Aromatase activity has been reported in bone from mixed cell populations derived from both sexes (Nawata *et al.*, 1995; Schweikert *et al.*, 1995; Sasano *et al.*, 1997) and from osteoblastic cell lines (Purohit *et al.*, 1992; Tanaka *et al.*, 1993; Nakano *et al.*, 1994). Aromatase expression in intact bone has also been documented by *in situ* hybridization and immunohistochemical analysis (Sasano *et al.*, 1997) (Table III). Aromatase mRNA is expressed predominantly in lining cells, chondrocytes, and some adipocytes, but there is no detectable expression in osteoclasts. At least in vertebral bone, the aromatase fibroblast (1b type) promoter is predominantly used (Sasano *et al.*, 1997). The enzyme kinetics in bone cells seem to be similar to those in other tissues, althoug the V_{max} may be increased by glucocorticoids (Tanaka *et al.*, 1993).

Aromatase can produce the potent estrogen estradiol but also can result in the weaker estrogen estrone from its adrenal precursors androstenedione and dehydroepiandrosterone (Nawata *et al.*, 1995). In addition to aromatase itself, osteoblasts contain enzymes that are able to interconvert estradiol and estrone (estradiol-17B hydroxysteroid dehydrogenase) and to hydrolyze estrone sulfate to estrone (estrone sulfatase) (Purohit *et al.*, 1992). Nawata *et al.* (1995) have reported that dexamethasone and 1α,25(OH)$_2$D$_3$ synergistically enhance aromatase activity and aromatase mRNA (P450$_{arom}$) expression in human osteoblast-like cells. There is no other information concerning the regulation of aromatase in bone, although this is an area of obvious interest given the potential importance of the enzyme and its regulation by a variety of mechanisms (including androgens and estrogens) in other tissues (Abdelgadir *et al.*, 1994; Simpson *et al.*, 1994). The finding of these enzymes in bone clearly raises the difficult issue of the origin of androgenic effects. Do they arise from direct androgen effects (as is suggested by the actions of nonaromatizable androgens) or to some extent from the local production of estrogenic intermediates?

The clinical impact of aromatase activity has recently been suggested by the reports of women (Conte *et al.*, 1994) and men (Morishima *et al.*, 1995; Carani *et al.*, 1997) with aromatase deficiencies who presented with a skeletal phenotype. The presentation of men with aromatase deficiency is very similar to that of a man with estrogen receptor-α deficiency, namely an obvious delay in bone age, lack of epiphyseal closure, and tall stature (Smith *et al.*, 1994), suggesting that aromatase (and thus estrogen action) has a substantial role to play during skeletal development in the male. In one case, estrogen therapy of a man with aromatase deficiency was associated with an increase in bone mass (Bilezikian *et al.*, 1998). Inhibition of aromatization in young growing orchidectomized males, with the nonsteroidal inhibitor vorozole, results in decreases in bone mineral density and changes in skeletal

TABLE III Confirmation by Recrystallization of the Identities of [³H]Dihydrotestosterone and [³H]Androstenedione Recovered after the Incubation of Normal and Osteoporotic Human Bone (Ground Spongiosa) with [1,2,76,7−³H]Testosterone

Crystallization	Solvent	Dihydrotestosterone			Androstenedione		
		³H (cpm/mg)	¹⁴C (cpm/mg)	³H/¹⁴C	³H (cpm/mg)	¹⁴C (cpm/mg)	³H/¹⁴C
1	Acetone	409	26	16	811	14	56
2	Benzene–heptane	408	25	16	811	14	57
3	Ethylacetate–cyclohexane	411	26	16	786	13	60
4	Ethylether–hexane	411	28	15	775	13	59
5	Methanol	393	26	15	791	16	48
Mother liquor		405	24	17	848	16	53

Pooled samples from 18 separate incubations of bone from various anatomical origin were chromatographed by preparative thin-layer chromatography. Material tentatively identified as [³H]dihydrotestosterone and [³H]androstenedione, respectively, was mixed with 200 mg of the appropriate carrier steroid and with ¹⁴C-labeled steroid for recrystallization as described in the text (Schweikert et al., 1980).

modeling, as does castration with resulting reduction in both androgens and estrogens. However, vorozole therapy induces less dramatic effects on bone turnover (Vanderschueren *et al.*, 1997). Inhibition of aromatization in older orchidectomized males resembles castration with similar increases in bone resorption and bone loss, suggesting that aromatase activity may also play a role in skeletal maintenance in males (Vanderschueren *et al.*, 1996). These studies herald the importance of aromatase activity (and estrogen) in the mediation of androgen action in bone.

Nevertheless, there is convincing evidence that some (if not most) of the impact of androgens in the skeleton are direct. For instance, as noted previously, both *in vivo* and *in vitro* systems reveal the effects of the nonaromatizable androgen DHT to be essentially the same as those of testosterone (*vida infra*). In addition, blockade of the androgen receptor with flutamide results in osteopenia apparently as a result of reduced bone formation (Goulding and Gold, 1993). These reports clearly indicate that androgens (independent of estrogenic metabolites) have primary effects on osteoblastic function, but the clinical reports of subjects with aromatase deficiency also highlight the relevance of androgen metabolism to bio-potent estrogens in bone. Obviously, the elucidation of the regulation of these events, and the mechanisms by which androgenic and estrogenic effects are coordinated, may have major physiological, pathophysiological, and therapeutic implications.

VII. Androgen Effects on Bone: Animal Studies

The effects of androgens on bone remodeling have been examined fairly extensively in animal models. Much of this work has been in species (rodents) not perfectly suited to reflect human bone metabolism, and certainly the field remains incompletely explored. Nevertheless, the animal models do provide valuable insights into the effects of androgens at organ and cellular levels. Most studies of androgen action have been performed in male rats, in which rapid skeletal growth occurs until about 4 months of age, at which time epiphyseal growth slows markedly (although never completely ceases at some sites). Because the effects of androgen deficiency may be different in growing and more mature animals (Vanderschueren and Bouillon, 1995), it is appropriate to consider the two situations independently.

A. Effects on Epiphyseal Function and Bone Growth during Skeletal Development

In most mammals there is a marked gender difference in morphology resulting in a sexually dimorphic skeleton. The mechanisms responsible for these differences are complex and presumably involve both androgenic and estrogenic actions. Estrogens are particularly important for the regulation of epiphyseal function and act to reduce the rate of longitudinal growth via influences on chondrocyte proliferation and action, as well as on the timing of epiphyseal closure (Turner *et al.*, 1994). Androgens appear to have somewhat opposite effects and tend to promote long bone growth, chondrocyte maturation, and metaphyseal ossification. Androgen deficiency retards those processes (Lebovitz and Eisenbarth, 1975). Nevertheless, excess concentrations of androgen will accelerate aging of the growth plate and reduce growth potential (Iannotti, 1990), possibly via conversion to estrogens.

Although the specific roles of sex steroids in the regulation of epiphyseal growth and maturation remain somewhat unresolved, there is evidence that androgens do have direct effects independent of those of estrogen. For instance, testosterone injected directly into the growth plates of rats increases plate width (Ren *et al.*, 1989). More specific evidence of androgen action comes from the *in vitro* studies described earlier. In a model of endochondral bone development based on the subcutaneous implantation of demineralized bone matrix in castrate rats, both testosterone and DHT increase the incorporation of calcium during osteoid formation (Kapur and Reddi, 1989). Interestingly, in this model androgens reduced the incorporation of [^{35}S]sulfate into glycosaminoglycans early in the developing cartilage. Certainly, androgens are known to interact considerably with the growth hormone–IGF system in the coordination of skeletal growth. Whereas androgens can affect a clear stimulation of growth in intact animals, in growth hormone deficiency that effect is essentially eliminated (Underwood and Van Wyk, 1992), underscoring the codependence of these two hormonal systems in the control of pubertal skeletal change. In sum, these data support the contention that androgens play a direct role in chondrocyte physiology, but how these actions are integrated with those of other regulators is unclear.

B. Effects on Bone Mass in Growing Male Animals

The most dramatic effect of androgens during growth may be on bone size. Male animals have larger bones, and particularly thicker cortices than females (Turner *et al.*, 1994; Kasra and Grynpas, 1995). The effects of androgens on bone mass maturation can to some extent be assessed by observing the results of androgen withdrawal. In most studies, orchiectomy in young rats results in a reduction in cortical bone mass within 2 to 4 weeks. Calcium content of the femur or tibia (Saville and Lieber, 1969; Schoutens *et al.*, 1984; Hock *et al.*, 1988; Vanderschueren *et al.*, 1994a; Kapitola *et al.*, 1995), whole femoral, tibial or body bone mineral density (Ongphiphadhanakul *et al.*, 1992; Kapitola *et al.*, 1995; Rosen *et al.*, 1995), and tibial diaphyseal cortical area (Turner *et al.*, 1990a) have been shown to be lower in castrated than in sham-operated controls. Similar trends have been reported in young, castrate male mice (Ornoy *et al.*, 1994). In animals followed for longer periods after castration (90 days), the density of cortical bone was

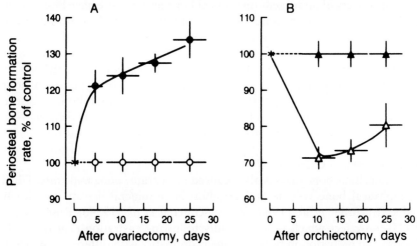

FIGURE 9   (A) The effect of ovariectomy (OVX) on periosteal bone formation rate. The mean ± SE (vertical bar) and tetracycline labeling period (horizontal line) for intact controls (-○-) and OVX (-●-) rats are shown as a function of time after OVX. $P < 0.01$ for all OVX time points compared to intact controls. (B) The effect of orchiectomy (ORX) on periosteal bone formation rate. The mean ± SE and tetracycline labeling period for intact controls (-▲-) and ORX (-△-) are shown as a function of time after ORX. $P < 0.01$ for all ORX time points compared to same labeling period in intact controls. Reprinted from Turner *et. al.,* 1990, with permission.

slightly (but not significantly) reduced, but bone area was clearly lessened in the diaphysis of the femur (Vanderschueren *et al.,* 1994b). At least in part, the reduction in cortical bone mass appears to result from a reduction in periosteal bone formation rate induced by gonadectomy in males (Turner *et al.,* 1989, 1990b). This response is distinctly different than that induced by oophorectomy, which results in an increase in periosteal apposition in the period immediately after surgery (Figure 9). This divergent trend in the periosteal response to castration in male and female animals abolishes the sexual dimorphism usually present in radial bone growth. Endosteal bone formation doesn't seem to be affected by orchiectomy (Turner *et al.,* 1989). As another indication that the cortical skeleton is affected by androgens, the characteristic acute increase in creatine kinase activity induced from diaphyseal bone by androgen treatment is abolished by orchiectomy (Sömjen *et al.,* 1994). For unclear reasons, it remains intact in epiphyseal specimens. Although castration in the male tends to slow growth and weight gain, the effects on cortical bone histomorphometry are present in pair-fed rats and in groups in which there was no difference in growth rates (Turner *et al.,* 1989, 1990b), indicating that the skeletal effects are not merely the indirect result of changes in body size or composition.

The effects of androgens on cortical bone architecture have biomechanical implications. For instance, in studies of long-term androgen administration to female primates, Kasra and Grynpas (1995) showed that cortical bone dimensions were increased and that tibia in treated animals were stronger, tougher, and stiffer. Thus, androgen deficiency during growth reduces cortical bone mass and strength, primarily by blunting periosteal bone apposition. The lack of significant change in bone density following castration suggests that there is not a major impact of androgen deficiency on cortical porosity. Whereas estrogens appear to increase endosteal bone apposition, androgens probably have little effect at that site (Turner et al., 1994; Kasra and Grynpas, 1995).

Cancellous bone mass is also reduced in castrate young male rats. Tibial metaphyseal bone volume and vertebral bone mineral density are clearly reduced (Turner et al., 1989; Vanderschueren et al., 1994a; Rosen et al., 1995), an effect which is seen rapidly following castration (Turner et al., 1989). The reduction in bone volume is dramatic, with differences between control and castrate of 40–50% appearing in 4–10 weeks (Wakley et al., 1991; Rosen et al., 1995). Rosen et al. (1995) showed that measures of trabecular bone volume and mineral density diverged much more than did areal measures of the proximal tibia or distal femur (by dual energy x-ray absorptiometry) and speculated that this difference reflected a more intense bone deficit from trabecular than from cortical compartments. An important issue that remains unresolved is whether the bone deficit is a result of actual loss of bone mass after castration, or whether the differences between castrate and control animals result from a failure of castrate animals to accrue bone normally. Nevertheless, bone changes after an orchiectomy occur in the presence of an increase in skeletal blood flow (Schoutens et al., 1984; Kapitola et al., 1995), osteoclast numbers and surface (Turner et al., 1989), serum and urine calcium levels (Turner et al., 1989), and increased serum tartrate-resistant acid phosphatase activity (Ongphiphadhanakul et al., 1992). All these findings strongly suggest an increase in bone remodeling and bone resorption. On the other hand, in one report, distal femoral bone loss after castration is accompanied by a reduction in bone remodeling (Tuukkanen et al., 1994). Parathyroid hormone concentrations have not been measured in these experiments, but vitamin D concentrations do not appear to be altered by orchiectomy (Turner et al., 1989). In sum, trabecular bone mass, as well as cortical mass, clearly depend on adequate androgen action in the growing male animal, but the specific mechanisms that mediate that effect are not well delineated.

C. Mature Male Animals

In mature rats androgen withdrawal also results in osteopenia. At a time when longitudinal growth has slowed markedly, pronounced differences between intact and castrate animals appear in cortical bone ash weight per

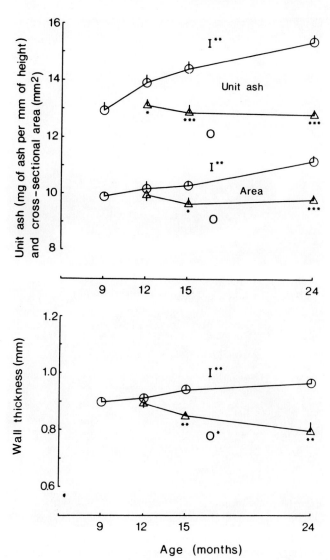

FIGURE 10   Bone mass, cross-sectional area, and wall thickness of the proximal femur cylinder form intact (I) and orchiectomized (O) rats (vertical bar ± SE). Comparison among mean values at the different ages for intact (I**) and castrated (O*) rats. *P < 0.05; *** P < 0.001. Reprinted from Danielsen *et al.,* 1992, with permission.

unit length, cross-sectional area, thickness, and bone mineral density (Wink and Felts, 1980; Verhas *et al.,* 1986; Danielsen *et al.,* 1992; Vanderschueren and Van Herck, 1992; Vanderschueren *et al.,* 1992; Gunness and Orwoll, 1995) (Figures 10 and 11). Periosteal bone accretion is reduced (Gunness

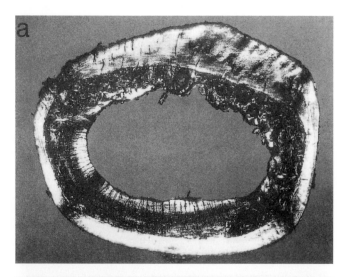

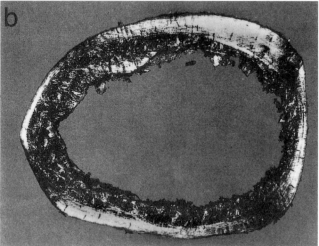

FIGURE 11   Microphotographs of 200 μm thick mid-diaphyseal cross sections from 24-month-old intact (a) and orchidectomized (b) rats taken in a polarization microscope. Original magnification ×14. Reprinted from Danielsen *et al.*, 1992, with permission.

and Orwoll, 1995), and endocortical bone loss is accelerated in orchiectomized animals (Danielsen *et al.*, 1992; Vanderschueren *et al.*, 1993b). As might be expected in light of these changes, the maximum compressive load is decreased in cortical bone; however, when corrected for cortical mass, there is no evidence of an abnormality in bone strength (Danielsen *et al.*, 1992). In addition to changes in bone size, increased intracortical resorption cavities are reported to result from orchiectomy (Wink and Felts, 1980).

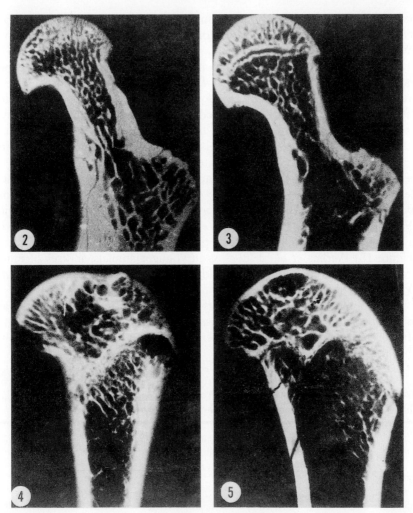

FIGURE 12   (2) Microradiograph of a mid-sagittal longitudinal section from the proximal end of a femur in a control rat, illustrating normal appearance of distribution of compact and spongy bone. Original magnification, ×7. (3) Microradiograph of a mid-sagittal longitudinal section from the proximal end of femur in a 4-months post-castrate rat. Much of the spongiosa has been lost. ×7 (4) Microradiograph of a mid-sagittal longitudinal section from the distal end of femur in a control rat. ×14. (5) Microradiograph of a mid-sagittal longitudinal section from the distal end of femur in a 4-months post-castrate rat. Metaphaseal spongiosa has almost disappeared and compacta is thin. ×14. Reprinted from Wink and Felts, 1980, with permission.

Cancellous bone volume is reduced rapidly after castration as well (Figure 12) (Wink and Felts, 1980; Gunness and Orwoll, 1995), and osteopenia becomes quite pronounced with time (Vanderschueren *et al.*, 1992). This bone loss appears to result in part from increases in bone resorption because it is associated with increased resorption cavities, osteoclasts, and blood flow (Wink and Felts, 1980; Verhas *et al.*, 1986; Gunness and Orwoll, 1995). Dynamic histomorphometric and biochemical measures of bone remodeling increase quickly (Vanderschueren *et al.*, 1992, 1994a), with evidence of increased osteoclast numbers only 1 week after castration (Gunness and Orwoll, 1995) (Table IV). These changes include an increase in osteoblastic activity, as well as increased bone resorption. In the SAMP6 mouse, a model of accelerated senescence in which osteoblastic function is impaired, the rise in remodeling after orchidectomy is blunted, which has been interpreted as evidence that the early changes after gonadectomy are dependent on osteoblast-derived signals (Weinstein *et al.*, 1997). Interestingly, this initial phase of increased bone remodeling activity appears to subside somewhat with time (Verhas *et al.*, 1986; Vanderschueren *et al.*, 1994a), and by 4 months there is evidence of a depression in bone turnover rates in some skeletal areas (Figure 13) (Verhas *et al.*, 1986). As in younger animals, indices of mineral metabolism are not altered by these changes in skeletal metabolism (Vanderschueren *et al.*, 1992).

    As a potential model for the effects of hypogonadism in humans, animal models therefore suggest an early phase of high bone turnover and bone loss after orchidectomy, followed by a later reduction in remodeling rates. How

TABLE IV   Static Histomorphometry of Proximal Tibial Metaphysis Cancellous Bone in Sham-Operated or Orchiectomized 4-Month-Old Male Rats after 1, 2, or 4 Weeks

	N	Bone volume[a] (%)	Trabecular number (n/mm)	Trabecular thickness (µm)	Osteoblast surface[b] (%)	Osteoclast surface[c] (%)	Numbers of osteoclasts[d] (n/mm)
1 week							
Sham	10	10 ± 1	2.6 ± 0.3	41.0 ± 2.6	4.9 ± 0.7	2.1 ± 0.3	0.67 ± 0.07
ORX	9	10 ± 1	2.4 ± 0.3	41.6 ± 2.7	3.8 ± 0.8	3.2 ± 0.7	1.03 ± 0.22
2 weeks							
Sham	9	9 ± 1	2.4 ± 0.3	39.8 ± 2.6	4.4 ± 1.0	1.7 ± 0.3	0.50 ± 0.1
ORX	9	7 ± 1	2.0 ± 0.4	38.6 ± 2.2	8.3 ± 2.8	2.8 ± 0.5	0.81 ± 0.1
4 weeks							
Sham	8	9 ± 1	2.2 ± 0.4	41.9 ± 4.0	$1.9 \pm 0.g$	2.0 ± 0.5	0.57 ± 0.2
ORX	12	6 ± 1	1.4 ± 0.2	41.8 ± 2.5	12.8 ± 2.2^a	3.8 ± 0.5	1.8 ± 0.1

Data expressed as mean $\pm$ SEM.
Significant treatment effect by two-way ANOVA: [a]$P < 0.02$; [c]$P < 0.001$, [d]$P < 0.002$.
Significant interaction effect by two-way ANOVA: [b]$P < 0.003$.
[a]Significantly different from sham, $P < 0.01$.
Reproduced from Gunness and Orwoll, *J. Bone Miner. Res.* 1995; 10:1735–1744 with permission of the American Society for Bone and Mineral Research.

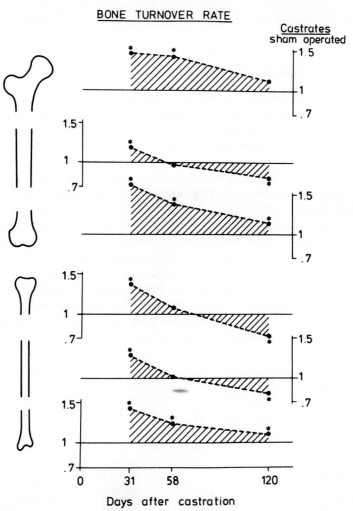

FIGURE 13 Evolution of the bone calcium turnover rate after castration (ratio of castrated/ sham-operated animals). * = $P < 0.05$. Reprinted from Verhas *et al.*, 1986, with permission.

long bone loss continues, and at what rate, is unclear. Both cortical and trabecular compartments are affected. The remodeling imbalance responsible for loss of bone mass appears complex because there are changes in rates of both bone formation and resorption and patterns that vary from one skeletal compartment to another. These changes are very similar to those noted in female animals after castration, in which a loss of estrogen has been associated with a stimulation of osteoblast progenitor differentiation, in turn inciting an increase in osteoclast numbers, bone resorption, and bone loss (Jilka *et al.*, 1998).

D. Androgens in the Female Animal

Of course androgens are present in females as well as males, and may affect bone metabolism. In castrate female rats, DHT administration suppresses elevated levels of markers of bone resorption, as well as increased osteocalcin levels (Mason and Morris, 1997). Interestingly, alkaline phosphatase concentrations increase further. Additional evidence to support the contention that androgens play a role in females includes the fact that antiandrogens are capable of evoking osteopenia in intact (i.e., fully estrogenized) female rats (Goulding and Gold, 1993; Lea *et al.*, 1996) (Figure 14). This obviously suggests that androgens provide crucial support to bone mass independent of estrogens. Of interest, the character of the bone loss induced by flutamide suggested that estrogen prevents bone resorption whereas androgens stimulate bone formation. In periosteal bone, dihydrotestosterone as well as testosterone appear to stimulate bone formation in orchidectomized young male rats, whereas in castrate females they suppress bone formation (Turner *et al.*, 1990b), perhaps reflecting an interaction or synergism between sex steroids and their effects on bone.

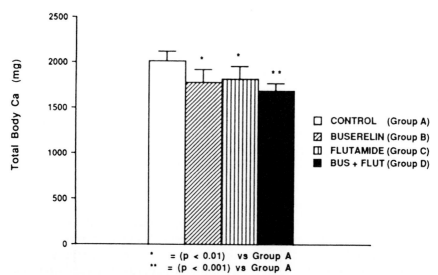

FIGURE 14   Effects of buserelin alone, flutamide alone, and buserelin and flutamide in combination on total-body calcium values after 4 weeks. Results are mean ± SD, $n = 7–8$. Reproduced from Goulding and Gold, *J. Bone Miner. Res.* 1993; 8:763–769 with permission of the American Society for Bone and Mineral Research.

E. Effects of Replacement Sex Steroids after Castration

Essentially all the alterations induced by orchiectomy (in both growing and mature animals) can be prevented by replacement with either testosterone or nonaromatizable androgens (Schoutens *et al.*, 1984; Turner *et al.*, 1990b; Wakley *et al.*, 1991; Vanderschueren *et al.*, 1993a; Sömjen *et al.*, 1994; Kapitola *et al.*, 1995) (Figures 15 and 16). These results strongly suggest that aromatization of androgens to estrogens cannot fully explain the actions of androgens on bone metabolism.

On the other hand, estrogens also seem to prevent bone loss after castration in male animals. Vanderschueren *et al.* (1992) reported that estradiol (and nandrolone) not only was capable of preventing the increase in biochemical indices stimulated by orchiectomy but was also able to prevent cortical and cancellous bone loss. In fact, estradiol resulted in an absolute increase in trabecular bone volume not achieved with androgen replacement. Similarly, estrogen was reported to antagonize the increase in blood flow resulting from castration and to increase bone ash weight more consistently than testosterone. Although the data thus far available are incomplete, these studies raise obvious questions of the overlap between the actions of androgens and estrogens in bone.

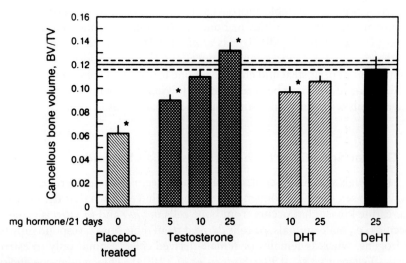

FIGURE 15 Cancellous bone volume (BV/TV) in control and androgen-treated ORX rats (vertical) compared to a reference group consisting of age-matched untreated intact rats of group 1 (horizontal lines). *$P < 0.05$. Reproduced from Wakley *et al.*, *J. Bone Miner. Res.* 1991; 6:325–330 with permission of the American Society for Bone and Mineral Research.

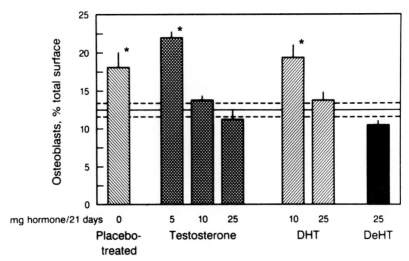

FIGURE 16   Osteoblast-lined cancellous bone surface (percentage of total surface) in control and androgen-treated ORX rats (vertical bars) compared to a reference group consisting of age-matched untreated intact rats of group 1 (horizontal lines). *$P < 0.05$. Reproduced from Wakley *et al., J. Bone Miner. Res.* 1991, 6:325–330 with permission of the American Society for Bone and Mineral Research.

The gender reverse of estrogen replacement in male animals is also instructive. Nonaromatizable androgens are capable of preventing or reversing osteopenia and abnormalities in bone remodeling in oophorectomized females (Turner *et al.*, 1990b; Tobias *et al.*, 1994). These actions apparently are the result of a suppression of cancellous bone resorption as well as a stimulation of periosteal and endosteal bone formation (Tobias *et al.*, 1994). Very similar results have been reported following treatment of oophorectomized animals with dehydroepiandrosterone (Turner *et al.*, 1990b).

F. Gender Specificity in the Actions of Sex Steroids

Although somewhat controversial, there seem to be gender-specific responses to sex steroids. Sömjen and colleagues have shown that the increase in creatine kinase that occurs from bone cells *in vivo* and *in vitro* is gender-specific (i.e., male animals, or cells derived from male bones, respond only to androgens, whereas females or female-derived cells respond only to estrogens) (Weisman *et al.*, 1993; Sömjen *et al.*, 1994). This gender specificity appears to depend on the previous history of exposure of animals to androgens (or estrogens). How such gender-specific effects might affect bone metabolism in the intact animal is completely unknown. Other gender-dependent effects on the skeleton have been reported in mice (Ornoy *et al.*,

1994), and as mentioned earlier, androgens appear to have gender-specific effects on periosteal bone formation (Turner *et al.*, 1990b).

G. The Animal Model of Androgen Resistance

The testicular feminized (TFM, androgen-receptor-deficient) male rate provides an interesting model for the study of the unique effects of androgens in bone. In these rats, androgens are presumed to be incapable of action, but estrogen and androstenedione concentrations are considerably higher than in normal males (Vanderschueren *et al.*, 1993b, 1994b). Clear alterations also exist in TFM male rats in serum levels of calcium and phosphorus (increased), IGF-1 (decreased), and osteocalcin (increased). Results of bone mass measures suggest that TFM rats have reduced longitudinal and radial growth rates, but that cancellous volume and density are similar to those of normal rats. In selected sites, measures of bone mass and remodeling were intermediate between normal male and female values. On the other hand, castration reduced bone volume markedly in TFM male rats, suggesting a major role for estrogens in skeletal homeostasis (Figure 17). This model indicates that androgens have an independent role to play in normal bone growth and metabolism, but the model is complex and not easily dissected.

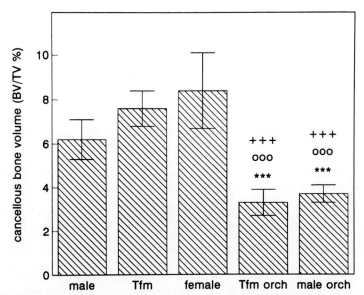

FIGURE 17   Cancellous bone volume (BV/TV in %) of the proximal metaphysis of the tibia in male, female, Tfm, and orchiectomized male rats. Reprinted from Vanderschueren *et al.*, 1994a, with permission.

VIII. Summary

The influences of androgens on bone are obviously pervasive and complex. They are particularly dramatic during growth in boys, but almost certainly play an important role during this period in girls as well. Throughout the rest of life, androgens affect skeletal function in both sexes. Nevertheless, relatively little has been done to unravel the mechanisms by which androgens contribute to the physiology and pathophysiology of bone, and there is still much to be learned about the roles of androgens at all levels. The interaction of androgens and estrogens, and how their respective actions can be used for specific diagnostic and therapeutic benefit, are important but unanswered issues. With an increase in the understanding of the nature of androgen effects will come greater opportunities to use their positive actions in the prevention and treatment of a wide variety of bone disorders.

References

Abdelgadir, S. E., Resko, J. A., Ojeda, S. R., Lephart, E. D., McPhaul, M. J., and Roselli, C. E. (1994). Androgens regulate aromatase cytochrome P450 messenger ribonucleic acid in rat brain. *Endocrinology (Baltimore)* **135**, 395–401.

Abu, E. O., Horner, A., Kusec, V., Triffitt, J. T., and Compston, J. E. (1997). The localization of androgen receptors in human bone. *J. Clin. Endocrinol. Metab.* **82**, 3493–3497.

Audi, L., Carrascosa, A., and Ballabriga, A. (1984). Androgen metabolism by human fetal epiphyseal cartilage and its condrocytes in primary culture. *J. Clin. Endocrinol. Metab.* **58**, 819–825.

Bellido, T., Jilka, R. J., Boyce, B. F., Girasole, G., Broxmeyer, H., Dalrymple, A., Murry, R., and Manolagas, S. C. (1995). Regulation of interleukin-6, osteoclastogenesis and bone mass by androgens: The role of the androgen receptor. *J. Clin. Invest.* **95**, 2886–2895.

Benz, D. J., Haussler, M. R., Thomas, M. A., Speelman, B., and Komm, B. S. (1991). High-affinity androgen binding and androgenic regulation of a_1(I)-procollagen and transforming growth factor-B steady state messenger ribonucleic acid levels in human osteoblast-like osteosarcoma cells. *Endocrinology (Baltimore)* **128**, 2723–2730.

Bilezikian, J. P., Morishima, A., Bell, J., and Grumbach, M. M. (1998). Increased bone mass as a result of estrogen therapy in a man with aromatase deficiency. *N. Engl. J. Med.* **339**, 599–603.

Bodine, P. V. N., Riggs, B. L., and Spelsberg, T. C. (1995). Regulation of c-fos expression and TGF-B production by gonadal and adrenal androgens in normal human osteoblastic cells. *J. Steroid Biochem. Mol. Biol.* **52**, 149–158.

Bruch, H.-R., Wolf, L., Budde, R., Romalo, G., and Schweikert, H.-U. (1992). Androstenedione metabolism in cultured human osteoblast-like cells. *J. Clin. Endocrinol. Metab.* **75**, 101–105.

Canalis, E., Centrella, M., and McCarthy, T. L. (1991). Regulation of insulin-like growth factor-II production in bone cultures. *Endocrinology (Baltimore)* **129**, 2457–2462.

Carani, C., Qin, K., Simoni, M., Faustini-Fustini, M., Serpente, S., Boyd, J., Korach, K. S., and Simpson, E. R. (1997). Effect of testosterone and estradiol in a man with aromatase deficiency. *N. Engl. J. Med.* **337**, 91–95.

Carracosa, A., Audi, L., Ferrandez, M. A., and Ballabriga, A. (1990). Biological effects of androgens and identification of specific dihydrotestosterone-binding sites in cultured human fetal epiphyseal chondrocytes. *J. Clin. Endocrinol. Metab.* **70**, 134–140.

Chang, C., Kokontis, J., and Liao, S. (1988). Structural analysis of complementary DNA and amino acid sequences of human and rat androgen receptors. *Proc. Natl. Acad. Sci. U.S.A.* **85**, 7211–7215.

Colvard, D., Spelsberg, T., Eriksen, E., Keeting, P., and Riggs, L. B. (1989a). Evidence of steroid receptors in human osteoblast-like cells. *Connec. Tissue Res.* **20**, 33–40.

Colvard, D. S., Eriksen, E. F., Keeting, P. E., Wilson, E. M., Lubahn, D. B., French, F. S., Riggs, B. L., and Spelsberg, T. C. (1989b). Identification of androgen receptors in normal human osteoblast-like cells. *Proc. Natl. Acad. Sci. U.S.A.* **86**, 854–857.

Conte, F. A., Grumbach, M. M., Ito, Y., Fisher, C. R., and Simpson, E. R. (1994). A syndrome of female pseudohermaphrodism, hypergonadotropic hypogonadism, and multicystic ovaries associated with missense mutations in the gene encoding aromatase (P450arom). *J. Clin. Endocrinol. Metab.* **78**, 1287–1292.

Corvol, M. T., Carracosa, A., Tsagris, L., Blanchard, O., and Rappaport, R. (1987). Evidence for a direct *in vitro* action of sex steroids on rabbit cartilage cells during skeletal growth: Influence of age and sex. *Endocrinology (Baltimore)* **120**, 1422–1429.

Danielsen, C. C., Mosekilde, L., and Andreassen, T. T. (1992). Long-term effect of orchidectomy on cortical bone from rat femur: Bone mass and mechanical properties. *Calcif. Tissue Int.* **50**, 169–174.

Fisher, L., Kogut, M. D., Moore, r. J., Goebelsmann, U., Weitzmann, J. J., Isaacs, H., Griffin, J. E., and Wilson, J. D. (1978). Clinical, endocrinological and enzymatic characterization of two patients with 5α-reductase deficiency: Evidence that a single enzyme is responsible for the 5α-reduction of cortisol and testosterone. *J. Clin. Endocrinol. Metab.* **47**, 653–664.

Fukayama, S., and Tashjian, H. J. (1989). Direct modulation by androgens of the response of human bone cells (SaOS-2) to human parathyroid hormone (PTH) and PTH-related protein. *Endocrinology (Baltimore)* **125**, 1789–1794.

Gill, R. K., Turner, R. T., Wronski, T. J., and Bell, N. H. (1998). Orchiectomy markedly reduced the concentration of the three isoforms of transforming growth factor β in rat bone, and reduction is prevented by testosterone. *Endocrinology (Baltimore)* **139**, 546–550.

Goulding, A., and Gold, E. (1993). Flutamide-mediated androgen blockade evokes osteopenia in the female rat. *J. Bone Miner. Res.* **8**, 763–769.

Gray, A., Feldman, H. A., McKinlay, J. B., and Longcope, C. (1991). Age, disease and changing sex hormone levels in middle-aged men: Results of the Massachusetts male aging study. *J. Clin. Endocrinol. Metab.* **73**, 1016–1025.

Gray, C., Colston, K. W., Mackay, A. G., Taylor, M. L., and Arnett, T. R. (1992). Interaction of androgen and 1,25-dihydroxyvitamin D3: Effects on normal rat bone cells. *J. Bone Miner. Res.* **7**, 41–46.

Gunness, M., and Orwoll, E. S. (1995). Early induction of alterations in cancellous and cortical bone histology after orchiectomy in mature rats. *J. Bone Miner. Res.* **10**, 1735–1744.

Hock, J. M., Gera, I., Fonseca, J., and Raisz, L. G. (1988). Human parathryoid hormone (1-34) increases bone mass in ovariectomized and orchidectomized rats. *Endocrinology (Baltimore)* **122**, 2899–2904.

Hofbauer, L. C., Hicok, K. C., Schroeder, M. J., Harris, S. A., Robinson, J. A., and Khosla, S. (1997). Development and characterization of a conditionally immortalized human osteoblastic cell line stably transfected with the human androgen receptor gene. *J. Cell. Biochem.* **66**, 542–551.

Iannotti, J. P. (1990). Growth plate physiology and pathology. *Orthop. Clin. North Am.* **21**, 1–17.

Jilka, R. L., Takahashi, K., Munshi, M., Williams, D. C., Roberson, P. K., and Manolagas, S. C. (1998). Loss of estrogen upregulates osteoblastogenesis in the murine bone marrow. *J. Clin. Invest.* **101**, 1942–1950.

Kapitola, J., Kubickova, J., and Andrle, J. (1995). Blood flow and mineral content of the tibia of female and male rats: Changes following castration and/or administration of estradiol or testosterone. *Bone* **16**, 69–72.

Kapur, S. P., and Reddi, A. H. (1989). Influence of testosterone and dihydrotestosterone on bond-matrix induced endochondral bone formation. *Calcif. Tissue Int.* **44**, 108–113.

Kasperk, C. H., Wergedal, J. E., Farley, J. R., Linkhart, T. A., Turner, R. T., and Baylink, D. J. (1989). Androgens directly stimulate proliferation of bone cells in vitro. *Endocrinology (Baltimore)* **124**(3), 1576–1578.

Kasperk, C., Fitzsimmons, R., Strong, D., Mohan, S., Jennings, J., Wergedal, J., and Baylink, D. (1990). Studies of the mechanism by which androgens enhance mitogenesis and differentiation in bone cells. *J. Clin. Endocrinol. Metab.* **71**, 1322–1329.

Kasperk, C., Helmboldt, A., Borcsok, I., Heuthe, S., Cloos, O., Niethard, F., and Ziegler, R. (1997a). Skeletal site-dependent expression of the androgen receptor in human osteoblastic cell populations. *Calcif. Tissue Int.* **61**, 464–473.

Kasperk, C. H., Wakley, G. K., Hierl, T., and Ziegler, R. (1997b). Gonadal and adrenal androgens are potent regulators of human bone cell metabolism in vitro. *J. Bone Miner. Res.* **12**, 464–471.

Kasra, M., and Grynpas, M. D. (1995). The effects of androgens on the mechanical properties of primate bone. *Bone* **17**, 265–270.

Kemppainen, J. A., Lane, M. V., Sar, M., and Wilson, E. M. (1992). Androgen receptor phosphorylation, turnover, nuclear transport, and transcriptional activation. *J. Biol. Chem.* **267**, 968–974.

Lea, C., Kendall, N., and Flanagan, A. M. (1996). Casodex (a nonsteroidal antiandrogen) reduces cancellous, endosteal, and periosteal bone formation in estrogen-replete female rats. *Calcif. Tissue Int.* **58**, 268–272.

Lebovitz, H. E., and Eisenbarth, G. S. (1975). Hormonal regulation of cartilage growth and metabolism. *Vitam. Horm. (N.Y.)* **33**, 575–648.

Lieberherr, M., and Grosse, B. (1994). Androgens increase intracellular calcium concentration and inositol 1,4,5-triphosphate and diacylglycerol formation via a pertussis toxin-sensitive G-protein. *J. Biol. Chem.* **269**, 7217–7223.

Lieberherr, M., Grosse, B., Kachkache, M., and Balsan, S. (1993). Cell signaling and estrogens in female rat osteoblasts: A possible involvement of unconventional nonnuclear receptors. *J. Bone Miner. Res.* **8**, 1365–1376.

Liesegang, P., Romalo, G., Sudmann, M., Wolf, L., and Schweikert, H.-U. (1994). Human osteoblast-like cells contain specific saturable, high-affinity glucocorticoid, androgen, estrogen and 1α,25-dihydroxycholecalciferol receptors. *J. Androl.* **15**, 194–199.

Lin, S.-C., Yamate, T., Taguchi, Y., Borba, V. Z. C., Girasole, G., O'Brian, C. A., Bellido, T., Abe, E., and Manolagos, S. C. (1997). Regulation of the gp80 and gp130 subunits of the IL-6 receptor by sex steroids in the murine bone marrow. *J. Clin. Invest.* **101**, 1942–1950.

Lubahn, D. B., Joseph, D. B., Sullivan, P. M., Willard, H. F., French, F. S., and Wilson, E. M. (1988). Cloning of human androgen receptor complementary DNA and localization to the X chromosome. *Science* **240**, 327–330.

Mahendroo, M. S., Cala, K. M., Landrum, C. P., and Russell, D. W. (1997). Fetal death in mice lacking 5α-reductase type I caused by estrogen excess. *Mol. Endocrinol.* **11**, 917–927.

Mason, R. A., and Morris, H. A. (1997). Effects of dihydrotestosterone on bone biochemical markers in sham and oophorectomized rats. *J. Bone Miner. Res.* **12**, 1431–1437.

Masuyama, A., Ouchi, Y., Sato, F., Hosoi, T., Nakamura, T., and Orimo, H. (1992). Characteristics of steroid hormone receptors in cultured MC3T3-E1 osteoblastic cells and effect of steroid hormones on cell proliferation. *Calcif. Tissue Int.* **51**, 376–381.

Meikle, A. W., Dorchuck, R. W., Araneo, B. A., Stringham, J. D., Evans, T. G., Spruance, S. L., and Daynes, R. A. (1992). The presence of a dehydroepiandrosterone-specific receptor binding complex in murine T cells. *J. Steroid Biochem. Mol. Biol.* **42**, 293–304.

Mizuno, Y., Hosoi, T., Inoue, S., Ikegami, A., Kaneki, M., Akedo, Y., Nakamura, T., Ouchi, Y., Chang, C., and Orimo, H. (1994). Immunocytochemical identification of androgen receptor in mouse osteoclast-like multinucleated cells. *Calcif. Tissue Int.* **54**, 325–326.

Morishima, A., Grumbach, M. M., Simpson, E. R., Fisher, C., and Qin, K. (1995). Aromatase deficiency in male and female siblings caused by a novel mutation and the physiological role of estrogens. *J. Clin. Endocrinol. Metab.* **80**, 3689–3698.

Nakano, Y., Morimoto, I., Ishida, O., Fujihira, T., Mizokami, A., Tanimoto, A., Yamagihara, N., Izumi, F., and Eto, S. (1994). The receptor, metabolism and effects of androgen in osteoblastic MC3T3-E1 cells. *Bone Miner.* **26**, 245–259.

Nawata, H., Tanaka, S., Takayanagi, R., Sakai, Y., Yanase, T., Ikuyama, S., and Haji, M. (1995). Aromatase in bone cell: Association with osteoporosis in postmenopausal women. *J. Steroid Biochem. Mol. Biol.* **53**, 165–174.

Ongphiphadhanakul, B., Alex, S., Braverman, L. F., and Baran, D. T. (1992). Excessive L-thyroxine therapy decreases femoral bone densities in the male rat: Effect of hypogonadism and calcitonin. *J. Bone Miner. Res.* **7**, 1227–1231.

Ornoy, A., Giron, S., Aner, R., Goldstein, M., Boyan, B. D., and Schwartz, Z. (1994). Gender dependent effects of testosterone and 17b-estradiol on bone growth and modelling in young mice. *Bone Miner.* **24**, 43–58.

Orwoll, E. S., Stribrska, L., Ramsay, E. E., and Keenan, E. (1991). Androgen receptors in osteoblast-like cell lines. *Calcif. Tissue Int.* **49**, 182–187.

Oursler, M. J., Osdoby, P., Pyfferoen, J., Riggs, B. L., and Spelsberg, T. C. (1991). Avian osteoclasts as estrogen target cells. *Proc. Natl. Acad. Sci. U.S.A.* **88**, 6613–6617.

Pilbeam, C. C., and Raisz, L. G. (1990). Effects of androgens on parathyroid hormone and interleukin-1-stimulated prostaglandin production in cultured neonatal mouse calvariae. *J. Bone Miner. Res.* **5**, 1183–1188.

Purohit, A., Flanagan, A. M., and Reed, M. J. (1992). Estrogen synthesis by osteoblast cell lines. *Endocrinology (Baltimore)* **131**, 2027–2029.

Raisz, L. G., Wiita, B., Artis, A., Bowen, A., Schwartz, S., Trahiotis, M., Shoukril, K., and Smith, J. (1996). Comparison of the effects of estrogen alone and estrogen plus androgen on biochemical markers of bone formation and resorption in postmenopausal women. *J. Clin. Endocrinol. Metab.* **81**, 37–43.

Ren, S. G., Malozowski, S., Sanchez, P., Sweet, D. E., Loriaux, D. L., and Cassorla, F. (1989). Direct administration of testosterone increases rat tibial epiphyseal growth plate width. *Acta Endocrinol. (Copenhagen)* **21**, 401–405.

Rosen, H. N., Tollin, S., Balena, R., Middlebrooks, V. L., Beamer, W. G., Donohue, L., R. Rosen, C., Turner, A., Holick, M., and Greenspan, S. L. (1995). Differentiating between orchiectomized rats and controls using measurements of trabecular bone density: A comparison among DXA, histomorphometry, and peripheral quantitative computerized tomography. *Calcif. Tissue Int.* **57**, 35–39.

Rosenberg, M. J., King, T. D. N., and Timmons, M. C. (1997). Estrogen-androgen for hormone replacement. *J. Reprod. Med.* **42**, 394–404.

Russell, D. W., and Wilson, J. D. (1994). Steroid 5α-reductase: Two genes/two enzymes. *Annu. Rev. Biochem.* **63**.

Sasano, H., Uzuki, M., Sawai, T., Nagura, H., Matsunaga, G., Kashimoto, O., and Harada, N. (1997). Aromatase in human bone tissue. *J. Bone Miner. Res.* **12**, 1416–1423.

Saville, P. D., and Lieber, C. S. (1969). Increases in skeletal calcium and femur cortex thickness in undernutrition. *J. Nutr.* **99**, 141–144.

Schoutens, A., Verhas, M., L'Hermite-Baleriaux, M., L'Hermite, M., Verschaeren, A., Dourov, N., Mone, M., Heilporn, A., and Tricot, A. (1984). Growth and bone haemodynamic responses to castration in male rats. Reversibility by testosterone. *Acta Endocrinol. (Copenhagen)* **107**, 428–432.

Schwartz, Z., Nasatzky, E., Ornoy, A., Brooks, B. P., Soskolne, W. A., and Boyan, B. D. (1994). Gender-specific, maturation-dependent effects of testosterone on chondrocytes in culture. *Endocrinology (Baltimore)* **134**, 1640–1647.

Schweikert, H.-U., Rulf, W., Niederle, N., Schafer, H. E., Kreck, E., and Kruck, F. (1980). Testosterone metabolism in human bone. *Acta Endocrinol. (Copenhagen)* **95**, 258–264.

Schweikert, H.-U., Wolf, L., and Romalo, G. (1995). Estrogen formation from androstenedione in human bone. *Clin. Endocrinol.* **43**, 37–42.

Simpson, E. R., Mahendroo, M. S., Means, G. D., Kilgore, M. W., Hinshelwood, M. M., Graham-Lorence, S., Amarneh, B., Ito, Y., Fisher, C. R., Michael, M. D., Mendelson, C. R., and Bulun, S. E. (1994). Aromatase cytochrome P450, the enzyme responsible for estrogen biosynthesis. *Endocr. Rev.* **15**, 342–355.

Smith, E. P., Boyd, J., Frank, G. R., Takahashi, H., Cohen, R. M., Specker, B., Williams, T. C., Lubahn, D. B., and Korach, K. S. (1994). Estrogen resistance caused by a mutation in the estrogen-receptor gene in a man. *N. Engl. J. Med.* **331**, 1056–1061.

Sömjen, D., Weisman, Y., Harell, A., Berger, E., and Kaye, A. M. (1989). Direct and sex-specific stimulation by sex steroids of creatine kinase activity and DNA synthesis in rat bone. *Proc. Natl. Acad. Sci. U.S.A.* **86**, 3361–3365.

Sömjen, D., Weisman, Y., Mor, Z., Harell, A., and Kaye, A. M. (1991). Regulation of proliferation of rat cartilage and bone by sex steroid hormones. *J. Steroid Biochem. Mol. Biol.* **40**, 717–723.

Sömjen, D., Mor, Z., and Kaye, A. M. (1994). Age dependence and modulation by gonadectomy of the sex-specific response of rat diaphyseal bone to gonadal steroids. *Endocrinology (Baltimore)* **134**, 809–814.

Takeuchi, M., Kakushi, H., and Tohkin, M. (1994). Androgens directly stimulate mineralization and increase androgen receptors in human osteoblast-like osteosarcoma cells. *Biochem. Biophys. Res. Commun.* **204**, 905–911.

Tanaka, S., Haji, M., Nishi, Y., Yanase, T., Takayanagi, R., and Nawata, H. (1993). Aromatase activity in human osteoblast-like osteosarcoma cell. *Calcif. Tissue Int.* **52**, 107–109.

Tobias, J. H., Gallagher, A., and Chambers, T. J. (1994). 5α-dihydrotestosterone partially restores cancellous bone volume in osteopenic ovariectomized rats. *Am. J. Physiol.* **267**, E853–E859.

Turner, R. T., Hannon, K. S., Demers, L. N., Buchanan, J., and Bell, N. (1989). Differential effects of gonadal function in bone histomorphometry in male and female rats. *J. Bone Miner. Res.* **4**, 557–563.

Turner, R. T., Bleiberg, B., Colvard, D. S., Keeting, P. E., Evans, G., and Spelsberg, T. C. (1990a). Failure of isolated rat tibial periosteal cells to 5α reduce testosterone to 5α-dihydrotestosterone. *J. Bone Miner. Res.* **5**, 775–779.

Turner, R. T., Wakley, G. K., and Hannon, K. S. (1990b). Differential effects of androgens on cortical bone histomorphometry in gonadectomized male and female rats. *J. Orthop. Res.* **8**, 612–617.

Turner, R. T., Riggs, B. L., and Spelsberg, T. C. (1994). Skeletal effects of estrogen. *Endocr. Rev.* **15**, 275–300.

Tuukkanen, J., Peng, Z., and Vaananen, H. K. (1994). Effect of running exercise on the bone loss induced by orchidectomy in the rat. *Calcif. Tissue Int.* **55**, 33–37.

Underwood, L. E., and Van Wyk, J. J. (1992). Normal and aberrant growth. *In* "Williams Textbook of Endocrinology" (J. D. Wilson and D. W. Foster, eds.), 8th ed., pp. 1079–1138. Saunders, Philadelphia.

Vanderschueren, D., and Bouillon, R. (1995). Androgens and bone. *Calcif. Tissue Int.* **56**, 341–346.

Vanderschueren, D., and Van Herck, E. (1992). Androgen deficiency effects in the rat skeleton. *Workshop Using Live Rate Skeletal Stud., 2nd,* Chicago.

Vanderschueren, D., Van Herck, E., Suiker, A. M. H., Visser, W. J., Schot, L. P. C., and Bouillon, R. (1992). Bone and mineral metabolism in aged male rats: Short and long term effects of androgen deficiency. *Endocrinology (Baltimore)* **130**, 2906–2916.

Vanderschueren, D., Van Herck, E., Schot, P., Rush, E., Einhorn, T., Geusens, P., and Bouillon, R. (1993a). The aged male rat as a model for human osteoporosis: Evaluation by nondestructive measurements and biomechanical testing. *Calcif. Tissue Int.* **53**, 342–347.

Vanderschueren, D., Van Herck, E., Suiker, A. M. H., Visser, W. J., Scot, L. P. C., Chung, K., Lucas, R. S., Einhorn, T. A., and Bouillon, R. (1993b). Bone and mineral metabolism in the androgen-resistant (testicular feminized) male rat. *J. Bone Miner. Res.* **8**, 801–809.

Vanderschueren, D., Jans, I., Van Herck, E., Moermans, K., Verhaeghe, J., and Bouillon, R. (1994a). Time-related increase of biochemical markers of bone turnover in androgen-deficient male rats. *Bone Miner.* **26**, 123–131.

Vanderschueren, D., Van Herck, E., Geusens, P., Suiker, A., Visser, W., Chung, K., and Bouillon, R. (1994b). Androgen resistance and deficiency have difference effects on the growing skeleton of the rat. *Calcif. Tissue Int.* **55**, 198–203.

Vanderschueren, D., Van Herck, E., De Coster, R., and Bouillon, R. (1996). Aromatization of androgens is important for skeletal maintenance of aged male rats. *Calcif. Tissue Int.* **59**, 179–183.

Vanderschueren, D., Van Herck, E., Nijs, J., and Ederveen, A. G. H. (1997). Aromatase inhibition impairs skeletal modeling and decreases bone mineral density in growing male rats. *Endocrinology (Baltimore)* **138**, 2301–2307.

Verhas, M., Schoutens, A., L'hermite-Baleriaux, M., Dourov, N., Verschaeren, A., Mone, M., and Heilporn, A. (1986). The effect of orchidectomy on bone metabolism in aging rats. *Calcif. Tissue Int.* **39**, 74–77.

Vermeulen, A. (1991). Clinical review 24: androgens in the aging male. *J. Clin. Endocrinol. Metab.* **73**, 221–224.

Vittek, J., Altman, K., Gordon, G. G., and Southren, A. L. (1974). The metabolism of 7α-³H-testosterone by rat mandibular bone. *Endocrinology (Baltimore)* **94**, 325–329.

Wakley, G. K., Schutte, H. D. J., Hannon, K. S., and Turner, R. T. (1991). Androgen treatment prevents loss of cancellous bone in the orchidectomized rat. *J. Bone Miner. Res.* **6**, 325–330.

Weinstein, R. S., Jilka, R. L., Parfitt, A. M., and Manolagas, S. C. (1997). The effects of androgen deficiency on murine bone remodeling and bone mineral density are mediated via cells of the osteoblastic lineage. *Endocrinology (Baltimore)* **138**, 4013–4021.

Weisman, Y., Cassoria, F., Malozowski, S., Krieg, R. J. J., Goldray, D., Kaye, A. M., and Sömjen, D. (1993). Sex-specific response of bone cells to gonadal steroids: Modulation in perinatally androgenized females and in testicular feminized male rats. *Steroids* **58**, 126–133.

Wilson, C. M., and McPhaul, M. J. (1994). A and B forms of the androgen receptor are present in human genital skin fibroblasts. *Proc. Natl. Acad. Sci. U.S.A.* **91**, 1234–1238.

Wink, C. S., and Felts, W. J. L. (1980). Effects of castration on the bone structure of male rats: A model of osteoporosis. *Calcif. Tissue Int.* **32**, 77–82.

Wiren, K. M., Zhang, X., Chang, C., Keenan, E., and Orwoll, E. (1997). Transcriptional upregulation of the human androgen receptor by androgen in bone cells. *Endocrinology (Baltimore)* **138**, 2291–2300.

Wrogemann, K., Podolsky, G., Gu, J., and Rosenmann, E. (1991). A 63-kDa protein with androgen-binding activity is not from the androgen receptor. *Biochem. Cell Biol.* **69**, 695–701.

Zhuang, Y. H., Blauer, M., Pekki, A., and Tuohimaa, P. (1992). Subcellular location of androgen receptor in rat prostate, seminal vesicle and human osteosarcoma MG-63 cells. *J. Steroid Biochem. Mol. Biol.* **41**, 693–696.

Chapter 13

Eric S. Orwoll

Bone and Mineral Unit
Oregon Health Sciences University
and the Portland VA Medical Center
Portland, Oregon

Androgens and Bone:
Clinical Aspects

I. Introduction

Androgens have myriad actions on the skeleton throughout life. During adolescence those effects clearly promote skeletal growth and the accumulation of mineral mass, and for many years there has been hope that these anabolic effects will be useful in the prevention and therapy of metabolic bone disease in later life. In fact, the essential nature of the effects of androgens in bone remains uncertain, and the clinical usefulness of androgens is clearly defined in only a few situations. Nevertheless, there is an increasing interest in how the actions of androgens are integrated into the broad scheme of bone metabolism and how those effects can be adapted for prevention and therapy.

II. Puberty

Adolescence is associated with profound increases in bone mass in both sexes. Both axial and appendicular bone mass increase (Gilsanz et al., 1988; Lu et al., 1994), with the addition of almost half of the total adult skeleton during this brief time. In boys, the rapid increase in indices of bone formation and skeletal mass during this period is closely linked to pubertal stage (Krabbe et al., 1979; Bonjour et al., 1991) (Figure 1) and to testosterone levels (Krabbe et al., 1979, 1984; Riis et al., 1985). These data are consistent with the precept that testicular androgen secretion plays a role in the genesis of the adolescent increase in bone mass. In addition, however, the increase in adrenal androgens that occurs in the prepubertal period (adrenarche) (Odell, 1989) may also affect bone mass. Longitudinal bone growth (via epiphyseal action) has been reported to accelerate during adrenarche (Parker, 1991). Bone mass accretion certainly occurs before sexual development begins (Slemenda et al., 1994) and could be influenced by the actions of adrenal androgens.

The overall result is a male skeleton that is larger in most dimensions, thus conferring a considerable biomechanical advantage. Total body mineral content is 25–30% greater in men (Rico et al., 1992). Both the diameter and cortical thickness (and hence the total mass and mineral content) of long bones is greater in men (Kelly et al., 1990b; Fehily et al., 1992). Vertebral size is also larger in men, even when other elements of body size (height, weight) are controlled (Gilsanz et al., 1994) (Table I). These gender differences in bone size are not matched by differences in the essential composition of bone because the true volumetric density of the bone in men and women is essentially the same (Bonjour et al., 1994).

That these pubertal changes in the male skeleton are related to androgen action is suggested by several kinds of evidence. Genetic males with complete androgen resistance appear to have low bone density (Soule et al., 1996) and a skeletal mass similar to that of women (Munoz-Torres et al., 1995). Moreover, the presence of androgen insufficiency, for instance in patients with isolated gonadotrophin deficiency, results in abnormally low bone mass even when corrected for bone age (Finkelstein et al., 1987). Treatment of these patients with testosterone before epiphyseal closure results in a rapid increase in bone mass (Finkelstein et al., 1989; Arisaka et al., 1991; Devogelaer et al., 1992). Finally, the short-term administration of testosterone to prepubertal boys quickly causes an increase in calcium retention and incorporation into bone (Mauras et al., 1994) (Figure 2). Nonaromatizable androgens have been reported to increase linear growth (Stanhope et al., 1988; Keenan et al., 1993), but their effects on bone density aren't yet clear.

Not only do androgens seem to be involved in normal bone mass development, but the actual timing of the onset of puberty is fundamentally important as well. It has been known that constitutionally delayed puberty can result in somewhat greater adult height (Uriarte et al., 1992), but bone mass

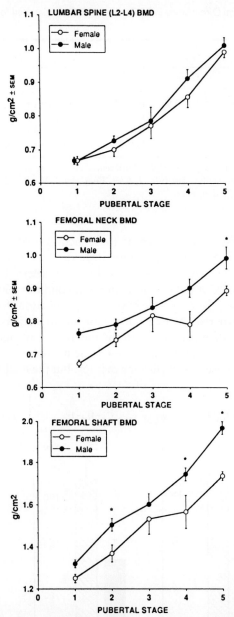

FIGURE I   Relation between BMD at the levels of the lumbar spine (I2–L4), FN, and FS and pubertal stages in female and male subjects. *, $P < 0.05$. Reproduced from Bonjour, J.-P., *et al.* (1991). Critical years and stages of puberty for spinal and femoral bone mass accumulation during adolescence. *J. Clin. Endocrinol. Metab.* **73**, 555–563, © The Endocrine Society, with permission.

TABLE I.   Vertebral Dimensions in 30 Boys and 30 Girls Matched for Age, Height, and Weight

	Cross-sectional area (cm²)			Height (cm)		
	Boys	Girls	P value	Boys	Girls	P value
L1	7.72 ± 1.24	6.69 ± 0.99	0.0001	1.83 ± 0.14	1.86 ± 0.18	NS
L2	8.33 ± 1.46	7.49 ± 0.99	0.0003	1.89 ± 0.14	1.93 ± 0.17	NS
L3	9.12 ± 1.46	8.12 ± 0.98	0.0001	1.94 ± 0.13	1.97 ± 0.16	NS
Mean	8.39 ± 1.35	7.50 ± 0.98	0.0001	1.89 ± 0.13	1.92 ± 0.17	NS

Reproduced from Gilsanz, V., *et al.* (1997). Differential effect of gender on the sizes of the bones in the axial and appendicular skeletons. *J. Clin. Endocrinol. Metab.* 82, 1603–1607, © The Endocrine Society, with permission.

is reduced in these patients even at the conclusion of sexual maturation (Finkelstein *et al.*, 1992, 1996) (Figure 3). In delayed puberty, bone density is also reduced even when adjusted for bone age (Bertelloni *et al.*, 1995). Constitutional delay of puberty is a common condition, and this reduction in peak adult bone mass may have important implications for eventual osteoporosis and fracture risk. More evidence for the importance of the timing of puberty comes from experience with the therapy of hypogonadal men who have not yet undergone puberty. In these patients, there is a brisk increase in bone mass in response to testosterone therapy, but the final bone mass devel-

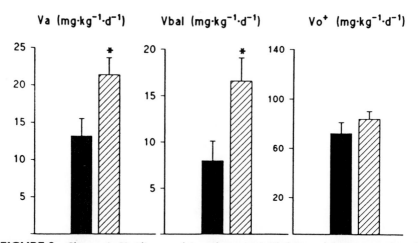

FIGURE 2   Changes in Va (dietary calcium absorption), Vbal (net calcium retention), and Vo+ (rate of bone accretion) in prepubertal children treated with testosterone (*n* = 6). Solid bars, before testosterone; hatched bars, after testosterone. *, *P* < 0.05. Reproduced from The Journal of Clinical Investigation, 1994, vol. 93, pp. 1014–1019 by copyright permission of the American Society for Clinical Investigation.

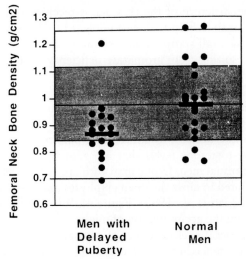

FIGURE 3   Femoral neck bone mineral density in 18 men with histories of delayed puberty and 24 normal men. The thick horizontal lines indicate the group means, and the shaded areas indicate the mean ± 1 SD and ± 2 SD for 24 normal men. The mean values in the two groups were significantly different ($P < 0.02$). Reproduced from Finkelstein, J. S., *et al.* (1996). A longitudinal evaluation of bone mineral density in adult men with histories of delayed puberty. *J. Clin. Endocrinol. Metab.* **81**, 1152–1155, © The Endocrine Society, with permission.

oped is impaired (Finkelstein *et al.*, 1989). A similar response is seen in boys with constitutional pubertal delay treated with testosterone (Bertelloni *et al.*, 1995).

All these findings support a crucial role of pubertal androgens in the development of adult bone mass in the male, probably as a result of both direct and indirect actions at the skeletal level. Because androgens are important in the development of peak bone mass, there is great potential for the use of androgens as therapeutic agents during this period of life. As is discussed elsewhere in this volume, the mechanisms by which androgens affect bone, particularly during growth, are probably integrally related to the effects of estrogens and the activity of aromatases.

III. Estrogens versus Androgens in Puberty

The dynamic interplay between androgens and estrogens at the skeletal level during puberty is not well understood but is probably quite important. That estrogen action is essential for the development of peak bone mass in men has been highlighted by reports of interesting young men with estrogen deficiency. Smith *et al.* (1994) described a young adult patient with an abnormality in the structure of the estrogen α-receptor (thus rendering him functionally estrogen-deficient, at least in regard to the α-receptor) who had a delayed bone age, tall stature, and profound osteopenia. Men with estrogen deficiency resulting from aromatase deficiency have also been recently noted to have a very similar phenotype (Morishima *et al.*, 1995; Bilezikian *et al.*, 1998). The common abnormalities in bone age and stature in these estrogen-deficient patients are to be expected because estrogens are essential for normal closure of growth plates in both sexes. The aberrations noted in bone mass are more difficult to understand, particularly because they exist in the face of testosterone levels that are actually higher (even strikingly higher) than in normal men. In one man with aromatase deficiency, estrogen treatment was noted to close the open epiphyses and result in an increase in bone mass (Bilezikian *et al.*, 1998) (Figure 4). Whether the increase in bone mass resulted from the accumulation of mineral at the growth plates or was the result of a general skeletal effect of estrogen is unknown, but it is of fundamental importance in the understanding of the respective roles of androgen and estrogen. If in fact the estrogen therapy resulted in an increase in bone mass unrelated to epiphyseal closure, estrogen would assume a more pivotal role in skeletal maturation in men and would shift therapeutic attention (for instance, in hypogonadal adolescents) to ensuring the adequacy of estrogen as well as androgen action.

IV. Age-Related Declines in Androgen Levels in Adult Men: Contribution to Bone Loss

Aging is associated with a clear decline in testicular and adrenal androgen levels in men (Gray *et al.*, 1991; Vermeulen, 1991), and there is considerable interest in the possibility that androgen replacement may attenuate that loss and reduce fracture rates in the elderly. Although there have been attempts to evaluate this hypothesis, most efforts have been indirect and less than conclusive. For instance, a variety of cross-sectional studies have examined the relationship between androgen levels and bone mass in older men. Some have suggested a significant association between androgen concentrations and bone mass (McElduff *et al.*, 1988; Kelly *et al.*, 1990b; Murphy *et al.*, 1993; Rudman *et al.*, 1994; Ongphiphadhanakul *et al.*, 1995), but others have not been able to substantiate an interaction between bone mass and either testosterone or adrenal androgens (Meier *et al.*, 1987; Barrett-Connor *et al.*, 1993; Drinka *et al.*, 1993; Wishart *et al.*, 1995). There continues to be much speculation about the role of the age-related decline in androgen levels in the development of bone loss in older men, and controversy surrounds the issue of whether androgen replacement is useful in the prevention of osteoporosis in older men.

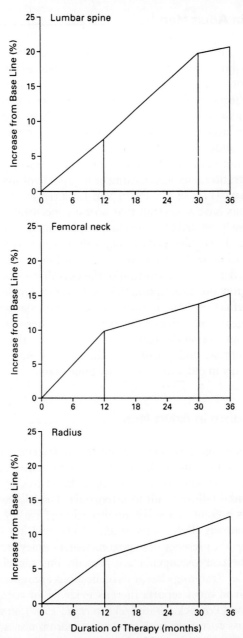

FIGURE 4   Changes in bone density during estrogen therapy. The percentage increase from baseline values is shown for each site. After the baseline determination, specific measurements were made at 12, 30, and 36 months. Reproduced from Bilezikian *et al.* (1998), Copyright © 1998 Massachusetts Medical Society. All rights reserved.

V. Estrogens in Adult Men

The possibility that there is an important role for estrogens in the maintenance of adult bone mass in men must be considered. It is feasible that estrogens function in men to maintain bone mass, presumably in concert with the direct effects of androgens. Recent data suggest that estrogen levels are significantly associated with bone mass in elderly men (Slemenda *et al.*, 1997) and that reduced estrogen levels may be related to the development of low bone mass in older men (Bernecker *et al.*, 1995). A fascinating series of male-to-female transsexuals indicates that in the presence of antiandrogen treatment or castration, estrogen treatment is capable of maintaining or increasing bone mass (Lips *et al.*, 1989; Van Kesteren *et al.*, 1996). In fact, recent publications have suggested that serum concentrations of estrogens may be more closely related to bone mass in older men than are androgens (Greendale *et al.*, 1997; Slemenda *et al.*, 1997). The correlations between estrogen levels and bone density were significant but were quite weak, and estrogen explained a minor proportion of the overall variation in bone density. Despite the previous assumption that androgens provided the dominant gonadal steroid effect on bone in men, this new information demands that the role of estrogens, and interactions between sex steroids, be further examined. These controversies remain unresolved and clearly affect the question of the usefulness, and possible mechanisms of action, of androgen replacement therapy in older men with low bone mass.

VI. Hypogonadism in Adult Men

After peak bone mass is achieved during adolescence, androgens continue to be vitally important in the maintenance of bone health. Abnormal gonadal function is well known to incur risk for bone loss, and a wide variety of causes of gonadal failure result in osteopenia (Orwoll and Klein, 1995). Hypogonadism is present in a substantial portion (15%) of men evaluated for severe osteoporosis (Kelepouris *et al.*, 1995), and hip fracture occurs more commonly in the presence of hypogonadism (Stanley *et al.*, 1991). Both cortical and trabecular osteopenia are present, but cancellous bone loss seems most intense. Resulting changes in cancellous architecture are not well characterized, but in most reports there is evidence of reduced trabecular number (Francis and Peacock, 1986; Jackson *et al.*, 1987). In some series, the degree of bone loss correlates with the level of serum testosterone (Foresta *et al.*, 1983; Horowitz *et al.*, 1992), but that is not a consistent finding. A threshold level of serum testosterone below which bone mass begins to decline, even in the absence of other skeletal stressors, has not been established. This issue is of considerable importance given the very wide range of testosterone levels in adult men and the lack of consensus concerning the definition of hypogonadism. Finally, because hypogonadism in men is usually characterized by at least some degree of estrogen as well as androgen deficiency, a component of hypogonadal bone disease may be related to a lack of estrogen action. Although this issue is not well understood, it remains likely that androgen deficiency is a major determinant of the observed changes in bone metabolism (*vide supra*).

Androgen insufficiency may be an important component of several other forms of metabolic bone disease as well. For instance, in subjects treated with glucocorticoids, testosterone levels can be substantially reduced (Reid *et al.*, 1985) and may contribute to bone loss. Similar interactions may result in remodeling alterations in patients with renal insufficiency, alcoholism, chemotherapy, and the like (Orwoll and Klein, 1995).

The mechanisms by which androgen withdrawal leads to bone loss in men have only begun to be explored. In the most direct assessment of the events following the onset of hypogonadism, Stepan *et al.* (1989) examined changes in bone mass and biochemical indices of remodeling in a group of men undergoing castration. In the 1 to 3 years these men were followed after orchidectomy, vertebral bone loss was rapid (~7%/year) (Figure 5) and progressed in conjunction with clear evidence of an increase in bone turnover. Essentially the same changes occur after the institution of GnRH agonist therapy in adult men (Goldray *et al.*, 1993). Thus in the early stages of hypo-

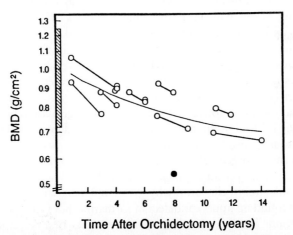

Time After Orchidectomy (years)

FIGURE 5   Scattergram of lumbar spinal BMD as a function of time after orchidectomy in 12 men. In eight patients the measurement was repeated after 1–3 years (_____). The line is a regression (second order). Deletion of the repeated measurements made no significant difference to the regression. The hatched bar indicates the normal range in men 25 to 45 years old for this laboratory. ●, A man who developed a hip fracture and died from its complications. Reproduced from Stepan, J. J., *et al.* (1989). Castrated men exhibit bone loss. *J. Clin. Endocrinol. Metab.* **69**, 523–527, © The Endocrine Society, with permission.

gonadism there appears to be an increase in remodeling and bone resorption, just as is seen in animal models of gonadal insufficiency. This concept is supported by the data indicating androgen action is important in the suppression of cytokines active in the stimulation of osteoclastogenesis (Bellido et al., 1995). Bone loss seems to be most intense in the several years after castration, with a subsequent slower phase of loss—a process remarkably similar to that seen in women after menopause. This pattern also is observed in castrate animals (Gunness and Orwoll, 1995). More information is needed concerning the histomorphometric character of acute androgen deficiency and the effects on specific skeletal compartments. For instance, it is unclear to what extent an androgen-dependent depression of bone formation accompanies the increase in bone resorption, especially in the slower phase of bone loss that probably follows the rapid loss that occurs immediately after the onset of hypogonadism. Whether abnormalities in cortical bone metabolism are as profound as those reported to occur in cancellous bone is also uncertain.

Commonly, the diagnosis of hypogonadism is made in the subacute or chronic phases of the disorder, and most evaluations of the nature of hypogonadal bone disease involve patients with long-standing reproductive abnormalities. In these patients the mechanisms responsible for osteopenia are particularly unclear, and the histological pattern of the bone disorder is not well described. There are some small retrospective series available, and most other reports are uncontrolled and involve men in whom the hypogonadism was of varied causation and duration. For example, in a study of 13 men with long-standing hypogonadism, Francis and Peacock (1986) found that bone remodeling and formation rates were reduced, and $1,25\text{-}(OH)_2$vitamin D levels and intestinal calcium absorption were low in those with fracture. With testosterone therapy, $1,25\text{-}(OH)_2$vitamin D levels increased, and there was a suggestion that indices of bone formation increased. Similarly, Delmas and Meunier (1981) found decreased rates of formation in a small group of hypogonadal men, and formation was low in a single case report by Baran (Baran et al., 1978), but vitamin D levels were not described. These contributions certainly raise the question of whether the osteopenia in patients with long-term androgen deficiency is, to a major extent, the result of a defect in bone formation. In contrast, Jackson et al. (1987) described the histomorphometric character of chronically hypogonadal men without vitamin D deficiency and found no apparent defect in formation but rather an increase in bone resorption. They suggested that earlier findings of a defect in bone formation were more the result of insufficient vitamin D action than of gonadal insufficiency. Actually, in all the available reports, there is considerable subject heterogeneity, and the nature of remodeling is quite variable. In the face of this considerable patient diversity, inadequate controls, and the presence of other confounding medical conditions, no firm conclusions can be drawn concerning the remodeling defect induced by long-standing hypogonadism in men. If it is similar to that in postmenopausal women, it would be expected that the initial period of increased remodeling would be followed by one of relatively lower remodeling rates and slower rates of change in bone mass. Since the descriptions of osteoporosis by Fuller Albright half a century ago, a reduction in bone formation has been postulated to be a primary cause of hypogonadal bone disease. In fact, this precept remains essentially unproved.

VII. Androgen Therapy: Potentially Useful Androgen Effects

Despite the relative paucity of research concerning androgen action in bone, there are several well-known effects, both direct and indirect, that may prove beneficial. An understanding of these actions was derived primarily from observations in animals or during human adolescence, but they have the potential to be translated into therapeutic terms.

A. Growth Promoting Effects

During adolescence, androgens appear to exert important effects on the skeleton. By the end of puberty, men have greater bone mass than women, a difference that is most marked in the cortical compartment (greater cortical diameter and thickness) (Martin, 1993; Bonjour *et al.*, 1994; van der Meulen *et al.*, 1996). Studies of the effects of testosterone on skeletal calcium accumulation during childhood strongly suggest that this is a direct effect of gonadal steroids (Mauras *et al.*, 1994), and in animals orchidectomy reduces periosteal bone formation, an effect which is reversed with androgen therapy (Turner *et al.*, 1990). The observation that, in genetic males with complete androgen insensitivity (androgen receptor dysfunction), skeletal size is similar to that in normal females strongly suggests that androgens play a major role (Vanderschueren, 1996). Nonaromatizable androgens promote skeletal growth (Stanhope *et al.*, 1988; Keenan *et al.*, 1993).

However, there may also be indirect effects that account for a larger skeleton in men. For instance, before and through puberty, boys have greater muscle and total body mass than do girls, and androgen therapy in adolescents with delayed puberty increase fat-free mass (Arslanian and Suprasongsin, 1997). The resultant increase in mechanical force exerted on the skeleton has been postulated to play a major role in the determination of bone mass (van der Meulen *et al.*, 1996; Gilsanz *et al.*, 1997). Androgens may also affect the growth hormone/IGF-1 axis (Parker *et al.*, 1984; Keenan *et al.*, 1993; Tai-Pang *et al.*, 1995; Benbassat *et al.*, 1997), that in turn may influence skeletal development. Finally, estrogen (derived from the aromatization of androgen) is very important for skeletal maturation (Smith *et al.*, 1994) and may contribute to male skeletal growth (Vanderschueren, 1996).

Because bone size and cortical thickness have profound effects on bio-mechanical strength and fracture resistance, these positive effects of androgens are of great potential use. The therapeutic impact of those actions may be more obvious during skeletal growth, for instance in the therapy of pubertal forms of hypogonadism in boys. However, if the potential for androgen action on cortical thickness or bone size continues into adulthood, those effects could be useful in the prevention and therapy of common age-related disorders as well (especially osteoporosis). That androgens may continue to exert those actions is suggested by the observation that long bone dimensions continue to increase during adulthood in men, presumably due to periosteal bone accretion, and that this increase is more marked in men than in women (Ruff and Hayes, 1988).

B. Suppression of Bone Resorption

In a manner that seems very similar to that of estrogen, androgens seem to exert a moderating effect on cancellous osteoclastic bone resorption. Increases in osteoclastic activity follow quickly after castration in males (Turner *et al.*, 1989, 1990; Gunness and Orwoll, 1995) and appear to be prevented by nonaromatizable androgens (Turner *et al.*, 1990). *In vitro*, androgens prevent the increases in cytokine generation that in large part mediate osteoclastogenesis and resorption after gonadectomy in males (Bellido *et al.*, 1995). Although there is considerable uncertainty about how the direct effects of androgens in bone cells are intertwined with the effects of estrogens derived from the aromatization of androgens, the effectiveness of nonaromatizable androgens in mediating these cellular effects points strongly to a primary androgen action.

C. Bone Formation

Androgens are the prototypical anabolic agents, and there has been considerable speculation that the effects of androgens in the skeleton may be in part the results of a stimulation of bone formation (Orwoll, 1996). There are androgen receptors in osteoblasts (Colvard *et al.*, 1989; Orwoll *et al.*, 1991) and evidence that androgens affect osteoblast activity (Fukayama and Tashjian, 1989; Kasperk *et al.*, 1990; Bellido *et al.*, 1995; Weinstein *et al.*, 1997). During pubertal development, and in the periosteal space, there is considerable support for the contention that androgens enhance bone formation (*vide supra*). In addition to possible effects on bone growth, some have speculated that androgens may promote increased osteoblastic new bone formation in cancellous areas. However, peak cancellous bone density is similar in males and females, and in most studies the benefits of androgen administration on trabecular bone mass has been modest. Certainly, there is yet little substantial evidence of a major anabolic effect. On the other hand, some reports suggest the possibility of impressive gains in bone density during androgen therapy of hypogonadal men. In view of the clear effects of androgens to reduce the increased rate of bone remodeling (and the rates of both resorption and formation) induced by castration, it is difficult to design experiments to examine directly the influence of androgens on bone formation in isolation. Thus the issue remains unresolved. If, in fact, androgens have positive effects on trabecular bone accumulation, there would be an obvious therapeutic potential.

D. Androgens and IGF-I

Androgens may exert many of their complex effects on bone metabolism via actions on cytokines and growth factors in the skeletal microenvironment. In addition, systemic levels of some of these substances are modulated by androgens (perhaps via conversion to estrogens) (Hobbs *et al.*, 1993; Weissberger and Ho, 1993), and may also affect bone health. IGF-1 has potent actions on bone, and serum levels are increased by androgens (Mauras *et al.*, 1987). If circulating IGF-1 levels have positive effects on bone, the increase stimulated by androgens may be beneficial.

E. Androgens and Muscle Strength

Muscle strength has long been considered responsive to androgens, and recent objective data support that contention. Because strength has been associated with increased bone mass and a reduction in fall propensity, this affect of androgens could be useful in reducing fracture risk. Certainly there remain unresolved issues (the effects of androgens on strength in physiologic concentrations, the usefulness of androgens in improving strength in the elderly, etc.), but the potential benefits of androgens acting on the skeleton via an effect on muscle may be substantial.

VIII. Androgen Replacement in Adolescent Hypogonadism

Because adolescence is such a critically important part of the process of attaining optimal peak bone mass, it is also especially vulnerable to disruption by alterations in gonadal function. Even constitutional pubertal delay is associated with a reduction in peak bone mass development, despite eventual full gonadal development (Finkelstein *et al.*, 1992, 1996). The impairment in bone mass in adolescence with organic hypogonadism (hypogonadotropic hypogonadism) is similar to patients with this form of hypogonadism studied later in life, suggesting that the detrimental effect suffered in adolescence is the major cause of osteopenia (Finkelstein *et al.*, 1987). In view of the major effects of androgens on the skeleton during growth (whether direct or indirect, as discussed earlier), the response to therapy of gonadal dysfunction during this time would be expected to be brisk. Although studies are few, this would appear to be the case (Arisaka *et al.*, 1995). Finkelstein *et al.* (1989) reported that treatment of hypogonadal men with testosterone elicited the most robust skeletal response in those who were skeletally immature (open epiphyses) (Figure 6). In young men considered to have constitutional delay of puberty, testosterone therapy results in a clear increase in bone mass, but whether this provides a solution to the problem of low peak bone mass in these patients is not yet known (Bertelloni *et al.*, 1995). All this information suggests that the diagnosis of frank hypogonadism during childhood or adolescence carries with it the risk of impaired skeletal development and that there is an opportunity to improve bone mass with androgen therapy. In fact, from a skeletal perspective, it appears that therapy should be initiated before epiphyseal closure to maximize bone mass accumulation. Issues that are unresolved include whether bone mass can be normalized with therapy, the most appropriate doses and timing of therapy, and the source of the beneficial effects (androgen versus estrogen, growth factor stimulation, etc.).

IX. Androgen Replacement in Hypogonadal Adult Men

Androgen therapy in hypogonadal men has been shown to affect bone mass positively, at least in most patient groups (Finkelstein *et al.*, 1989; Diamond *et al.*, 1991; Devogelaer *et al.*, 1992; Orwoll and Klein, 1995). For instance, Katznelson *et al.* recently reported an increase in spinal BMD of 5–6% in a group of adult men with hypogonadism treated with testosterone for 18 months (Katznelson *et al.*, 1996), although there was an insignificant increase in radial BMD (Figure 7). As in the experience reported by Katznelson *et al.*, the increase in density following testosterone replacement generally appears to be most apparent in cancellous bone (e.g., lumbar spine), although the literature is not particularly consistent in this regard. Most reports indicate that the increase in bone mass with testosterone therapy can be expected to be modest in the short term (up to 24 months), but Behre *et al.* (1997) noted an increase in spinal trabecular BMD of >20% in the first year of testosterone therapy in a group of hypogonadal men, with further increases thereafter (Figure 8). The most marked increases were observed in those with the lowest testosterone levels before therapy. In men treated for at least 3 years, bone density was found to be at levels normally expected for their ages. Although the experience remains small, there is a suggestion that, in older men with hypogonadism, the response to therapy can be expected to be similar to that in younger adult patients (Morley *et al.*, 1993; Behre *et al.*, 1997).

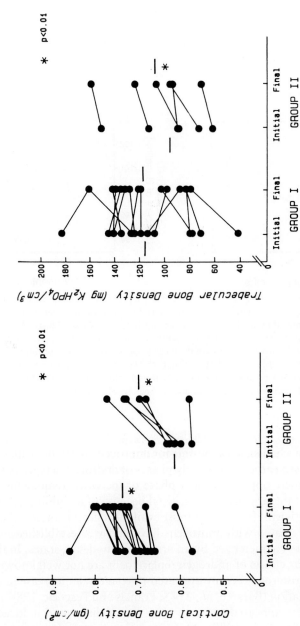

FIGURE 6 Cortical bone density before and after treatment of men with isolated GnRH deficiency who initially had fused epiphyses (group I) or who initially had open epiphyses (group II). The solid lines represent the mean cortical bone density, which increase significantly after treatment in both groups I and II ($P < 0.01$). Cortical bone density increased more in group II than in group I ($P < 0.05$). Increases in bone density during treatment of men with idiopathic hypogonadotropic hypogonadism. *J. Clin. Endocrinol. Metab.* **69**, 776–783, © The Endocrine Society, with permission.

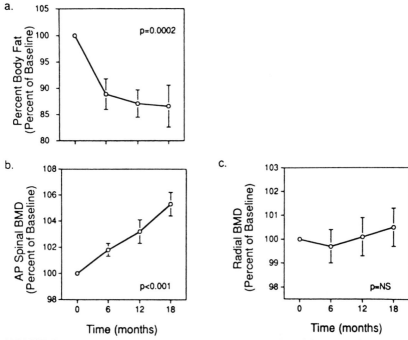

FIGURE 7   Changes in percent body fat and BMD in hypogonadal men receiving testosterone replacement therapy. (a) Percent body fat determined by bioelectric impedance analysis. (b) AP spinal BMD determined by dual energy x-ray absorptiometry. (c) Radial BMD determined by single photon absorptiometry. Data are represented as the mean + SEM percentage of the baseline. Statistical significance for analysis of the mean slope is shown in the bottom right-hand corner of each figure. Reproduced from Katznelson, L. (1996). Increase in bone density and lean body mass during testosterone administration in men with acquired hypogonadism. *J. Clin. Endocrinol. Metab.* **81**, 4358–4365, © The Endocrine Society, with permission.

The cellular mechanisms responsible for improvements in bone mass are unclear. As discussed earlier, in the early phases of androgen deficiency (e.g., after castration) there appears to be a phase of increased remodeling and resorption, so that therapy may be beneficial because of an inhibitory effect on osteoclastic activity. However, in most available clinical studies, the patient populations treated with androgens have had well-established hypogonadism and were characterized by an array of remodeling states. In these subjects the cellular effects of androgen replacement are not well known. In some reports, testosterone therapy appeared to result in an increase in cancellous bone formation (Baran *et al.*, 1978; Francis and Peacock, 1986), but in other series there appeared to be no clear remodeling trend induced by therapy (Finkelstein *et al.*, 1989). Most recently, several groups have reported that biochemical indices of remodeling decline in response to tes-

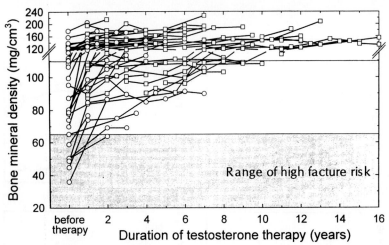

FIGURE 8 Increase in spinal BMD during long-term testosterone substitution therapy up to 16 years in 72 hypogonadal patients. Circles indicate hypogonadal patients with first quantitative computed tomography (QCT) measurement before institution of therapy, squares show those patients already receiving therapy at the first QCT. The dark shaded area indicates the range of high fracture risk, the unshaded area shows the range without significant fracture risk, and the light shaded area indicates the intermediate range where fractures may occur. Reproduced from Behre, H. M., et al. (1997). Long-term effect of testosterone therapy on bone mineral density in hypogonadal men. J. Clin. Endocrinol. Metab. **82**, 2386–2390, © The Endocrine Society, with permission.

tosterone replacement (Katznelson et al., 1996; Wang et al., 1996b) (Figure 9), which is what might be predicted if sex steroid deficiency results in an increase in remodeling, with bone loss on that basis. Interestingly, some reports also suggest that osteocalcin and/or alkaline phosphatase levels may increase with androgen therapy (Morley et al., 1993; Wang et al., 1996b; Guo et al., 1997), perhaps signaling an increase in bone formation (Figure 10).

In addition to the generally positive effects of androgen replacement therapy in hypogonadal men, additional benefits may be gained from the increases that have been noted in strength and lean body mass in these patients (Morley et al., 1993; Katznelson et al., 1996; Wang et al., 1996b; Sih et al., 1997). Because lean body mass and strength have been correlated with bone mass and a reduced propensity to fall, they may further serve to promote bone health and reduce fracture risk.

Despite the generally positive tenor of most studies of the skeletal effects of testosterone replacement, in some patient groups (for instance those with Kleinfelter's syndrome), the advantage associated with androgen therapy is questionable. The available studies report very mixed results (Kubler et al., 1992; Wong et al., 1993). This may be because the level of androgen defi-

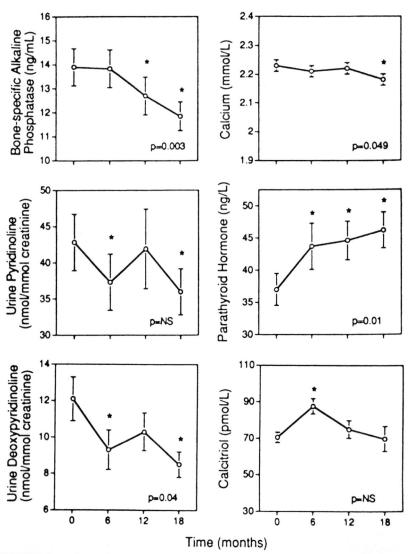

FIGURE 9   Indexes of bone turnover, calcium regulatory hormones, and calcium in hypo-gonadal men receiving testosterone replacement therapy. Data are expressed as the mean ± SEM. Statistical significance for analysis of the mean slope is shown in the bottom right-hand corner of each figure. *$P < 0.05$ compared to the baseline value, by paired t test analysis. Reproduced from Katznelson, L., *et al.* (1996). Increase in bone density and lean body mass during testosterone administration in men with acquired hypogonadism. *J. Clin. Endocrinol. Metab.* 81, 4358–4365, © The Endocrine Society, with permission.

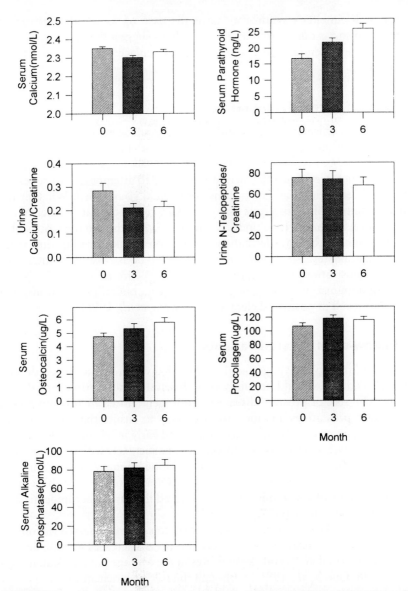

FIGURE 10   Serum and urinary bone marker levels in hypogonadal men before (0 months; hatched bar) and after 3 months (shaded bar) and 6 months (open bar) of SLT (5.0 mg, three times per day) treatment. See text for significance levels. The urinary calcium/creatinine ratio is expressed as millimoles/millimoles, and the urinary *N*-telopeptide/creatinine ratio is expressed as nanomoles of BCE/millimoles of creatinine. Reproduced from Wang, C., *et al.* (1996). Sublingual testosterone replacement improves muscle mass and strength, decreases bone resorption, and increases bone formation markers in hypogonadal men. *J. Clin. Endocrinol. Metab.* **81,** 3654–3662, © The Endocrine Society, with permission.

ciency in Kleinfelter's syndrome (as in the case of some other causes of hypogonadism) is quite variable. These findings suggest the need to consider carefully the potential benefits of androgen replacement in each patient individually.

A. Doses/Routes of Administration

The most efficacious doses and routes of androgen administration for the prevention/therapy of bone loss in hypogonadal men remain uncertain. In part, this is because the specific testosterone levels necessary for an optimal effect have not been defined. Current practice is to attempt to ensure testosterone concentrations similar to those of normal young men. Whether the pulsatile pattern of testosterone exposure characteristic of intramuscular administration is more or less conducive to skeletal health than the more stable pattern produced by transdermal administration is unknown. In some studies, transdermal testosterone therapy appeared to be as effective as intramuscular administration in promoting bone mass (Behre *et al.*, 1997). Novel routes of administration are being examined (e.g., buccal preparations) and appear to result in positive skeletal effects (Wang *et al.*, 1996b).

B. Follow-up of Treated Patients

The follow-up of hypogonadal men treated with testosterone, although not well codified, should certainly include careful monitoring for adverse effects. The risk of prostate disease in androgen-treated men is unknown, but regular prostate evaluations are necessary to ensure that any development of benign or malignant disease is detected early in its course. The development of errythrocytosis is not uncommon, particularly with intramuscular testosterone administration, and complete blood counts at 6 to 12 month intervals are useful to detect its appearance. Other problems that have been postulated to be of concern in androgen-treated men are hyperlipidemia and sleep apnea (Swerdloff and Wang, 1993).

In terms of skeletal effects, therapeutic success may be assessed via follow-up bone mass measures. In view of recent reports, increases in bone density can be anticipated at several skeletal sites in the average patient (Katznelson *et al.*, 1996; Guo *et al.*, 1997). Although the role of biochemical markers of remodeling is controversial, the available data suggest that an adequate androgen effect should be accompanied by a fall in indices of bone resorption, an effect that should be especially useful if resorption markers are increased at base line (Katznelson *et al.*, 1996; Wang *et al.*, 1996b; Guo *et al.*, 1997). Markers of bone formation may be more difficult to use at present in routine clinical situations; some reports suggest that increases follow therapy, whereas others support a decline (Katznelson *et al.*, 1996; Wang *et al.*, 1996a; Guo *et al.*, 1997). The response may depend on the specific marker. Clearly, clinicians deciding on a follow-up strategy must be aware of the uncertainty currently inherent in the field and the vagaries of using the tools available (i.e., issues of measurement precision).

C. Unresolved Issues

There remain many additional unresolved issues concerning the role of androgen treatment in the prevention/therapy of osteoporosis in hypogonadal men, including:

• The degree of hypogonadism (level of testosterone) at which adverse skeletal effects begin to occur is undefined, and hence it is difficult to decide upon the usefulness of therapy in many men with borderline levels of serum testosterone.

• Because hypogonadism in men results in deficiencies of estrogen as well as testosterone, and because testosterone therapy results in increases in serum estrogen (as well as androgen) levels, the relative roles of estrogen versus testosterone in affecting skeletal health in hypogonadal men are unclear. It is unknown whether it is useful to assess estrogen concentrations in the diagnosis of hypogonadal bone disease in men, or whether using estrogen levels to monitor the success of testosterone therapy is beneficial.

• In general, the available treatment studies are of relatively short duration, and it is unclear how long any increases in bone mass can be sustained and what eventual treatment effect can be expected.

• The increase in bone mass that appears to accompany testosterone therapy is of uncertain usefulness in preventing fractures.

• Whether pretreatment age, duration of hypogonadism, degree of osteopenia, remodeling character, and associated medical conditions affect the therapeutic response is relatively unknown.

• Potential adverse effects of androgen therapy (e.g., prostate, lipid) are not well delineated.

X. Androgen Replacement in Aging Men

Old age is associated with a panoply of physical changes in men, many of which have been speculated to be related, either directly or indirectly, to the decline in androgens that accompanies aging (Lamberts *et al.*, 1997). A few small trials of androgen administration in older men have suggested that there may be beneficial effects (increased strength and improved body composition) (Tenover, 1992; Morley *et al.*, 1993; Sih *et al.*, 1997), and some reports, as of yet inconclusive, indicate that bone mass or biochemical indices of remodeling may improve (Tenover, 1992; Morley *et al.*, 1993). Whether androgen replacement therapy can prevent or reverse bone loss in aging men is of enormous importance, but it remains uncertain. Until there is more definitive data available concerning both advantages and disadvantages, testosterone replacement should not be used in elderly patients unless there is convincing evidence for androgen deficiency. This decision is difficult in many older men who have symptoms that can be associated with androgen deficiency but that are also common in the aged regardless of gonadal status (weakness, loss of libido or sexual ability, etc.). The identification of hypogonadism in this group is made especially challenging by the expected decline in androgen levels with age and the dirth of data concerning the levels (threshold concentrations) that are associated with adverse effects on bone.

XI. Androgen Therapy in Eugonadal Men

It has been hypothesized that androgens may have positive effects on bone formation and resorption (*vida supra*). The threshold level of androgens necessary to provide maximal skeletal benefits is unknown, and some have speculated that testosterone supplementation would benefit osteoporotic men even in the face of normal testosterone levels. The experience with this approach has been very limited, but Anderson *et al.* (1997) recently found in an uncontrolled trial that testosterone supplementation was associated with an increase in bone density and a reduction in biochemical markers of remodeling in a group of osteoporotic, eugonadal men. This approach remains very much of uncertain benefit, and until its advantages are documented in controlled trials, it cannot be recommended. This is particularly true in view of the lack of knowledge concerning the potential adverse effects that may be associated with testosterone supplementation.

XII. Androgen Therapy in Secondary Forms of Metabolic Bone Disease in Men

A variety of systemic illnesses and medications are associated with lowered testosterone levels (Gray *et al.*, 1991), and it has been postulated that relative hypogonadism may contribute to the bone loss that also accompanies many of these conditions. For instance, renal insufficiency, glucocorticoid excess, post-transplantation, malnutrition, and alcoholism are all associated with osteopenia and with low testosterone concentrations. Although there is little experience with testosterone supplementation in these patients, it may offer advantages to skeletal health as well as to other tissues (muscle, red cells, etc.). In a randomized study of crossover design, Reid *et al.* (1996) reported that testosterone therapy apparently improved bone density (and body composition) in a small group of men receiving glucocorticoids. Similarly, testosterone therapy apparently improved forearm bone mass in a small group of men with hemochromatosis (treated simultaneously with venesection) (Diamond *et al.*, 1991). The number of patients affected by conditions associated with low testosterone levels is potentially quite large, and more information is needed to understand the role of androgen replacement in the prevention/therapy of concomitant bone loss.

XIII. Therapy with Other Androgens

Several androgenic compounds may have effects on bone mass, and of most current interest are adrenal androgens. DHEA has become widely available as a supplement and has been the source of considerable recent debate. DHEA levels fall dramatically with aging in both sexes (Lamberts *et al.*, 1997), and because DHEA can act as a precursor for both androgens and estrogens, there is some reason to expect that its administration may have effects on bone metabolism and bone mass. A variety of attempts have been made to link those changes with alterations in bone mass associated with age (Barrett-Connor *et al.*, 1993), but to date the information available is both inconclusive and incomplete. Labrie *et al.* (1997) reported that cutaneous DHEA therapy in post-menopausal women was associated with an increase in spinal bone density, with reductions in some markers of bone remodeling (but increases in others). Similar studies are available in animals. There remains no long-term, well-controlled trials of DHEA supplementation in any coherent subject group, and until that information is available, no confident recommendations can be made. Of concern, there is also no available data concerning the potential risks associated with long-term therapy.

XIV. Research Directions

The skeleton is an androgen-responsive tissue, and theoretically there are a number of mechanisms by which androgen action may be important for skeletal health in both men and women. Clinical studies show that androgen therapy provides benefit for the prevention and therapy of bone loss in hypogonadal men, and added gain may result from increases in muscle strength, particularly in older men at risk for falls. Nevertheless, the potential usefulness of androgen therapy, even in men, remains unclear. Major issues to be clarified include the appropriate criteria for patient selection, the specifics of dosing and drug delivery, the nature of short- and long-term adverse effects, and the impact of therapy on fracture rates. Some of these issues can be clarified only with large-scale intervention trials. Androgens may have usefulness in women as well, but adverse effects loom as a more difficult problem. In both men and women, a greater understanding of the molecular mechanisms of androgen action in the skeleton may provide means to harness the beneficial effects of androgens without the disadvantages, for instance by the development of compounds with tissue-specific actions.

References

Anderson, F. H., Francis, R. M., Peaston, R. T., and Wastell, H. J. (1997). Androgen supplementation in eugonadal men with osteoporosis: Effects of six months' treatment on markers of bone formation and resorption. *J. Bone Miner. Res.* **12**, 472–478.

Arisaka, O., Arisaka, M., Hosaka, A., Shimura, N., and Yabuta, K. (1991). Effect of testosterone on radial bone mineral density in adolescent male hypogonadism. *Acta Paediatr. Scand.* **80**, 378–380.

Arisaka, O., Arisaka, M., Nakayama, Y., Fujiwara, S., and Yabuta, K. (1995). Effect of testosterone on bone density and bone metabolism in adolescent male hypogonadism. *Metabol. Clin. Exp.* **44**, 419–423.

Arslanian, S., and Suprasongsin, C. (1997). Testosterone treatment in adolescents with delayed puberty: Changes in body composition, protein, fat, and glucose metabolism. *J. Clin. Endocrinol. Metab.* **82**, 3213–3220.

Baran, D. T., Bergfeld, M. A., Teitelbaum, S. L., and Avioli, L. V. (1978). Effect of testosterone therapy on bone formation in an osteoporotic hypogonadal male. *Calcif. Tissue Res.* **26**, 103–106.

Barrett-Connor, E., Kritz-Silverstein, D., and Edelstein, S. L. (1993). A prospective study of dehydroepiandrosterone sulfate (DHEAS) and bone mineral density in older men and women. *Am. J. Epidemiol.* **137**, 201–206.

Behre, H. M., Kliesch, S., Leifke, E., Link, T. M., and Nieschlag, E. (1997). Long-term effect of testosterone therapy on bone mineral density in hypogonadal men. *J. Clin. Endocrinol. Metab.* **82**, 2386–2390.

Bellido, T., Jilka, R. J., Boyce, B. F., Girasole, G., Broxmeyer, H., Dalrymple, A., Murry, R., and Manolagas, S. C. (1995). Regulation of interleukin-6, osteoclastogenesis and bone mass by androgens: The role of the androgen receptor. *J. Clin. Invest.* **95**, 2886–2895.

Benbassat, C. A., Maki, K. C., and Unterman, T. G. (1997). Circulating levels of insulin-like growth factor (IGF) binding protein-1 in aging men: Relationships to insulin, glucose, IGF, and dehydroepiandrosterone sulfate levels and anthropometric measures. *J. Clin. Endocrinol Metab.* **82**, 1482–1491.

Bernecker, P. M., Willvonseder, R., and Resch, H. (1995). Decreased estrogen levels in male patients with primary osteoporosis. *Abstr. 17th Annu. Meet. Am. Soc. Bone Mine. Res.*

Bertelloni, S., Baroncelli, G. I., Battini, R., Perri, G., and Saggese, G. (1995). Short-term effect of testosterone treatment on reduced bone density in boys with constitutional delay of puberty. *J. Bone Miner. Res.* **10**, 1488–1495.

Bilezikian, J. P., Morishima, A., Bell, J., and Grumbach, M. M. (1998). Increased bone mass as a result of estrogen therapy in a man with aromatase deficiency. *N. Engl. J. Med.* **339**, 599–603.

Bonjour, J.-P., Theintz, G., Buchs, B., Slosman, D., and Rizzoli, R. (1991). Critical years and stages of puberty for spinal and femoral bone mass accumulation during adolescence. *J. Clin. Endocrinol. Metab.* **73**, 555–563.

Bonjour, J.-P., Theintz, G., Law, F., Slosman, D., and Rizzoli, R. (1994). Peak bone mass. *Osteoporosis Int.* **1**, S7–S13.

Colvard, D. S., Eriksen, E. F., Keeting, P. E., Wilson, E. M., Lubahn, D. B., French, F. S., Riggs, B. L., and Spelsberg, T. C. (1989). Identification of androgen receptors in normal human osteoblast-like cells. *Proc. Natl. Acad. Sci. U.S.A.* **86**, 854–857.

Delmas, P., and Meunier, P. J. (1981). L'ostéoporose au cours du syndrome de Klinefelter. Données histologiques osseuses quantitatives dans cinq cas. Relation avec la carence hormonale. *Nouv. Presse Med.* **10**, 687.

Devogelaer, J. P., De Cooman, S., and de Deuxchaisnes, C. N. (1992). Low bone mass in hypogonadal males. Effect of testosterone substitution therapy, a densitometric study. *Maturitas* **15**, 17–23.

Diamond, T., Stiel, D., and Posen, S. (1991). Effects of testosterone and venesection on spinal and peripheral bone mineral in six hypogonadal men with hemochromatosis. *J. Bone Miner. Res.* **6**, 39–43.

Drinka, P. J., Olson, J., Bauwens, S., Voeks, S., Carlson, I., and Wilson, M. (1993). Lack of association between free testosterone and bone density separate from age in elderly males. *Calcif. Tissue Int.* **52**, 67–69.

Fehily, A. M., Coles, R. J., Evans, W. D., and Elwood, P. C. (1992). Factors affecting bone density in young adults. *Am. J. Clin. Nutr.* **56**, 579–586.

Finkelstein, J. S., Klibanski, A., Neer, R. M., Greenspan, S. L., Rosenthal, D. I., and Crowley, W. F. J. (1987). Osteoporosis in men with idiopathic hypogonadotropic hypogonadism. *Ann. Intern. Med.* **106**, 354–361.

Finkelstein, J. S., Klibanski, A., Neer, R. M., Doppelt, S. H., Rosenthal, D. I., Serge, G. V., and Crowley, W. F. (1989). Increases in bone density during treatment of men with idiopathic hypogonadotropic hypogonadism. *J. Clin. Endocrinol. Metab.* **69**, 776–783.

Finkelstein, J. S., Neer, R. M., Biller, B. M. K., Crawford, J. D., and Klibanski, A. (1992). Osteopenia in men with a history of delayed puberty. *N. Engl. J. Med.* **326**, 600–604.

Finkelstein, J. S., Klibanski, A., and Neer, R. M. (1996). A longitudinal evaluation of bone mineral density in adult men with histories of delayed puberty. *J. Clin. Endocrinol. Metab.* **81**, 1152–1155.

Foresta, C., Ruzza, G., Mioni, R., Meneghello, A., and Baccichetti, C. (1983). Testosterone and bone loss in Klinefelter's syndrome. *Horm. Metab. Res.* **15**, 56–67.

Francis, R. M., and Peacock, M. (1986). Osteoporosis in hypogonadal men: Role of decreased plasma 1,25-dihydroxyvitamin D, calcium malabsorption, and low bone formation. *Bone* **7**, 261–268.

Fukayama, S., and Tashjian, H. J. (1989). Direct modulation by androgens of the response of human bone cells (SaOS-2) to human parathyroid hormone (PTH) and PTH-related protein. *Endocrinology (Baltimore)* **125**, 1789–1794.

Gilsanz, V., Dibbens, D. T., Roe, T. F., Carlson, M., Senac, M. O., Boechat, M. I., Huang, H. K., Schulz, E. E., Libanati, C. R., and Cann, C. C. (1988). Vertebral bone density in children: Effect of puberty. *Radiology* **166**, 847–850.

Gilsanz, V., Boechat, M. I., Gilsanz, R., Loro, M. L., Roe, T. F., and Goodman, W. G. (1994). Gender differences in vertebral sizes in adults: Biomechanical implications. *Radiology* **190**, 678–682.

Gilsanz, V., Kovanlikaya, A., Costin, G., Roe, T. F., Sayre, J., and Kaufman, F. (1997). Differential effect of gender on the sizes of the bones in the axial and appendicular skeletons. *J. Clin. Endrocrinol. Metab.* **82**, 1603–1607.

Goldray, D., Weisman, Y., Jaccard, N., Merdler, C., Chen, J., and Matzkin, H. (1993). Decreased bone density in elderly men treated with the gonadotropin-releasing hormone agonist decapeptyl (D-Trp⁶-GnRH). *J. Clin. Endocrinol. Metab.* **76**, 288–290.

Gray, A., Feldman, H. A., McKinlay, J. B., and Longscope, C. (1991). Age, disease and changing sex hormone levels in middle-aged men: Results of the Massachusetts male aging study. *J. Clin. Endocrinol. Metab.* **73**, 1016–1025.

Greendale, G. A., Edelstein, S., and Barrett-Connor, E. (1997). Endogenous sex steroids and bone mineral density in older women and men: The Rancho Bernardo Study. *J. Bone Miner. Res.* **12**, 1833–1843.

Gunness, M., and Orwoll, E. S. (1995). Early induction of alterations in cancellous and cortical bone histology after orchiectomy in mature rats. *J. Bone Miner. Res.* **10**, 1735–1744.

Guo, C.-Y., Jones, H., and Eastell, R. (1997). Treatment of isolated hypogonadotropic hypogonadism effect on bone mineral density and bone turnover. *J. Clin. Endocrinol. Metab.* **82**, 658–665.

Hobbs, C. J., Plymate, S. R., Rosen, C., and Adler, R. A. (1993). Testosterone administration increases insulin-like growth factor-1 levels in normal men. *J. Clin. Endocrinol. Metab.* **77**, 776–779.

Horowitz, M., Wishart, J. M., O'Loughlin, P. D., Morris, H. A., Need, A. G., and Nordin, B. E. C. (1992). Osteoporosis and Kleinefelter's syndrome. *Clin. Endocrinol. (Oxford)* **36**, 113–118.

Jackson, J. A., Kleerekoper, M., Parfitt, A. M., Sukhaker Rao, D., Villanueva, A. R., and Frame, B. (1987). Bone histomorphometry in hypogonadal and eugonadal men with spinal osteoporosis. *J. Clin. Endocrinol. Metab.* **65**, 53–58.

Kasperk, C., Fitzsimmons, R., Strong, D., Mohan, S., Jennings, J., Wergedal, J., and Baylink, D. (1990). Studies of the mechanism by which androgens enhance mitogenesis and differentiation in bone cells. *J. Clin. Endocrinol. Metab.* **71**, 1322–1329.

Katznelson, L., Finkelstein, J. S., Schoenfeld, D. A., Rosenthal, D. I., Anderson, E. J., and Klibanski, A. (1996). Increase in bone density and lean body mass during testosterone administration in men with acquired hypogonadism. *J. Clin. Endocrinol. Metab.* **81**, 4358–4365.

Keenan, B. S., Richards, G. E., Ponder, S. W., Dallas, J. S., Nagamani, M., and Smith, E. R. (1993). Androgen-stimulated pubertal growth: The effects of testosterone and dihydrotestosterone on growth hormone and insulin-like growth factor-I in the treatment of short stature and delayed puberty. *J. Clin. Endocrinol. Metab.* **76**, 996–1001.

Kelepouris, N., Harper, K. D., Gannon, F., Kaplan, F. S., and Haddad, J. G. (1995). Severe osteoporosis in men. *Ann. Intern. Med.* **123**, 452–460.

Kelly, P. J., Pocock, N. A., Sambrook, P. N., and Eisman, J. A. (1990a). Dietary calcium, sex hormones, and bone mineral density in men. *Br. Med. J.* **300**, 1361–1364.

Kelly, P. J., Twomey, L., Sambrook, P. N., and Eisman, J. A. (1990b). Sex differences in peak adult bone mineral density. *J. Bone Miner. Res.* **5**, 1169–1175.

Krabbe, S., Christiansen, C., Rodbro, P., and Transbol, I. (1979). Effect of puberty on rates of bone growth and mineralisation. *Arch. Dis. Child.* **54**, 950–953.

Krabbe, S., Hummer, L., and Christiansen, C. (1984). Longitudinal study of calcium metabolism in male puberty. *Acta Paediatr. Scand.* **73**, 750–755.

Kubler, A., Schulz, G., Cordes, U., Beyer, J., and Krause, U. (1992). The influence of testosterone substitution on bone mineral density in patients with Klinefelter's syndrome. *Exp. Clin. Endocrinol.* **100**, 129–132.

Labrie, F., Diamond, P., Cusan, L., Gomez, J., Bélanger, A., and Candas, B. (1997). Effect of 12-month dehydroepiandrosterone replacement therapy on bone, vagina, and endometrium in postmenopausal women. *J. Clin. Endocrinol. Metab.* **82**, 3498–3505.

Lamberts, S. W. J., van den Beld, A. W., and van der Lely, A. (1997). The endocrinology of aging. *Science* **278**, 419–424.

Lips, P., Asscheman, H., Uitewaal, P., Netelenbos, J. C., and Gooren, J. (1989). The effect of cross-gender hormonal treatment on bone metabolism in male-to-female transsexuals. *J. Bone Miner. Res.* **4**, 657–662.

Lu, P. W., Briody, J. N., Ogle, G. D., Morley, K., Humphries, I. R. J., Allen, J., Howman-Giles, R., and Sillence, D. (1994). Bone mineral density of total body, spine, and femoral neck in children and young adults: A cross-sectional and longitudinal study. *J. Bone Miner. Res.* **9**, 1451–1458.

Martin, B. (1993). Aging and strength of bone as a structural material. *Calcif. Tissue Int.* **53**,(Suppl. 1), S34–S40.

Mauras, N. R., Blizzard, R. M., Link, K., Johnson, M. L., Rogol, A. D., and Velduis, J. D. (1987). Augmentation of growth hormone secretion during puberty: Evidence for a pulse amplitude-modulated phenomenon. *J. Clin. Endocrinol. Metab.* **64**, 596–601.

Mauras, N., Haymond, M. W., Darmaun, D., Vieira, N. E., Abrams, S. A., and Yergey, A. L. (1994). Calcium and protein kinetics in prepubertal boys. Positive effect of testosterone. *J. Clin. Invest.* **93**, 1014–1019.

McElduff, A., Wilkinson, M., Ward, P., and Posen, S. (1988). Forearm mineral content in normal men: Relationship to weight, height and plasma testosterone concentrations. *Bone* **9**, 281–283.

Meier, D. E., Orwoll, E. S., Keenan, E. J., and Fagerstrom, R. M. (1987). Marked decline in trabecular bone mineral content in healthy men with age: Lack of association with sex steroid levels. *J. Am. Geriatr. Soc.* **35**, 189–197.

Morishima, A., Grumbach, M. M., Simpson, E. R., Fisher, C., and Qin, K. (1995). Aromatase deficiency in male and female siblings caused by a novel mutation and the physiological role of estrogens. *J. Clin. Endocrinol. Metab.* **80**, 3689–3698.

Morley, J. E., Perry, H. M., III, Kaiser, F. E., Kraenzel, D., Jensen, J., Houston, K., Mattammal, M., and Perry, H. M., Jr. (1993). Effects of testosterone replacement therapy in old hypogonadal males: A preliminary study. *J. Am. Geriatr. Soc.* **41**, 149–152.

Munoz-Torres, M., Jodar, E., Quesada, M., and Escobar-Jimenez (1995). Bone mass in androgen-insensitivity syndrome: Response to hormonal replacement therapy. *Calcif. Tissue Int.* **57**, 94–96.

Murphy, S., Khaw, K.-T., Cassidy, A., and Compston, J. E. (1993). Sex hormones and bone mineral density in elderly men. *Bone Miner.* **20**, 133–140.

Odell, W. D. (1989). Puberty. In "Endocrinology" (L. J. DeGroot, ed.). Saunders, Philadelphia.

Ongphiphadhanakul, B., Rajatanavin, R., Chailurkit, L., Paiseu, N., Teerarungsikul, K., Sirisriro, R., Komindr, S., and Puavilai, G. (1995). Serum testosterone and its relation to bone mineral density and body composition in normal males. *Clin. Endocrinol.* **43**, 727–733.

Orwoll, E. S. (1996). Androgens as anabolic agents for bone. *Trends Endocrinol. Metab.* **7**, 77–84.

Orwoll, E. S., and Klein, R. F. (1995). Osteoporosis in men. *Endocr. Rev.* **16**, 87–116.

Orwoll, E. S., Stribrska, L., Ramsay, E. E., and Keenan, E. (1991). Androgen receptors in osteoblast-like cell lines. *Calcif. Tissue Int.* **49**, 182–187.

Parker, L. N. (1991). Adrenarche. *Endcrinol. Metab. Clin. North Am.* **20**, 71–83.

Parker, M. W., Johanson, A. J., and Rogol, A. D. (1984). Effect of testosterone on somatomedin C concentrations in prepubertal boys. *J. Clin. Endocrinol. Metab.* **58**, 87–90.

Reid, I. R., France, J. T., Pybus, J., and Ibbertson, H. K. (1985). Plasma testosterone concentrations in asthmatic men treated with glucocorticoids. *Br. Med. J.* **291**, 574.

Reid, I. R., Wattie, D. J., Evans, M. C., and Stapleton, J. P. (1996). Testosterone therapy in glucocorticoid-treated men. *Arch. Intern. Med.* **156**, 1173–1177.

Rico, H., Revilla, M., Hernandez, E. R., Villa, L. F., and Alvarez del Buergo, M. (1992). Sex differences in the acquisition of total bone mineral mass peak assessed through dual-energy x-ray absorptiometry. *Calcif. Tissue Int.* **51**, 251–254.

Riis, B. J., Krabbe, S., Christiansen, C., Catherwood, B. D., and Deftos, L. J. (1985). Bone turnover in male puberty: A longitudinal study. *Calcif. Tissue Int.* **37**, 213–217.

Rudman, D., Drinka, P. J., Wilson, C. R., Mattson, D. E., Scherman, F., Cuisinier, M. C., and Schultz, S. (1994). Relations of endogenous anabolic hormones and physical activity to bone mineral density and lean body mass in elderly men. *Clin. Endocrinol.* **40**, 653–661.

Ruff, C. B., and Hayes, W. C. (1988). Sex differences in age-related remodeling of the femur and tibia. *J. Orthop. Res.* **6**, 886–896.

Sih, R., Morley, J. E., Kaiser, F. E., Perry, H. M. I., Patrick, P., and Ross, C. (1997). Testosterone replacement in older hypogonadal men: A 12-month randomized controlled trial. *J. Clin. Endocrinol. Metab.* **82**, 1661–1667.

Slemenda, C. W., Resiter, T. K., Hui, S. L., Miller, J. Z., Christian, J. C., and Johnston, C. J. (1994). Influences on skeletal mineralization in children and adolescents: Evidence for varying effects of sexual maturation and physician activity. *J. Pediatr.* **125**, 201–207.

Slemenda, C. W., Longscope, C., Zhou, I., Hui, S., Peacock, M., and Johnston, C. C. (1997). Sex steroids and bone mass in older men. Positive associations with serum estrogens and negative associations with androgens. *J. Clin. Invest.* **100**, 1755–1759.

Smith, E. P., Boyd, J., Frank, G. R., Takahashi, H., Cohen, R. M., Specker, B., Williams, T. C., Lubahn, D. B., and Korach, K. S. (1994). Estrogen resistance caused by a mutation in the estrogen-receptor gene in a man. *N. Engl. J. Med.* **331**, 1056–1061.

Soule, S. G., Conway, G., Prelevic, G. M., Prentice, M., Ginsburg, J., and Jacobs, H. S. (1996). Osteopenia is a feature of the androgen insensitivity syndrome. *Clin. Endrocrinol.* **43**, 671–675.

Stanhope, R., Buchanan, C. R., Fenn, G. C., and Preece, M. A. (1988). Double blind placebo controlled trial of low dose oxandrolone in the treatment of boys with constitutional delay of growth and puberty. *Arch. Dis. Child.* **63**, 501–505.

Stanley, H. L., Schmitt, B. P., Poses, R. M., and Deiss, W. P. (1991). Does hypogonadism contribute to the occurrence of a minimal trauma hip fracture in elderly men? *J. Am. Geriatr. Soc.* **39**, 766–771.

Stepan, J. J., Lachman, M., Zverina, J., Pacovsky, V., and Baylink, D. J. (1989). Castrated men exhibit bone loss: Effect of calcitonin treatment on biochemical indices of bone remodeling. *J. Clin. Endocrinol. Metab.* **69**, 523–527.

Swerdloff, R. S., and Wang, C. (1993). Androgen deficiency and aging in men. *West. J. Med.* **159**, 579–585.

Tai-Pang, I., Hoffman, D. M., O'Sullivan, A. J., Kin-Chuen, L., and Ho, K. K. Y. (1995). Do androgens regulate growth hormone-building protein in adult men? *J. Clin. Endocrinol. Metab.* **80**, 1278–1282.

Tenover, J. S. (1992). Effects of testosterone supplementation in the aging male. *J. Clin. Endocrinol. Metab.* **75**, 1092–1098.

Turner, R. T., Hannon, K. S., Demers, L. N., Buchanan, J., and Bell, N. (1989). Differential effects of gonadal function in bone histomorphometry in male and female rats. *J. Bone Miner. Res.* **4**, 557–563.

Turner, R. T., Wakley, G. K., and Hannon, K. S. (1990). Differential effects of androgens on cortical bone histomorphometry in gonadectomized male and female rats. *J. Orthop. Res.* **8**, 612–617.

Uriarte, M. M., Baro, J., Garcia, H. B., Barnes, K. M., Loriaux, D. L., and Cutler, G. B. J. (1992). The effect of pubertal delay on adult height in men with isolated hypogonadotropic hypogonadism. *J. Clin. Endocrinol. Metab.* **74**, 436–440.

van der Meulen, M. C. H., Ashford, M. W., Kiratli, B. J., Bachrach, L. K., and Carter, D. R. (1996). Determinants of femoral geometry and structure during adolescent growth. *J. Orthop. Res.* **14**, 22–29.

Vanderschueren, D. (1996). Androgens and their role in skeletal homeostasis. *Horm. Res.* **46**, 95–98.

Van Kesteren, P., Lips, P., Deville, W., Popp-Snijders, C., Asscheman, H., Megens, J., and Gooren, L. (1996). The effect of one-year cross-sex hormonal treatment on bone metabolism and serum insulin-like growth factor-1 in transsexuals. *J. Clin. Endocrinol. Metab.* **81**, 2227–2232.

Vermeulen, A. (1991). Androgens in the aging male. *J. Clin. Endocrinol. Metab.* **73**, 221–224.

Wang, C., Eyre, D. R., Clark, D., Kleinberg, C., Newman, C., Iranmanesh, A., Veldhuis, J., Dudley, R. E., Berman, N., Davidson, T., Barstow, T. J., Sinow, R., Alexander, G., and Swerdloff, R. S. (1996b). Sublingual testosterone replacement improves muscle mass and strength, decreases bone resorption, and increases bone formation markers in hypogonadal men—A clinical research center study. *J. Clin. Endocrinol. Metab.* **81**, 3654–3662.

Weinstein, R. S., Jilka, R. L., Parfitt, A. M., and Manolagas, S. C. (1997). The effects of androgen deficiency on murine bone remodeling and bone mineral density are mediated via cells of the osteoblastic lineage. *Endocrinology (Baltimore)* **138**, 4013–4021.

Weissberger, A. J., and Ho, K. K. Y. (1993). Activation of the somatotropic axis by testosterone in adult males: Evidence for the role of aromatization. *J. Clin. Endocrinol. Metab.* **76**, 1407–1412.

Wishart, J. M., Need, A. G., Horowitz, M., Morris, H. A., and Nordin, B. E. C. (1995). Effect of age on bone density and bone turnover in men. *Clin. Endocrinol.* **42**, 141–146.

Wong, F. H. W., Pun, K. K., and Wang, C. (1993). Loss of bone mass in patients with Klinefelter's syndrome despite sufficient testosterone replacement. *Osteoporosis Int.* **7**, 281–287.

Chapter 14

Patrick M. Doran*
Russell T. Turner†
B. Lawrence Riggs*
Sundeep Khosla*

*Endocrine Research Unit
Division of Endocrinology and Metabolism
†Department of Orthopedics
Mayo Clinic and Mayo Foundation
Rochester, Minnesota

Estrogens and Bone Health

I. Introduction

In 1941, Fuller Albright was the first to note the importance of estrogen in bone metabolism. Since then, estrogen deficiency has clearly been identified as the major factor contributing to involutional osteoporosis in women, and the effects of estrogen on the skeleton have been the subject of intensive investigation. Moreover, while androgens clearly have significant effects on the male skeleton, recent genetic and epidemiologic evidence suggests that estrogen may also play an important role in bone metabolism in men. This chapter will review our current understanding of estrogen effects on the skeleton at the cellular level as well as at the physiological level in animals and humans.

II. Cellular and Molecular Effects of Estrogen on Bone ⎯⎯⎯⎯

Estrogen deficiency is characterized by an acceleration of bone turnover, with both an increase in the frequency of activation of remodeling units and a loss of balance between osteoblastic and osteoclastic activity in favor of the latter at each of these units (Parfitt, 1979). This process results in more numerous and deeper resorption spaces, with perforation of trabecular plates and loss of other architectural elements, ultimately weakening bone and increasing fracture risk (Parfitt *et al.*, 1983). The identification of estrogen receptors on human osteoblasts (Eriksen *et al.*, 1988) (Figure 1) led to the notion that estrogen likely had direct skeletal effects, as opposed to previous concepts invoking changes in calcitropic hormones as mediators of the skeletal effects of estrogen deficiency.

A. Estrogen Effects on Osteoclasts

The main action of estrogen on bone remodeling is to decrease bone resorption (Turner *et al.*, 1994a). Indeed, the presence of estrogen receptors in human osteoclast-like cells (Oursler *et al.*, 1994) and the ability of estrogen to inhibit osteoclastic resorptive activity *in vitro* suggest that at least some of the effects of estrogen on bone resorption are mediated directly through osteoclastic cells. In addition, estrogen increases transforming

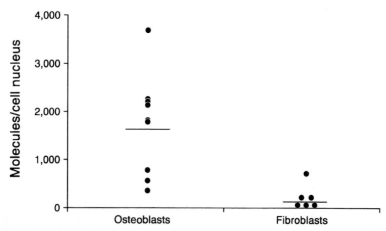

FIGURE 1   Nuclear binding assay specific for estrogen receptors in human fibroblasts and in seven strains of human osteoblast-like cells from normal women. Reproduced with Modifications, with permission from Eriksen, E. F., Colvard, D. S., Berg, N. J., Graham, M. L., Mann, K. G., Spelsberg, T. C., and Riggs, B. L. (1988). Evidence of estrogen receptors in normal human osteoblast-like cells. *Science* **241**, 84–86. Copyright 1988 American Association for the Advancement of Science.

growth factor beta (TGF-β) production by osteoclasts which, in turn, may inhibit osteoclastic bone resorption in an autocrine fashion (Robinson *et al.*, 1996). Finally, recent studies indicate that estrogen promotes apoptosis (i.e., programmed cell death) of osteoclasts, and that this effect may also be mediated by TGF-β (Hughes *et al.*, 1996).

In addition to possible direct effects of estrogen on osteoclasts, estrogen may also regulate the production of cytokines by osteoblasts or bone marrow cells, which would then affect osteoclastic activity by a paracrine mechanism (Rodan and Martin, 1981; Manolagas and Jilka, 1995). Thus, the estrogen-induced decrease in bone turnover could be due to the stimulation of the release of osteoclast inhibitory factors and/or by the inhibition of the production of osteoclast stimulatory factors. For example, in addition to stimulating osteoclastic TGF-β production, estrogen also increases the secretion of active TGF-β by osteoblasts (Oursler *et al.*, 1991), which may then inhibit osteoclastic activity in a paracrine fashion.

A number of other cytokines, including interleukin (IL)-1, tumor necrosis factor α (TNF-α), macrophage-colony stimulating factor (M-CSF), IL-6, and prostaglandins may also be potential candidates for mediating the bone loss following estrogen deficiency. Pacifici *et al.* (1991) initially reported that IL-1 production by peripheral blood monocytes was increased in oophorectomized women, and this was suppressed by estrogen replacement therapy. Subsequently, Kimble *et al.* (1994) reported that the administration of IL-1 receptor antagonist (IL-1ra), a specific competitive inhibitor of IL-1, to ovariectomized rats decreased bone resorption and bone loss. In addition to IL-1, Kitazawa *et al.* (1994) have provided evidence that TNF-α may also mediate the effects of estrogen deficiency. Thus, they showed that administration of a soluble type I TNF receptor that binds to TNF-α and inhibits TNF action prevented the increase in bone resorption and bone loss following ovariectomy in rats. In addition, Ammann *et al.* (1997) found that transgenic mice expressing soluble TNF receptor were protected against bone loss following ovariectomy.

Another potential cytokine involved in mediating the effects of estrogen deficiency on the skeleton is M-CSF, a potent stimulator of the proliferation and differentiation of osteoclast precursors (Tanaka *et al.*, 1993a). Thus, stromal cells from ovariectomized mice have been shown to produce greater amounts of M-CSF than cells from control mice, and *in vivo* treatment with either estrogen or a combination of IL-1 receptor antagonist and TNF binding protein abolishes the *in vitro* increase in M-CSF production by stromal cells from the ovariectomized mice (Kimble *et al.*, 1996). Therefore, it appears that enhanced production of IL-1 and TNF from bone marrow mononuclear cells following ovariectomy may lead to expansion of a high M-CSF-secreting bone marrow stromal cell population.

Other studies indicate, however, that IL-6 may also play a key role in mediating bone loss following estrogen deficiency. Girasole *et al.* (1992)

showed that estrogen suppressed IL-1 or TNF-α induced IL-6 production by murine bone marrow stromal and osteoblastic cells. Subsequently, Jilka *et al.* (1992) demonstrated that an IL-6 neutralizing antibody could prevent the increase in osteoclastogenesis induced by ovariectomy in rats. Moreover, Kassem *et al.* (1996a) showed that estrogen inhibited the production of IL-6 mRNA and protein induced by IL-1 and TNF-α in human osteoblastic cells stably transfected with the human ER-α gene. Finally, Poli *et al.* (1994) found that IL-6 knockout mice were protected against ovariectomy-induced bone loss.

Thus, there are a number of candidate cytokines that might mediate the effects of estrogen on regulating bone resorption, and, in fact, it appears likely that multiple cytokines may be involved and act cooperatively. Miyaura *et al.* (1995) found, for example, that IL-6 neutralizing antibody only partially inhibited the bone resorbing activity of bone marrow supernatants from ovariectomized mice. Also, the bone resorbing activity was decreased by indomethacin, indicating that prostaglandins may also mediate, in part, the bone resorption induced by estrogen deficiency. In addition, Kawaguchi *et al.* (1995) found that marrow supernatants from ovariectomized mice stimulated cyclooxygenase (COX)-2 mRNA expression and prostaglandin E synthesis in mouse calvarial cultures. Simultaneous treatment with submaximal doses of IL-1α, IL-6, and soluble IL-6 receptor (which enhances IL-6 action) resulted in a marked induction *in vitro* in osteoclast formation and COX-2-mediated PGE synthesis. These data are thus consistent with the hypothesis that several bone-resorbing cytokines, such as IL-1, TNF-α, IL-6, prostaglandins, and probably others, act cooperatively in inducing bone resorption after estrogen deficiency (Figure 2). This may account for the fact that clinical investigative studies comparing either peripheral serum (McKane *et al.*, 1994) or marrow plasma (Kassem *et al.*, 1996b) concentrations of these cytokines in estrogen-depleted or estrogen-replaced postmenopausal women have failed to detect any consistent differences in any of these cytokines. It is likely that, *in vivo*, multiple cytokines are involved, and the changes in individual cytokines are of a magnitude that are difficult to detect in clinical-investigative studies.

B. Estrogen Effects on Osteoblasts

In addition to direct and indirect effects on osteoclasts, estrogen likely also has direct effects on osteoblasts, although these effects may be quite model-dependent. Gray *et al.* (1987, 1989), for example, found that estrogen treatment transiently inhibited proliferation and increased alkaline phosphatase activity in a rat osteogenic sarcoma cell line, UMR-106. In contrast, Ernst *et al.* (1989) found that estrogen treatment of cultured osteoblast-like cells derived from fetal rat calvaria increased cell proliferation, mRNA for type I procollagen, and synthesis of collagenase-digestable protein. Studies

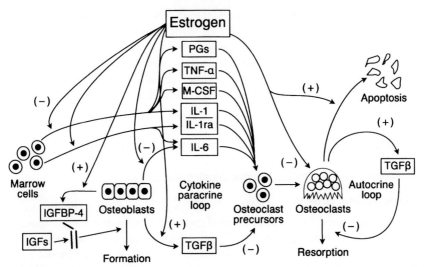

FIGURE 2   Schematic representation of the mediators of estrogen effects on bone cells. IL, interleukin; IL-1ra, interleukin-1 receptor antagonist; TNF, tumor necrosis factor; PGs, prostaglandins; M-CSF, macrophage-colony stimulating factor; IGF, insulin-like growth factor; IGFBP, insulin-like growth factor binding protein; TGFβ, transforming growth factor beta. See text for discussion.

using a conditionally immortalized human fetal osteoblast cell line (hFOB/ ER9) that expresses high levels of ER-α, however, have found a consistent inhibitory effect of estrogen on proliferation (Kassem *et al.,* 1996c; Robinson *et al.,* 1997). This has been associated with an increase in insulin-like growth factor (IGF) binding protein (IGFBP)-4 levels, which inhibits IGF action (Ernst *et al.,* 1989). Estrogen treatment of these cells also resulted in an increase in alkaline phosphatase mRNA and activity, a decrease in osteocalcin mRNA, and no effects on type I collagen protein levels or osteonectin steady-state mRNA levels (Robinson *et al.,* 1997). In addition, estrogen also induced the mRNA for bone morphogenetic protein 6 (BMP-6) in these cells, but not other BMPs (Rickard *et al.,* 1998). Because BMP-6 is expressed in the hypertrophic cartilage in the developing fetal skeleton (Lyons *et al.,* 1989), these data suggest that estrogen may regulate skeletal development, at least in part, through BMP-6. These data thus indicate that estrogen does directly regulate osteoblast proliferation and differentiation, although the net effect of estrogen on osteoblasts likely depends on a number of factors, including species differences, cellular heterogeneity, incomplete differentiation, and/or low or variable ER content among the various cell lines and primary cultures. Figure 2 summarizes the potential mediators of estrogen action on osteoblasts, in addition to estrogen effects on osteoclasts, via its action on osteoblasts and marrow mononuclear cells.

Preliminary evidence also suggests that the osteocyte may also be a target for estrogen action. Estrogen withdrawal associated with GnRH therapy has, for example, been shown to induce apoptosis of osteocytes in iliac bone (Tomkinson *et al.*, 1997). Because osteocytes may be involved in mechano-sensing and transducing loading responses (Pitsillides *et al.*, 1995), these effects of estrogen deficiency could impair the skeletal response to loading.

III. Effects of Estrogen on Laboratory Animals ──────────

A. Sexual Dimorphism of the Skeleton

I. Longitudinal Growth

There are sex differences in skeletal growth in many, but not all, species. The rates of growth and ultimate length of long bones in females are less than males in rats (Hansson *et al.*, 1972) and mice (Lopez *et al.*, 1986), but the opposite is the case in other strains of mice and in many raptors (Audubon, 1831). Estrogen acts in concert with other hormones and systemic factors to influence longitudinal growth. Because of the interaction between multiple factors, the specific actions of estrogen on the growth plate are only partially characterized.

Ovariectomy slows the age-related decrease in longitudinal bone growth in rats (Stenström *et al.*, 1982; Turner *et al.*, 1994b). As expected, estrogen treatment shows a dose-dependent inhibition of longitudinal growth in ovariectomized rats (Turner *et al.*, 1994b) and mice (Herbai, 1971) suggesting that the steroid is the principal ovarian hormone active on growth plate cartilage. This conclusion is supported by studies showing that administration of estrogen during the prenatal (Migliaccio *et al.*, 1992), early postnatal (Ostadalova, 1976), and prepubertal periods (Budy *et al.*, 1952) results in limb shortening. Furthermore, the longitudinal bone growth rate is cyclic during the estrus cycle in the normal adolescent female rat, with the slow phase of bone growth occurring when estrogen levels are maximal and the fast phase occurring when estrogen levels are minimal (Whitson *et al.*, 1978).

The mechanism of action of estrogen on growth plate cartilage is poorly understood. It is clear, however, that estrogen stimulates maturation of cartilage without increasing the growth rate. At the cellular level, estrogen inhibits cell division by cartilage cells in the proliferative zone of the growth plate (Whitson *et al.*, 1978; Strickland and Sprinz, 1973; Gustafsson *et al.*, 1975). The age-related decrease in size of the hypertrophic chondrocytes is accentuated by estrogen (Gustafsson *et al.*, 1975). It is not clear which, if any, of these effects are direct actions of the hormone. It is especially interesting that the potent antiestrogen, ICI 182, 780, has no effect on longitudinal bone growth in either ovariectomized or ovary-intact rats (Sibonga *et al.*, 1998).

Some of the effects of estrogen on longitudinal bone growth are not mediated by direct actions on the growth plate cartilage cells. The growth rate is determined by chondrocyte cell proliferation, hypertrophy, and secretion of extracellular matrix. The magnitude by which vascular invasion exceeds cartilage growth controls epiphyseal closure and depends upon chondroclast recruitment and activity. Chondrocyte proliferation and chondroclast recruitment are both inhibited by estrogen, but to different degrees (Turner *et al.*, 1994b; Gustafsson *et al.*, 1975).

2. Bone Architecture

In addition to their effects on longitudinal growth, sex steroids influence skeletal architecture in many vertebrates by modifying intramembranous bone formation in flat bones, as well as radial growth, modeling, and remodeling of tubular (long) bones. Radial growth results from addition of new bone onto periosteal surfaces by secondary intramembranous bone formation. Modeling involves regional bone formation and/or bone resorption with a subsequent change in overall bone shape (e.g., enlargement of marrow cavity with age). In contrast, remodeling is characterized by sequential periods of bone resorption and bone formation at the same location with little or no net change in bone architecture (Frost, 1986).

Many factors, including sex steroids, influence bone turnover. Sex differences in the architecture of the skull, pelvis, and long bones have been shown to result from differential growth and modeling rates (Dahinten and Pucciarelli, 1986; Aceitero *et al.*, 1987). The cancellous osteopenia which occurs in growing rats after ovariectomy is largely due to increased resorption of calcified cartilage by chondroclasts in the zone of vascular invasion (Turner *et al.*, 1994b) and to increased resorption of the secondary spongiosa (Wronski *et al.*, 1988a, 1989a).

All stages of skeletal development and maturation appear to be influenced by estrogen. Calcification of the femoral head epiphysis occurs earlier in female rats than in males; administration of estradiol leads to earlier calcification in both sexes (Koshino and Olsson, 1975) and increases peak bone density, but not bone mass, in rabbits when given from 6 weeks of age to maturity (Gilsanz *et al.*, 1988). Neonatal exposure to the synthetic estrogen diethylstilbestrol (DES) induces permanent changes in skeletal tissue in mice, including shorter and denser long bones (Breur *et al.*, 1991).

The injection of female neonatal rats with testosterone diminishes the sex-based difference in pelvic size (Hughes and Tanner, 1974). Transplantation of pelves from female to male mice resulted in a male morphology, whereas bones from male and female mice gonadectomized at birth or transplanted from male to female have a female morphology (Crelin, 1960; Dahinten and Pucciarelli, 1986). Normal cranial maturation is increased in rats by ovariectomy and decreased by estradiol treatment, findings suggesting that estradiol in females counteracts testosterone-mediated sexual dimorphism (Dahinten and Pucciarelli, 1986).

There are profound sex differences in longitudinal and radial growth of rat long bones whereby males grow more rapidly and have a much larger final cross-sectional area than females. Gonadectomy results in decreased radial bone growth in males and increased radial growth in females such that the sex difference is largely eliminated. The sex difference is reestablished in gonadectomized rats by administering estrogens to females and androgens to males (Turner et al., 1987a, 1989, 1990a).

The volume of the medullary canal in rat tibiae is enlarged following ovariectomy due to a net increase in bone resorption (Dahinten and Pucci-arelli, 1986; Kalu et al., 1989). Osteoclast number is increased (Turner et al., 1987b) and bone formation remains unchanged or increased (Turner et al., 1987a,b, 1989, 1990a). As a result of the opposing changes in radial growth and endocortical modeling, the cortical bone volume decreases very slowly in ovariectomized rats (Turner et al., 1987b, 1989, 1990a,b). It may, in fact, increase in growing rats because the increase in periosteal addition of bone exceeds the increase in endocortical resorption (Turner et al., 1990b).

The compartment-specific changes in cortical bone which accompany estrogen deficiency and repletion result from alterations in cell number and activity. Ovariectomy results in increases in osteoclast number on the endo-cortical surface of long bone in rats, whereas estrogen treatment of ovariec-tomized rats prevents the osteoclast-mediated increase in medullary area (Turner et al., 1987a,b). Ovariectomy increases and estrogen replacement decreases periosteal bone formation in long bones of rats (Turner et al., 1987a,b, 1989). Also, estrogen treatment decreases osteoblast number and size and the bone formation rate in calvarial periosteum (Turner et al., 1992). mRNA levels for bone matrix proteins were uniformly decreased in perios-teum from tibiae, femora, and calvariae (Turner et al., 1990c, 1992), sug-gesting a similar mode of action of the hormone on each of these bones. Importantly, DES dramatically decreased the number of preosteoblasts in S-phase of the cell cycle in rat calvarial periosteum, indicating that the hor-mone inhibits the differentiation of preosteoblasts to osteoblasts (Turner et al., 1992). Thus, estrogen appears to inhibit recruitment as well as synthetic activity of osteoblasts.

No clear sex difference in cancellous bone architecture has been docu-mented in growing animals. Because estrogens (Urist et al., 1948; Lindquist et al., 1960) and androgens (Swanson and VanDerWerffTenBosch, 1963) have important effects on endochondral ossification, bone turnover, and maintenance of cancellous bone volume in the metaphysis of growing ani-mals, it is likely that detailed studies would also reveal sex differences in cancellous bone. Importantly, estrogen in female rats (Wronski et al., 1988a, 1989a; Turner et al., 1988) and androgens in males (Turner et al., 1989; Wakley et al., 1991) are essential for maintenance of normal cancellous bone volume.

In summary, sex steroids are responsible for the sexual dimorphism of the skeleton. Estrogen and androgens have activities which differ from one another. Estrogen has clearly been demonstrated to have an important role in the growth and maturation of the female skeleton. Its role in the male skeleton is much less certain.

B. Maintenance of Bone Mass

I. Effects on Bone Volume

Estrogen is essential for maintenance of normal bone volume. Ovariectomy leads to a deficit in ash weight and bone mineral density in adult rats and monkeys (Jordan *et al.*, 1987; Saville, 1969; Lindsay *et al.*, 1978; Mazess *et al.*, 1987; Jayo *et al.*, 1990). These changes are due to endocortical bone resorption and net resorption of cancellous bone (Wronski *et al.*, 1988a, 1989a; Turner *et al.*, 1987a; Nyda *et al.*, 1948); they are prevented by estrogen replacement. Similar comparable changes occur in rats (Goulding and Gold, 1989) and monkeys (Mann *et al.*, 1990) following administration of GnRH agonists, a nonsurgical intervention which results in serum estradiol levels comparable with ovariectomy (Goulding and Fisher, 1991). Similarly, administration of ICI 182, 780 (an antiestrogen with minimal estrogen agonistic activity) to ovary-intact rats results in cancellous osteopenia (Gallagher *et al.*, 1993).

2. Site-Specific Actions on Bone Turnover

Ovariectomy results in elevated serum osteocalcin in rats (Ismail *et al.*, 1988), suggesting that there is a global increase in bone turnover. However, there are also site-specific effects on the skeleton, as shown in Figure 3 for the differences between cortical and cancellous bone. In addition, ovariectomy results in differential rates of cancellous osteopenia. For example, bone is lost from rat vertebrae but the time course for the response is prolonged compared to long bones (Wronski *et al.*, 1985, 1988a, 1989b). There are also differences between long bones; osteopenia develops more rapidly in tibiae than humeri. Finally, cancellous osteopenia develops in the proximal tibial metaphysis but not the proximal epiphysis, suggesting that there are also important regional differences within individual bones. The site-specific differences in the skeletal response to estrogen deficiency may be related to differences in metabolic activity, blood supply, osteoprogenitor cell populations, baseline levels of bone turnover, and/or the magnitude of the mechanical strain experienced by bone cells (Westerlind *et al.*, 1997).

The more rapid longitudinal bone growth in rats after ovariectomy (compared to age-matched ovary-intact animals) does not result in increased cancellous bone volume despite the increased synthesis of calcified cartilage. Parallel increases in chondroclast number in the zone of vascular invasion in ovariectomized rats reduces the volume of the primary spongiosa and cancels the effects of increased synthesis. Estrogen treatment increases mineralized cartilage in the primary spongiosa by reducing chondroclast number. As a consequence of the effects of estrogen to alter the rate of growth and to

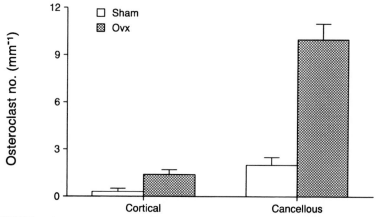

FIGURE 3   The site-specific effects of ovariectomy on osteoclast number is illustrated for rat tibia. Osteoclast number was increased following ovariectomy (OVX) on endocortical as well as cancellous bone surfaces. However, osteoclasts were much more prevalent on cancellous bone surfaces in both intact and OVX rats. These differences may explain why cancellous bone is lost more rapidly than cortical bone following OVX. Reproduced, with modifications, from Turner, R. T., Riggs, B. L., and Spelsberg, T. C. (1994). Skeletal effects of estrogen. *Endocrine Reviews* 15(3), 275–300, © The Endocrine Society, with permission.

inhibit production of chondroclasts and osteoclasts during the course of an experiment, many of the changes in cancellous bone volume reported for the tibial metaphysis of young estrogen-treated rats result from altered bone maturation and growth rates rather than from decreased bone turnover as formerly believed (Turner *et al.*, 1994b; Lindquist *et al.*, 1960).

Ovariectomy results in severe cancellous osteopenia in long bones and vertebrae of rats (Wronski *et al.*, 1985, 1989b) and vertebrae of monkeys (Jerome *et al.*, 1986; Longcope *et al.*, 1989). The response to ovariectomy in dogs has been less consistent with no change (Snow and Anderson, 1986) and bone loss (Martin *et al.*, 1987) reported. Ovariectomy results in increases in osteoblast-lined perimeter, osteoclast-lined perimeter, and osteoclast size in long bones of rats (Turner *et al.*, 1988; Wronski *et al.*, 1985, 1986). There are simultaneous increases in the mineral apposition and bone formation rates, suggesting that ovariectomy results in chronic high bone turnover. Cancellous bone turnover remains elevated in rats for at least 1 year following ovariectomy (Wronski *et al.*, 1988a, 1989a). Bone formation is increased in ovariectomized monkeys (Jerome *et al.*, 1994), suggesting that the bone loss in nonhuman primates is also associated with increased bone turnover.

3. Effects on Cancellous Bone Formation

The cellular mechanism of estrogen action on cancellous bone turnover is controversial. On one hand, there is universal agreement that estrogen inhibits bone resorption in rats (Turner *et al.*, 1988; Anderson *et al.*, 1970; Wronski *et al.*, 1988b; Yamamoto and Rodan, 1990). On the other hand, estrogen has been reported to inhibit (Wronski *et al.*, 1988b; Kalu *et al.*, 1991) and stimulate (Yamamoto and Rodan, 1990; Chow *et al.*, 1992) cancellous bone formation.

Doses of estrogen reported to stimulate bone formation showed a time-dependent inhibition of incorporation of ^{3}H-proline into bone matrix, a decreased recruitment of osteoblasts from marrow cell precursors, a decreased osteoblast number, and no change or decreased mRNA levels for bone matrix proteins (Turner *et al.*, 1993; Westerlind *et al.*, 1993; Salih *et al.*, 1993). Also, estrogen was shown to "increase" fluorochrome-labeled perimeter in rat tibia by inhibiting osteoclast-mediated resorption of bone matrix containing the fluorochrome (Turner *et al.*, 1993; Westerlind *et al.*, 1993), suggesting that the putative anabolic effects of estrogen on bone formation may be artifactual.

4. Role of Estrogen on Bone Physiology in Male Laboratory Animals

Estrogen receptor-alpha and estrogen receptor-beta mRNA has been detected in cortical and cancellous bone from rats (Westerlind *et al.*, 1995; Onoe *et al.*, 1997). The mRNA for estrogen receptor-beta was reported to be expressed at similar levels in bone from male and female rats (Onoe *et al.*, 1997). Estrogen administered to growing male rats had effects on cortical and cancellous bone which were similar to those reported in females (Wakley *et al.*, 1997). These included decreases in bone growth and turnover. Longitudinal growth was suppressed as was periosteal and cancellous bone formation and mineral apposition rates; while bone dimensions were decreased, cancellous bone density was increased.

In sexually mature male rats, tamoxifen reduced disuse osteopenia in rat long bones by inhibiting bone resorption (Wakley *et al.*, 1988). A similar inhibition in bone resorption was observed in immobilized female rats following treatment with diethylstilbestrol (DES) (Cavolina *et al.*, 1997).

Preliminary results suggest that disruption of estrogen receptor-alpha by homologous recombination in mice (Korach *et al.*, 1996) resulted in decreases in bone density in male and female mice. The effects of estrogen on the skeleton of growing mice is unclear. In male mice, neonatal exposure to DES reduced the ash weight of the pelvis and femur (Fukazawa *et al.*, 1996). In contrast, treatment of orchiectomized weanling mice treated with 17β-estradiol resulted in increases in tibial bone weight, ash, weight, and Ca and P content (Ornoy *et al.*, 1994).

In summary, administered estrogen has effects on the mature male skeleton which differ from androgens and are similar, if not identical, to actions on the female skeleton. The physiological relevance, however, is unclear at this time.

IV. Effects of Estrogen on Human Bone Metabolism and Calcium Homeostasis

A. Bone Loss Patterns over Life

After achieving peak bone mass in young adulthood, bone mineral density (BMD) generally remains constant until middle life in both sexes. It has been suggested that the gradual deterioration of ovarian function after about age 35 may influence bone remodeling prior to overt menopause and cause, at least in some individuals, significant bone loss. However, by far the most dramatic changes occur at the time of menopause per se. With its onset, estrogen concentrations fall to 10–20% of their premenopausal levels, and women undergo a transient, accelerated phase of bone loss which, after about a decade, merges asymptotically with an underlying late phase of slow bone loss that persists indefinitely. This slow, continuous phase also begins in middle life and is equally present in men. These patterns are shown schematically in Figure 4.

B. Accelerated Phase of Bone Loss in Women

This transient phase of bone loss clearly results from estrogen deficiency because it coincides with the onset of menopause, ovariectomy, or any other form of ovarian failure and because it can be prevented by estrogen replacement. The accelerated phase subsides after approximately 15 years and ac-

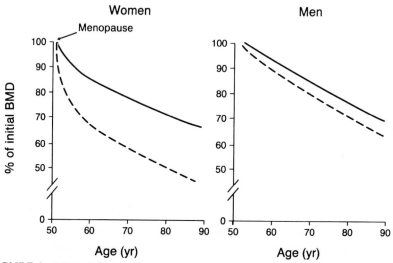

FIGURE 4   Schematic representation of changes in bone mass over life in cancellous (broken line) and cortical (solid line) bone in women (left panel) and men (right panel) from age 50 onward. See text for description.

counts for losses of from 20 to 30% of cancellous bone and from 5 to 10% of cortical bone (Riggs and Melton, 1986). As discussed in Section I, bone loss at menopause occurs through the loss of estrogen's tonic restraining effects on bone turnover. A reflection of these changes was seen in a population-based study in which menopause produced a 45% increase in formation markers and a 90% rise in resorption indices (Garnero et al., 1996). It is noteworthy that this type of change in turnover markers persists well beyond the accelerated phase, as will be discussed in the next section. Estrogen deficiency increases bone sensitivity to parathyroid hormone (PTH) (Cosman et al., 1993) and, possibly, to other resorption-inducing agents that further enhance the resorption defect. Compensatory increases in urinary calcium excretion (Heaney et al., 1978; McKane et al., 1995) and decreases in intestinal calcium absorption (Gennari et al., 1990) prevent the resultant skeletal outflow of calcium into the extracellular fluids from producing hypercalcemia. Consequently, serum intact PTH levels tend to remain within normal limits in early menopause, although there is a trend toward slightly reduced levels with respect to comparable women treated with estrogen replacement therapy (ERT) (Prince et al., 1990, 1991).

C. Continuous Phase of Bone Loss

In contrast to the accelerated phase which results mostly from a direct disinhibition of bone turnover caused by estrogen deficiency, the bone loss in the protracted, age-related phase is predominantly caused by changes in extraskeletal calcium metabolism and secondary hyperparathyroidism. This phase accounts for losses of about 20 to 30% of cancellous bone and about 20 to 30% of cortical bone, in men as well as in women (Riggs and Melton, 1986). Numerous studies have now demonstrated an age-related increase in serum parathyroid hormone levels and in bone turnover (Ledger et al., 1995) in both men and in women (Epstein et al., 1986; Khosla et al., 1998). Moreover, suppression of PTH secretion by intravenous calcium infusion abolishes the differences in bone resorption markers between young and elderly women (Ledger et al., 1995), strongly suggesting that the increase in bone resorption in aging women is PTH-dependent. Finally, a number of randomized studies have shown that dietary calcium supplementation in elderly women reverses age-associated hyperparathyroidism (McKane et al., 1996) and reduces bone loss (Elders et al., 1994; Reid et al., 1995).

Recent studies indicate that estrogen therapy, likely due to effects on extra-skeletal calcium homeostasis, can reverse or prevent the secondary hyperparathyroidism in aging women (Riggs et al., 1998). Thus, even though intestinal calcium absorption is reduced in elderly women (Bullamore et al., 1970; Ireland and Fordtran, 1973), ERT in postmenopausal women with osteoporosis has been shown to increase both serum total and free 1,25 dihydroxyvitamin D (1,25 $(OH)_2D$) levels and calcium absorption (Gallagher et al., 1979; Cheema et al., 1989). In addition, in perimenopausal women before and 6 months after oophorectomy, the expected increase in calcium absorption in response to 1,25 $(OH)_2D$ treatment was blunted in the presence of estrogen deficiency, suggesting also a direct enhancing effect of estrogen on intestinal calcium absorption (Gennari *et al.*, 1990), possibly through a preservation of 1,25 $(OH)_2D$ receptor numbers (Horst *et al.*, 1990).

In addition to effects on intestinal calcium absorption, estrogen may also have significant effects on renal calcium handling, resulting in improved calcium balance. McKane *et al.*, (1995), for example, assessed renal calcium transport directly at baseline and during administration of a saturating dose of PTH in postmenopausal women before and after 6 months of ERT. They demonstrated a PTH-independent increase in tubular calcium absorption in the estrogen replete compared with the estrogen deficient women, whereas tubular reabsorption of other cations was unaffected; these observations are consistent with a direct effect of estrogen on renal calcium conservation.

Finally, estrogen may have direct effects on PTH secretion. Thus, Cosman *et al.* (1994) found that ERT in postmenopausal women decreased PTH secretion in response to EDTA-induced hypocalcemia, suggesting that estrogen also acts directly on the parathyroid gland to reduce PTH secretion. Corroborating this conclusion, the parathyroid gland has been found to contain estrogen receptors by some (Navey-Many *et al.*, 1992), although not by others (Prince *et al.*, 1991).

These extra-skeletal effects of estrogen, then, may prevent the age-related increase in serum PTH levels in elderly postmenopausal women by improving overall calcium homeostasis. In support of this, recent studies comparing young adult premenopausal women, untreated older women, and older women on ERT have found that once estrogen deficiency was corrected, serum PTH and bone resorption markers were similar in the elderly, estrogen-treated and the young women (McKane *et al.*, 1997; Khosla *et al.*, 1997). Moreover, short-term ERT of women over 80 years of age reduced bone turnover markers significantly (Prestwood *et al.*, 1994).

In summary, the slow bone loss in later menopause seems to be predominantly caused by hyperparathyroidism secondary to multiple changes in extra-skeletal calcium homeostasis. In turn, these changes appear tightly associated with estrogen deficiency, can be reversed with ERT, and the bone-preserving effects of ERT appear to reach well into the ninth decade, possibly even later. Finally, whether estrogen (or testosterone) has similar, extra-skeletal effects on calcium homeostasis in men is unclear and needs further investigation.

D. Gender Comparison and the Role of Estrogen in Bone Metabolism in Males

During their lifetimes, despite the absence of a menopause equivalent, men still undergo two-thirds of the bone loss incurred by women (Riggs *et al.*,

1981). Also, after accounting for the lack of this rapid phase, the pattern of the continuous phase of bone loss and the increase in serum PTH and bone resorption markers in aging men are virtually superimposable upon those occurring in women (Epstein *et al.*, 1986; Prince *et al.*, 1995; Khosla *et al.*, 1998).

Conventional thought holds that skeletal mass is maintained mainly by estrogen in women and testosterone in men, given the similar rapid bone loss that follows oophorectomy (Genant *et al.*, 1982) and orchiectomy (Stepan *et al.*, 1989), respectively. However, because both testosterone and estrogen are produced by the testes and because both their concentrations fall to extremely low levels after orchiectomy, these studies do not quantitate the relative contribution of testosterone versus estrogen in this male equivalent of early menopausal, high-turnover bone loss.

An important source of circulating estrogens in men and in postmeno-pausal women is the conversion of androgens to estrogens, which results from the action of the enzyme aromatase cytochrome P450. The aromatase enzyme is encoded by the CYP19 gene on chromosome 15 (Nebert *et al.*, 1989), and this gene is widely expressed throughout the body, including the placenta and blastocyst, the ovary, the Leydig cells of the testis, adipose tissue, the liver, muscle, hair follicles, and the brain, including the hypothal-amus (Simpson *et al.*, 1994).

Although osteoblasts contain androgen receptors, there is also evidence that tissue-level aromatization may mediate at least some of the skeletal effects of androgens. Indeed, significant aromatase activity has been detected in human osteoblastic cell lines in culture (Purohit *et al.*, 1992; Tanaka *et al.*, 1993b; Schweikert *et al.*, 1995). Specific aromatase inhibitors also arrested estrogen formation in these cells (Schweikert *et al.*, 1995).

Some of the most compelling arguments for a key role of estrogen in male bone metabolism were found in so-called "experiments of nature." In 1994, Smith *et al.* described a 28-year-old man with homozygous null mu-tations in the estrogen receptor gene who, despite normal total and free testosterone and elevated estrogen levels, had unfused epiphyses, eunuchoid habitus, marked osteopenia, and elevated bone turnover indices. Subse-quently, a similar skeletal phenotype was described in two males with ho-mozygous null mutations of the aromatase gene (Morishima *et al.*, 1995; Carani *et al.*, 1997). In both instances, BMD was significantly reduced, and bone turnover markers were markedly increased despite normal androgen levels. Testosterone treatment in one patient did not significantly affect bone turnover (Carani *et al.*, 1997), but estrogen replacement markedly increased BMD in both patients (Morishima *et al.*, 1997). These individuals and their response to treatment suggest that, in males, estrogen is essential for epi-physeal closure and attainment of maximal bone mass, as well as mainte-nance of the equilibrium between bone formation and resorption. However, these observations still do not exclude a role for androgens in these processes.

In addition to these rare individuals, recent epidemiologic evidence is also consistent with an important role for estrogen in skeletal metabolism in older males, even though earlier reports have failed to detect an association between estrogen and BMD in men (Meier *et al.*, 1987; Kelly *et al.*, 1990). Slemenda *et al.* (1997), for example, found that serum estradiol, but not testosterone levels, were positively associated with BMD in men over age 65 years. Bernecker *et al.* (1995) determined that mean serum estradiol, rather than testosterone, was significantly reduced in 56 men (mean age 61.2 ± 1.5 years) with established idiopathic osteoporosis as compared to age-matched control subjects. Finally, Greendale *et al.* (1997) found that in men within a similar age range, serum bioavailable [or non-sex hormone binding globulin (SHBG)-bound] estrogen was more strongly associated with BMD than bioavailable testosterone.

In an effort to further define the relative contributions of estrogen versus testosterone toward determining bone mineral density in men, Khosla *et al.* (1998) studied a population-based, age-stratified sample of men ($n = 346$) as well as a comparable group of women ($n = 304$) aged 21 to 94 years. From age 25 to 85 years, serum total testosterone and estrogen levels decreased in the men by 30% and 12%, but bioavailable testosterone and estrogen levels decreased by 64% and 47%, respectively. By multivariate analysis, serum bioavailable estrogen was the consistent independent predictor of BMD in both men and in postmenopausal women. Collectively, these data are thus consistent with the hypothesis that age-related decreases in estrogen availability may, at least in part, account for the fall in BMD in aging men, although more work clearly needs to be done to better define the role of estrogen versus testosterone deficiency in causing age-related bone loss in men.

V. Summary

Estrogen has long been recognized as an important regulator of bone metabolism and acts via complex cellular and molecular mechanisms, likely involving cytokines, that have both autocrine and paracrine effects. The skeletal effects of estrogen in laboratory animals are evident in several aspects of growth as well as in maintenance of bone mass. Estrogen deficiency mediates postmenopausal bone loss initially by its acceleration of bone turnover, and then later perhaps by effects on calcium homeostasis that lead to secondary hyperparathyroidism. The recent descriptions of rare disorders of estrogen synthesis and action have indicated that estrogen may play a key role in bone metabolism not just in females but also in males. This hypothesis has been strengthened by several epidemiologic studies showing a stronger association between bone mass and estrogen levels as compared to testosterone levels in men. Future work will undoubtedly shed new light on the relative contributions of estrogen versus androgens toward bone metabolism in men, both in the attainment of peak bone mass and in the pathogenesis of age-related bone loss.

Acknowledgments

Supported by Research Grants AG-04875 and AR-30582 from the National Institutes of Health, U.S. Public Health Service.

References

Aceitero, J., Gaytan, F., and Ranz, F. B. (1987). Effects of neonatal estrogenization on rat bone development: A histomorphometric study. *Calcif. Tiss. Int.* **40,** 189–193.

Ammann, P., Rizzoli, R., Bonjour, J., Bourrin, S., Meyer, J., Vassaili, P., and Garcia, I. (1997). Transgenic mice expressing soluble tumor necrosis factor-receptor are protected against bone loss caused by estrogen deficiency. *J. Clin. Invest.* **99,** 1699–1703.

Anderson, J. J. B., Greenfield, J. W., Posada, J. R., and Crackel, W. C. (1970). Effect of estrogen on bone mineral turnover in mature female rats as measured by Strontium-85. *Proc. Soc. Exp. Biol. Med.* **135,** 883–886.

Audubon, J. J. (1831). "Ornithological Biography." Adam Black, Edinburgh.

Bernecker, P. M., Willvonseder, R., and Resch, H. (1995). Decreased estrogen levels in male patients with primary osteoporosis. *J. Bone Miner. Res.* **10,** S445.

Breur, G. J., VanEnkevort, B. A., Farnum, C. E., and Wilsman, N. J. (1991). Linear relationship between the volume of hypertrophic chondrocytes and the rate of longitudinal bone growth in growth plates. *J. Orthop. Res.* **9,** 348–359.

Budy, A. M., Urist, M. R., and McLean, F. C. (1952). The effect of estrogens on the growth apparatus of the bones of immature rats. *Am. J. Path.* **28,** 1143–1153.

Bullamore, J. R., Gallagher, J. C., Wilkinson, R., Nordin, B. E. C., and Marshall, D. H. (1970). Effects of age on calcium absorption. *Lancet* **2,** 535–537.

Carani, C., Qin, K., Simoni, M., Faustini-Fustini, M., Serpente, S., Boyd, J., Korach, K. S., and Simpson, E. R. (1997). Effect of testosterone and estradiol in a man with aromatase deficiency. *N. Engl. J. Med.* **337,** 91–95.

Cavolina, J. M., Evans, G. L., Harris, S. A., Zhang, M., Westerlind, K. C., and Turner, R. T. (1997). The effects of orbital spaceflight on bone histomorphometry and mRNA levels for bone matrix proteins and skeletal signaling peptides in ovariectomized growing rats. *Endocrinology (Baltimore)* **138,** 1567–1576.

Cheema, C., Grant, B. F., and Marcus, R. (1989). Effects of estrogen circulating "free" and total 1,25-dihydroxyvitamin D and on the parathyroid-vitamin D axis in postmenopausal women. *J. Clin. Invest.* **83,** 537–542.

Chow, J., Tobias, J. H., Colston, K. W., and Chambers, T. J. (1992). Estrogen maintains trabecular bone volume in rats not only by suppression of bone resorption but also by stimulation of bone formation. *J. Clin. Invest.* **89,** 74–78.

Cosman, F., Shen, V., Xie, F., Seibel, M., Ratcliffe, A., and Lindsay, R. (1993). Estrogen protection against bone resorbing effects of parathyroid hormone infusion. *Ann. Intern. Med.* **118,** 337–343.

Cosman, F., Nieves, J., Horton, J., Shen, V., and Lindsay, R. (1994). Effects of estrogen on response to edetic acid infusion in postmenopausal osteoporotic women. *J. Clin. Endocrinol. Metab.* **78,** 939–943.

Crelin, E. S. (1960). The development of bony pelvic sexual dimorphism in mice. *Ann. N.Y. Acad. Sci.* **84,** 479–512.

Dahinten, S. L., and Pucciarelli, H. M. (1986). Variations in sexual dimorphism in the skulls of rats subjected to malnutrition, castration, and treatment with gonadal hormones. *Am. J. Phys. Anthrop.* **71,** 63–67.

Elders, P. J. M., Lips, P., Netelenbos, J. C., van Ginkel, F. C., Khoe, E., van der Vijgh, W. J. F., and van der Stelt, P. F. (1994). Long-term effect of calcium supplementation on bone loss in perimenopausal women. *J. Bone Miner. Res.* **9,** 963–970.

Epstein, S., Bryce, G., Hinman, J. W., Miller, O. N., Riggs, B. L., Hui, S. L., and Johnston, C. C., Jr. (1986). The influence of age on bone mineral regulating hormones. *Bone* **7,** 421–425.

Eriksen, E. F., Colvard, D. S., Berg, N. J., Graham, M. L., Mann, K. G., Spelsberg, T. C., and Riggs, B. L. (1988). Evidence of estrogen receptors in normal human osteoblast-like cells. *Science* **241,** 84–86.

Ernst, M., Heath, J. K., and Rodan, G. A. (1989). Estradiol effects on proliferation, messenger ribonucleic acid for collagen and insulin-like growth factor-1, and parathyroid hormone-stimulated adenylate cyclase activity in osteoblastic cells from calvariae and long bones. *Endocrinology (Baltimore)* **125,** 825–833.

Frost, H. M. (1986). "Intermediary Organization of the Skeleton." CRC Press, Boca Raton, FL.

Fukazawa, Y., Nobata, S., Katoh, M., Tanaka, M., Kobayashi, S., Ohta, Y., Hayashi, Y., and Iguchi, T. (1996). Effect of neonatal exposure to diethylstilbestrol and tamoxifen on pelvis and femur in male mice. *Anat. Rec.* **244,** 416–422.

Gallagher, A., Chambers, T. J., and Tobias, J. H. (1993). The estrogen antagonist ICI 182,780 reduces cancellous bone volume in female rats. *Endocrinology (Baltimore)* **133,** 2787–2791.

Gallagher, J. C., Riggs, B. L., Eisman, J., Hamstra, A., Arnaud, S. B., and DeLuca, H. F. (1979). Intestinal calcium absorption and serum vitamin D metabolites in normal subjects and osteoporotic patients: Effects of age and dietary calcium. *J. Clin. Invest.* **64,** 729–736.

Garnero, P., Sornay-Rendu, E., Chapuy, M., and Delmas, P. D. (1996). Increased bone turnover in late postmenopausal women is a major determinant of osteoporosis. *J. Bone Miner. Res.* **11,** 337–349.

Genant, H. K., Cann, C. E., Ettinger, B., and Gordan, G. S. (1982). Quantitative computed tomography of vertebral spongiosa: A sensitive method for detecting early bone loss after oophorectomy. *Ann. Intern. Med.* **97,** 699–705.

Gennari, C., Agnusdei, D., Nardi, P., and Civitelli, R. (1990). Estrogen preserves a normal intestinal responsiveness to 1,25-dihydroxyvitamin D3 in oophorectomized women. *J. Clin. Endocrinol. Metab.* **71,** 1288–1293.

Gilsanz, V., Roe, T. F., Gibbens, D. T., Schulz, E. E., Carlson, M. E., Gonzalez, O., and Boechat, M. I. (1988). Effect of sex steroids on peak bone density of growing rabbits. *Am. J. Physiol.* **255,** E416–E421.

Girasole, G., Jilka, R. L., Passeri, G., Boswell, S., Boder, G., Williams, D. C., and Manolagas, S. C. (1992). 17beta-estradiol inhibits interleukin-6 production by bone marrow-derived stromal cells and osteoblasts *in vitro:* A potential mechanism for the antiresorptive effect of estrogen. *J. Clin. Invest.* **9,** 883–891.

Goulding, A., and Fisher, L. (1991). 17b-estradiol protects rats from osteopenia associated with administration of the luteinising hormone release hormone (LHRH) agonist, buserelin. *Bone Miner.* **13,** 47–53.

Goulding, A., and Gold, E. (1989). A new way to induce oestrogen-deficiency osteopenia in the rat: Comparison of the effect of surgical ovariectomy and administration of the LHRH agonist buserelin on bone resorption and composition. *J. Endocrinol.* **121,** 293–298.

Gray, T. K., Flynn, T. C., Gray, K. M., and Nabell, L. M. (1987). 17beta-estradiol acts directly on the clonal osteoblastic cell line UMR106. *Proc. Natl. Acad. Sci. U.S.A.* **84,** 6267–6271.

Gray, T. K., Mohan, S., Linkhart, T. A., and Baylink, D. J. (1989). Estradiol stimulates *in vitro* the secretion of insulin-like growth factors by the clonal osteoblastic cell line, UMR106. *Biochem. Biophys. Res. Commun.* **158,** 407–412.

Greendale, G. A., Edelstein, S., and Barrett-Connor, E. (1997). Endogenous sex steroids and bone mineral density in older women and men: The Rancho Bernardo Study. *J. Bone Miner. Res.* **12**, 1833–1843.

Gustafsson, P. O., Kasström, H., Lindberg, L., and Olsson, S. E. (1975). Growth and mitotic rate of the proximal tibial epiphyseal plate in hypophysectomized rats given estradiol and human growth hormone. *Acta Radiol. Suppl.* **344**, 69–74.

Hansson, L. I., Menander-Sellman, K., Stenström, A., and Thorngren, K.-G. (1972). Rate of normal longitudinal bone growth in the rat. *Calcif. Tiss. Res.* **10**, 238–251.

Heaney, R. P., Recker, R. R., and Saville, P. D. (1978). Menopausal changes in calcium balance performance. *J. Lab. Clin. Med.* **92**, 953–963.

Herbai, G. (1971). Studies on the site and mechanism of action of the growth inhibiting effects. *Acta Physiol. Scand.* **83**, 77–90.

Horst, R. L., Goff, J. P., and Reinhardt, T. A. (1990). Advancing age results in reduction of intestinal and bone 1,25-dihydroxyvitamin D receptor. *Endocrinology (Baltimore)* **126**, 1053–1057.

Hughes, D. E., Dai, A., Tiffee, J. C., Li, H. H., Mundy, G. R., and Boyce, B. F. (1996). Estrogen promotes apoptosis of murine osteoclasts mediated by TGF-beta. *Na. Med.* **2**, 1132–1136.

Hughes, P. C. R., and Tanner, J. M. (1974). The effect of a single neonatal sex hormone injection on the growth of the rat pelvis. *Acta Endocrinol. (Stockholm)* **77**, 612–624.

Ireland, P., and Fordtran, J. S. (1973). Effects of dietary calcium and age on jejunal calcium absorption in humans studied by intestinal perfusion. *J. Clin. Invest.* **64**, 729–736.

Ismail, F., Epstein, S., Fallon, M. D., Thomas, S. B., and Reinhardt, T. A. (1988). Serum bone Gla protein and the vitamin D endocrine system in the oophorectomized rat. *Endocrinology (Baltimore)* **122**, 624–630.

Jayo, M. J., Weaver, D. S., Adams, M. R., and Rankin, S. E. (1990). Effects on bone of surgical menopause and estrogen therapy with or without progesterone replacement in cynomolgus monkeys. *Am. J. Obstet. Gynecol.* **193**, 614–618.

Jerome, C. P., Kimmel, D. B., McAlister, J. A., and Weaver, D. S. (1986). Effects of ovariectomy on iliac trabecular bone in baboons *(Papio anubis). Calcif. Tiss. Int.* **39**, 206–208.

Jerome, C. P., Carlson, C. S., Register, T. C., Bain, F. T., Jayo, M. J., Weaver, D. S., and Adams, M. R. (1994). Bone functional changes in intact, ovariectomized, and ovariectomized, hormone-supplemented adult cynomologus monkeys *(Macaca fuscicularis)* evaluated by serum markers and dynamic histomorphometry. *J. Bone Miner. Res.* **9**, 527–540.

Jilka, R. L., Hangoc, G., Girasole, G., Passeri, G., Williams, D. C., Abrams, J. S., Boyce, B., Broxmeyer, H., and Manolagas, S. C. (1992). Increased osteoclast development after estrogen loss: Mediation by interleukin-6. *Science* **257**, 88–91.

Jordan, V. C., Phelps, E., and Lindgren, J. V. (1987). Effects of antiestrogens on bone in castrated, and intact female rats. *Breast Cancer Res. Treat.* **10**, 31–35.

Kalu, D. N., Liu, C. C., Hardin, R. R., and Hollis, B. W. (1989). The aged rat model of ovarian hormone deficiency bone loss. *Endocrinology (Baltimore)* **124**, 7–16.

Kalu, D. N., Liu, C. C., Solerno, E., Hollis, B., Echon, R., and Ray, M. (1991). Skeletal response of ovariectomized rats to low and high doses of 17b-estradiol. *Bone Min.* **14**, 175–187.

Kassem, M., Harris, S. A., Spelsberg, T. C., and Riggs, B. L. (1996a). Estrogen inhibits interleukin-6 production and gene expression in a human osteoblastic cell line with high levels of estrogen receptors. *J. Bone Miner. Res.* **11**, 193–199.

Kassem, M., Khosla, S., Spelsberg, T. C., and Riggs, B. L. (1996b). Cytokine production in the bone marrow microenvironment: Failure to demonstrate estrogen regulation in early post-menopausal women. *J. Clin. Endocrinol. Metab.* **81**, 513–518.

Kassem, M., Okazaki, R., De Leon, D., Harris, S. A., Robinson, J. A., Spelsberg, T. C., Conover, C. A., and Riggs, B. L. (1996c). Potential mechanism of estrogen-mediated decrease in bone formation: Estrogen increases production of inhibitory insulin-like growth factor-binding protein-4. *Proc. Assoc. Am. Physicians* **108**, 155–164.

Kawaguchi, H., Pilbeam, C. C., Vargas, S. J., Morse, E. E., Lorenzo, J. A., and Raisz, L. G. (1995). Ovariectomy enhances and estrogen replacement inhibits the activity of bone marrow factors that stimulate prostaglandin production in cultured mouse calvaria. *J. Clin. Invest.* **96**, 539–548.

Kelly, P. J., Pocock, N. A., Sambrook, P. N., and Eisman, J. A. (1990). Dietary calcium, sex hormones, and bone mineral density in men. *Br. Med. J.* **300**, 1361–1364.

Khosla, S., Atkinson, E. J., Melton, L. J., III, and Riggs, B. L. (1997). Effects of age and estrogen status on serum parathyroid hormone levels and biochemical markers of bone turnover in women: A population based study. *J. Clin. Endocrinol. Metab.* **82**, 1522–1527.

Khosla, S., Melton, L. J., III, Atkinson, E. J., O'Fallon, W. M., Klee, G. G., and Riggs, B. L. (1998). Relationship of serum sex steroid levels and bone turnover markers with bone mineral density in men and women: A key role for bioavailable estrogen. *J. Clin. Endocrinol. Metab.* **83**, 2266–2274.

Kimble, R. B., Vannice, J. L., Bloedow, D. C., Thompson, R. C., Hopfer, W., Kung, V. T., *et al.* (1994). Interleukin-1 receptor antagonist decreases bone loss and bone resorption in ovariectomized rats. *J. Clin. Invest.* **93**, 1959–1967.

Kimble, R. B., Srivastava, S., Ross, P. F., Matayoshi, A., and Pacifici, R. (1996). Estrogen deficiency increases the ability of stromal cells to support murine osteoclastogenesis via an interleukin-1 and tumor necrosis factor-mediated stimulation of macrophage colony stimulating factor production. *J. Biol. Chem.* **271**, 28890–28897.

Kitazawa, R., Kimble, R. B., Vannice, J. L., Kung, V. T., and Pacifici, R. (1994). Interleukin-1 receptor antagonist and tumor necrosis factor binding protein decrease osteoclast formation and bone resorption in ovariectomized mice. *J. Clin. Invest.* **94**, 2397–2406.

Korach, K. S., Couse, J. F., Curtis, S. W., Washburn, T. F., Lindzey, J., Kimbro, K. S., Eddy, E. M., Migliaccio, S., Snedeker, S. M., Lubahn, D. B., Schomberg, D. W., and Smith, E. P. (1996). Estrogen receptor gene disruption: Molecular characterization and experimental and clinical phenotypes. *Recent Prog. Horm. Res.* **51**, 159–186.

Koshino, T., and Olsson, S. E. (1975). Normal and estradiol induced calcification of the femoral head in rats. *Acta Radiol. Suppl.* **344**, 47–52.

Ledger, G. A., Burritt, M. F., Kao, P. C., O'Fallon, W. M., Riggs, B. L., and Khosla, S. (1995). Role of parathyroid hormone in mediating nocturnal and age-related increases in bone resorption. *J. Clin. Endocrinol. Metab.* **80**, 3304–3310.

Lindquist, B., Budy, A. M., McLean, F. C., and Howard, J. L. (1960). Skeletal metabolism in estrogen-treated rats studied by means of Ca^{45}. *Endocrinology (Baltimore)* **66**, 100–111.

Lindsay, R., Aitken, J. M., Hart, D. M., and Purdie, D. (1978). The effect of ovarian sex steroids on bone mineral status in the oophorectomized rat and in the human. *Postgrad. Med. J.* **54**, 50–58.

Longcope, C., Hoberg, L., Steuterman, S., and Baran, D. (1989). The effect of ovariectomy on spine bone mineral density in Rhesus monkeys. *Bone* **10**, 341–344.

Lopez, A., Ventanas, J., and Burgos, J. (1986). Oestradiol and testosterone binding sites in mice tibiae and their relationship with bone growth. *Exp. Clin. Endocrinol.* **88**, 31–38.

Lyons, K. M., Pelton, R. W., and Hogan, B. L. (1989). Patterns of expression of murine Vgr-1 and BMP-2a RNA suggest that TGFb-like genes co-ordinately regulate aspects of embryonic development. *Genes Dev.* **3**, 1657–1668.

Mann, D. R., Gould, K. G., and Collins, D. C. (1990). A potential primate model for bone loss resulting from medical oophorectomy or menopause. *J. Clin. Endocrinol. Metab.* **71**, 105–110.

Manolagas, S. C., and Jilka, R. L. (1995). Bone marrow, cytokines, and bone remodeling. Emerging insights into the pathophysiology of osteoporosis. *N. Engl. J. Med.* **332**, 305–311.

Martin, R. B., Butcher, R. L., Sherwood, L. L., Buckendahl, P., Boyd, R. D., Farris, D., Sharkey, N., and Dannucci, G. (1987). Effects of ovariectomy in beagle dogs. *Bone* **8**, 23–31.

Mazess, B., Vetter, J., and Weaver, D. S. (1987). Bone changes in oophorectomized monkeys: CT findings. *J. Comp. Assist. Tomogr.* **11**, 302–305.

McKane, W. R., Khosla, S., Peterson, J. M., Egan, K., and Riggs, B. L. (1994). Circulating levels of cytokines that modulate bone resorption: Effects of age and menopause in women. *J. Bone Miner. Res.* **9**, 1313–1318.

McKane, W. R., Khosla, S., Burritt, M. F., Kao, P. C., Wilson, D. M., Ory, S. J., and Riggs, B. L. (1995). Mechanism of renal calcium conservation with estrogen replacement therapy in women in early postmenopause—a clinical research center study. *J. Clin. Endocrinol. Metab.* **80**, 3458–3464.

McKane, W. R., Khosla, S., Egan, K. S., Robins, S. P., Burritt, M. F., and Riggs, B. L. (1996). Role of calcium intake in modulating age-related increases in parathyroid function and bone resorption. *J. Clin. Endocrinol. Metab.* **81**, 1699–1703.

McKane, R. W., Khosla, S., Risteli, J., Robins, S. P., Muhs, J. M., and Riggs, B. L. (1997). Role of estrogen deficiency in pathogenesis of secondary hyperparathyroidism and increased bone resorption in elderly women. *Proc. Assoc. Am. Physicians* **109**, 174–180.

Meier, D. E., Orwoll, E. S., Keenan, E. J., and Fagerstrom, R. M. (1987). Marked decline in trabecular bone mineral content in healthy men with age: Lack of association with sex steroid levels. *J. Am. Geriatr Soc.* **35**, 189–197.

Migliaccio, S., Newbold, R. R., Bullock, B. C., McLachlan, J. A., and Korach, K. S. (1992). Developmental exposure to estrogens induces persistent changes in skeletal tissue. *Endocrinology (Baltimore)* **130**, 1756–1758.

Miyaura, C., Kusano, K., Masuzawa, T., Chaki, O., Onoe, Y., Aoyagim, M., *et al.* (1995). Endogenous bone-resorbing factors in estrogen deficiency: Cooperative effects of IL-1 and Il-6. *J. Bone Miner Res.* **10**, 1365–1373.

Morishima, A., Grumbach, M. M., Simpson, E. R., Fisher, C., and Qin, K. (1995). Aromatase deficiency in male and female siblings caused by a novel mutation and the physiological role of estrogens. *J. Clin. Endocrinol. Metab.* **80**, 3689–3698.

Morishima, A., Grumbach, M. M., and Bilezikian, J. P. (1997). Estrogen markedly increases bone mass in an estrogen deficient young man with aromatase deficiency. *J. Bone Miner. Res.* **12** (Suppl. 1), S126.

Navey-Many, T., Almogi, G., Livni, N., and Silver, J. (1992). Estrogen receptors and biologic response in rat parathyroid tissue and C cells. *J. Clin. Invest.* **90**, 2434–2438.

Nebert, D. W., Nelson, D. R., Adesnik, M., *et al.* (1989). The P450 gene superfamily and recommended nomenclature. *DNA* **8**, 1–13.

Nyda, M. J., DeMajo, S. F., and Lewis, R. A. (1948). The effect of ovariectomy and physiologic doses of estradiol upon body weight, linear growth and fat content of the female albino rat. *Bull. Johns Hopkins Hosp.* **83**, 279–287.

Onoe, Y., Miyaura, C., Ohta, H., Nozawa, S., and Suda, T. (1997). Expression of estrogen receptor beta in rat bone. *Endocrinology (Baltimore)* **138**, 4509–4512.

Ornoy, A., Giron, S., Aner, R., Goldstein, M., Boyan, B. D., and Schwartz, Z. (1994). Gender dependent effects of testosterone and 17 beta-estradiol on bone growth and modeling in young mice. *Bone Miner.* **24**, 43–58.

Ostadalova, I. (1976). The effect of single dose of oestrogens administered during the early postnatal period on the DNA content of rat bone epiphyses. *Physiol. Bohemoslov.* **25**, 97–102.

Oursler, M. J., Cortese, C., Keeting, P., Anderson, M. A., Bonde, S. K., Riggs, B. L., and Spelsberg, T. C. (1991). Modulation of transforming growth factor-beta production in normal human osteoblast-like cells by 17 beta-estradiol and parathyroid hormone. *Endocrinology (Baltimore)* **129**, 3313–3320.

Oursler, M. J., Pederson, L., Fitzpatrick, L. A., and Riggs, B. L. (1994). Human giant cell tumors of the bone (osteoclastomas) are estrogen target cells. *Proc. Natl. Acad. Sci. U.S.A.* **91**, 5227–5231.

Pacifici, R., Brown, C., Puscheck, E., Friedrick, E., Slatopolsky, E., Maggio, D., *et al.* (1991). Effect of surgical menopause and estrogen replacement on cytokine release from human blood mononuclear cells. *Proc. Natl. Acad. Sci. U.S.A.* **88**, 5134–5138.

Parfitt, A. M. (1979). Quantum concept of bone remodeling and turnover: Implications for the pathogenesis of osteoporosis. *Calcif. Tissue Int.* **28**, 1–5.

Parfitt, A. M., Mathews, C. H. E., Villaneuva, A. R., Kleerekoper, M., Frame, B., and Rao, D. S. (1983). Relationships between surface, volume and thickness of iliac trabecular bone in aging and in osteoporosis. *J. Clin. Invest.* **72**, 1396–1409.

Pitsillides, A., Rawlinson, S., Suswillo, R., Bourrin, S., Zaman, G., and Lanyon, L. (1995). Mechanical strain-induced NO production by bone cells: A possible role in adaptive bone (re)modelling. *FASEB J* **9**, 1614–1622.

Poli, V., Balena, R., Fattori, E., Markatos, A., Yamamoto, A., Tanaka, H., *et al.* (1994). Interleukin-6 deficient mice are protected from bone loss caused by estrogen depletion. *EMBO* **13**, 1189–1196.

Prestwood, K. M., Pilbeam, C. C., Burleson, J. A., Woodiel, F. N., Delmas, P. D., Deftos, L. J., and Raisz, L. G. (1994). The short term effects of conjugated estrogens on bone turnover in older women. *J. Clin. Endocrinol. Metab.* **79**, 366–371.

Prince, R. L., Schiff, I., and Neer, R. M. (1990). Effects of transfermal estrogen replacement on parathyroid hormone secretion. *J. Clin. Endocrinol. Metab.* **71**, 1284–1287.

Prince, R. L., MacLaughlin, D. T., Gaz, R. D., and Neer, R. M. (1991). Lack of evidence for estrogen receptors in human and bovine parathyroid tissue. *Clin. Endocrinol. Metab.* **72**, 1226–1228.

Prince, R., Dick, I., Devine, A., Price, R. Gutteridge, D., Kerr, D., Criddle, A., Garcia-Webb, P., and St. John, A. (1995). The effects of menopause and age on calcitropic hormones: A cross-sectional study of 655 healthy women aged 35 to 90. *J. Bone Miner. Res.* **10**, 835–842.

Purohit, A., Flanagan, A. M., and Reed, M. J. (1992). Estrogen synthesis by osteoblast cell lines. *Endocrinology (Baltimore)* **131**, 2027–2029.

Reid, I. R., Ames, R. W., Evans, M. C., Gamble, G. D., and Sharpe, S. J. (1995). Long-term effects of calcium supplementation on bone and fractures in postmenopausal women: A randomized controlled trial. *Am. J. Med.* **98**, 331–335.

Rickard, D. J., Hofbauer, L. C., Bonde, S. K., Gori, F., Spelsberg, T. C., and Riggs, B. L. (1998). Bone morphogenetic protein-6 production in human osteoblastic cell lines. Selective regulation by estrogen. *J. Clin. Invest.* **101**, 413–422.

Riggs, B. L., and Melton, L. J., III (1986). Involutional osteoporosis. *N. Engl. J. Med.* **314**, 1676–1686.

Riggs, B. L., Wahner, H. W., Dunn, W. L., Mazess, R. B., Offord, K. P., and Melton, L. J., III (1981). Differential changes in bone mineral density of the appendicular skeleton with aging: relationship to spinal osteoporosis. *J. Clin. Invest.* **67**, 328–335.

Riggs, B. L., Khosla, S., and Melton, L. J., III (1998). A unitary model for involutional osteoporosis: Estrogen deficiency causes both type I and type II osteoporosis in postmenopausal women and contributes to bone loss in aging men. *J. Bone Miner. Res.* **13**, 763–773.

Robinson, J. A., Riggs, B. L., Spelsberg, T. C., and Oursler, M. J. (1996). Osteoclasts and transforming growth factor-b: Estrogen-mediated isoform-specific regulation of production. *Endocrinology (Baltimore)* **137**, 615–621.

Robinson, J. A., Harris, S. A., Riggs, B. L., and Spelsberg, T. C. (1997). Estrogen regulation of human osteoblastic cell proliferation and differentiation. *Endocrinology (Baltimore)* **138**, 2919–2927.

Rodan, G. A., and Martin, T. J. (1981). Role of osteoblasts in hormonal control of bone resorption—a hypothesis. *Calcif. Tissue Int.* **33**, 344–351.

Salih, M. A., Liu, C.-C., Arjmandi, B. H., and Kalu, D. N. (1993). Estrogen modulates the mRNA levels for cancellous bone protein of ovariectomized rats. *Bone Miner.* **23**, 285–299.

Saville, P. D. (1969). Changes in skeletal mass and fragility with castration in the rat: A model of osteoporosis. *J. Am. Geriatr. Soc.* **17**, 155–166.

Schweikert, H.-U., Wolf, L., and Romalo, G. (1995). Oestrogen formation from androstenedione in human bone. *Clin. Endocrinol.* **43**, 37–42.

Sibonga, J. D., Dobnig, H., Harden, R. M., and Turner, R. T. (1998). Effect of the high affinity estrogen receptor ligand ICI 182,780 on the rat tibia. *Endocrinology* **139**, 3736–3742.

Simpson, E. R., Mahendroo, M. S., Means, G. D., Kilgore, M. W., Hinshelwood, M. M., Graham-Lorence, S., Amarneh, B., Ito, Y., Fisher, C. R., Michael, M. D., Mendelson, C. R., and Bulun, S. E. (1994). Aromatase cytochrome p450, the enzyme responsible for estrogen biosynthesis. *Endocr. Rev.* **15**, 342–355.

Slemenda, C. W., Longcope, C., Zhou, L., Hui, S. L., Peacock, M., and Johnston, C. C. (1997). Sex steroids and bone mass in older men. Positive associations with serum estrogens and negative associations with androgens. *J. Clin. Invest.* **100**, 1755–1759.

Smith, E. P., Boyd, J., Frank, G. R., Takahashi, H., Cohen, R. M., Specker, B., Williams, T. C., Lubahn, D. B., and Korach, K. S. (1994). Estrogen resistance caused by a mutation in the estrogen receptor gene in a man. *N. Engl. J. Med* **331**, 1056–1061.

Snow, G. R., and Anderson, C. (1986). The effect of 17b-estradiol and progestagen on trabecular bone remodeling in oophorectomized dogs. *Calcif. Tiss. Int.* **39**, 198–205.

Stenström, A., Hansson, L. I., and Thorngren, K. G. (1982). Effect of ovariectomy on longitudinal bone growth. *Anat. Embryol.* **164**, 9–18.

Stepan, J. J., Lachman, M., Zverina, J., and Pacovsky, V. (1989). Castrated men exhibit bone loss: Effects of calcitonin treatment on biochemical indices of bone remodeling. *J. Clin. Endocrinol. Metab.* **69**, 523–527.

Strickland, A. L., and Sprinz, H. (1973). Studies of the influence of estradiol and growth hormone on the hypophysectomized immature rate epiphyseal cartilage growth plate. *Am. J. Obstet. Gynecol.* **115**, 471–477.

Swanson, H. E., and VanDerWerffTenBosch, J. J. (1963). Sex differences in growth of rats, and their modification by a single injection of testosterone propionate shortly after birth. *J. Endocrin.* **26**, 197–207.

Tanaka, S., Takahashi, N., Udagawa, N., Tamura, T., Akatsu, T., Stanley, E. R., *et al.* (1993a). Macrophage colony stimulating factor is indispensable for both proliferation and differentiation of osteoclast progenitors. *J. Clin. Invest.* **91**, 257–263.

Tanaka, S., Haji, M., Nishi, Y., Yamase, T., Takanayagi, R., and Nawata, H. (1993b). Aromatase activity in human osteoblast-like osteosarcoma cell. *Calcif. Tissue Int.* **52**, 107–109.

Tomkinson, A., Reeve, J., Shaw, R. W., and Noble, B. S. (1997). The death of osteocytes via apoptosis accompanies estrogen withdrawl in human bone. *J. Clin. Endocrinol. Metab.* **82**, 3128–3135.

Turner, R. T., Vandersteenhoven, J. J., and Bell, N. H. (1987a). The effects of ovariectomy and 17b-estradiol on cortical bone histomorphometry in growing rats. *J. Bone Min. Res.* **2**, 115–122.

Turner, R. T., Wakley, G. K., Hannon, K. S., and Bell, N. H. (1987b). Tamoxifen prevents the skeletal effects of ovarian hormone deficiency in rats. *J. Bone Min. Res.* **2**, 449–456.

Turner, R. T., Wakley, G. K., Hannon, K. S., and Bell, N. H. (1988). Tamoxifen inhibits osteoclast-mediated resorption of trabecular bone in ovarian hormone deficient rats. *Endocrinology (Baltimore)* **122**, 1146–1150.

Turner, R. T., Hannon, K. S., Demers, L. M., Buchanan, J., and Bell, N. H. (1989). Differential effects of gonadal function on bone histomorphometry in male and female rats. *J. Bone Min. Res.* **4**, 557–563.

Turner, R. T., Wakley, G. K., and Hannon, K. S. (1990a). Differential effects of androgens on cortical bone histomorphometry in gonadectomized male and female rats. *J. Orthop. Res.* **8**, 612–617.

Turner, R. T., Lifrak, E. T., Beckner, M., Wakley, G. K., Hannon, K. S., and Parker, L. N. (1990b). Dehydroepiandrosterone reduces cancellous bone osteopenia in ovariectomized rats. *Am. J. Physiol.* **258**, E673–E677.

Turner, R. T., Colvard, D. S., and Spelsberg, T. C. (1990c). Estrogen inhibition of periosteal bone formation in rat long bones: Down-regulation of gene expression for bone matrix proteins. *Endocrinology (Baltimore)* **127**, 1346–1351.

Turner, R. T., Backup, P., Sherman, P. J., Hill, E., Evans, G. L., and Spelsberg, T. C. (1992). Mechanism of action of estrogen on intramembranous bone formation: Regulation of osteoblast differentiation and activity. *Endocrinology (Baltimore)* **131**, 883–889.

Turner, R. T., Evans, G. L., and Wakley, G. K. (1993). Mechanism of action of estrogen on cancellous bone balance in tibiae of ovariectomized growing rats: Inhibitioin of indices of formation and resorption. *J. Bone Min. Res.* **8**, 359–366.

Turner, R. T., Riggs, B. L., and Spelsberg, T. C. (1994a). Skeletal effects of estrogen. *Endocr. Rev.* **15**, 275–300.

Turner, R. T., Evans, G. L., and Wakley, G. K. (1994b). Reduced chondroclast differentiation results in increased cancellous bone volume in estrogen-treated growing rats. *Endocrinology (Baltimore)* **134**, 461–466.

Urist, M. R., Budy, A. M., and McLean, F. C. (1948). Species differences in the reaction of the mammalian skeleton to estrogen. *Proc. Soc. Exp. Biol. Med.* **68**, 324–326.

Wakley, G. K., Baum, R. L., Hannon, K. S., and Turner, R. T. (1988). Tamoxifen treatment reduces osteopenia induced by immobilization in the rat. *Calcif. Tissue Int.* **43**, 383–388.

Wakley, G. K., Shutte, D. E., Hannon, K. S., and Turner, R. T. (1991). The effects of castration and androgen replacement therapy on bone: A histomorphometric study in the rat. *J. Bone Miner. Res.* **6**, 325–330.

Wakley, G. K., Evans, G. L., and Turner, R. T. (1997). Short-term effects of high dose estrogen on tibiae of growing male rats. *Calcif. Tissue Int.* **60**, 37–42.

Westerlind, K. C., Wakley, G. K., Evans, G. L., and Turner, R. T. (1993). Estrogen does not increase bone formation in growing rats. *Endocrinology (Baltimore)* **133**, 2924–2934.

Westerlind, K. C., Sarkar, G., Bolander, M. E., and Turner, R. T. (1995). Estrogen receptor mRNA is expressed *in vivo* in rat calvarial periosteum. *Steroids* **60**(8), 484–487.

Westerlind, K. C., Wronski, T. J., Ritman, E. L., Luo, Z.-P., An, K.-N., Bell, N. H., and Turner, R. T. (1997). Estrogen regulates the rate of bone turnover but bone balance in ovariectomized rats is modulated by prevailing mechanical strain. *Proc. Natl. Acad. Sci. U.S.A.* **94**, 4199–4204.

Whitson, S. W., Dawson, L. R., and Jee, W. S. S. (1978). A tetracycline study of cyclic longitudinal bone growth in the female rat. *Endocrinology (Baltimore)* **103**, 2006–2010.

Wronski, T. J., Lowry, P. L., Walsh, C. C., and Ignaszewski, L. A. (1985). Skeletal alterations in ovariectomized rats. *Calcif. Tiss. Int.* **37**, 324–328.

Wronski, T. J., Walsh, C. C., Ignaszewski, L. A. (1986). Histologic evidence for osteopenia and increased bone turnover in ovariectomized rats. *Bone* **7**, 119–123.

Wronski, T. J., Cintron, M., and Dann, L. M. (1988a). Temporal relationship between bone loss and increased bone turnover in ovariectomized rats. *Calcif. Tiss. Int.* **43**, 179–183.

Wronski, T. J., Cintron, M., Doherty, A. L., and Dann, L. M. (1988b). Estrogen treatment prevents osteopenia and depresses bone turnover in ovariectomized rats. *Endocrinology (Baltimore)* **123**, 681–686.

Wronski, T. J., Dann, L. M., Scott, K. S., and Cintron, M. (1989a). Long-term effects of ovariectomy and aging on the rat skeleton. *Calcif. Tiss. Int.* **45**, 360–366.

Wronski, T. J., Dann, L. M., and Horner, S. L. (1989b). Time course of vertebral osteopenia in ovariectomized rats. *Bone* **10**, 295–301

Yamamoto, T. T. Y., and Rodan, G. A. (1990). Directs effects of 17b-estradiol on trabecular bone in ovariectomized rats. *Proc. Natl. Acad. Sci. U.S.A.* **87**, 2172–2176.

Chapter 15

Torben Steiniche and Erik F. Eriksen

University Department of Endocrinology
Aarhus Amtssygehus and
University Department of Pathology
Aarhus Kommunehospital
DK-8000 Aarhus C., Denmark

Age-Related Changes in Bone Remodeling

I. Introduction

Three basic mechanisms are involved in the turnover and development of bone: (a) longitudinal growth, (b) modeling and (c) remodeling. Longitudinal growth ceases with closure of the epiphyseal plates at the end of the growing period. During the growth phase a continuous adaptation of the macroscopic shape of the bone takes place. Some surfaces are under continuous resorption and others under continuous formation, a process called modeling. Modeling serves to alter the amount of bone that is present and to determine its geometry and size (Frost, 1969) but is not a factor of importance in the pathogenesis of acquired metabolic bone disease in adults. On the other hand, remodeling is a process that starts with fetal osteogenesis and continues throughout life. It results in turnover of lamellar bone without

Osteoporosis in Men

299

causing large changes in its quantity, geometry, or size (Frost, 1969). By the process of remodeling, bone is renewed through internal reorganization by localized osteoclastic resorption followed by osteoblastic formation in a coordinated sequence of events (Fig. 1). After activation (A), osteoclasts start to erode and form a resorption cavity (R). When a certain resorption depth is reached, mononuclear cells that complete the resorption replace the osteoclasts. The resorption period (RP) lasts for about 4–6 weeks, resulting in the creation of a resorption lacuna with a certain final resorption depth. After completion of resorption, preosteoblasts invade the cavity, differentiate to osteoblasts, and start bone matrix formation (F). After a certain period (the initial mineralization lag time) bone matrix is subsequently mineralized to form lamellar bone. Osteoblasts thereby refill the lacuna with lamellar bone, in essence repairing the resorption-mediated defect. During this process some osteoblasts will be incorporated in the matrix, and later in mineralized bone, as osteocytes, which are connected to one another and to surface lining cells, by canaliculi. The duration of the bone formation period (FP) is about 3 months, with the final result a new bone structural unit (BSU), characterized by a certain mean wall thickness.

In cortical bone similar events proceed as part of Haversian remodeling with osteoclasts forming the so-called "cutting cone" and osteoblasts subsequently filling the tunnel formed by osteoclastic resorption ("closing cone") (Fig. 1).

As described above, resorption and formation are closely associated with each other both temporarily (time) and spatially (space) (Eriksen et al., 1984a,b; Frost, 1969; Parfitt, 1976). In the normal remodeling process resorption will always be followed by formation, and formation will always be preceded by resorption. The frequency by which a given site on the trabecular bone surfaces undergoes remodeling is termed the activation frequency.

Cancellous and cortical bone are continuously renewed by these processes to adjust architecture to changes in prevailing mechanical forces, to preserve the viability of the embedded osteocytes, and to avoid stress fractures. The remodeling process may further be essential for microfracture repair. Several systemic hormones and local cytokines (Watrous and Andrews, 1989) regulate the remodeling process.

A. Variation in Bone Remodeling

Bone turnover due to remodeling displays substantial regional variations between different skeletal sites (Podenphant and Engel, 1987). Furthermore, there exist variations in bone remodeling (turnover) and balance between different bone envelopes (cancellous, endocortical, intracortical, and pericortical). In general, the bone balance seems to be negative at the cancellous and endocortical envelope (Han et al., 1996), whereas the bone balance seems to be zero or even slightly positive at the pericortical envelope.

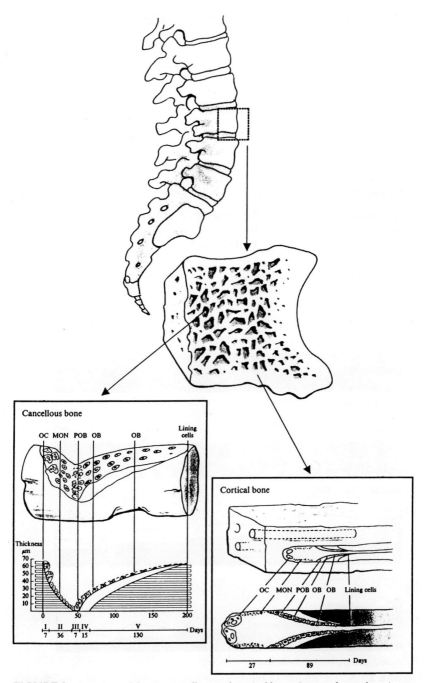

FIGURE 1   Bone remodeling in cancellous and cortical bone. See text for explanations.

Ethnicity also seems to influence the remodeling process. Both Han *et al.* (1996) and Weinstein and Bell (1988) found that the rate of bone turnover was lower in blacks than in whites. Potential differences between the two sexes and how age influences the remodeling process are discussed later.

B. Bone Loss due to Remodeling

By the remodeling process bone may be gained or lost by three mechanisms: reversible bone loss/gain, irreversible bone loss/gain by changes in bone balance at the BMU level, and loss of trabecular elements.

I. Reversible Bone Loss/Gain

The remodeling space is the amount of bone that has been removed by osteoclasts and not yet reformed by the osteoblasts during the remodeling sequence (Parfitt, 1983) (Fig. 2). The total remodeling space within the skeleton depends on the number of ongoing remodeling cycles, the duration of the resorptive and formative periods, and the depths of the resorption lacunae. In normal individuals, the remodeling space constitutes 6–8% of the

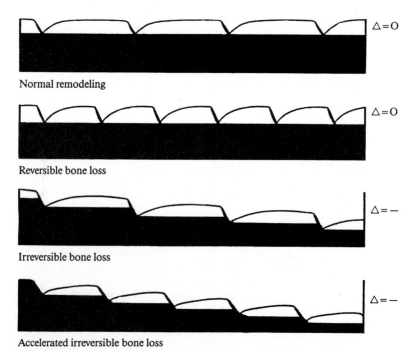

FIGURE 2 Normal remodeling and reversible bone loss due to increased remodeling space. Irreversible bone loss due to imbalance between resorption and formation and accelerated irreversible bone loss due to high turnover accompanied by remodeling imbalance.

skeletal volume (Parfitt, 1983). An increase in activation frequency leads to an increase in the number of ongoing remodeling cycles (Fig. 2). This will increase the remodeling space and by that proportionally decrease the amount of bone. Obviously, the opposite effect is seen if the activation frequency is decreased. The process is reversible because the remodeling space, and thereby the bone volume, returns to normal when the metabolic challenge to the bone is removed and the activation frequency returns to normal.

2. Irreversible Bone Loss/Gain by Changes in Bone Balance

In normal young adults, the amount of bone formed by the osteoblasts at the remodeling site is equal to the amount of bone previously resorbed. However, a negative balance may occur, leading to a thinning of the trabeculae and osteopenia (Fig. 2). The loss rate will increase if the remodeling imbalance is accompanied by increased activation frequency. An increase in trabecular thickness will occur if the bone balance per remodeling site is positive.

3. Irreversible Loss of Whole Trabecular Elements

A very deep resorption lacuna may perforate a trabecular plate, removing the basis for the subsequent bone formation and, by that, cause the loss of a structural element, adding to the disintegration of the trabecular network (Parfitt, 1984). The risk of trabecular plate perforations depends on the activation frequency, resorption depth, and trabecular thickness. Although the loss of bone volume by this mechanism may be limited, the effect on the biomechanical competence (strength) is pronounced (Parfitt, 1987). As mentioned below, the female skeleton is subjected to more profound disintegration of trabecular structure due to perforations than the male skeleton (Fig. 3).

II. Bone Mass and Structure

Age-related bone loss is an inescapable consequence of bone remodeling after the growth phase, affecting all groups studied, whether defined by sex, race, economic development, geographic location, or historical epoch. Due to the remodeling process described above, both men and women lose bone with age and experience a certain deterioration of the bone architecture. The rate of bone loss and the effect of this loss on bone architecture may differ between the two sexes. It seems that bone density in women is slightly higher than in men at the end of the growth phase, whereas the opposite is found after the age of 60 (Melsen et al., 1978). Mosekilde (1989, 1990) found that in men there is a greater cross-sectional area of the vertebral body and an increase in this with age, leading to better biomechanical competence (Mosekilde, 1990). This observation is supported by Feik et al. (1996), who

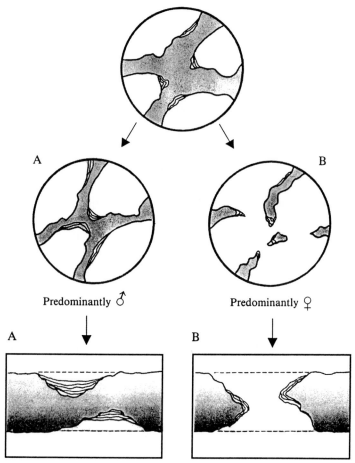

FIGURE 3 Differences between bone loss mechanisms operating in men and women. Women tend to have a higher degree of trabecular perforations and consequently more disintegration of trabecular architecture than men, who tend to have a higher degree of trabecular thinning.

found a fairly uniform increase in the subperiosteal area in the femoral mid-shaft in men from around the third to the seventh decade. Thus, men seem to have a positive balance at the periosteal surface. Women displayed two distinct phases during this period: relative stability until around the meno-pause and then a marked increase in the superiosteal area and medullary area (Feik *et al.*, 1996). In another study, Mosekilde (1989) found that both men and women undergo age-related loss of vertebral trabecular bone mass and structure with an increase in the distance between the horizontal trabec-ulae in both sexes, but in individuals older than 75 years, this increase was significantly higher for females than for males (Mosekilde, 1989).

The star volume is a stereologic parameter that can, in an unbiased way, describe structural changes of cancellous bone. It is defined as the mean volume of all the parts of an object that can be seen unobscured in all directions from a particular point inside the object. Vesterby (1990) found a significant increase in marrow space star volume with age in the iliac crest and the first lumbar vertebra in both men and women. From these data, Vesterby concluded that the age-related reduction in cancellous bone is accompanied by loss of whole bone structures. The increase in marrow space star volume in the first lumbar vertebra was, moreover, significantly greater for women than for men (Vesterby, 1990) (Fig. 4). Compston *et al.* (1987) performed a study on iliac crest bone biopsies from 90 subjects using a computerized method that automatically identifies and quantifies nodes, free ends, and a number of topologically defined struts and found that loss of trabeculae resulting in decreased interconnectedness of the normal bone structural pattern plays an important role in age-related bone loss in females. Removal of trabeculae also occurs in males but is less prominent, implying that trabecular thinning makes a greater contribution to age-related bone loss in males (Compston *et al.*, 1987). In a study by Aaron *et al.* (1987) on biopsies from the ilium of 86 women and 98 men aged 20–90 years the same conclusion was drawn.

Thus, men and women lose bone in different ways. Women lose bone predominantly by trabecular perforations and men predominantly by trabecular thinning (Fig. 3). As a consequence, one would expect differences in the remodeling process between the two sexes or differences in bone structure at the end of the growth phase.

III. Age-Related Changes in Bone Turnover (Activation Frequency) and Differences between Men and Women _____

Histomorphometric analyses of bone biopsy obtained from the iliac crest after tetracycline double labeling is still the only method where the whole remodeling process can be evaluated. The results concerning bone turnover changes with age and the differences between sexes are however somewhat conflicting.

A. Bone Remodeling in Healthy Men

In rather extensive analyses of bone biopsies obtained from the iliac crest after tetracycline labeling, both Dahl *et al.* (1988) and Melsen and Mosekilde (1978) found no changes in static (extend of osteoid and eroded surfaces) or dynamic (labeled surfaces, mineral appositional rate, adjusted appositional rate or bone formation rate) parameters in men with age. In iliac crest samples obtained postmortem from 43 young men and 49 elderly men Nordin *et al.* (1984) found a significant reduction in osteoid surfaces (forming sur-

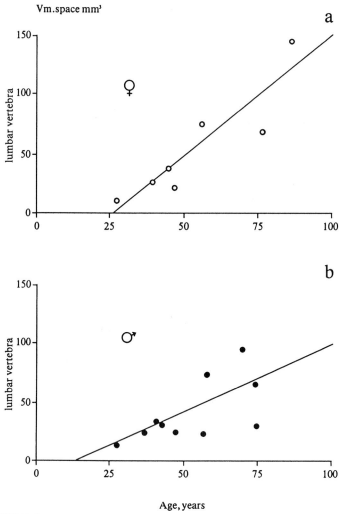

FIGURE 4   Age-dependent changes in marrow star volume in men and women. Note the more pronounced increase with age in women. Reproduced with permission from Vesterby (1990).

faces) in elderly men compared to the younger men, whereas no significant difference was observed in the extent of resorptive surfaces. In bone biopsies from 43 healthy men, aged 20–80 years, Clarke *et al.* (1996) found a decrease in osteoblast–osteoid interface by 19.2%, double-labeled osteoid 18.6% and single-labeled osteoid 18.0% over this age span. None of the other static or dynamic histomorphometric parameters changed with age in this population sample of healthy men (Clarke *et al.*, 1996). In summary, the bone turnover in healthy men, as reflected in static and dynamic histomorpho-metric data, seems to be either constant with age or decrease only slightly.

B. Bone Remodeling in Healthy Women

In healthy women the data available are also conflicting. In a study of 29 women aged 19–53 years Melsen and Mosekilde (1978) found a decrease in bone remodeling with age expressed by a significant decrease in labeled surfaces, adjusted appositional rate, and bone formation rate. On the other hand, Dahl *et al.* (1988) found that in 46 women aged 21–81 years, all mea-sured formation indices except mineral appositional rate increased with age, as did the calculated surface-based bone formation rate. Eastell *et al.* (1988) assessed bone formation in 12 young and 11 older women (ages 30–41 and 55–73, respectively) using biochemical bone markers, calcium kinetics, and bone histomorphometry. Bone formation (mean $\pm$ SE) was higher in the older women than in the younger women based on measurements of serum osteocalcin (1.67 $\pm$ 0.07 versus 1.14 $\pm$ 0.10 nmol/L; $p < 0.01$) and serum bone-specific alkaline phosphatase (388 $\pm$ 42 versus 223 $\pm$ 22 nkatal/L; $p < 0.01$) (Fig. 5). Bone formation rate by histomorphometry also revealed increased bone formative activity in older women (31.1 $\pm$ 4.9% versus 15.1 $\pm$ 2.7%/yr in the younger group [$p < 0.01$]) (Fig. 5), but was similar in the two groups when calcium accretion rates were assessed kinetically (5.9 $\pm$ 1.0 versus 7.5 $\pm$ 1.2). This latter discrepancy may have been the result of several age-related factors, especially reduced mineralization of com-pleted osteons. Han *et al.* (1997) studied 142 healthy women aged 20–74 years, and reported bone formation and resorption indices to be significantly higher in the postmenopausal compared to the premenopausal subjects, re-flecting a 33% increase in activation frequency. The results from Recker *et al.* (1988), who studied bone biopsies from 34 healthy postmenopausal women aged 45–74 years, complicated the topic further. Their values for the extent of eroded (resorptive) and osteoid (formative) surfaces, mineral appositional rate, and comparable dynamic variables (as, for example, bone formation rate) were nearly identical with the data from young women (ages 19–53, mean age 29) presented by Melsen and Mosekilde (1978) and described earlier. Furthermore, Recker *et al.* (1988) found a decrease in mineral ap-positional rate with age in the postmenopausal women, whereas all other measured and derived static and dynamic parameters showed no correlation with age.

The divergent results reported may to some degree reflect differing pro-portions of premenopausal and postmenopausal women and, in the post-menopausal group, differences in the distribution of women regarding number of years past menopause. Furthermore, the two studies by Melsen and Dahl did not calculate volume referent bone formation rate, as was the case in the study of Eastell *et al.* If the data are cautiously interpreted, there seems to be

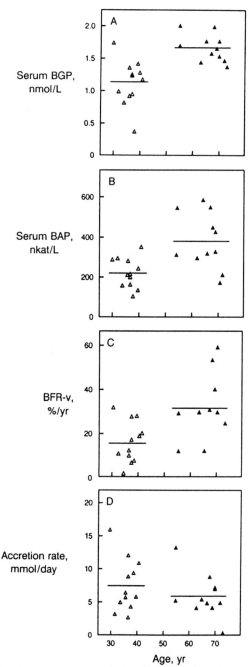

FIGURE 5 Differences in bone turnover in young (open triangles) and old women (closed triangles). Biochemical markers (S-osteocalcin [BGP] and S-bone alkaline phosphatase [BAP]) and bone histomorphometric assessment of the osteoblastic bone volume referent formation rate (BFR-v) show increases in old women. These increases are not, however, reflected in the calcium kinetic accretion rate. Reproduced with permission from Eastell *et al.* (1988), Bone formation rate in older normal women, *J. Clin. Endocrinol. Metab.* **67**, 741–748, © The Endocrine Society.

a reduction in bone remodeling in women from a young age to the time of menopause (Melsen and Mosekilde, 1978). After menopause an increase in bone turnover ensues, which explains the findings of an increased activation frequency in postmenopausal women by Han *et al.* (1997) and Eastell *et al.* (1988). In older women, bone turnover may again decrease to similar, or even lower, levels than those noted in premenopausal women. Nevertheless, in some studies a persistent increase in bone turnover persists in older post-menopausal women.

C. Bone Remodeling in Healthy Men Compared with Healthy Women

Studies comparing bone remodeling in men and women in different decades are few. In 72 healthy Norwegians (46 women) aged 21–81 years, Dahl *et al.* (1988) found more extensive osteoid and labeled surfaces, as well as a higher bone formation rate, in men compared with women. The same high level of osteoid and labeled surfaces and bone formation rate was found by Melsen and Mosekilde (1978) in men compared with women in a group of 41 normal Danes (12 males and 29 females) aged 19–56 years.

D. Age-Related Changes in the Amount of Bone Resorbed (Resorption Depth) and Reformed (Wall Thickness) during the Remodeling Cycle: Differences between Men and Women

The amount of bone reformed during the remodeling cycle (wall thickness) decreases in men and women with age (Kragstrup *et al.*, 1983; Lips *et al.*, 1978; Qiu *et al.*, 1990). Mean wall thickness in young individuals averages 60–65 μm and decreases to values of 35–40 μm in the very old. However, no gender differences have been noted either in wall thickness or in the slope of the decrease in wall thickness with age (Kragstrup *et al.*, 1983).

Two groups have studied the relation between resorption depth, sex, and age (Croucher *et al.*, 1991; Eriksen *et al.*, 1985). Eriksen *et al.* (1985) determined resorption depth by counting the number of lamellae from the trabecular surfaces to the bottom of preosteoblast-like cell lacunae (lacunae where resorption had terminated—final resorption depth), while Croucher *et al.* (1991) assessed resorption cavities by a computerized technique in which the eroded bone surface was reconstructed and measurements made interactively. The latter method does not measure final erosion depth. These methodological differences may explain the somewhat different results reported. Eriksen *et al.* (1985) found a decrease in resorption depth with age in both sexes (Fig. 6). Furthermore, the mean final resorption depth was larger in females aged 30–60 years than in men of the same age. Croucher *et al.*

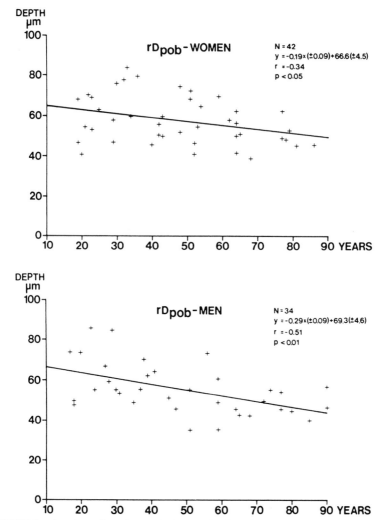

FIGURE 6 Age-dependent changes in erosion depth with age in men and women. Reproduced with permission from Eriksen *et al.* (1985).

(1991) reported no significant correlation between maximum and mean cavity depth and age in either sex.

The reduction in final resorption depth with age is parallel to the decrease in mean thickness of completed walls previously described (Eriksen *et al.*, 1985; Kragstrup *et al.*, 1983), leading to a slight negative bone balance per remodeling cycle in both men and women. The balance may be slightly more negative in women aged 30–60 years because of the increase in final resorption depth found in this age period (Eriksen *et al.*, 1985).

IV. Conclusion _____

In men, a rather constant rate of bone turnover/remodeling with age, combined with a slightly negative bone balance per remodeling cycle, may explain the slight but steady age-related decrease in bone volume. This is consistent with the observation that men lose bone primarily as a result of trabecular thinning. In contrast, women more often experience loss of whole trabecular elements. In women the increase in bone turnover in the early postmenopausal period, combined with an increase in resorption depth at age 30–60, leads to an increased risk for trabecular perforations and loss of whole trabecular elements. Thus, gender variations in adult bone turnover, resorption depth, and bone balance very well explain the observed differences in bone structure in elderly women and men.

References _____

Aaron, J. E., Makins, N. B., and Sagreiya, K. (1987). The microanatomy of trabecular bone loss in normal aging men and women. *Clin. Orthop.* 260–271.

Clarke, B. L., Ebeling, P. R., Jones, J. D., Wahner, H. W., O'Fallon, W. M., Riggs, B. L., and Fitzpatrick, L. A. (1996). Changes in quantiative bone histomorphometry in aging healthy men. *J. Clin. Endocrinol. Metab.* **81**, 2264–2270.

Compston, J. E., Mellish, R. W., and Garrahan, N. J. (1987). Age-related changes in iliac crest trabecular microanatomic bone structure in man. *Bone* **8**, 289–292.

Croucher, P. I., Garrahan, N. J., Mellish, R. W., and Compston, J. E. (1991). Age-related changes in resorption cavity characteristics in human trabecular bone. *Osteoporos. Int.* **1**, 257–261.

Dahl, E., Nordal, K. P., Halse, J., and Attramadal, A. (1988). Histomorphometric analysis of normal bone from the iliac crest of Norwegian subjects. *Bone Miner.* **3**, 369–377.

Eastell, R., Delmas, P. D., Hodgson, S. F., Eriksen, E. F., Mann, K. G., and Riggs, B. L. (1988). Bone formation rate in older normal women: Concurrent assessment with bone histomorphometry, calcium kinetics, and biochemical markers. *J. Clin. Endocrinol. Metab.* **67**, 741–748.

Eriksen, E. F., Melsen, F., and Mosekilde, L. (1984a). Reconstruction of the resorptive site in iliac trabecular bone: A kinetic model for bone resorption in 20 normal individuals. *Metab. Bone Dis. Relat. Res.* **5**, 235–242.

Eriksen, E. F., Gundersen, H. J., Melsen, F., and Mosekilde, L. (1984b). Reconstruction of the formative site in iliac trabecular bone in 20 normal individuals employing a kinetic model for matrix and mineral apposition. *Metab. Bone Dis. Relat. Res.* **5**, 243–252.

Eriksen, E. F., Mosekilde, L., and Melsen, F. (1985). Trabecular bone resorption depth decreases with age: Differences between normal males and females. *Bone* **6**, 141–146.

Feik, S. A., Thomas, C. D., and Clement, J. G. (1996). Age trends in remodeling of the femoral midshaft differ between the sexes. *J. Orthop. Res.* **14**, 590–597.

Frost, H. M. (1969). Tetracycline-based histological analysis of bone remodeling. *Calcif. Tissue Res.* **3**, 211–237.

Han, Z. H., Palnitkar, S., Rao, D. S., Nelson, D., and Parfitt, A. M. (1996). Effect of ethnicity and age or menopause on the structure and geometry of iliac bone. *J. Bone Miner. Res.* **11**, 1967–1975; errata: *Ibid.*, **12**(5), 867 (1997).

Han, Z. H., Palnitkar, S., Rao, D. S., Nelson, D., and Parfitt, A. M. (1997). Effects of ethnicity and age or menopause on the remodeling and turnover of iliac bone: Implications for mechanisms of bone loss. *J. Bone Miner. Res.* **12**, 498–508.

Kragstrup, J., Melsen, F., and Mosekilde, L. (1983). Thickness of bone formed at remodeling sites in normal human iliac trabecular bone: Variations with age and sex. *Metab. Bone Dis. Relat. Res.* **5**, 17–21.

Lips, P., Courpron, P., and Meunier, P. J. (1978). Mean wall thickness of trabecular bone packets in the human iliac crest: changes with age. *Calcif. Tissue Res.* **26**, 13–17.

Melsen, F., and Mosekilde, L. (1978). Tetracycline double-labeling of iliac trabecular bone in 41 normal adults. *Calcif. Tissue Res.* **26**, 99–102.

Melsen, F., Melsen, B., Mosekilde, L., and Bergmann, S. (1978). Histomorphometric analysis of normal bone from the iliac crest. *Acta Pathol. Microbiol. Scand., Sect. A* **86**, 70–81.

Mosekilde, L. (1989). Sex differences in age-related loss of vertebral trabecular bone mass and structure—biomechanical consequences. *Bone* **10**, 425–432.

Mosekilde, L. (1990). Sex differences in age-related changes in vertebral body size, density and biomechanical competence in normal individuals. *Bone* **11**, 67–73.

Nordin, B. E., Aaron, J., Speed, R., Francis, R. M., and Makins, N. (1984). Bone formation and resorption as the determinants of trabecular bone volume in normal and osteoporotic men. *Scott. Med. J.* **29**, 171–175.

Parfitt, A. M. (1976). The actions of parathyroid hormone on bone: Relation to bone remodeling and turnover, calcium homeostasis, and metabolic bone disease. Part I of IV parts: Mechanisms of calcium transfer between blood and bone and their cellular basis: Morphological and kinetic approaches to bone turnover. *Metab., Clin. Exp.* **25**, 809–844.

Parfitt, A. M. (1983). Bone histomorphometry: Techniques and interpretation. *In* "The Physiologic and Clincal Significance of Bone Histomorphometric Data" (R. R. Recker, ed.), pp. 143–224. CRC Press, Boca Raton, FL.

Parfitt, A. M. (1984). Age-related structural changes in trabecular and cortical bone: Cellular mechanisms and biomechanical consequences. *Calcif. Tissue Int.* **36**(Suppl. 1), S123-8.

Parfitt, A. M. (1987). Trabecular bone architecture in the pathogenesis and prevention of fracture. *Am. J. Med.* **82**, 68–72.

Podenphant, J., and Engel, U. (1987). Regional variations in histomorphometric bone dynamics from the skeleton of an osteoporotic woman. *Calcif. Tissue Int.* **40**, 184–188.

Qiu, M. C., Wang, J. Y., Li, W. S., Qi, Q. L., Shao, Q., Liu, W., Gao, Z. H., and Li, S. L. (1990). Dynamic study on iliac trabeculae of normal Chinese. *Chin. Med. J. (Engl. Transl.)* **103**, 363–368.

Recker, R. R., Kimmel, D. B., Parfitt, A. M., Davies, K. M., Keshawarz, N., and Hinders, S. (1988). Static and tetracycline-based bone histomorphometric data from 34 normal postmenopausal females. *J. Bone Miner. Res.* **3**, 133–144.

Vesterby, A. (1990). Star volume of marrow space and trabeculae in iliac crest: Sampling procedure and correlation to star volume of first lumbar vertebra. *Bone* **11**, 149–155.

Watrous, D. A., and Andrews, B. S. (1989). The metabolism and immunology of bone. *Semin. Arthritis Rheum.* **19**, 45–65.

Weinstein, R. S., and Bell, N. H. (1988). Diminished rates of bone formation in normal black adults. *N. Engl. J. Med.* **319**, 1698–1701.

Chapter 16

Lis Mosekilde

Department of Cell Biology
Institute of Anatomy
University of Aarhus
Aarhus, Denmark

Trabecular Microarchitecture and Aging

I. Introduction

Vertebral fracture incidence has increased three- to fourfold for women and more than fourfold for men during the last 30 years (Bengnér *et al.,* 1988). The other major fragility fracture—the proximal femoral fracture—has shown a similar pattern, with a two- to threefold increase in incidence for both men and women. The data are age-adjusted and therefore highlight the decrease in bone mass or bone quality from generation to generation (Obrant *et al.,* 1989). However, the described changes in the incidence of vertebral and femoral neck fracture cannot be related to the menopause because the increase is more pronounced for men than for women. Therefore, other etiological factors must be considered. In order to do this, basic knowledge of normal age- and gender-related changes in bone structure and function is crucial. A description of the pattern of the remodeling process in the load-bearing trabecular network is essential for understanding these age- and gender-related changes and for choosing the most appropriate therapeutic and preventive avenue.

Until recently, age- and gender-related changes in trabecular bone microarchitecture have mainly been derived from study of iliac crest bone biopsies. Dynamic and static histomorphometry have been used to describe the remodeling process per se, and two- and three-dimensional methods were employed to identify remodeling-based changes in cancellous microarchitecture. The two- and three-dimensional analyses that have been used are (1) parallel-plate model (Parfitt *et al.*, 1983; Kleerekoper *et al.*, 1985); (2) node-strut analysis (Compston *et al.*, 1987, 1989); (3) trabecular bone pattern factor (Hahn *et al.*, 1992); (4) marrow space star volume (Vesterby, 1990); and (5) connectivity density (Thomsen *et al.*, 1996) but they have not been able to provide any conclusive answer concerning age- and gender-related changes in trabecular microarchitecture. Importantly, they have not been able to provide a final answer concerning the relationship between microarchitecture and strength (Odgaard, 1997). Recently, it has been shown that only connectivity shows any age-related gender-specific changes, although these could not be translated into a significantly different bone mass/strength relationship between men and women (Thomsen *et al.*, 1998). Many of these studies have focused not only on age- and gender-related differences in microarchitecture, but also on the influence of hormones and drugs on trabecular bone structure. Special attention has been paid to changes in remodeling and microarchitecture in women around the menopause.

In the following, another approach to the problem will be explored. Special emphasis will be placed on the load-bearing cancellous network of the spine, rather than the iliac crest, and it will be considered as an integral part of the whole vertebral body with surrounding soft tissues such as disc, muscle, and connective tissue fibers and also blood supply. Finally, the importance of loading/disuse for this integrated network will be emphasized. Thereby, the normal age- and gender-related changes in a load-bearing cancellous network will be described in a broader perspective.

II. The Human Spine

A. Peak Bone Mass and Strength

Half of vertebral bone mass is found in the vertebral body, the load-bearing part of the vertebra. When peak bone mass has been attained (at the age of 25 to 30 years), the vertebral body consists of a central cancellous network that is sharply demarcated by a bony shell approximately 400–500 μm thick (Vesterby *et al.*, 1991) and vertebral endplates with a thickness of 300–400 μm. The central cancellous network is isotropic in the horizontal plane but anisotropic in all other directions (Mosekilde *et al.*, 1985). The trabecular bone volume (BV/TV) is 15–20% with an ash-density of 0.200–0.250 g/cm³ (Mosekilde, 1989). This special microarchitecture provides great strength with minimum bone mass. In young individuals, the load-bearing capacity of a lumbar vertebral body is 800–1200 kg, or even more (Mosekilde and Mosekilde, 1990). (See Table I.)

Peak bone mass is 25–30% higher in men than in women, mainly because vertebral size (cross-sectional area) is larger in men than in women (Mosekilde and Mosekilde, 1990) (See Figure 1.) There is no gender difference in cancellous bone density (Mosekilde, 1989). Peak bone mass is determined by genetic factors and also by physical activity (loading) during childhood and adulthood (Gilsanz et al., 1988).

B. Normal Age-Related Changes

From the age of 25 to 35 years, there is a continuous loss of vertebral trabecular bone mass and microarchitecture due to a negative balance during the remodeling process (1–3 μm is lost during completion of each cycle) (Eriksen, 1986). These changes seem to start in the center of the vertebral body (the vascular region) and progress superiorly and inferiorly from there. Furthermore, there is an age-related thinning of the endplates and of the "cortical" shell due to the remodeling-based endosteal bone resorption (Ritzel et al., 1997). Concomitantly, cross-sectional area increases, partly due to periosteal bone formation (modeling) (Mosekilde and Mosekilde, 1990; Frost, 1988) and partly due to osteophyte formation (Schmorl and Junghanns, 1988). This reduces the vertebral body load-bearing capacity of 800–1200 kg in young individuals to only 150–250 kg in the elderly (Mosekilde and Mosekilde,

TABLE I   *In Vitro* Data Concerning Human Vertebral Body Characteristics in Relation to Age

	Age (years)		
	20–40	70–80	Osteoporotic
Trabecular bone volume, BV/TV (%)	15–20	8–12	4–8
Ash density (g/cm³)	0.200–0.250	0.100–0.150	0.060–0.090
Microarchitecture:			
1. Anisotropy	2:1	4:1	?
2. Horizontal, trab. thickness (μm)	150–160	90–110	?
3. Distance between horiz. trab. (μm)	500–700	1200–1800	?
Cortical thickness (μm)	400–500	200–300	120–150
Load-bearing capacity (kg)	800–1200	150–250	60–150
Load-bearing capacity of cortical rim as % of total	25–30	70–80	80–90

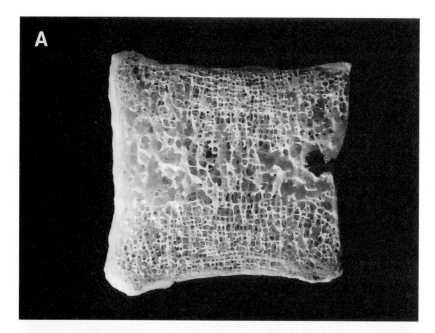

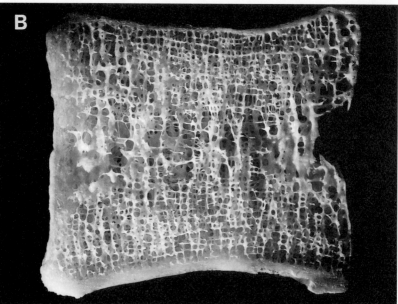

FIGURE I   Vertebral bodies (L_2) from young individuals: (A) young woman; (B) young man. The trabecular network is dense, with a "perfect" architecture in both. The main gender-related difference is vertebral size. Normal photograph—same magnification × 2.6.

1990). (See Table 1.) These age-related changes will, if they become pro-nounced, cause fragility fractures of the vertebral bodies (Figure 2).

III. Structural Determinants of Vertebral Strength and Mechanisms for Loss of Strength with Age ————————

The strength of the vertebral body is determined by several key factors of which vertebral body cross-sectional area, thickness of the "cortical rim", thickness of the endplates, and density (combined with the microarchitecture of the central cancellous network), are the most important. The exact roles of each of these factors have never been determined. This is due partly to the complexity of the structure and partly to the fact that each factor changes independently with age, menopause, loading, disuse, metabolic bone diseases, and other conditions such as disc degeneration or osteophyte formation.

A. Cross-Sectional Area

The cross-sectional area of the vertebral body is directly correlated with the load-bearing capacity of the vertebral body during both pure compression and bending loads—the two dominant forces on the vertebral body during normal, daily activity (Biggemann *et al.*, 1988; Brinckmann *et al.*, 1989). Vigorous exercise exerts a direct effect on the vertebral body cross-sectional area (Block *et al.*, 1986), possibly as a result of direct periosteal stimulation, as shown by Pead *et al.* (1988). As a result of genetic, hormonal, or mechanical influences, the cross-sectional area of vertebral bodies in men is 20–30% greater than in women. This size difference will, of itself, result in a 20–30% higher load-bearing capacity than seen in female vertebral bodies. In many *in vivo* bone density measurements, this important size factor has been neglected.

The cross-sectional area of vertebral bodies seems to increase with age in men but not in women (Mosekilde and Mosekilde, 1990). This age-related increase, seen solely in male vertebral bodies, can partly offset the concomitant decline in material properties (that is seen in both sexes) and is therefore an important compensatory mechanism for the age-related decline in bone density. At other skeletal sites, for example the long bones, an age-related increase in cross-sectional area has been demonstrated to be greater in men, and a direct stimulatory effect of loading on periosteal expansion has been suggested (Ruff and Hayes, 1983, 1988).

B. Thickness of the "Cortical" Shell

The thickness of the cortical ring in relation to age has been directly measured in very few human studies (Vesterby *et al.*, 1991; Ritzel *et al.*,

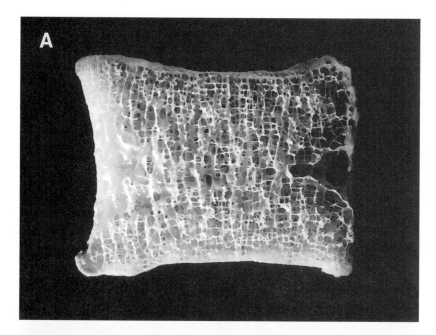

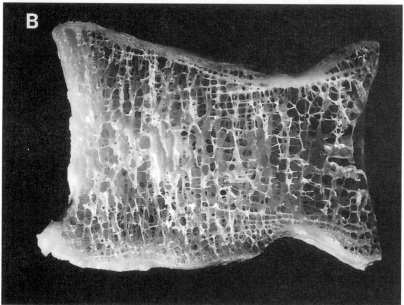

FIGURE 2   Vertebral bodies from elderly individuals: (A) elderly woman; (B) elderly man. Trabecular bone density has decreased, and many perforations are seen in both genders. The man has suffered endplate depressions. The main gender-related difference is again the size. Normal photograph—same magnification × 2.6.

1997). However, even in young persons the cortical ring is very thin and usually consists of what appears to be condensed cancellous bone, rather than real cortical bone with Haversian systems. Occasionally, a few Haversian osteons have been noticed in the shell in younger individuals (Ritzel *et al.*, 1997). The study by Ritzel *et al.* (1997) failed to identify any age-related gender-specific differences in cortical thickness.

The amount of cortical bone and its importance for the load-bearing capacity of the vertebral body is a matter of debate. The conventional view has been that the vertebral body consists of approximately 70% cancellous bone and 30% cortical bone (Eastell *et al.*, 1990). However, Nottestad *et al.* (1990) showed the opposite: 30–40% cancellous bone and 60–70% cortical bone. Both view points could be correct, because the cancellous bone mass in the central part of the vertebral body declines much faster than cortical bone with age (Cann, 1988). Therefore, a shift in cancellous bone mass dominates in vertebral bodies in younger individuals, cortical bone seems to dominate in the very old. The relative prominence of the cortical shell therefore increases with age. This is also true in biomechanical terms (Rockoff *et al.*, 1969). In young individuals, the load-bearing capacity of the cortical rim is only 20–25% of the total capacity of the vertebral body (Mosekilde and Mosekilde, 1990). With age, the cortical ring becomes thinner in both men and women, and at the age of 80–90 years it has a thickness of only 200–300 μm^3 (Ritzel *et al.*, 1997). Despite the thinness of the cortical shell in elderly individuals, it might at this age contribute some 70–80% of the load-bearing capacity of the vertebral body, as the loss of trabecular network has become proportionately greater (Mosekilde and Mosekilde, 1990) (Table I).

In both men and women, thinning of the cortical shell is caused by endosteal resorption, but in men there is also a significant modeling of the cortical shell caused by slow periosteal apposition, as mentioned earlier. The vertebral periosteal surface seems to be very rough, with collagen fibers (from the deep abdominal muscles) attaching directly onto the bone surface (Figure 3, see color insert). During normal aging, as the cortical shell becomes thinner, large defects develop in the shell. In part, this may be due to the arterial changes in the human vertebral body associated with aging. In children and young adults, there is only one type of artery (central), but with aging the number of peripheral arteries increases, and these have to enter the vertebral body through defects in the shell (Ratcliffe, 1986). In addition, the collagen fibers enter the vertebral body through the same defects and attach themselves to trabecular structures within (Figure 4, see color insert). The fibers seem to pull on these fragile structures, move them, and perhaps slowly destroy them.

C. Endplates

In young individuals, the endplates have a thickness of 200–400 μm. They are thin structures perforated by vessels entering the fibrocartilage of the discs from the vertebral bodies. The endplates can also be described as condensed cancellous bone, and are often double-layered—a phenomenon sometimes seen in normal x-rays of the spine. On their external side, the endplates have fibrocartilaginous tissue and discs, but on the internal face, they are supported directly by the cancellous network. However, the endplates are not solid structures, and the many perforations mean that disc tissue (cartilage) is in direct contact with the marrow tissue inside the vertebral body. This special construction might be an optimization of the shock absorption capacity of the spine (Figure 5, see color insert). Direct measurements of age-related changes in the endplates have not been performed, and no data exist concerning gender-specific differences.

In young individuals, the discs can absorb and distribute stresses and strains applied to the vertebrae (Hansson and Roos, 1981), but with age the intervertebral discs lose elasticity and height and thereby their capacity to absorb and distribute loads (Hansson and Roos, 1981). Forces, even trivial, therefore tend to reach very high values at small, localized areas and can thereby cause endplate depressions with herniation of disc tissue or formation of biconcave vertebrae. This is further facilitated in elderly individuals, where the endplate lacks support because of little remaining cancellous connectivity (Figure 6). The delicate contact between the disc tissue and the cancellous bone in the vertebral body pinpoints that the disc status is a very important factor concerning vertebral deformities and clinical vertebral fractures.

D. Vertebral Trabecular Network

The vertebral cancellous network in younger individuals is dense and well connected. The volumetric density of the whole cancellous network is identical for young men and young women: the ash-density is approximately 0.200 g/cm³, and the trabecular bone volume is 15–20% (Mosekilde, 1989) (Table I).

Hemopoietic marrow fills the space between the trabeculae and has an internal hydraulic effect (Kazarian and Graves, 1977). The marrow remains hemopoietic throughout life, although with age there is a slight increase in fat cells. Fat cells seem to replace both hemopoietic cells, sinusoids, and bone tissue during normal aging (Burkhardt et al., 1987). Direct histomorphometric measurements have shown age-related increases from 14 to 33% in fat cells with no gender-specific differences (Burkhardt et al., 1987). Several of the bone cells involved in the remodeling process are directly recruited from the hemopoietic bone marrow or from the abundant sinusoidal capillaries in the marrow. Therefore, the close connection between red marrow and bone tissue in the vertebral bodies is responsible for the high turnover (remodeling) at this site (Parfitt, 1983). The same high bone turnover is seen in the iliac crest (Parfitt, 1983). However, at other skeletal sites where there has been a shift from hemopoietic to fat marrow in young adulthood (e.g., the

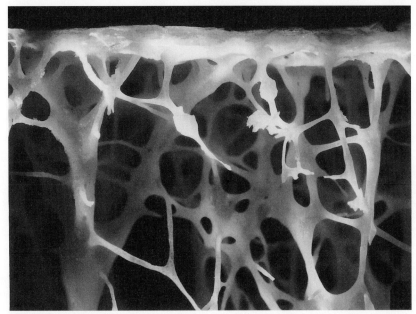

FIGURE 6   Endplate with "supporting" cancellous network. Several perforations of horizontal struts are seen, and two microcalluses are present on vertical trabeculae. Normal photograph.

diaphyses of the long bones), the bone turnover (remodeling activity) is much lower.

The slightly negative balance of 1–3 μm inherent in the remodeling process has as its primary result the thinning of horizontal struts in the load-bearing vertebral trabecular network and, secondarily, osteoclastic perforations of trabecular (Mosekilde, 1990). Resorption lacunae normally reach a depth of 45–50 μm (Eriksen, 1986) (Figure 7), and thus one resorption cavity covering more than half the circumference of a thin trabecula, or two resorption cavities (one on each side of a trabecular structure), would therefore easily perforate a 90–110 μm thick horizontal trabecula (Mosekilde, 1988) (Figure 8).

The decline in trabecular bone mass, the decline in trabecular thickness, and the perforations in the network are all caused by the remodeling process and contribute to age-related changes in vertebral character. This pattern, with selective thinning and perforation of horizontal struts, is seen in both men and women during normal aging (Atkinson, 1967; Pugh *et al.*, 1973, 1974; Mosekilde, 1989). However, due to the increased activation frequency associated with the menopause (Eriksen, 1986) women seem to have an increased number of perforations (Thomsen *et al.*, 1994). The specific removal

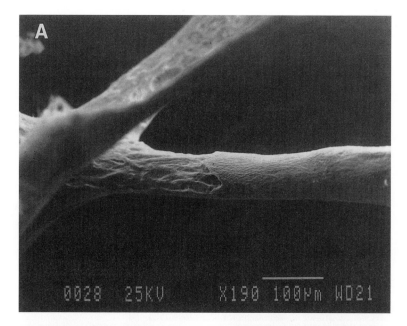

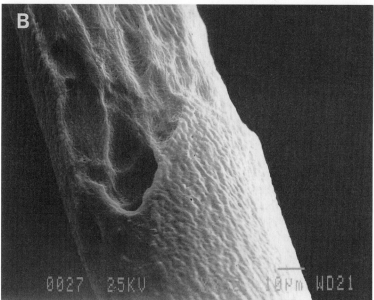

FIGURE 7   Scanning electron microscopy (SEM) photographs demonstrating the work pattern of the remodeling process on a horizontal strut in the network. Such a remodeling process covering more than half of a thin trabecula or a process on each side of a trabecula would be able to cause perforation. Magnifications × 190 and × 390.

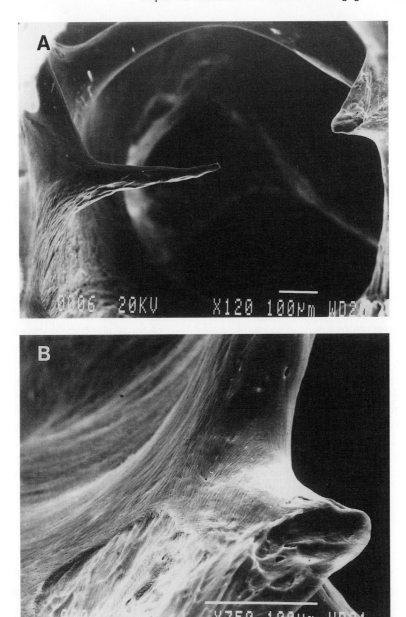

FIGURE 8 SEM photographs of a perforated trabecular strut. Osteoclastic footprints are seen at the end of the horizontal strut. Magnifications × 120 and × 350.

of horizontal struts increases the anisotropic properties of the cancellous network with aging. The anisotropy index increases from 2:1 to 4:1 or even more (Mosekilde et al., 1985).

The biomechanical consequences of the disruption of the load-bearing vertebral network are far-reaching. Because the strength of a trabecular structure is exponentially proportional to its radius, thinning of the vertical structures has therefore a tremendous influence on their strength (Bell et al., 1967; Townsend et al., 1975). The situation is similar concerning the length between supporting, horizontal struts: the compressive strength of the network is proportional to the square of the distance between the supporting struts (Bell et al., 1967; Mosekilde et al., 1987). For these reasons, the relationship between cancellous bone density and strength will not be a linear function, but rather a power function (Carter and Hayes, 1977; Mosekilde et al., 1987; Ebbesen et al., 1997).

It should be recognized that not only is bone strength dependent on trabecular size and number, but also on connectivity. The loss of connectivity in the load-bearing network seems irreversible. Remodeling sites on disconnected and unloaded structures show no sign of bone formation (uncoupling) (Mosekilde, 1990) (Figure 9), perhaps because strain or stress applied to bone seems essential to enable osteoblasts to form new bone on existing surfaces (Parfitt, 1984, 1987, 1988). In the absence of a framework upon which to form new bone, the osteoblasts are unable to refill the gaps in the network that result from trabecular loss. Therefore, even though the negative balance during each remodeling process will cause (in theory) a reversible bone loss, the osteoclastic perforations will cause an irreversible loss of bone mass, connectivity, and strength (Figure 10). The thin, horizontal struts in the load-bearing network which have been perforated are now unloaded and will therefore be resorbed by osteoclasts (Mosekilde, 1990). It is doubtful whether such a perforated structure with no contact between the ends will ever be able to be reconnected.

IV. Gender-Specific Differences in the Aging Process

Cross-sectional studies on human autopsy cases have clearly shown that age is the major determinant of vertebral bone mass, strength, and structure. When gender-specific differences are investigated, three different contributing factors can be identified.

1. At the age of 20 to 30 years, men have a higher peak bone mass and strength than women (20–30% higher).
2. Men show an age-related compensatory increase in bone size (cross-sectional area of the vertebral bodies) that is not as pronounced in women. Furthermore, women with osteoporosis have been shown in

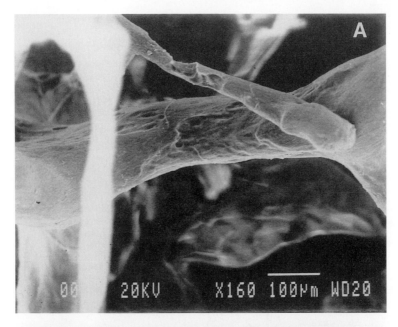

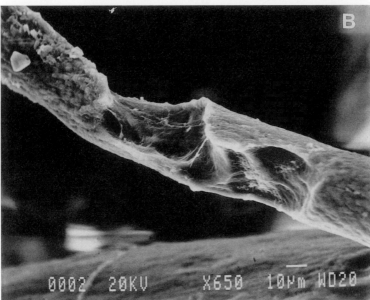

FIGURE 9   SEM photographs of a perforated and unloaded horizontal strut in the vertebral trabecular network. The structure is being removed by osteoclastic resorption. Magnifications × 160 and × 650.

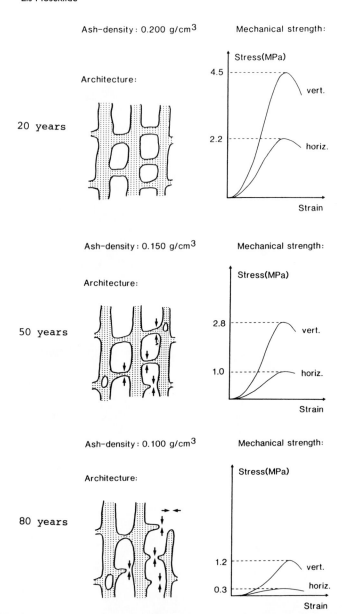

FIGURE 10 Schematic drawing of the typical age-related changes in bone density, architecture, and strength in vertebral trabecular bone.

clinical studies to have very small vertebral bodies and thereby low
load-bearing capacity (Gilsanz *et al.*, 1995).

3. After the age of 50 years (presumably as a result of the menopause),
   women show a higher degree of disconnection of the horizontal
   trabecular struts, and this leads to a more pronounced deterioration
   of the network (Mosekilde, 1989).

Very little research attention has been paid to the first two points: peak bone
mass and changes in cross-sectional area. These are two factors closely related to physical activity (loading). Menopause-related changes have at-
tracted almost all the attention and research effort.

V. The Role of These Age-Related Changes in Fracture Causation—Osteoporosis

In osteoporosis the normal remodeling-based age-related changes in cortical thickness, cancellous bone density, and connectivity become even more
pronounced. The sum of these changes causes a pronounced weakening of the
vertebral bodies. The load-bearing capacity of whole lumbar vertebrae will
often decline to values of approximately 80–90 kg (Table 1). In osteoporotic
patients, cortical thickness (endplate and rim) is reduced to around 120–150
μm. The trabecular network ash-densities can be as low as 0.6–0.9 mg/cm^3,
and trabecular bone volume BV/TV is typically 4–8% (Mosekilde, 1989).
At the same time, most of the horizontal struts in the network will be very
thin and often perforated, and the risk of microdamage will increase. These
changes in trabecular bone density and microarchitecture cause a pronounced
decline in strength of the central cancellous bone, and loaded vertebral structures fail through buckling instead of through compression (Bell *et al.*, 1967).

The vertical trabeculae which break during loading will heal by normal
fracture repair processes (in cartilage and woven bone formation) and microcalluses will form, but this normal healing process will occur only if the two
ends of the fracture remain in contact (Figure 11). These microcalluses are
typically found just underneath the endplates (sometimes several hundred in
one vertebral body) (Vernon-Roberts and Pirie, 1973) and will later be
smoothed by the remodeling process (Figure 11B). The number of microcalluses increases with age, but gender-specific differences have not been shown.

VI. Osteophyte Formation and Bone Structure and Strength

Osteophyte formation is a normal age-related phenomenon. Schmorl
and Junghanns (1988) found that in a large autopsy series (4253 subjects
aged 50 years or more), 60% of women and 80% of men had osteophytes.

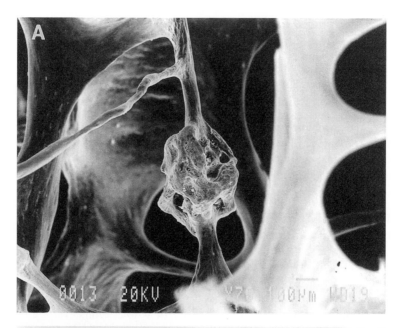

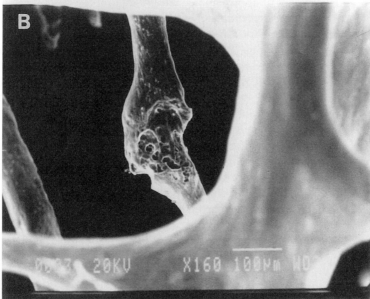

FIGURE 11   (A) SEM photograph showing microcallus formed on vertical trabecula. Magnification × 70. (B) SEM photograph of a microcallus at a later stage. The microcallus is being smoothed by the remodeling process. Magnification × 160.

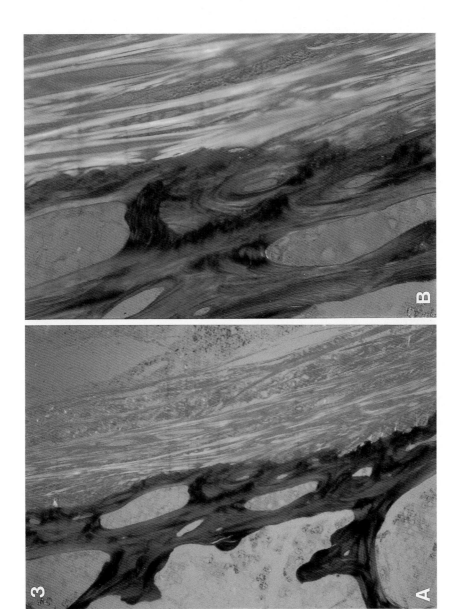

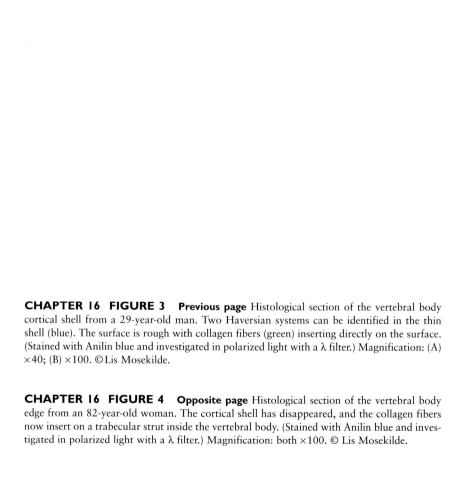

CHAPTER 16 FIGURE 3 **Previous page** Histological section of the vertebral body cortical shell from a 29-year-old man. Two Haversian systems can be identified in the thin shell (blue). The surface is rough with collagen fibers (green) inserting directly on the surface. (Stained with Anilin blue and investigated in polarized light with a λ filter.) Magnification: (A) ×40; (B) ×100. ©Lis Mosekilde.

CHAPTER 16 FIGURE 4 **Opposite page** Histological section of the vertebral body edge from an 82-year-old woman. The cortical shell has disappeared, and the collagen fibers now insert on a trabecular strut inside the vertebral body. (Stained with Anilin blue and investigated in polarized light with a λ filter.) Magnification: both ×100. © Lis Mosekilde.

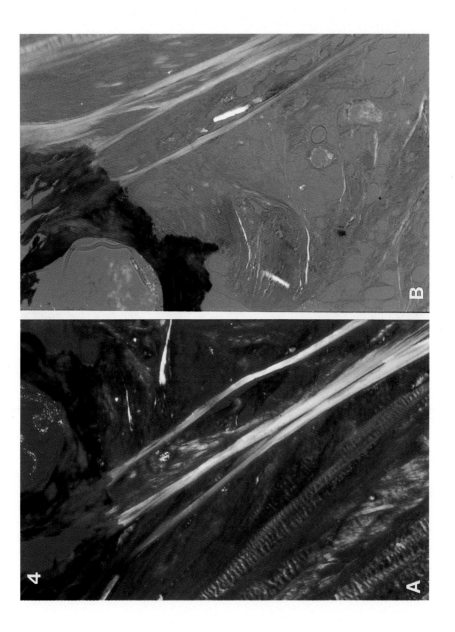

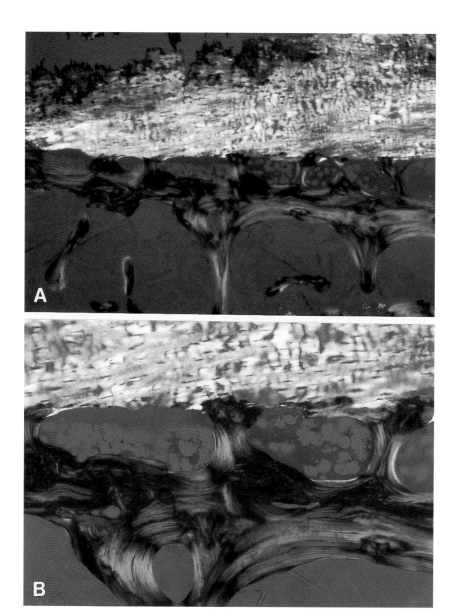

CHAPTER 16 FIGURE 5 Histological section of the endplate from the vertebral body of a 29-year-old man. The endplate (blue) does not form a solid layer. The disc tissue (white) is in direct contact with the bone marrow. (Stained with Anilin blue and investigated in polarized light with a λ filter.) Magnification: (A) × 40, (B) × 100. © Lis Mosekilde.

Osteophytes add bone to the periosteal surface of the vertebral bodies. This added bone tissue can best be described as very dense cancellous bone and is always in contact with the cancellous bone in the vertebral body itself. Usually, this is not weight-bearing bone, so it adds to vertebral mass without increasing bone strength or bone quality. In more advanced stages, osteophytes from one vertebral body will merge with osteophytes from a neighboring vertebral body and thereby become weight-bearing. The osteophytes thereby move loads on the spine away from the vertebral body to the outer "bridge" of osteophytes. This shift in load-pattern can be recognized in the central trabecular network, both in normal individuals and in patients with osteoporosis (Figure 12). In individuals with normal bone density, the trabecular structures near the osteophyte migrate toward the osteophyte and therefore seem to radiate from it into the central cancellous network (Figure 12B). This pattern suggests that mechanical loading is important for the microarchitecture of bone and that micromodeling and thickening of trabeculae are possible (Frost, 1988). The same trabecular pattern associated with osteophytes can be identified in individuals with osteoporosis (Figure 12C), demonstrating that loading is important and trabecular modeling drift is possible in these patients. In fact, these may be changes more pronounced in patients with osteoporosis (Figure 12A).

VII. Avenues for Future Research

Much has been learned about the microarchitectural changes associated with aging and disease. In several areas, additional information is necessary.

1. More *in vitro* studies describing the normal age-related changes in bone mass, size, density, microarchitecture, and strength in both men and women are needed. These studies should focus especially on load-bearing bone (spine, femoral neck), and they should treat bone as an integral part of the musculoskeletal system.
2. Densitometry is being used as the "gold standard," but still very little is known concerning the relationship between conventional measures of density and bone mass, size, cortical thickness, microarchitecture, and bone strength. This is an area that needs further *in vitro* investigation in both males and females.
3. Physical activity plays an important role in skeletal growth, modeling, and remodeling. The effectiveness of physical activity in the prevention of age-related microarchitural changes deserves more attention.
4. The methods available for quantification of cancellous bone microarchitecture should be expanded. Ideally, noninvasive methods should be developed to assess trabecular characteristics in clinical situations.

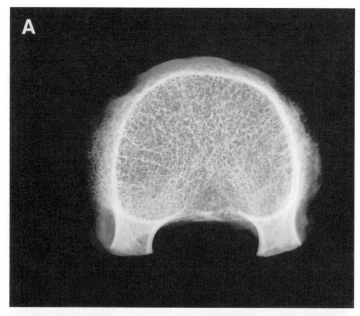

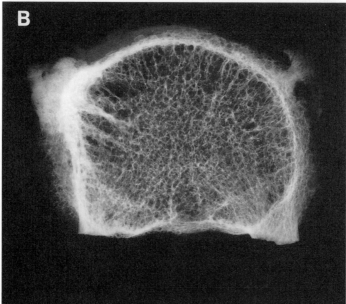

FIGURE 12 Contact radiograph of horizontal sections through vertebral bodies. (A) Normal vertebral body from individual without osteophytes or osteoporosis. (B) Vertebral body from 91-year-old man with osteophyte formation. (C) Vertebral body from 79-year-old woman with osteoporosis and also osteophyte formation.

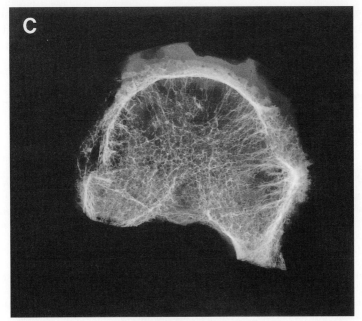

FIGURE 12   *Continued*

VIII. Conclusions

Only very recently has it been acknowledged that men have a high incidence of fragility fractures, and that this incidence is increasing at a faster rate than it is in women. Age-related changes in load-bearing cancellous microarchitecture cannot be considered separately from that of the surrounding tissues. Loading plays an important role in the achievement of peak bone mass, in the maintenance of trabecular microarchitecture (through the remodeling process), and in the orientation of the trabeculae and the periosteal apposition (through the modeling process). Loading is therefore important throughout life for the maintenance of bone mass and strength during normal aging—for women as for men. Spinal bone strength is determined by several factors: cortical thickness, bone size, trabecular bone density, and microarchitecture. All these factors change with age as a result of the remodeling process. When the changes become pronounced, fragility fractures occur. The general pattern, for both men and women, is of an extreme (70–80%) decline in vertebral bone strength during normal aging, but there is a slightly different aging pattern for men and women. Men achieve a higher peak bone mass than women (mainly because of a larger cross-sectional area of their bones), they do not experience an accelerated loss of bone and connectivity in middle age, and they seem to be able to compensate for loss of bone material strength by increasing their vertebral cross-sectional area with age. As a result, the decline in bone strength is much less pronounced (35–45%) in men and may be more frequently offset by osteophyte formation.

References

Atkinson, P. J. (1967). Variation in trabecular structure of vertebrae with age. *Calcif. Tissue Res.* 1, 24–32.

Bell, G. H., Dunbar, O., Beck, J. S., and Gibb, A. (1967). Variations in strength of vertebrae with age and their relation to osteoporosis. *Calcif. Tissue Res.* 1, 75–86.

Bengnér, U., Johnell, O., and Redlund-Johnell, I. (1988). Changes in incidence and prevalence of vertebral fractures during 30 years. *Calcif. Tissue Int.* 42, 293–296.

Biggemann, M., Hilweg, D., and Brinckmann, P. (1988). Prediction of the compressive strength of vertebral bodies of the lumbar spine by quantitative computed tomography. *Skeletal Radiol.* 17, 264–269.

Block, J. E., Genant, H. K., and Black, D. (1986). Greater vertebral bone mineral mass in exercising young men. *West J. Med.* 145, 39–42.

Brinckmann, P., Biggemann, M., and Hilweg, D. (1989). Prediction of the compressive strength of human lumbar vertebrae. *Spine* 14, 606–610.

Burkhardt, R., Kettner, G., Böhm, W., Schmidmeier, M., Schlag, R., Frisch, B., Mallmann, B., Eisenmenger, W., and Gilg, T. (1987). Changes in trabecular bone, hematopoiesis and bone marrow vessels in aplastic anemia, primary osteoporosis, and old age: A comparative histomorphometric study. *Bone* 8, 157–164.

Cann, C. E. (1988). Quantitative CT for determination of bone mineral density: A review. *Radiology* 166, 509–522.

Carter, D. R., and Hayes, W. C. (1977). The compressive behavior of bone as a two-phase porous structure. *J. Bone Jt. Surg. Am.* Vol. 59A(7), 954–962.

Compston, J. E., Mellish, R. W. E., and Garrahan, N. J. (1987). Age-related changes in iliac crest trabecular microanatomic bone structure in man. *Bone* 8, 289–292.

Compston, J. E., Mellish, R. W. E., Croucher, P., Newcombe, R., and Garrahan, N. J. (1989). Structural mechanisms of trabecular bone loss in man. *Bone Miner.* 6, 339–350.

Eastell, R., Mosekilde, Li., Hodgson, S. F., and Riggs, B. L. (1990). Proportion of human vertebral body bone that is cancellous. *J. Bone Miner. Res.* 5, 1237–1241.

Ebbesen, E. N., Thomsen, J. S., and Mosekilde, Li. (1997). Nondestructive determination of iliac crest cancellous bone strength by pQCT. *Bone* 21(6), 535–540.

Eriksen, E. F. (1986). Normal and pathological remodeling of human trabecular bone: Three dimensional reconstruction of the remodeling sequence in normals and in metabolic bone disease. *Endocr. Rev.* 7, 379–408.

Frost, H. M. (1988). Editorial: Vital biomechanics: Proposed general concepts for skeletal adaptations to mechanical usage. *Calcif. Tissue Int.* 42, 145–156.

Gilsanz, V., Gibbens, D. T., Carlson, M., Boechat, M. I., Cann, C. E., and Schulz, E. E. (1988). Peak trabecular vertebral density: A comparison of adolescent and adult females. *Calcif. Tissue Int.* 43, 260–262.

Gilsanz, V., Loro, M. L., Roe, T. F., Sayre, J., Gilsanz, R., and Schulz, E. E. (1995). Vertebral size in elderly women with osteoporosis: Mechanical implications and relationship to fractures. *J. Clin. Invest.* 95, 2332–2337.

Hahn, M., Vogel, M., Pompesius-Kempa, M., and Delling, G. (1992). Trabecular bone pattern factor; A new parameter for simple quantification of bone microarchitecture. *Bone* 13, 327–330.

Hansson, T., and Roos, B. (1981). The relation between bone mineral content, experimental compression fractures, and disc degeneration in lumbar vertebrae. *Spine* 6, 147–153.

Kazarian, L., and Graves, G. A. (1977). Compressive strength characteristics of the human vertebral centrum. *Spine* **2,** 1–14.

Kleerekoper, M., Villanueva, A. R., Stanciu, J., Sudhaker Rao, D., and Parfitt, A. M. (1985). The role of three dimensional trabecular microstructure in the pathogenesis of vertebral compression fractures. *Calcif. Tissue Int.* **37,** 594–597.

Mosekilde, Li. (1988). Age related changes in vertebral trabecular bone architecture—Assessed by a new method. *Bone* **9,** 247–250.

Mosekilde, Li. (1989). Sex differences in age-related loss of vertebral trabecular bone mass and structure—biomechanical consequences. *Bone* **10,** 425–432.

Mosekilde, Li., and Mosekilde, Le. (1990). Sex differences in age-related changes in vertebral body size, density and biomechanical competence in normal individuals. *Bone* **11,** 67–73.

Mosekilde, Li., Viidik, A., and Mosekilde, Le. (1985). Correlation between the compressive strength of iliac and vertebral trabecular bone in normal individuals. *Bone* **6,** 291–295.

Mosekilde, Li. (1990). Consequences of the remodeling process for vertebral trabecular bone structure—A scanning electron microscopy study (uncoupling of unloaded structures). *Bone Miner.* **10,** 13–35.

Mosekilde, Li., Mosekilde, Le., and Danielsen, C. C. (1987). Biomechanical competence of vertebral trabecular bone in relation to ash density and age in normal individuals. *Bone* **79,** 85.

Obrant, K. J., Bengnér, U., Johnell, O., Nilsson, B. E., and Sernbo, I. (1989). Editorial: Increasing age-adjusted risk of fragility fractures: A sign of increasing osteoporosis in successive generations? *Calcif. Tissue Int.* **44,** 157–167.

Odgaard, A. (1997). Three-dimensional methods for quantification of cancellous bone architecture. *Bone* **20,** 315–328.

Nottestad, S. Y., Baumel, J. J., Kimmel, D. B., Recker, R. R., and Heaney, R. P. (1990). The properties of trabecular bone in human vertebrae. *J. Bone Miner. Res.* **2,** 221–229.

Parfitt, A. M. (1983). The physiologic and clinical significance of bone histometry data. *In* "Bone Histomorphometry: Techniques and Interpretation" (R. R. Recker, ed.), pp. 143–221. CRC Press, Boca Raton, FL.

Parfitt, A. M. (1984). Age-related structural changes in trabecular and cortical bone: Cellular mechanisms and biomechanical consequences. *Calcif. Tissue Int.* **36,** 37–45.

Parfitt, A. M. (1987). Trabecular bone architecture in the pathogenesis and prevention of fracture. *Am. J. Med.* **82,** 68–72.

Parfitt, A. M. (1988). Bone remodeling: Relationship to the amount and structure of bone, and the pathogenesis and prevention of fractures. *In* "Osteoporosis: Etiology, Diagnosis and Management" (B. L. Riggs and L. J. Melton, III, eds.), pp. 45–93. Raven Press, New York.

Parfitt, A. M., Mathews, H. E., Villanueva, A. R., Kleerekoper, M., Frame, B., and Rao, D. S. (1983). Relationships between surface, volume, and thickness of iliac trabecular bone in aging and in osteoporosis. *J. Clin. Invest.* **72**(4), 1396–1409.

Pead, M. J., Skerry, T. M., and Lanyon, L. E. (1988). Direct transformation from quiescence to bone formation in the adult periosteum following a single brief period of bone loading. *J. Bone Miner. Res.* **3,** 647–656.

Pugh, J. W., Rose, R. M., and Radin, E. L. (1973). Elastic and viscoelastic properties of trabecular bone: Dependence on structure. *J. Biomech.* **6,** 475–485.

Pugh, J. W., Radin, E. L., and Rose, R. M. (1974). Quantitative studies of human subchondral cancellous bone. *J. Bone Jt. Surg., Am Vol.* **56A**(2), 313–321.

Ratcliffe, J. F. (1986). Arterial changes in the human vertebral body associated with aging: The ratios of peripheral to central arteries and arterial coiling. *Spine* **11**(3), 235–240.

Ritzel, H., Amling, M., Pösl, M., Hahn, M., and Delling, G. (1997). The thickness of human vertebral cortical bone and its changes in aging and osteoporosis: A histomorphometric analysis of the complete spinal column from thirty-seven autopsy specimens. *J. Bone Miner. Res.* **12**(1), 89–95.

Rockoff, S. D., Sweet, E., and Bleustein, J. (1969). The relative contribution of trabecular and cortical bone to the strength of human lumbar vertebrae. *Calcif. Tissue Res.* **3,** 163–175.

Ruff, C. B., and Hayes, W. C. (1983). Cross-sectional geometry of Pecos Pueblo femora and tibiae—A biomechanical investigation: II. Sex, age and side differences. *Am. J. Phys. Anthropol.* **60**, 383–400.

Ruff, C. B., and Hayes, W. C. (1988). Sex differences in age-related remodeling of the femur and tibia. *J. Orthop. Res.* **6**, 886–896.

Schmorl, G., and Junghanns, H. (1988). Development, growth, anatomy and function of the spine. *In* "The Human Spine in Health and Disease II" (E. F. Besemann, ed.), pp. 6–9. Grune & Stratton, New York and London.

Thomsen, J. S., Mosekilde, Li., Boyce, R. W., and Mosekilde, E. (1994). Stochastic simulation of vertebral trabecular bone remodeling. *Bone* **15**, 655–666.

Thomsen, J. S., Barlach, J., and Mosekilde, Li. (1996). Determination of connectivity density in human iliac crest bone biopsies assessed by a computerized method. *Bone* **18**(5), 459–465.

Thomsen, J. S., Ebbesen, E. N., and Mosekilde, Li. (1998). Relationships between static histomorphometry and bone strength measurements in human iliac crest bone biopsies. *Bone* **22**(2), 153–163.

Townsend, P. R., Rose, R. M., and Radin, E. L. (1975). Buckling studies of single human trabeculae. *J. Biomech.* **8**, 199–201.

Vernon-Roberts, B., and Pirie, C. J. (1973). Healing trabecular microfractures in the bodies of lumbar vertebrae. *Ann. Rheum. Dis.* **32**, 406–412.

Vesterby, A. (1990). Star volume of marrow space and trabeculae in iliac crest: Sampling procedure and correlation to star volume of first lumbar vertebrae. *Bone* **11**, 149–155.

Vesterby, A., Mosekilde, Li., Gundersen, H. J. G., Melsen, F., Mosekilde, Le., Holme, K., and Sørensen, L. (1991). Biologically meaningful determinants of the *in vitro* strength of lumbar vertebra. *Bone* **12**, 219–224.

Chapter 17

Tuan V. Nguyen[1]
John A. Eisman

Bone and Mineral Research Division
Garvan Institute of Medical Research
St. Vincent's Hospital
Sydney, NSW 2010, Australia

Risk Factors for Low Bone Mass in Men

I. Introduction

With aging, bone is gradually lost and its microarchitectural quality deteriorates, resulting in increased susceptibility to fracture with minimal trauma, which is referred to as osteoporosis. Osteoporosis is a dimorphic condition, affecting both men and women. From adolescence to middle age, the incidence of fractures in males is greater than females (Anerson *et al.*, 1988; Melton and Cummings, 1987). However, among the elderly, this trend is reversed: fractures in elderly men being approximately one third of that reported in women (Jones *et al.*, 1994a; Cummings *et al*, 1985; Wolinsky *et al.*, 1997). Osteoporosis is increasingly becoming prevalent in the general population, consistent with the expected aging of contemporary populations around the world. In a recent projection (Gullberg *et al.*, 1997), the

---

[1]Present address: Wright State University School of Medicine, Dayton, Ohio 45387.

incidence of hip fracture, the most serious single consequence of osteoporosis, is expected to increase more than three times within the next 50 years. Interestingly, there is geographic variation in the incidence of fractures between as well as within European, North American, and Asian regions. Caucasian women are generally at greater risk of fractures than Asian women, who, in turn, are at greater risk than African women. Apart from differences in criteria for ascertainment of fractures, other factors such as genetic and life-style factors are likely responsible for the interracial and interregional differences. Osteoporosis is considered to be a multifactorial disease, resulting from a multiplicity of genetic and environmental factors. One of the common denominators of risks for osteoporotic fractures is bone mass. For any given age group, fracture subjects have lower bone mass than nonfracture subjects. However, some subjects with low bone mass escape fracture, whereas subjects with relatively higher bone mass suffer fracture. Thus, other factors, including fall-related factors, are likely to be involved in the pathophysiology and etiology of fractures.

Osteoporosis has increasingly been recognized as one of the major public health concerns in contemporary society, due to its impact on morbidity, mortality, and costs to the community. Proposals for mass screening and intervention have been discussed. However, the discussions have been based on the pathophysiology and etiology, derived from studies in women, and much remains to be explored in men. There are a number of issues of osteoporosis in men that need to be addressed:

- How prevalent is osteoporosis for any given age group?
- How many fractures in men are attributable to osteoporosis?
- How large is the contribution of major risk factors?
- How do these factors interact to produce a fracture risk?

II. Prevalence of Osteoporosis and Low Bone Mass

From an epidemiological viewpoint, a disease can be characterized by its distribution and its determinants in the general population setting. The distribution of osteoporosis can be assessed in terms of its incidence and prevalence. Incidence is defined as the number of persons who suffer at least one episode of the disease during a defined period, divided by the average number of persons exposed to the risk of the disease during that period. Prevalence is defined as the number of persons who have had at least one episode attributable to the disease at a given point in time divided by the number of persons exposed to risk at that time.

Prevalence can also be defined in quantitative terms of bone mass or density because this is the major bone-related determinant of fracture risk. In a recent World Health Organization consensus, a quantitative definition of osteoporosis has been proposed based on the distribution of bone mineral density (BMD) (Kanis and the WHO Study Group, 1994). Three facts are known about the distribution of BMD: first, at any given age, it is normally distributed; second, the mean of BMD possibly reaches its peak at the ages of 20 to 30; and third, its standard deviation remains virtually constant across age groups. According to the World Health Organization definition, a subject is classified as having "osteoporosis" if his/her bone mineral density is 2.5 standard deviation (SD) below the young normal mean, taken as aged between 20 and 30 years old. A subject is classified as having low bone mass, if his/her bone mineral density is between 1 SD and 2.5 SD below the young normal mean. The prevalence of low bone density and osteoporosis in men has been estimated using data from the NHANES III study (Looker *et al.*, 1997). In that study, low bone density was observed in 33% and osteoporosis in 6% of men aged 50 years old or above. Melton (1995), based on BMD at the spine, hip, or midradius, estimated that the prevalence of osteoporosis among women aged 50+ years was 30%.

Based on the areal femoral neck BMD data from the Dubbo Osteoporosis Epidemiology Study (DOES) subjects, the overall prevalence of low bone density was estimated at 42% in men and 51% in women aged 60 or above. In women, there was tendency of decreasing prevalence with advancing age, whereas in men, there was no systematic variation between age groups (Table I). The overall prevalence of osteoporosis was 27% in women and 11% in men. In contrast to that of low bone density, the prevalence of osteoporosis increased linearly with advancing age. For example, in women aged 60 to 64, the prevalence was 13% and increased progressively to almost 63% among those aged 80 or above. A similar, but smaller increase was observed in men: from less than 10% among those aged 70 years old or less to almost 30% among those aged 80 years old or above (Table I). On the average, every 5-year increase in age was associated with a 5.5% increase in the prevalence of osteoporosis in men compared with an 11% increase in women. The prevalence of bone density of more than one SD below young normal

TABLE I   Prevalence of Low Bone Mass (osteopenia) and Osteoporosis among Men and Women Aged 60 or Above

Age	Low bone mass (%)		Osteoporosis (%)	
	Men	Women	Men	Women
60–64	37.4	51.2	5.1	12.6
65–69	44.2	59.9	7.9	15.5
70–74	38.9	50.0	9.6	32.7
75–79	52.7	46.9	20.0	40.1
80+	42.1	31.8	28.1	62.9
All	42.4	50.5	10.9	27.2

Source: The Dubbo Osteoporosis Epidemiology Study.

values (of the same sex) was consistently lower in men compared to that in women. Nine of 10 women over the age of 75 years had either low bone density or osteoporosis; the corresponding figure for men was 7 out of 10.

However, common densitometric methods do not completely correct for the size of bone, which is greater in men than in women. In preliminary analysis of DOES data, when bone size is taken into account, volumetric femoral neck BMD (g/cm^3) in men was similar to that in women (manuscript in preparation). The similarity was observed in both fracture and nonfracture cases. Moreover, using the volumetric data, prevalence of osteoporosis between men and women was similar. Classification of osteoporosis based on volumetric BMD could avoid some of the bias caused by differential bone size between men and women.

The diagnoses of osteoporosis and low bone density based on a surrogate measurement such as BMD is certainly not without limitation. It has been pointed out that different criteria for men and racial populations may be required (Elandt-Johnson and Lester, 1995; Kanis, 1997). Furthermore, different bone densitometers have different levels of "peak" bone density, which can confound the diagnostic criteria (Pocock *et al.*, 1992). More importantly, BMD, like any other physical parameters, is measured with error. This random error can induce diagnostic misclassification. It has been estimated that for the criteria proposed by the WHO, almost 20% of subjects are expected to be misclassified as having "osteoporosis," even with a coefficient of reliability of 0.98 for femoral neck BMD (Nguyen *et al.*, 1997).

III. Incidence of Fractures ─────────────────────────────

The incidence of fractures in the general population varies with age. It is greatest in the young and very old (Cummings *et al.*, 1985; Garraway *et al.*, 1979; Donaldson *et al.*, 1990). Among the age group of 0 to 44 years, the incidence is higher in males than in females, possibly related to trauma in adolescent males with more aggressive, risk-taking activities than in adolescent females. However, this trend is reversed among those aged 55 or older, when incidence in females is higher than in males.

In the Dubbo study, among men and women over the age of 60 years, almost 30% of all fractures occurred in men. Among both sexes, 50 and 31% of fracture cases were observed in subjects aged 75+ and 80+ years, respectively. The overall incidence of fracture among men aged 60 years or older was 218 per 10,000 person-years, about half in women (421 per 10,000 person-years). However, most of this difference was attributable to the higher female-male ratio in the 60-70 age range. Among the older men and women (>70 years), the difference between sexes was not large. For both sexes, the incidence increases exponentially with age, particularly among the 80+ years age group (Figure 1). In men, it was estimated that the

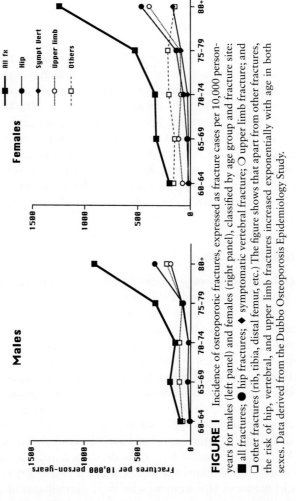

FIGURE I Incidence of osteoporotic fractures, expressed as fracture cases per 10,000 person-years for males (left panel) and females (right panel), classified by age group and fracture site: ■ all fractures; ● hip fractures; ◆ symptomatic vertebral fracture; ○ upper limb fracture; and □ other fractures (rib, tibia, distal femur, etc.) The figure shows that apart from other fractures, the risk of hip, vertebral, and upper limb fractures increased exponentially with age in both sexes. Data derived from the Dubbo Osteoporosis Epidemiology Study.

remaining life-time risk of fracture (at any site) for subjects surviving at the age of 60 and 70 was 26% and 21%, respectively (Nguyen et al., 1996).

A. Hip Fracture

Hip fracture is one of the most serious consequences of osteoporosis. It has been estimated that approximately one third of total hip fractures worldwide occur in men (Cooper et al., 1992). In DOES, hip fracture accounted for 20 and 23% of total fractures among men and women, respectively. However, the overall incidence of hip fracture in women was more than twice that in men (98 versus 45 per 10,000 population). In both sexes, an exponential increase in risk with age was observed, such that the number of hip fractures among persons aged 80 or above accounted for more than 50% of total hip fractures. The incidence was 467 and 340 per 10,000 population in women and men, respectively. These figures are comparable to the incidence among the American male Caucasian population as recently reported (Lauderdale et al., 1997). In that study, it was also noted that the age-specific incidence of hip fractures among Asian American males was lower than among the African-American and Caucasian American males, consistent with other observations (Bacon et., 1996; Ross et al., 1991; Silverman and Madison, 1988).

B. Vertebral Fractures

In the Dubbo Osteoporosis Epidemiology Study, symptomatic vertebral fracture accounted for 12 and 16% of total fractures among women and men, respectively; the incidence was 50 and 34 per 10,000 population. A majority (more than 64%) of symptomatic vertebral fractures occurred in subjects aged 75 years or older. Even though the incidence increased exponentially with age in women, no such trend was observed in men. However, in both sexes, incidence of vertebral fracture among subjects aged 75+ years was three-fold higher than those aged between 60 and 75 years old.

Vertebral fractures assessed according to quantitative vertebral morphometric criteria can be asymptomatic (Cooper et al., 1993); hence the term "vertebral deformity" is more accurate than "fracture," even in prevalence estimates. A number of criteria have been developed using stringent criteria 3 or 4 SD change from expected values (Eastell et al., 1991). A random sample of 113 men and 187 women, who were participants of DOES, were studied using the criteria proposed by Eastell et al (1991). The prevalence of deformity increased with advancing age and was higher in men than in women (Jones et al., 1996). The prevalence in men was estimated at 25%, which is higher than in females (20%). Similar prevalence has been reported from the United States (Davies et al., 1993) and Europe (O'Neil et al., 1993). Criteria for diagnosis are also important; it has been shown that the 4-SD reduction in vertebra-specific anterior-to-posterior ratio, middle-to-posterior ratio of posterior height alone correlates well with clinically diagnosed vertebral fractures and significant back pain (Ettinger *et al.*, 1992), whereas the 3-SD criterion could give rise to a 22-28% misclassification rate (Jones *et al.*, 1996).

C. Upper Limb Fractures

Fractures of the upper limb have not generally been recognized as osteoporotic fractures in studies in men. However, using the criterion of low trauma fractures, in the DOES, fractures at the upper limb (e.g., distal forearm, proximal humerus, and wrist) accounted for 17 and 30% of total fractures in men and women, respectively. The overall incidence of these fractures among men (38 per 10,000 person-years) was approximately one-third that of women (125 per 10,000 population). In men, there was a steady increase in the incidence of fractures with advancing age, whereas no such systematic variation with age was observed in women. Nevertheless, in both sexes, subjects aged 80 years or older had the highest incidence of fracture.

IV. Risk Factors for Fractures ⎯⎯⎯⎯⎯⎯⎯⎯⎯⎯⎯⎯⎯

Risk factors for fractures have been studied extensively in the past 30 years, mainly in older women. Risk factors that emerged from these studies can be broadly grouped into those associated with BMD and those associated with falls. The BMD-related factors are old age, low body weight, estrogen deficiency, smoking, excessive alcohol intake, low calcium intake, inadequate physical activity, vitamin D deficiency, and reproductive history. Fall-related factors include impaired balance and gait, poor vision, muscle weakness, psychotropic medication, history of falls, and environmental hazards. A familial history of fracture may not be accounted for by these factors, possibly suggesting distinct genetic contribution to fracture risk.

A. Bone Mineral Density

Case-control studies have suggested that BMD in men with hip fracture is about 10% lower than those without fractures (Grisso *et al.*, 1991; Greenspan *et al.*, 1994a). A large-scale longitudinal study has further shown that femoral neck BMD in men with hip, vertebral, and upper limb fractures are 24% (or 0.22g/cm^2), 12% (0.10g/cm^2), and 12% (0.10 g/cm^2), respectively, lower than nonfracture subjects (Nguyen *et al.*, 1996). A decrease of 1-SD in femoral neck BMD was associated with a 2.3 (95% CI: 1.7 to 3.2), 1.9 (95% CI: 1.5 to 2.6), and 1.5 (95% CI: 1.1 to 1.9) increase in odds of fracture in the hip, vertebral, and upper limbs, respectively. These relative risk figures are highly comparable to those reported in women (Cummings *et al.*, 1990; Melton *et al.*, 1993).

B. Fractures Attributable to Osteoporosis

Based on the WHO definition of osteoporosis, with a known relative risk (RR) of fracture associated with osteoporosis and the known prevalence (p) of osteoporosis in the population, it is possible to estimate the proportion of fractures which are attributable to osteoporosis by the formulation $AR = p(RR - 1)/[p(RR - 1) + 1]$. In this formulation, attributable risk (AR) is thus the proportion by which the incidence rate of fracture in the population would be reduced if exposure to the risk factors (measured by p) were eliminated.

Men and women with "osteoporosis" were, respectively, associated with a 19- and 8-fold increase in the risk of fracture at the hip (Table II). Thus, approximately two-thirds of hip fractures in both men and women were attributable to osteoporosis. Risk of vertebral fractures among osteoporotic men $(RR 9.6)$ was comparatively higher than that in osteoporotic women (8.8), but the proportion of osteoporosis-attribution was lower in men (48%) compared to that in women (68%). Upper limb fractures that could be attributable to osteoporosis in men (44%) was higher than those in

TABLE II. Relative Risk of Fractures Due to Osteoporosis and Proportion of Fractures Attributable to Osteoporosis in Elderly Subjects

	Men	*Women*
Prevalence of osteoporosis (%)	10.9	27.2
Relative risk of fractures associated with osteoporosis[a]		
Hip	19.0	8.3
Vertebral	9.6	8.8
Upper limbs	7.1	2.7
Attributable proportion (%)[b]		
Hip	66.2	66.7
Vertebral	48.3	68.0
Upper limbs	40.0	31.6

Source: The Dubbo Osteoporosis Epidemiology Study.
[a]Based on WHO classification (i.e., areal femoral neck BMD of 2.5-SD below the young normal mean).
[b]Attributable proportion is the proportion by which the incidence of fractures would be reduced if osteoporosis were eliminated (see text for details).

women (32%), and the relative risk of these fractures in "osteoporotic" men was more than twice to that in "osteoporotic" women ($RR7.1$ versus 2.7).

C. Falls and Fall-Related Factors

Apart from BMD, fall is a major determinant of fractures. Poor *et al* (1995) found that 76% of hip fractures were associated with a fall indoors. However, not all falls result in a fracture because the nature and direction of a fall is also an important determinant (Greenspan *et al.*, 1994b; Nevitt and Cummings, 1993). Falling in men and women is associated with muscle weakness, high postural instability (Brocklehurst *et al.*, 1982; Fernies *et al.*, 1982), poor balance, and taking more than four medications (Robbins *et al.*, 1989). High body sway (Nguyen *et al.*, 1993) and low quadriceps strength (Nguyen *et al.*, 1993; Cooper *et al.*, 1988) are also predictive of fractures, mainly in men. Furthermore, a history of fall (in the previous 12 months) was a strong predictor of subsequent hip fracture risk; every previous fall being associated with 3.5-fold (95% CI: 1.5 to 7.8), 3.6-fold (95% CI: 1.4 to 9.0), and 1.3-fold (95% CI: 1.1 to 1.6) increase in the risk of hip, vertebral, and upper limb fractures, respectively.

The prevalence of falls increases with advancing age in both men and women (Nguyen *et al.*, 1996; Nevitt and Cummings, 1993; Prudham and Evans, 1981; Lord *et al.*, 1994). Falls were reported in 1 in 5 men and 1 in 3 women and appeared to increase with age to reach one in three among men and 40% among women aged 80+ years (Figure 2). Those who fell once had a higher risk of recurrent falls. These observations are similar to that of

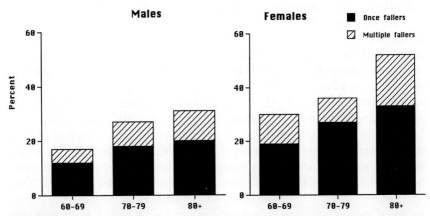

FIGURE 2   Incidence of falls in males (left panel) and females (right panel), classified by age group. The figure shows that women had a higher risk of falling than males; however, in both sexes, the risk increased linearly with advancing age. Data derived from the Dubbo Osteoporosis Epidemiology Study.

Prudham and Evans (1981), who also observed that falls were more common in women than in men (34% versus 19%).

V. Bone Mineral Density in Men

Whereas much research effort and attention have been directed toward identification of determinants for BMD in women, there have been few studies in men. There are four major epidemiological studies in elderly men: the Rotterdam study (Burger *et al.*, 1994), Rancho Bernardo (Edelstein and Barrett-Connor, 1993), the Framingham study (Hannan *et al.*, 1992), and the Dubbo Osteoporosis Epidemiology Study (Nguyen *et al.*, 1993, 1996). From these few studies, there are different patterns in BMD between men and women, despite similar determinants.

A. Age-Related Change in BMD

Bone mineral density in later decades of life is dependent on the peak bone mass achieved during growth and its subsequent rate of loss. It has been estimated that, over a lifetime, a woman loses about half of her trabecular and one third of her cortical bone (Riggs *et al.*, 1982). In men, such estimates are not available. However, given that men and women have similar peak bone density levels (Kelly *et al.*, 1990c) and that femoral neck BMD among elderly men is 15 to 20% higher than in women (Burger *et al.*, 1994; Edelstein and Barrett-Connor, 1993; Hannan *et al.*, 1992; Nguyen *et al.*, 1994), it could be inferred that bone loss in men is slower than in women. Indeed, cross-sectional data from the DOES (Nguyen *et al.*, 1994) and the Rotterdam study (Burger *et al.*, 1994) indicated that in elderly men, there was no apparent decline in lumbar spine BMD with age. In fact, there was a nonsignificant trend of increase with age. This upward trend and even the lack of a decline despite decreases at other bone sites has been taken as related to osteoarthritis, artifically elevating lumbar spine BMD measurements. This is a factor in both men and women over the age of 50 years. In women in the DOES study, there was a decline in spinal BMD with advancing age such that women aged 80 or above had about 10% lower BMD than those in the 60- to 64-years age group. This trend was confirmed in two major longitudinal studies (Jones *et al.*, 1994b; Ensrud *et al.*, 1995) in which there was an overall increase in lumbar spine BMD ($0.4 \pm 0.1\%$ per year; mean $\pm$ SE), whereas in women, there was a slight decrease ($-0.2 \pm 0.07\%$ per year; $n = 878$). In a longitudinal study (Jones *et al.*, 1994b), the higher degree of osteophytosis in men was associated with higher and significant increase in lumbar spine BMD. Subjects with any degree of osteophytosis had higher BMD (21%) compared to those without osteophytosis. There was, however, no such effect observed in femoral neck BMD.

In contrast to the lumbar spine, there is a clear decrease in BMD at the femoral neck in both men and women, although men experience a less pronounced reduction. For example, cross-sectionally, the average decrement was 6.4% per 10 years in men, and 10.2% per 10 years in women (Nguyen *et al.*, 1994). Longitudinal studies (Jones *et al.*, 1994b; Ensrud *et al.*, 1995) have also shown progressive loss of femoral neck BMD in both men (0.6% per year) and women (1% per year). However, not all subjects lose bone. During a 2.5 years of follow-up, only 5% of men had a decrease in femoral neck BMD of more than 2% per year; a further 27% had a reduction of between 1 and 2% per year, and 68% of men had unchanged or even increased BMD. In women, 25% had BMD reduced by more than 2% per year, another 30% had a reduction of between 1 and 2% per year, and 45% of women experienced unchanged or an increased BMD (Jones *et al.*, 1994b). When measurement error was taken into account [i.e., when a change of 0.07 g/cm² between two measurements was considered to be significant (Nguyen *et al.*, 1997)], only 24% of women and 17% of men experienced significant bone loss at the femoral neck.

B. Body Size

Obesity is associated with lower risk of fractures in men (Nguyen *et al.*, 1996; Grisso *et al.*, 1991; Poor *et al.*, 1995), but the association is not independent of BMD (Nguyen *et al.*, 1996). In women, weight is highly related to BMD, and the same, albeit somewhat weaker, relationship is also observed in men (Edelstein and Barrett-Connor, 1993; Hannan *et al.*, 1992; Nguyen *et al.*, 1994; Seeman *et al.*, 1993; Felson *et al.*, 1998). Higher weight is also associated with reduced bone loss (Jones *et al.*, 1994b). In cross-sectional data from DOES, variation in weight accounts for 10 and 17% of total variance of BMD at the lumbar spine and femoral neck, respectively. In men, every 10 kg increase in weight was associated with a 0.07 g/cm² increase in BMD (at both the lumbar spine and femoral neck sites). Body weight is predominantly made up of two components—lean body mass and fat mass—and which of the components is related to bone mass is a subject of much contention. Reid *et al.* (1992) found that bone mass was associated with fat mass in women, but not in men, whereas lean mass was not significantly associated with bone mass in either sex. In contrast, Edelstein and Barrett-Connor (1993) found that bone mass in elderly men and women was related to both lean and fat mass. These discrepancies may be related to the statistical problem of collinearity. Because lean mass and fat mass are related (when they are treated as independent factors in a multiple linear regression model), it is difficult to separate the specific effect of each factor. However, after controlling for the collinearity, the discrepancy in findings is likely due to the way in which bone mass is expressed. For example, fat mass was found to be the main determinant when bone mass was expressed as

volumetric density (g/cm³), whereas lean mass was the independent determinant when bone mass was expressed as areal density (g/cm²) (Nguyen
et al., 1998).

Heavier subjects have thick soft tissue which could alter edge detection
and/or bone mass determination. Tothill and Pye (1992) have demonstrated
that nonuniform distribution of fat could artificially elevate spinal BMD
between 3% (in men) to 6% (in women), which is likely due to the nonlinear
relationship between BMD and BMC with thickness (Tothill and Avenell,
1994). On the other hand, *in vivo* studies have demonstrated the nonsignificant effect of fat on BMD (Wallister *et al.*, 1993). However, the effect of fat
distribution on BMD measurement is more pronounced at the lumbar spine
and not significant at the femoral neck. Taking these observations together,
it could be inferred that the association between BMD and weight is attributable to both underlying biological mechanisms and artifact.

C. Physical Activity

Although exercise is often advocated in the prevention of osteoporosis,
there are many unresolved questions regarding its effect on bone density.
Because most, if not all, studies have been on women, there are no data
relating to exercise and bone loss in men. However, indirect evidence tends
to point to a positive association between physical activity and bone density
in men (Dalen and Olsson, 1974; Kelly *et al.*, 1990a; Brewer *et al.*, 1983;
Krall and Dawson-Hughes, 1994; Drinkwater, 1993). These studies also appear to indicate that the effect of physical activity and quadriceps strength
on bone density is more consistent and stronger at the weight-bearing site.
Quadriceps strength and physical activity were each associated with higher
bone density at the femoral neck (Glynn *et al.*, 1995; Need *et al.*, 1995). This
finding is also consistent with a larger epidemiological study (Nguyen *et al.*,
1994) and the positive correlation between grip strength and forearm BMD
(Bevier *et al.*, 1990). In the DOES study, for example, subjects in the high
physical activity group (assessed by using the Framingham questionnaire;
Kannel and Sorlie, 1979) had higher bone density at the femoral neck, but
not at the lumbar spine. At the femoral neck, the difference between those in
the lowest and highest quartile of physical activity index was 4.5% (or 0.03
g/cm²). However, the maximum proportion of variance of femoral neck
BMD attributable to physical activity index was 1.3%. Similarly, men with
higher muscle strength had higher bone density (Nguyen *et al.*, 1994). Men
in the top quartile of quadriceps strength (>44 kg) had 8% higher femoral
neck BMD than those in the lowest quartile (<25 kg). Variation in quadriceps strength explained a maximum of 4.5% of variance of BMD (mainly at
the femoral neck). Thus, the combination of indices of muscle strength and
physical activity modestly contributed to the total variance of BMD in elderly men and women.

D. Dietary Calcium Intake

Studies examining the relationship between calcium intake and bone mass have produced inconsistent findings. An epidemiological study (Matkovic et al., 1977) in Yugoslavia has found a positive association between bone mass and dietary calcium intake. A weak relationship between bone mass and calcium intake was also observed in a survey in the United States (Garn et al., 1981). Dietary calcium intake was also reported to be associated with peak bone mass in men (Kelly et al., 1990a,b) but not in women (Kelly et al., 1990b). In the Dubbo study (Nguyen et al., 1994), the median dietary calcium intake for the men was 572 mg/day, with 75% of subjects having intake levels lower than 800 mg/day, the recommended daily allowance for maintenance of mineral balance (Morley, 1996). In these men, as in Kroger and Laitinen (1992), a positive association between dietary calcium intake and BMD was observed in the femoral neck and lumbar spine. The difference between the lowest quartile ($\leqslant$400 mg/day) and highest quartile (>800 mg/d) was 0.08 g/cm^2 after adjusting for age. At the femoral neck, the association was significant in men, before or after adjusting for age and weight. However, the effect was modest, as the maximum proportion of variance attributable to variation in dietary calcium intake was only 2%. However, other studies have not found such a relationship (Marcus, 1982; Yano et al., 1985; Freudenheim et al., 1986; Ooms et al., 1993; Bauer et al., 1993).

Studies of the association between dietary calcium intake and bone loss in interventional trials have produced equally varied results. Calcium supplementation was associated with a significant increase in BMD at the femoral neck, but not in other areas of the femur nor in the lumbar spine (Haines et al., 1995). However, there is a general consensus that there is a modest effect of dietary calcium in the rates of cortical bone loss (Horsman et al., 1977; Ettinger et al., 1987; Recker, 1993; Riis et al., 1987). Although higher dietary calcium intake was reported to be associated with lower risk of fracture in both men and women (Cooper et al., 1988; Lau et al., 1988), this relationship was not independent of BMD (Nguyen et al., 1996).

There are several possible reasons for those variable findings, including confounding life-style factors such as smoking and alcohol. Dietary calcium intake variation between studies due to the measurement techniques or the populations themselves may have confounded some analyses. Variations in experimental designs and population characteristics, past and present level of calcium intake, as well as complex interactions of calcium metabolism with various hormones such as estrogen may also contribute to the variability in findings.

E. Smoking

Smoking is also a risk factor for osteoporosis. A recent meta analysis of 29 studies indicates that smoking is associated with both lower bone density and greater risk of fractures (Law and Hackshaw, 1997). Women who smoke have lower cortical bone mass than those who do not smoke (Avioli, 1981; Daniell, 1976; Paganini-Hill *et al.*, 1991; Lindsay, 1981). Smokers typically have 0.5 to 1-SD lower BMD compared to nonsmokers (Nguyen *et al.*, 1994; Daniell, 1976; Sowers *et al.*, 1990). The effect of smoking was convincingly demonstrated by using the twin model (Hopper and Seeman, 1994; Kelly *et al.*, 1990a). These two studies found that within twin pairs, the heavier smoking twin had about 9 to 6% lower BMD at the spine and femoral neck, respectively, and the effect appeared to be dose-dependent. Smoking has been associated with high bone loss at the radius (Krall and Dawson-Hughes, 1991), although not at the lumbar spine or femoral neck (Slemenda *et al.*, 1989).

A detrimental effect of smoking was also reported in two other cross-sectional studies in premenopausal women (Hollenbach *et al.*, 1993; Franceschi *et al.*, 1996), and this adverse effect seemed to be stronger in men. On the other hand, Glynn *et al.* (1995) found no significant effect of current cigarette smoking on BMD, and in this study, no association between BMD and alcohol consumption, current leisure-time physical activity or dietary calcium intake. In DOES, approximately 15% men and 9% women reported to be current smokers. In both sexes, the prevalence was higher in younger age groups (<70 years) than in the older age group (>80 years old). In men, smoking was associated with lower BMD at the femoral neck (-0.05 g/cm^2) and lumbar spine (-0.06 g/cm^2). This effect was independent of age and weight. There are no studies on whether discontinuation of smoking alters rates of bone loss or fractures in men.

The mechanism of smoking effect on BMD in men remains largely unknown. However, animal studies suggest an impaired bone formation upon exposure to nicotine (Riebel *et al.*, 1995). Thus, smoking could exert its toxic effect directly on bone or via its effect on calcium absorption (Krall and Dawson-Hughes, 1991).

F. Alcohol

Prolonged high intake of alcohol is associated with adverse effects in skeletal integrity in men (Bikle *et al.*, 1985; Laitinen and Valimaki, 1991; Moniz, 1994), with evidence of reduced bone mass in iliac crest, calcaneus, and hip and vertebral column, all areas with high proportion of metabolically active trabecular bone (Bikle *et al.*, 1985; Seeman *et al.*, 1983; Feitelberg *et al.*, 1987; Crilly and Richardson-Delaquerriere, 1990; Crilly *et al.*, 1988; Spencer *et al.*, 1986; Lindsell *et al.*, 1982; Israel *et al.*, 1980; Diamond *et al.*, 1989; Hernandez-Avilia *et al.*, 1991; Gonzalez-Calvin *et al.*, 1993). Habitual consumption of alcohol was also associated with increased bone loss in longitudinal studies (Slemenda *et al.*, 1992; Saville, 1965; Nilsson and Westlin, 1973; Dalen and Lamke, 1976; Johnell *et al.*, 1982; DeVernejoul *et al.*, 1983). On the other hand, some large-scale studies (Nguyen *et al.*, 1994;

Holbrook and Barrett-Connor, 1993) have found that moderate alcohol intake was actually associated with increased bone density.

The association between alcohol abuse and the incidence of fracture is not well documented and often contradictory. Alcoholism is associated with increased risk of falling (Waller, 1978) and increased risk for hip fracture (Hutchinson *et al.*, 1979; Paganini-Hill *et al.*, 1981). An interaction between age and alcohol intake in the risk of vertebral fracture has been reported, with a 2.4-fold increase in risk of vertebral fractures among men aged 60 years or older, but not among younger men (Seeman *et al.*, 1983). On the other hand, Felson *et al.* (1988) found no significant increased risk hip fracture associated with alcohol intake, whether moderate or heavy, in either men and women. For both sexes combined, a relative risk of 1.3 (95% CI: 1.1 to 1.8) for 7 ounces per week consumption among subjects aged 65 years or less; this effect was not observed among older subjects. Hemenway *et al.* (1994) also found no significant association between alcohol or smoking and forearm fracture risk in men. Confounding factors associated with alcohol use such as poor nutrition, liver disease, and increased falls limit ascribing a causal association between alcohol intake and osteoporotic fractures through effects on bone per se.

G. Genetic Factors

Numerous studies have been carried out to estimate the heritability of bone density, particularly in twins. The twin design is based on the concept that monozygotic (MZ) twins share 100% of their genotypes, whereas dizygotic twins share an average of 50% of their genotypes. Thus, a comparison of correlations between MZ and DZ twins should shed light on the relative contribution of genetic and environmental factors. These analyses depend upon a number of assumptions such as equality of common environmental correlation between MZ and DZ twins, no gene-gene or gene-environmental interaction (Kempthorne and Osborne, 1961), which may or may not be justifiable in practical situations.

Based on the radiographic examination of metacarpals among siblings, the heritability of bone mass was proposed more than 30 years ago (Garn *et al.*, 1964). Smith *et al.* (1973) and Moller *et al.* (1978) observed a greater correlation of forearm BMD among MZ (0.70) than among DZ pairs (0.45) and estimated heritability of 49%. However, for the adolescent twins (less than 18 years old), the authors estimated the heritability of 75%. This observation was later confirmed by a study in a small number of MZ and DZ twins (Seeman *et al.*, 1996). The investigators inferred that environmental influence may be greater in the late decades of life, and thus genetic effect is predominantly exerted in the attainment of peak bone mass.

In most twin studies in the 1980s and 1990s, it seems clear that the proportion of variance of BMD accounted by genetic factors is around 65 to

92% in women (Nguyen *et al.*, 1998; Seeman *et al.*, 1996; Dequeker *et al.*, 1987, Pocock *et al.*, 1987; Christian *et al.*, 1989; Slemenda *et al.*, 1991; Young *et al.*, 1995), and this effect persists even in the late decades of life (Flicker *et al.*, 1995). Sibling studies also yielded similar estimate of heritability (Lutz and Tesar, 1990; Tylavsley *et al.*, 1989; Evans *et al.*, 1988; Krall and Dawson-Hughes, 1993). However, in one small study of 34 mother-daughter pairs, familial resemblance in BMD was not observed (Sowers *et al.*, 1986).

Studies on genetics of bone density in men are scarce. Christian *et al.* (1989) studied a group of 38 MZ and 42 DZ twins aged between 44 and 55 years old and found that the intraclass correlation in radial bone mass for MZ and DZ was 0.70 and 0.45, respectively, making the index of heritability of 50%. Data from 28 MZ and 23 DZ male twin pairs, as part of the original study of Pocock *et al.* (1987), indicate that the heritability of bone mass in men is similar to that in women (85% for lumbar spine and 79% for femoral neck).

H. Candidate Genes

Even though the relative contribution of genetic factors to the determination of BMD has been established, the search for spcific genes that are involved in the genetic regulation has not always been easy and less than successful. Based on the observation of an association between serum osteocalcin, a bone turnover marker, and polymorphisms of the vitamin D receptor (VDR) gene (Morrison *et al.*, 1992), a linkage between this gene and BMD in twins was reported (Morrison *et al.*, 1994). It was shown further in an association analysis that higher BMD was associated with the Bsm-1 *b* allele and that the association was co-dominant such that subjects with *bb* genotype had, on the average, 1-SD (0.12 g/cm^2) higher lumbar spine BMD than subjects with *BB* genotypes. However, this strength of association was reduced substantially after correcting for misgenotyping (Morrison *et al.*, 1997). Numerous studies in the last 3 years have been conflicting, some confirming (either in the same or opposite direction) and some unable to corroborate the relationship (Cooper and Umbach, 1996; Eisman, 1995; Peacock, 1995).

Other studies have attempted to search for additional genes such as collagen 1 alpha 1 (Coll1α1) (Grant *et al.*, 1996), estrogen receptor (ER) (Qi *et al.*, 1994; Sano *et al.*, 1995), and interleukin-6 (IL-6) genes (Murray *et al.*, 1997), which are hypothesized to be involved in the determination of BMD. Following the initial report of association between BMD and polymorphisms at the Coll1α1 gene, several studies have reported conflicting results, either confirming (Garnero *et al.*, 1997; Uitterlinden *et al.*, 1997; Roux *et al.*, 1997) or refuting the reported association (Vandevyver *et al.*,

1997; Hustmyer *et al.*, 1997). Similar conflicting data have also been reported on the role of the ER gene in the genetic regulation of BMD (Han *et al.*, 1997). In all studies, where significant association was found, the contribution of these genes' alleles to total variation in BMD is modest (less than 5%).

There are many, but not specific, reasons for the discrepancies of findings in different ethnic and regional populations. First, there could be interaction of any gene allelic differences with the genetic or environmental backgrounds. For instance, dietary calcium intake, a possible contributor to BMD, varies widely between Asian and Caucasian populations and between studies. This mechanism was examined in the studies of Ferrari *et al.* (1994) and Krall *et al.* (1995). In the former study, subjects who were carriers of *Bb* genotype responded to calcium intake, i.e. no significant bone loss, whereas subjects with *bb* or *BB* experienced significant bone loss regardless of dietary calcium intake. In the second study (Krall *et al.*, 1995), at low dietary calcium intake, subjects with *BB* genotype responded to calcium supplementation, whereas the *bb* or *Bb* subjects did not.

Importantly, many of these studies have been based on relatively small sample sizes and thus may not have sufficient power to detect a true association or to exclude one with reasonable confidence. However, it is worth noting that almost all studies so far on the relationship between VDR gene and BMD have been based on association, rather than linkage, analysis. There are crucial differences between these two approaches. Association studies test whether a phenotype and an allele show correlated occurrence in a population, whereas linkage analysis tests whether they show transmission within a pedigree. Importantly, linkage can exist, but not be apparent in association studies, when there are many trait-causing chromosomes in a population so that association with any particular allele is weak. Alternatively, it may be possible to show an association but not linkage, when allele frequencies are high in affected subjects, for example at the insulin locus which may show strong association but weak linkage to NIDDM (Thomson *et al.*, 1989).

In the last 3 years, with the exception of the study by Morrison *et al.* (1994), all other studies on candidate genes have been association-based investigations, which cannot directly address a linkage relationship. Association can result when a certain allele is actually responsible for the regulation of BMD or is in linkage disequilibrium with a nearby causative gene locus. However, association can be due to a random, artifact of population admixture. Moreover, true association due to linkage disequilibrium can yield seemingly contradictory results, since linkage disequilibrium depends on a population's evolutionary history, as has been pointed out by Cooper and Clayton (1988). Thus, pooling data from many genetically different populations can obscure a true association, due to, for example, differing linkage phase between these populations.

VI. Summary and Future Directions _____

A. Summary

From a demographic viewpoint, one of the striking features of the 20th century is the worldwide changes in the population structure. The proportion of the elderly population (aged 65 years or above) in the world is projected to increase from 6.8% in 2001 to 14.4% by the year 2041. Even though the proportion may increase twofold, the actual number of people would increase by 3.4 times (from 376 million in 1996 to 1.27 billion in 2041). This increase will place a higher dependence on the working population well into the 21st century. At present, there are about 9 wage earners for every retiree; by the year 2041, this ratio is projected to be 4.4 : 1. Thus, in the next 50 years or so, among men, the worldwide incidence of fractures, and the hip in particular, is projected to triple, whereas the incidence in women will increase 2.4 times (Gullberg *et al.*, 1997). With the morbidity and economic and social impacts of fractures, this increase will place a great strain on health resource and will be supported by an increasingly smaller productive population.

Osteoporosis and low bone density are common in the elderly population. Importantly, in contrast to popular belief, fractures in men account for at least one third of total fractures in the elderly. However, the *risk* of fracture in men was half that of women. On the other hand, among the old (80+ years), the incidence of fractures, particularly at the hip and vertebrae, in men approaches that in women. Because men tend to have a lower life expectancy than women, it could thus be argued that the risk of fractures in men with increasing life expectancy will progressively increase.

During the past 30 years or so, a variety of risk factors have been identified for osteoporotic fractures, such as age, thin body build, estrogen deficiency, vitamin D deficiency, sedentary life-style, immobilization, cigarette use, alcohol abuse, some medications, poor dietary calcium intake, as well as certain ethnic backgrounds. However, low bone density and fall-related factors appeared to be the major and common determinants of fracture risk in both men and women in the DOES study. It has been estimated that more than 90% of the risk of hip fracture (in both men and women) was attributable to a combination of low femoral neck BMD (more than 2.5-SD below young normal), a history of falls and body sway (higher than the 75th percentile level). On the other hand, for vertebral fracture, the contribution of lumbar spine BMD, falls, and old age accounted for more than 80 and 50% of risk in women and men, respectively. For upper limb (proximal humerus and distal forearm) fractures, more than 50 and 72% of risk in women and men, respectively, were attributable to low femoral neck BMD, a history of falls, and height loss in women and low dietary calcium intake in men.

Although most fractures (>90%) are associated with a fall, only 5% of fallers suffer a fracture. In DOES, as in other studies, the incidence of falls increased with advancing age and was higher in women than in men. A history of falls was associated with a clear increase in the risk of subsequent fracture, particularly at the hip. This contribution appears to be greater in men ($RR = 3.9$) than in women ($RR = 2.4$).

Bone loss in the elderly, in both men and women, does not stop or reduce but accelerates with advancing age. The accelerated bone loss partially explains the increased risk of fractures among elderly women, as bone loss itself is a predictor of fracture risk.

B. Future Directions

In the past 50 years or so, there has been a shift of focus from disease treatment toward risk identification and disease prevention. From the population viewpoint, intervention aimed at modification of environmental factors could reduce the prevalence of osteoporosis. Thus, the identification of principal risk factors for osteoporosis and clarification of their relative strength in men should be a priority. Comprehensive and well-controlled studies are required to address a number of issues relating to the roles of physical activity, dietary calcium, and other nutrients in peak bone mass and rates of bone loss in elderly men. Although the prevalence of falls in men is lower than in women, it is one of the principle predictors of fractures in men and deserves more careful study.

Although the majority of variance of bone density being attributable to genetic factors, environmental factors account for up to one third of the variance of BMD and one sixth of the variance of bone loss in the elderly. It is yet to be determined whether genetic factors that determine BMD in women also regulate BMD in men and whether the mode of inheritance of fracture risk in men is the same as in women. Moreover, gene-environment interactions are yet to be studied adequately in men or women. Thus, the challenge of future research in the genetics of osteoporosis will be to identify major genes in which their modes of transmission and genetic architecture underlying the observed variation in bone density and its change as well as possible gene-environment or gene-gene interactions. Given the problems of interpretation of results from association studies, and since many genes and environmental factors are expected to be involved in determining bone density, future genetic research should concentrate on linkage studies (Carey and Williamson, 1991; Risch, 1990a,b; Risch and Zhang, 1995, 1996).

Once genetic loci, environmental factors, and their interactions have been identified, it is logical to develop strategies for prevention. The goal of prevention of osteoporosis is to reduce fracture incidence, to reduce premature mortality, and to maintain or improve quality of life. The need and criteria for implementation of preventative medicine (Lawrence and Mickalide, 1987) could be justified from a standpoint of current knowledge of the relationships between bone density and fracture risk (i.e., bone density-atttributable risk of fracture is relatively high, the measurement of bone density is reliable and accurate, measurement of BMD is cost-effective in considering hormone replacement therapy, and treatment is available).

However, controversies exist as to whether preventive approaches should be based on the population at large (low-risk) or selected (high-risk) individuals. The former strategies depend on changes in diet, exercise, and life-style habits for the entire population, whereas the latter depend on identification of high-risk individuals for targeted intervention. Although life-style modification has been proposed as an approach to prevent osteoporosis, there is insufficient evidence that any such modifications have long-term efficacy in terms of fracture prevention or that such modifications could be implemented in population at large with reasonable compliance. On the other hand, a major argument against the high-risk strategy has been based on the inability of present methods to detect such patients with high sensitivity and specificity and on the unfavorable cost-benefit ratio of case-finding for adequate individuals in the general population.

In summary, from the clinical as well as economic points of view, aggressive measures to detect osteoporosis in men at earlier stages may be warranted. However, much operational research is needed to define the roles of genes, environments, and their interactions more clearly to develop more effective preventive programs for osteoporosis.

References

Anerson, T. J., Melton, L. J., Lewallen, D. G., and O'Fallon, W. M. (1988). Epidemiology of disphyseal and distal forearm fractures in Rochester, Minnesota 1965–1984. *Clin. Orthop. Relat. Res.* **234**, 188–194.

Avioli, L. V. The endocrinology of involutional osteoporosis. *In* "Osteoporosis: Recent Advances in Pathogenesis and Treatment" (H. F. DeLuca, H. M. Frost, W. S. S. Jee, eds.) (1981) pp. 343–351. University Park Press, Baltimore, MD.

Bacon, W. E., Maggi, S. M., Looker, A. *et al.* (1996). International comparison of hip fracture rates in 1988–1989. *Osteoporosis Int.* **6**, 69–75.

Bauer, D. C., Browner, W. S., Cauley, J. A., Orwoll, E. S., Scott, J. C., Black, D. M., Tao, J. L., and Cummings, S. R. (1993). Factors associated with appendicular bone mass in older women: The Study of Osteoporotic Fractures Research Group. *Ann. Intern. Med.* **118**, 657–665.

Bevier, W. C., Wiswell, R. A., Pyka, G., Kozak, K. C., Newhall, K. M., and Marcus, R. (1990). Relationship of body composition, muscle strength and aerobic capacity to bone mineral density in older men and women. *J. Bone. Miner. Res.* **4**, 421–432.

Bikle, D. D., Genant, H. K., and Cann, C. E. (1985). Bone disease in alcohol abuse. *Ann. Intern. Med.* **103**, 42–48.

Brewer, V., Meyer, B. M., Keele, M. S., Upton, S. J., and Hagan, R. D. (1983). Role of exercise in prevention of involutional bone loss. *Med. Sci. Sports Exercise* **15**, 445–449.

Brocklehurst, J. C., Robertson, D., and James-Groom, P. (1982). Clinical correlates of sway in old age—sensory modalities. *Age Ageing* **11**, 1–10.

Burger, H., van Daele, P. L. A., Algra, D., van den Ouweland, F. A., Grobbee, D. E., Hofman, A., van Kujik, C., Schutte, H. E., Birkenhager, J. C., and Pols, H. A. P. (1994). The association between age and bone mineral density in men and women aged 55 years and over: The Rotterdam Study. *Bone Miner.* **25**, 1–13.

Carey, G., and Williamson, J. (1991). Linkage analysis of quantitative traits: Increasing power by using selected samples. *Am. J. Hum. Genet.* **49**, 786–796.

Christian, J. C., Yu, P., Slemenda, C. W., and Johnston, C. C. (1989). Heritability of bone mass: A longitudinal study in aging male twins. *Am. J. Hum. Genet.* **44**, 429–433.

Cooper, C., Barker, D. J. P., and Wickham, C. (1988). Physical activity muscle strength and calcium intake in fracture of the proximal femur in Britain. *Br. Med. J.* **297**, 1443–1446.

Cooper, C., Campion, G., and Melton, L. J., III. (1992). Hip fractures in the elderly: A World-wide projection. *Osteoporosis Int.* **2**, 285–289.

Cooper, C., O'Neill, T., and Silman, A. (1993). The epidemiology of vertebral fractures. *Bone* **14**, S89–S97.

Cooper, D. N., and Clayton, J. F. (1988). DNA polymorphism and the study of disease associations. *Hum. Genet.* **78**, 299–312.

Cooper, G. S., and Umbach, D. M. (1996). Are vitamin D receptor polymorphisms associated with bone mineral density? A meta analysis. *J. Bone Miner. Res.* **11**, 1841–1849.

Crilly, R. G., and Richardson-Delaquerriere, L. (1990). Current bone mass and body weight changes in alcoholic males. *Calcif. Tissue Int.* **46**, 169–172.

Crilly, R. G., Anderson, C., and Hogan, D. (1988). Bone histomorphometry, bone mass and related parameters in alcoholic males. *Calcif. Tissue Int.* **43**, 269–276.

Cummings, S. E., Kelsey, J. L., Nevitt, M. C., and O'Dowd, K. J. (1985). Epidemiology of osteoporosis and osteoporotic hip fractures. *Epidemiol. Rev.* **7**, 178–208.

Cummings, S. R., Black, D. M., Nevitt, M. C., Browner, W. S., Cauley, J. A., Genant, H. K., Mascioli, S. R., Scott, J. C., Seeley, D. G., Steiger, P., and Vogt, T. M. (1990). Appendicular bone density and age predict hip fracture in women. *JAMA, J. Am. Med. Assoc.* **263**, 665–668.

Dalen, N., and Lamke, B. (1976). Bone mineral losses in alcoholics. *Acta Orthop. Scand.* **47**, 469–471.

Dalen, N., and Olsson, K. E. (1974). Bone mineral content and physical activity. *Acta Orthop. Scand.* **45**, 170–174.

Daniell, H. W. (1976). Osteoporosis of the slender smokers: Vertebral compression fractures and loss of metacarpal cortex in relation to postmenopausal cigarette smoking and lack of obesity. *Arch. Intern. Med.* **136**, 298–304.

Davies, K. M., Stegman, M. R., and Recker, R. R. (1993). Preliminary vertebral deformity analysis for a rural population of older men and women. *J. Bone Miner. Res.* **8**, S331.

Dequeker, J., Nijs, J., Verstraeten, A., Geusens, P., and Gevers, G. (1987). Genetic determinants of bone mineral content at the spine and radius. *Bone* **8**, 207–209.

DeVernejoul, M. C., Bielakoff, J., Herve, M., Gueris, J., Hott, M., Modrowski, D., Kuntz, D., Miravet, L., and Ryckewaert, A. (1983). Evidence for defective osteoblastic function: A role for alcohol and tobacco consumption in osteoporosis in middle aged men. *Clin. Orthop.* **179**, 107–115.

Diamond, T., Stiel, D., Lunzer, M., Wilkinson, M., and Posen, S. (1989). Ethanol reduced bone formation and may cause osteoporosis. *Am. J. Med.* **86**, 282–288.

Donaldson, L. J., Cook, A., and Thomson, R. G. (1990). Incidence of fractures in a geographically defined population. *J. Epidemiol. Commun. Health* **44**, 241–245.

Drinkwater, B. L. (1993). Exercise in the prevention of osteoporosis. *Osteoporosis Int.* **1** (Suppl.), S169–S171.

Eastell, R., Cedell, S. L., Wahner, H. W., Riggs, B. L., and Melton, L. J., III (1991). Classification of vertebral fractures. *J. Bone Miner. Res.* **6**, 207–213.

Edelstein, S. L., and Barrett-Connor, E. (1993). Relation between body size and bone mineral density in elderly men and women. *Am. J. Epidemiol.* **138**, 160–169.

Eisman, J. A. (1995). Vitamin D receptor gene akkekes and osteoporosis: An affirmative view. *J. Bone Miner. Res.* **9**, 1289–1293.

Elandt-Johnson, R. C., and Lester, G. E. (1995). A mathematical approach to the definition of osteoporosis. *J. Bone Miner. Res.* **11**, 1199–1200.

Ensrud, K. E., Palermo, L., Black, D. M., Cauley, J. A., Jergas, M., Orwoll, E. S., Nevitt, M. C., Fox, K. M., and Cummings, S. R. (1995). Hip and calcaneous bone loss increase with advancing age: Longitudinal results from the Study of Osteoporotic Fracture. *J. Bone Miner. Res.* **10**, 1778–1787.

Ettinger, B., Genant, H. K., and Cann, C. E. (1987). Postmenopausal bone loss is prevented by treatment with low dosage estrogen and calcium. *Ann. Intern. Med.* **106**, 40–45.

Ettinger, B., Black, D. M., Nevitt, M. C. et al. (1992). Contribution of vertebral deformities to chronic back pain and disability. *J. Bone Miner. Res.* **7**, 449–456.

Evans, R. A., Marel, G. M., Lancaster, E. K., Kos, S., Evans, M., and Wong, S. Y. P. (1988). Bone mass is low in relatives of osteoporotic patients. *Ann. Intern. Med.* **109**, 870–873.

Feitelberg, S., Epstein, S., and Insmail, F. (1987). Deranged bone mineral metabolism in chronic alcoholism. *Metab. Clin. Exp.* **36**, 322–326.

Felson, D. T., Kiel, D. P., Anderson, J. J., and Kannel, W. B. (1988). Alcohol consumption and hip fractures: The Framingham Study. *Am. J. Epidemiol.* **128**, 1102–1110.

Felson, D. T., Zhang, Y., Hannan, M. T., and Anderson, J. J. (1998). Effects of weight and body mass index on bone mineral density in men and women: The Framingham Study. *J. Bone Miner. Res.* **8**, 567–572.

Fernies, G. R., Gryfe, C. I., Holliday, P. J., and Llewellyn, A. (1982). The relationship of postural sway in standing to the incidence of falls in geriatric subjects. *Age Ageing* **11**, 11–16.

Ferrari, S., Rizzoli, R., Chevalley, T., Slosman, D., Eisman, J. A., and Bonjour, J. P. (1994). Vitamin D receptor gene polymorphisms and the rate of change of lumbar spine bone mineral density in elderly men and women. *Lancet* **345**, 423–424.

Flicker, L., Hopper, J. L., Rogers, L., Kaymacki, B., Green, R. M., and Wark, J. D. (1995). Bone mineral density determinants in elderly women: A twin study. *J. Bone Miner. Res.* **10**, 1607–1613.

Franceschi, S., Schinella, D., Bidoli, E., Dal Maso, L., La Vecchia, C., Parazzini, F., and Zecchin, R. (1996). The influence of body size, smoking, and diet on bone density in pre- and postmenopausal women. *Epidemiology* **7**, 411–414.

Freudenheim, J. L., Johnson, N. E., and Smith, E. L. (1986). Relationships between usual nutrient intake and bone mineral content of women 35–65 years of age: Longitudinal and cross-sectional analysis. *Am. J. Clin. Nutr.* **44**, 863–876.

Garnero, P., Borel, O., Grant, S. F. A., Ralston, S. H., and Delmas, P. D. (1997). SP1 binding site polymorphism in the collagen type I a1 gene, peak bone mass, postmenopausal bone loss and bone turnover: The OFELY Study. *J. Bone Miner. Res.* **12**, S490 (abstr. S548).

Garn, S. M., Pao, E. M., and Rihl, M. E. (1964). Compact bone in Chinese and Japanese. *Science* **143**, 1439–1440.

Garn, S. M., Solomon, M. A., and Friedl, J. (1981). Calcium intake and bone quality in elderly. *Ecol. Food Nutr.* **10**, 131–133.

Garraway, W. M., Stauffer, R. N., Kurland, L. T., and O'Fallon, W. M. (1979). Limb fractures in a defined community. I. Frequency and distribution. *Mayo Clin. Proc.* **54**, 701–707.

Glynn, N. W., Meilahn, E. N., Charron, M., Anderson, S. J., Kuller, L. H., and Cauley, J. A. (1995). Determinants of bone mineral density in older men. *J. Bone Miner. Res.* **10**, 1769–1777.

Gonzalez-Calvin, J. L., Garcia-Sanchez, A., and Bellot, V. (1993). Mineral metabolism, osteoblastic function and bone mass in chronic alcoholism. *Alcohol Alcohol.* **28**, 571–579.

Grant, S. F. A., Reid, D. M., Blake, G., Herd, R., Fogelman, I., and Ralston, S. H. (1996). Reduced bone density and osteoporotic fracture associated with a polymorphic Sp1 binding site in the collagen type I a 1 gene. *Na. Genet.* **14**, 203–205.

Greenspan, S. L., Myers, E. R., Maitland, L. A., Kido, T. H., Krasnow, M. B., and Hayes, W. C. (1994a). Trochanteric bone mineral density is associated with type of hip fracture in the elderly. *J. Bone Miner. Res.* **12**, 1889–1894.

Greenspan, S. L., Myers, E. R., Maitland, L. A., Resnick, N. M., and Hayes, W. C. (1994b). Fall severity and bone mineral density as risk factors for hip fracture in ambulatory elderly. *JAMA, J. Am. Med. Assoc.* **271**, 128–133.

Grisso, J. A., Chiu, G. Y., Maislin, G., Steinmann, W. C., and Portale, J. (1991). Risk factors for hip fractures in men: A preliminary study. *J. Bone Miner. Res.* **6**, 865–868.

Gullberg, B., Johnell, O., and Kanis, J. A. (1997). World-wide projections for hip fracture. *Osteoporosis Int.* **7**, 407–413.

Haines, C. J., Chung, T. K., Leung, P. C., Hsu, S. Y., and Leung, D. H. (1995). Calcium supplementation and bone mineral density in postmenopausal women using estrogen replacement therapy. *Bone* **16**, 529–531.

Han, K. O., Moon, I. G., Kang, Y. S., Chung, H. Y., Min, H. K., and Han, I. K. (1997). Non-association of estrogen receptor genotypes with bone mineral density and estrogen responsiveness to hormone replacement therapy. *J. Clin. Endocrinol. Metab.* **82**, 991–995.

Hannan, M. T., Felson, D. T., and Anderson, J. J. (1992). Bone mineral density in elderly men and women: Results from the Framingham Osteoporosis Study. *J. Bone Miner. Res.* **7**, 547–553.

Hemenway, D., Azrael, D. R., Rimm, E. B., Feskanich, D., and Willett, W. C. (1994). Risk factors for wrist fracture: Effect on age, cigarettes, alcohol, body height, relative weight and handedness on the risk for distal forearm fractures in men. *Am. J. Epidemiol.* **140**, 361–367.

Hernandez-Avilia, M. Colditz, G. A., and Stampger, M. J. (1991). Caffeine, moderate alcohol intake and risk of fractures of the hip and forearm in middle-aged women. *Am. J. Clin. Nutr.* **54**, 157–163.

Holbrook, T. L., and Barrett-Connor, E. (1993). A prospective study of alcohol consumption and bone mineral density. *Br. Med. J.* **306**, 1506–1509.

Hollenbach, K. A., Barrett-Connor, E., Edelstein, S. L. and Holbrook, T. (1993). Cigarette smoking and bone mineral density in older men and women. *Am. J. Public Health* **83**, 1265–1270.

Hopper, J. L., and Seeman, E. (1994). Bone density in twins discordant for tobacco use. *N. Engl. J. Med.* **330**, 477–480.

Horsman, A., Gallagher, J. C., Simpson, M., and Nordin, B. E. C. (1977). Prospective trial of estrogen and calcium in postmenopausal bone loss. *Br. Med. J.* **2**, 789–792.

Hustmyer, F. G., Liu, G., Christian, J. C., Johnston, C. C., and Peacock, M. (1997). Is the polymorphism at the Sp1 binding site in the collagen 1 gene associated with bone mineral density? *J. Bone Miner. Res.* **12**, S 490 (abstr. S551).

Hutchinson, T. A., Polansky, S. M., and Feinstein, A. R. (1979). Postmenopausal estrogen protect against fractures of hip and distal radius: A case-control study. *Lancet* **2**, 705–709.

Israel, Y., Orrego, H., and Hold, S. (1980). Identification of alcohol abuse: Thoracic fractures on routine chest X-rays as indicators of alcoholism. *Alcoholism* **4**, 420–422.

Johnell, O., Nilsson, B. E., and Wiklund, P. E. (1982). Bone morphometry in alcoholics. *Clin. Orthp.* **165**, 253–258.

Jones, G., Nguyen, T., Sambrook, P. N., Kelly, P. J., Gilbert, C. and Eisman, J. A. (1994a). Symptomatic fracture incidence in elderly men and women: The Dubbo Osteoporosis Epidemiology Study. *Osteoporosis Int.* **4**, 277–282.

Jones, G., Nguyen, T. V., Sambrook, P. N., Kelly, P. J., and Eisman, J. A. (1994b). Progressive femoral neck bone loss in the elderly: Longitudinal findings from the Dubbo Osteoporosis Epidemiology Study. *Br. Med. J.* **309**, 691–695.

Jones, G., White, C., Nguyen, T. V., Sambrook, P. N., Kelly, P. J., and Eisman, J. A. (1996). Prevalent vertebral deformities: Relationship to bone mineral density and spinal osteophytosis in elderly men and women. *Osteoporosis Int.* **6**, 399–406.

Kanis, J. A. (1997). Diagnosis of osteoporosis. *Osteoporosis Int.* **7** (Suppl. 3), S108–S116.

Kanis, J. A., and the WHO Study Group (1994). Assessment of fracture risk and its application to screening for postmenopausal osteoporosis. Synopsis of a WHO report. *Osteoporosis Int.* **4**:368–381.

Kannel, W. B., and Sorlie, P. D. (1979). Some health benefits of physical activity: The Framingham Study. *Arch. Intern. Med.* **139**, 857–861.

Kelly, P. J., Eisman, J. A., Stuart, M. C., *et al.,* (1990a). Somatomedin-C, physical fitness and bone density. *J. Clin. Endocrinol. Metab.* **70**, 718–723.

Kelly, P. J., Pocock, N. A., Sambrook, P. N., and Eisman, J. A. (1990b). Dietary calcium, sex hormones and bone mineral density in normal men. *Br. Med. J.* **300**, 1361–1364.

Kelly, P. J., Twomey, L., Sambrook, P. N., and Eisman, J. A. (1990c). Sex differences in peak adult bone mineral density. *J. Bone Miner. Res.* **5**, 1169–1175.

Kempthorne, O., and Osborne, R. H. (1961). The interpretation of twin data. *Am. J. Hum. Genet.* **13**, 320–339.

Krall, E. A., and Dawson-Hughes, B. (1991). Smoking and bone loss among postmenopausal women. *J. Bone Miner. Res.* **6**, 331–338.

Krall, E. A., and Dawson-Hughes, B. (1993). Heritability and life-style determinants of bone mineral density. *J. Bone Miner. Res.* **8**, 1–9.

Krall, E. A., and Dawson-Hughes, B. (1994). Walking is related to bone density and rate of bone loss. *Am. J. Med.* **96**, 20–26.

Krall, E. A., Parry, P., Lichter, J. B., and Dawson-Hughes, B. (1995). Vitamin D receptor alleles and rates of bone loss: Influences of years since menopause and calcium intake. *J. Bone Miner. Res.* **10**, 978–984.

Kroger, H., and Laitinen, K. (1992). Bone mineral density measured by dual x-ray absorptiometry in normal men. *Eur. J. Clin. Invest.* **22**, 454–460.

Laitinen, K., and Valimaki, M. (1991). Alcohol and bone. *Calcif. Tissue Int.* **49** (Suppl.), S70–S73.

Lau, E., Donnan, S., Barker, D. J. P., and Cooper, C. (1988). Physical activity and calcium intake in fracture of the proximal femur in Hong Kong. *Br. Med. J.* **297**, 1441–1443.

Lauderdale, D. S., Jacobsen, S. J., Furner, S. E., Levy, P. S., Brody, J. A., and Goldberg, J. (1997). Hip fracture incidence among elderly Asian-American populations. *Am. J. Epidemiol.* **146**, 502–509.

Law, M. R., and Hackshaw, A. K. (1997). A meta analysis of cigarette smoking, bone mineral density and risk of hip fracture: Recognition of a major effect. *Br. Med. J.* **315**, 841–846.

Lawrence, R. S., and Mickalide, A. D. (1987). Preventive services in clinical practices: Designing the periodic health examination. *JAMA, J. Am. Med. Assoc.* **257**, 2205–2207.

Lindsay, R. (1981). The influence of cigarette smoking on bone mass and bone loss. *In* "Osteoporosis: Recent Advances in Pathogenesis and Treatment." H. F. DeLuca, H. M. Frost, S. S. J. Webster, eds. University Park Press, Baltimore, MD.

Lindsell, D. R., Wilson, A. G., and Maxwell, J. D. (1982). Fractures on the chest radiograph in detection of alcoholic liver disease. *Br. Med. J.* **285**, 597–599.

Looker, A. C., Orwoll, E. S., Johnston, C. C., Lindsay, R. L., Wahner, H. W., Dunn, W. L., Calvo, M. S., Harris, T. B., and Heyse, S. P. (1997). Prevalence of low femoral bone density in older adults from NHANES III. *J. Bone Miner. Res.* **12**, 1761–1768.

Lord, S. R., Clark, R. D., and Webster, I. W. (1991). Physiological factors associated with falls in an elderly population. *J. Am. Geriatr. Soc.* **39**, 1194–1200.

Lord, S. R., Sambrook, P. N., Gilbert, C., Kelly, P. J., Nguyen, T., Webster, I. W., and Eisman, J. A. (1994). Postural stability, fall and fractures in the elderly, results from the Dubbo Osteoporosis Epidemiology Study. *Med. J. Aust.* **160**, 684–691.

Lutz, J., and Tesar, R., (1990). Mother-daughter pairs: Spinal and femoral bone densities and dietary intakes. *Am. J. Clin. Nutr.* **52**, 872–877.

Marcus, R. (1982). The relationship of dietary calcium to the maintenance of skeletal integrity in man: An interface of endocrinology and nutrition. *Metab. Clin. Exp.* **31**, 93–102.

Matkovic, V., Kostial, K., Simonovic, I., Brodarec, A., and Buzina, R. (1977). Influence of calcium intake, age and sex on bone. *Calcif. Tissue Res.* **22** (Suppl.), 393–396.

Melton, L. J., III, and Cummings, S. R. (1987). Heterogeneity of age-related fractures: Implications for epidemiology. *Bone Miner.* **2**, 321–331.

Melton, L. J., III, Atkinson, E. J., O'Fallon, M., Wahner, H. W., and Riggs, B. L. (1993). Long-term fracture prediction by bone mineral assessed at different sites. *J. Bone Miner. Res.* **8**, 1227–1233.

Moller, M., Horsman, A., Harvald, B., Hauge, M., Henningsen, K., and Nordin, B. E. C. (1978). Metacarpal morphometry in monozygotic and dizygotic twin studies. *Calc. Tissue Res.* **25**, 197–201.

Moniz, C. (1994). Alcohol and bone. *Br. Med. Bull.* **50**, 67–75.

Morley, J. E. (1996). Nutritional status of the elderly. *Am. J. Med.* **81**, 679–695.

Morrison, N. A., Yeoman, R., Kelly, P. J., and Eisman, J. A. (1992). Contribution of trans-acting factor alleles to normal physiological variability: Vitamin D receptor gene polymorphisms and circulating osteocalcin. *Proc. Natl. Acad. Sci. U. S. A.* **89**, 6665–6669.

Morrison, N. A., Qi, J. C., Tokita, A., Kelly, P., Croft, L., Nguyen, T. V., Sambrook, P. N., and Eisman, J. A. (1994). Prediction of bone density by vitamin D receptor alleles. *Nature (London)* **367**, 284–287.

Morrison, N. A., Qi, J. C., Tokita, A., Kelly, P., Croft, L., Nguyen, T. V., Sambrook, P. N., and Eisman, J. A. (1997). Prediction of bone density by vitamin D receptor alleles: Corrections. *Nature (London)* **387**, 106.

Murray, R. E., McGuigan, F., Grant, S. F. A., Reid, D. M., and Ralston, S. H. (1997). Polymorphisms of the interleukin–6 gene are associated with bone density. *Bone* **21**, 89–92.

Need, A. G., Wishart, J. M., Scopacasa, F., Horowitz, M., Morris, H. A., and Nordin, B. E. C. (1995). Effect of physical activity on femoral bone density in men. *Br. Med. J.* **310**, 1501–1502.

Nevitt, M. C., and Cumming, S. R. (1993). Type of fall and risk of hip and wrist fractures: The Study of osteoporotic fractures. *J. Am. Geriatr. Soc.* **52**, 192–198.

Nguyen, T., Sambrook, P., Kelly, P., Jones, G., Lord, S., Freund, J., and Eisman, J. (1993). Prediction of osteoporotic fractures by postural instability and bone density. *Br. Med. J.* **307**, 1111–1115.

Nguyen, T. V., Kelly, P. I., Sambrook, P. N., Gilbert, C., Pocock, N. A., and Eisman, J. A. (1994). Life-style factors and bone density in the elderly: Implications for osteoporosis prevention. *J. Bone Miner. Res.* **9**, 1339–1346.

Nguyen, T. V., Eisman, J. A., Kelly, P. J., and Sambrook, P. N. (1996). Risk factors for osteoporotic fractures in men. *Am. J. Epidemiol.* **144**, 255–263.

Nguyen, T. V., Sambrook, P. N., and Eisman, J. A. (1997). Source of variability in bone density: Implication for study design and analysis. *J. Bone Miner. Res.* **12**, 124–135.

Nguyen, T. V., Howard, G., Kelly, P. J., and Eisman, J. A. (1998). Bone mass, lean mass, fat mass: Same genes or same environment. *Am. J. Epidemiol.* **147**, 3–16.

Nilsson, B. E., and Westlin, N. E., (1973). Changes in bone mass in alcoholics. *Clin. Orthop.* **90**, 229–232.

O'Neil, T. W., Valow, J., and Cooper, C. (1993). Differences in vertebral deformity indices between three European populations. *J. Bone Miner. Res.* **8**, S149.

Ooms, M. D., Lips, P. Van Lingen, A., and Valkenburg, H. A. (1993). Determinants of bone mineral density and risk factors for osteoporosis in healthy elderly women. *J. Bone Miner. Res.* **8**, 669–675.

Paganini-Hill, A., Ross, A. K., Gerkins, J. R. et al. (1981). Menopausal estrogen therapy and hip fractures. *Ann. Intern. Med.* **95**, 28–31.

Paganini-Hill, A., Chao, A. Ross, H. K., and Henderson, B. E. (1991). Exercise and other factors in the prevention of hip fracure: The Leisure World Study. *Epidemiology* **2**, 16–25.

Peacock, M. (1995). Vitamin D receptor gene alleles and osteoporosis: A contrasting view. *J. Bone Miner. Res.* **9**, 1294–1297.

Pocock, N. A., Eisman, J. A., Hopper, J. L., Yeates, M. G., Sambrook, P. N., and Eberl, S. (1987). Genetic determinants of bone mass in adults: A twin study. *J. Clin. Invest.* **80**, 706–710.

Pocock, N., Sambrook, P. N., Nguyen, T. V., Kelly, P. J., Freund, J., and Eisman, J. A. (1992). Assessment of spinal and femoral bone density by dual x-ray absorptionmetry: Comparison of Lunar and Hologic instruments. *J. Bone Miner. Res.* **7**, 1081–1085.

Poor, G., Atkinson, E. J., O'Fallon, W. M., and Melton, L. J., III (1995). Predictors of hip fractures in elderly men. *J. Bone Miner. Res.* **10**, 1900–1907.

Prudham, D., and Evans, J. G. (1981). Factors associated with falls in the elderly: A community study. *Age Ageing* **10**, 141–146.

Qi, J. C., Morrison, N. A., Nguyen, T. V., White, C. P., Kelly, P. J., Sambrook, P. N., and Eisman, J. A. (1994). Estrogen receptor genotypes and bone mineral density in women and men. *J. Bone Miner. Res.* **10**, S170.

Recker, R. R. (1993). Prevention of osteoporosis: Calcium nutrition. *Osteoporosis Int.* **3** (Suppl. 1), 163–165.

Reid, I. R., Plank, L. D., and Evans, M. C. (1992). Fat massis an important determinant of whole body bone density in premenopausal women but not in men. *J. Clin. Endocrinol. Metab.* **75**, 779–782.

Riebel, B. L., Boden, S. D., Whitesides, T. E., Hutton, W. C. (1995). The effect of nicotine on incorporation of cancellous bone graft in an animal model. *Spine* **20**, 2198–2202.

Riggs, B. L., Wahner, H. W., Seeman, E. et al. (1982). Changes in bone mineral density of the proximal femur and spine with aging: Differences between the postmenopausal and senile osteoporosis syndromes. *J. Clin. Invest.* **70**, 716–723.

Riis, B., Thomsen, K., and Christiansen, C. (1987). Does calcium supplementation prevent bone loss? A double-blind controlled clinical study. *N. Engl. J. Med.* **316**, 173–177.

Risch, N. (1990a). Linkage strategis for genetically complex trait I. Multilocus models. *Am. J. Hum. Genet.* **46**, 222–228.

Risch, N. (1990b). Linkage strategis for genetically complex trait II. The power of affected relative pairs. *Am. J. Hum. Genet.* **46**, 229–241.

Risch, N., and Zhang, H. (1995). Extreme discordant sib pairs for mapping quantitative trait loci in human. *Science* **268**, 1584–1589.

Risch, N., and Zhang, H. (1996). Mapping quantitative trait loci with extreme discordant sib pairs: Sampling considerations. *Am. J. Hum. Genet.* **58**, 836–843.

Robbins, A. S., Rubenstein, L. Z., Josephson, K. K. et al. (1989). Predictors of falls among elderly people. *Arch. Intern. Med.* **149**, 1628–1632.

Ross, P. D., Norimatsu, H., Davis, J. W., Yano, K., Wasnich, R. D., Fujiwara, S., Hosoda, Y., and Melton, L. J., III (1991). A comparison of hip fracture incidence among native Japanese, Japanese-Americans and American Caucasians. *Am. J. Epidemiol.* **133**, 801–809.

Roux, C., Dougados, M., Abel, L., Mercier, G., and Lucotte, G. (1997). Association of a polymorphism in the collagen I a1 gene with osteoporosis in French women (Letter). *Arthritis Rheum.* **18**, 187–188.

Sano, M., Inoue, S., Hosoi, T., Ouchi, Y., Emi, M., Shiraki, M., and Orimo, H. (1995). Association of estrogen receptor dinucleotide repeat polymorphism with osteoporosis. *Biochem. Biophys. Res. Commun.* **217**, 378–383.

Saville, P. D. (1965). Changes in bone mass with age and alcoholism. *J. Bone Jnt. Surg. Am. Vol.* **47A**, 492–499.

Seeman, E., Melton, L. J., III, O'Fallon, W. M., and Riggs, B. L. (1983). Risk factors for osteoporosis in men. *Am. J. Med.* **75**, 977–982.

Seeman, E., Young, N., Szmukler, G., Tsalamandris, C., and Hopper, J. L. (1993). Risk factors for osteoporosis. *Osteoporosis Int.* **3** (Suppl. 1), 40–43.

Seeman, E., Hopper, J. L., Young, N. R., Formica, C., Goss, P., and Tsakamandris, C. (1996). Do genetic factors explain associations between muscle strength, lean mass, and bone density? A twin study. *Am. J. Physiol.* **270**, E320–E327.

Silverman, S. L., and Madison, R. E. (1988). Decreased incidence of hip fracture in Hispanics, Asian and Blacks: California Hospital Discharge Data. *Am. J. Public Health* **78**, 1482–1483.

Slemenda, C. W., Hui, S. L., Longcope, C., and Johnston, C. C., Jr. (1989). Cigarette smoking, obesity, and bone mass. *J. Bone Miner. Res.* **4**, 737–741.

Slemenda, C. W., Christian, J. C., Williams, C. J., Norton, J. A., and Johnston, C. C. (1991). Genetic determinants of bone mass in adult women: A reevaluation of the twin model and the potential importance of gene interaction on heritability estimates. *J. Bone Miner. Res.* **6**, 561–567.

Slemenda, C. W., Christian, J. C., Reed, T., Reister, T. K., Williams, C. J., and Johnston, C. C., Jr. (1992). Long-term bone loss in men. *Ann. Intern. Med.* **117**, 286–291.

Smith, D. M., Nance, W. E., Kang, K. W., Christian, J. C., and Johnston, C. C. (1973). Genetic factors in determining bone mass. *J. Clin Invest.* **52**, 2800–2808.

Sowers, M. F., Burns, T. L., and Wallace, R. B. (1986). Familial resemblance of bone mass in adult women. *Genet. Epidemiol.* **3**, 85–93.

Sowers, M. F., Shapiro, B., Gilbraith, M. A. et al. (1990). Health and hormonal characteristics of women with low premenopausal bone mass. *Calcif. Tissue Int.* **47**, 130–135.

Spencer, H., Rubio, N., and Rubio, E. (1986). Chronic alcoholism: Frequently overlooked cause of osteoporosis in men. *Am. J. Med.* **80**, 393–397.

Thomson, G., Robinson, W. P., Kuhner, M. K., Joe, S., and Klitz, W. (1989). HLA and insulin gene association with IDDM. *Genet. Epidemiol.* **6**, 155–160.

Tothill, P., and Avenell, A. (1994). Errors in dual-energy X-ray absorptiometry of the lumbar spine owing to fat distribution and soft tissue thickness during weight change. *Br. J. Radiol.* **67**, 71–75.

Tothill, P., and Pye, D. W. (1992). Errors due to non-uniform distribution of fat in dual X-ray absorptiometry of the lumbar spine. *Br. J. Radiol.* **65**, 807–813.

Tylavsky, F. A., Bortz, A. D., Hancock, R. L., and Anderson, J. J. (1989). Familial resemblance of radial bone mass between pre-menopausal mothers and their college age daughters. *Calcif. Tissue Int.* **45**, 265–272.

Uitterlinden, A. G., Burger, H., Huang, Q., Grant, S. F. A., Hofman, A., Ralston, S. H., van Leeuwen, J. P. T. M., and Pols, H. A. P. (1997). Collagen 1a1 Sp1 polymorphism predict bone mass, bone loss and fracture. *J. Bone Miner. Res.* **12**, S119 (abstr. 66).

Vandevyver, C., Philippaerts, L., Cassiman, J. J., Raus, J., and Geusens, P. (1997). Bone mineral density in postmenopausal women is not associated with type I collagen I and collagen 2 dimorphisms. *J. Bone Miner. Res.* **12**, S490 (abstr. S550).

Waller, J. (1978). Falls among the elderly: Human and environmental factors. *Accid. Anal. Prev.* **10**, 21–33.

Wallister, J., Nieves, J., Cosman, F., and Lindsay, R. (1993). Fat mass does not interfere with measurement of lumbar spine BMD by DXA in thin or obese subjects. *J. Bone Miner. Res.* **8** (Suppl. 1), S351.

Wolinsky, F. D., Fitzgerald, J. F., and Stump, T. E. (1997). The effect of hip fracture on mortality, hospitalization and functional status: A prospective study. *Am. J. Public Health* **87**, 398–403.

Yano, K., Heilbrun, L. K., Wasnich, R. D., Hankin, J. H., and Vogel, J. M. (1985). The relationship between diet and bone mineral content of multiple skeletal sites in elderly Japanese-American men and women living in Hawaii. *Am. J. Clin. Nutr.* **42**, 877–888.

Young, D., Hopper, J. L., Nowsen, C. A., Green, R. M., Sherwin, J., Kaymacki, B., Smid, M., Guest, G. S., Larkins, R. G., and Wark, J. D., (1995). Determinants of bone mass in 10 to 26 years old females: A twin study. *J. Bone Miner. Res.* **10**, 558–567.

Chapter 18

Jane A. Cauley
Joseph M. Zmuda

Department of Epidemiology
Graduate School of Public Health
University of Pittsburgh
Pittsburgh, Pennsylvania

Risk Factors for Fractures in Men

I. Introduction

Age-adjusted incidence rates of hip fractures have stabilized in women (Melton *et al.*, 1987; Naessen *et al.*, 1989) but continue to increase in men (Boyce and Vessey, 1985; Obrant *et al.*, 1989) such that the incidence rate in men is nearing that observed several decades ago in women. As the population ages, more hip fractures will occur in both men and women, but the proportionate increase may be greater in men. Mortality after a hip fracture may actually be greater in men than women. More than half of men who suffer a hip fracture are discharged to a nursing home, and 79% of these men who survive at 1 year reside in nursing homes or intermediate care facilities (Poor *et al.*, 1995a). Only 41% of survivors return to their prefracture level of functioning, and about 60% have difficulty with ambulation (Poor *et al.*, 1995a). Vertebral fractures are the most common fracture in men and are also associated with morbidity and functional impairment

(Burger *et al.*, 1997). The total health care expenditures attributed to osteo-porotic fractures in men in the United States is $2.7 billion per year (Ray *et al.*, 1997).

Given the magnitude of the problem and its growing public health im-pact, it is essential to understand which risk factors predispose men to osteo-porotic fractures so that preventive steps can be taken. In general, risk factors for fractures in men have been poorly defined. Here, we review the current knowledge about risk factors for hip fractures, vertebral fractures, wrist frac-tures, and all clinical fractures in men. We concentrated our review on studies which reported results for men separate from women. Studies which pooled results on both genders were not considered because for the most part, only a small proportion of the fractures occurred in men.

A. Prospective Cohort Studies of Fracture in Men

Retrospective studies of risk factors for fractures have a number of im-portant biases which limit their interpretation: selection bias of cases, non-response bias, survival bias, choice of inadequate or unrepresentative controls, referral bias, and recall bias of exposures prior to the fracture. The fracture itself or the treatment for the fracture may also influence the risk factor of interest. The most important limitation, however, is the inability to estab-lish the temporal sequence of events necessary to establish a cause-effect relationship.

Prospective studies avoid many of these potential biases: risk factors are measured prior to the occurrence of the fracture, thereby establishing the time sequence for a cause-effect relationship. We have summarized the prospective studies in Table I. To our knowledge there have been nine published prospec-tive reports of a select number of risk factors and the risk of hip fracture; five of these studies are from the United States. The three prospective studies of all clinical fractures include one from Australia and two from Sweden. One prospective study has been reported on risk factors for wrist fractures.

B. Risk Factors for Hip Fracture

I. Age and Ethnicity

Older age is a major risk factor for hip fracture in men (Jacobsen *et al.*, 1990). This increased risk continues into the tenth decade of life (Figure 1). The incidence of hip fracture is greater for white men than black men: the age-adjusted incidence of femoral neck fracture was 2.18 and 1.23 [per 1000 person-years (PY)] in white and black men, respectively, and 2.28 and 1.24 for trochanteric fractures in white and black men, respectively (Karagas *et al.*, 1996b). The incidence of hip fracture among white men age 65 was 0.9 per 1000 PY, increasing exponentially to 26.0 per 1000 PY among white

TABLE I Prospective Cohort Studies of Fracture in Men

Author (year)	Cohort (country)	No. of Men	Characteristics	Follow-up	Fracture outcome (number) (ascertainment method)	Risk factors examined
Felson et al. (1988)	Framingham (USA)	1,089	Age 28–62 yr Caucasian	35 yr	Hip fractures (43) (50% validated by medical records)	Alcohol consumption
Forsen et al. (1994)	Nord-Jrondelag County (Norway)	18,198	Age 50+ yr; 20%, age ≥ 75 yr Caucasian	3 yr	Hip fracture (421) (validated by medical record)	Age, smoking, physical activity, body weight, ill-health
Gardsell et al. (1990)	Malmo (Sweden)	654	Age 30–89 yr	11 yr	All clinical fractures (165) (32 hip fractures) (all validated by x-ray)	Age, BMC, width of radial, height, weight, grip strength
Hemenway et al. (1994a)	Health Professional Follow-up Study (USA)	49,897	Age 40–75 yr 97% Caucasians	6 yr	Wrist fractures (271) (self report)	Age, height, BMI, cigarette smoking, alcohol intake
Hemenway et al. (1994b)	Health Professional Follow-up Study (USA)	49,895	Age 40–75 yr 97% Caucasians	6 yr	Hip fractures (67) (all validated by medical record)	Age, height, BMI, cigarette smoking, alcohol intake
Holbrook et al. (1988)	Rancho Bernardo (USA)	426	Age 50–79 yr 100% Caucasians	14 yr	Hip fractures (15) (death certificates or validated by telephone interview)	Nutrient intake: calcium, protein, total fat, total carbohydrate, fiber, caffeine, vitamin D, vitamin C, magnesium, copper, zinc, total calories
Joakimsen et al. (1998)	Tromso Study (Norway)	9,012	Age 32–66 yr	7 yr	All nonspine fractures (661) Hip fractures (13) (validated by X-ray)	Physical activity: leisure time and occupational; change in physical activity
Langlois et al. (1998)	Established populations for Epidemiologic Study of the Elderly (USA)	2,413	Age 67–104 yr 100% Caucasian	8 yr	Hip fractures (72) (Medicare hospitalization files)	Weight, weight & height age 50; BMI age 50, weight change since age 50, number of medical conditions, low mental status score, physical disability, physical activity, cigarette smoking, alcohol

(continues)

TABLE I Prospective Cohort Studies of Fracture in Men *(continued)*

Author (year)	Cohort (country)	No. of Men	Characteristics	Follow-up	Fracture outcome (number) (ascertainment method)	Risk factors examined
Meyer et al. (1997)	National Health Screening (CVD) (Norway)	27,015	Age 35–49 yr Caucasian	14 yr	Hip fracture (64) (excluded traumatic and pathologic fractures) (validated by medical records)	Height, weight, BMI, physical activity, diabetes, stroke, disability, marital status, smoking
Meyer et al. (1997)	National Health Screening (CVD) (Norway)	20,035	Age 35–49 yr Caucasians	14 yr	Hip fracture (55) (validated by medical record)	Subset of above cohort with nutrient data: milk, calcium, animal protein, coffee, height, BMI
Meyer et al. (1995)	National Health Screening (tuberculosis) (Norway)	209,351	Age 50–89 yr Caucasians	16 yr	Fatal hip fracture (2,043) (death certificates)	Height, BMI
Mussolino et al. (1998)	National Health and Nutrition Examination Survey I (USA)	2,879	Age 45–74 yr 100% Caucasian	13.9 yr	Hip fractures (71) (validated by medical record)	Age, previous fracture, BMI, smoking, alcohol, physical activity, weight loss, calcium, caloric intake, protein consumption, no. of chronic diseases, BMD
Nyquist et al. (1998)	Malmo (Sweden)	242	Age 50–80 yr	7 yr	All clinical fractures (31) (validated by medical record)	Age, weight, height, BMD, testosterone, SHBG, skinfold thickness, alcohol abuse marker
Nguyen et al. (1996)	Dubbo (Australia)	820	Age 60+ yr; 25%, age ≥ 75 yr	5 yr	All clinical fractures (166) (31 hip fracture) (all validated) 32 symptomatic vertebral fractures)	Age, BMD, muscle strength, body weight, previous falls and fractures, height, weight, alcohol, physical activity, thiazide
Ross et al. (1996)	Honolulu (USA)	996	Not reported	6.4 yr	New vertebral fractures (42) on serial radiographs (15% reduction)	BMD

Note: BMI, body mass index; BMC, bone mineral content; BMD, bone mineral density.

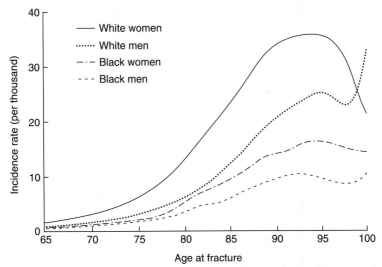

FIGURE 1 Annual age-specific incidence of hip fracture among the elderly: population-based rates by race and sex for 1984–1987, United States. Lines represent a smoothed curve based on the calculated age-, race-, and sex-specific incidence rates. Reproduced with permission from Jacobsen *et al.* (1990). *Am. J. Public Health* **80,** 871–872. Copyright APHA.

men age 96. This exponential rise in hip fracture with age was not observed for black males. The increased incidence with age was more linear in black males and appears to level off after age 90 (Jacobsen *et al.*, 1990). The incidence of hip fracture in Asian men is about half that in Caucasian men (Ling *et al.*, 1996; Ross *et al.*, 1991). Similar findings were observed for Hispanic men (Silverman and Madison, 1988; Bauer, 1988).

2. Skeletal Status

Four case-control studies have reported lower bone mineral density (BMD) measurements in male hip fracture patients compared to controls (Table II). Hip BMD was about 1 to 1.5 standard deviations (SD) lower among the cases. In one study, the hip fracture cases had significantly lower body weight, body mass index (BMI, wt/ht^2), fat and lean mass. Adjustment for BMI attenuated the differences in spine BMD but the differences in hip BMD remained statistically significant.

Cross-sectionally, the average (± 1 SD) femoral neck BMD among men of age 60 to 64 was 0.888 ± 0.12 g/cm^2 and, among men of age 80 to 84, 0.829 ± 0.139 g/cm^2, about a 7% decline. This age-related decline in BMD was estimated to be associated with a 60% increased (95% confidence intervals: 1.3 to 1.8) relative risk of hip fracture (De Laet *et al.*, 1997).

Two prospective studies examined the risk of hip fracture by BMD. A 54% sample of the 2879 men in the National Health and Nutrition

TABLE II Bone Density Measurements in Male Hip Fracture Patients and Controls

Author	No. of cases	No. of controls (source)	Measurement of BMD	BMD site	Results (g/cm²) Cases	Results (g/cm²) Controls	Comments
Karllson et al. (1993)	26	50 (community controls)	DXA (Lunar DPX-L)	Femoral neck Trochanter Whole body Spine	0.76 0.71 1.02 1.01	0.88* 0.88** 1.11 1.17*	After adjusting for body weight, spine differences were no longer significant
Boonen et al. (1997)	40	40 (community controls)	DXA (Lunar DPX-L)	Femoral neck Trochanter	0.61 0.51	0.95** 0.90**	Cases had significantly lower body weight, but no adjustment made
Thiebaud et al. (1997)	43	44 (hospital controls)	DXA (Hologic 1000)	Total hip Femoral neck Trochanter	0.70 0.64 0.55	0.92** 0.79** 0.71**	Hip fracture cases had significantly lower BMI, but no adjustments were made
Center et al. (1998)	13	65 (Dubbo cohort)	DXA (Lunar DPX-L)	Femoral neck	0.67	0.89**	Age-matched cases and controls

* $p < 0.05$; ** $p < 0.001$.

Examination Survey (NHANES) I and the Epidemiologic Follow-up to this survey had BMD measurements using radiographic absorptiometry (RA) of the left hand. The multivariate-adjusted relative risk of hip fracture per 1 SD decrease in phalangeal BMD was 1.73 (1.11 to 2.68) (Mussolino *et al.*, 1998). Within the Dubbo Osteoporosis Epidemiology Study, a 1 SD decrease in femoral neck BMD was associated with a relative risk of 3.2 (1.6 to 6.4) of hip fracture (Center *et al.*, 1998; Nguyen *et al.*, 1996). These relative risks are consistent with a meta-analysis of prospective studies in women of the relationship between BMD and fractures: 1 SD decrease in hip BMD was associated with a 2.6 *RR* of hip fracture; forearm BMD, a 1.4 *RR* of hip fracture; and spine BMD, a 1.8 *RR* of hip fracture (Marshall *et al.*, 1996).

BMD is not the only determinant of skeletal strength. Bone strength also depends on the microarchitectural properties of bone including the orientation and thickness, number and spacing of the trabeculae (Myers and Wilson, 1997). Quantitative ultrasound is a promising tool for assessing these qualitative properties in addition to and distinct from bone mass (Brandenburger, 1993) and, at least in women, predict the risk of hip fracture independent of BMD (Bauer *et al.*, 1997). There are no studies of quantitative ultrasound (QUS) and hip fractures in men.

In women, measures of hip geometry predict the risk of hip fracture independent of BMD (Faulkner *et al.*, 1993). Two studies of hip fracture in men included a measure of hip axis length from dual energy x-ray absorptiometry (DXA) scans. In one study, the average hip axis length was similar in 33 men with a hip fracture compared to controls (61.2 ± 4.6 mm versus 61.0 ± 3.6 mm, respectively) (Karlsson *et al.*, 1996). This study was limited because the DXA scans were obtained within 2 weeks of the fracture, and positioning errors may have occurred because of postoperative pain.

In the Dubbo Osteoporosis Epidemiology Study, femoral neck axis length was measured in a nested case-control design in 13 men who subsequently developed a hip fracture and two sets of controls: age-matched and height-matched (Center *et al.*, 1998). One standard deviation increase in femoral neck axis length was associated with an odds ratio (95% confidence interval) of hip fracture of 1.1 (0.8 to 1.6) among age-matched controls and 2.11 (1.2 to 3.6) among height-matched controls. In the final multivariate model, femoral neck axis length was not an independent predictor of hip fractures. Measurements of femoral neck axis length do not include structures proximal to the femoral neck (the acetabular width) and are not directly comparable to studies of hip axis length.

Cross-sectional studies of the geometric characteristics of the femoral neck demonstrated in women a decline in femoral neck cross-sectional area and the cross-sectional moment of inertia, a geometric index of bone rigidity with increasing age (Beck *et al.*, 1992). In men, there was a compensatory increase in the width of the femoral neck such that the cross-sectional moment of inertia showed no change. These results suggest that characteristics of hip geometry may not contribute to hip fractures in older men because of these compensatory changes, although there are no data to confirm this speculation. However, these data are cross-sectional, and estimates of change based on cross-sectional data may be biased. A recent 20-year longitudinal study of women reported an actual expansion of the femoral neck with age in women (Heaney *et al.*, 1997). This latter study did not include men. Future longitudinal studies of changes in skeletal dimensions and their role in hip fractures in men are needed.

Finally, markers of bone turnover, specifically pyridinoline and deoxypyridinoline were found to be almost twice as high in male hip fracture patients compared to controls (Boonen *et al.*, 1997). There was no significant difference in osteocalcin levels. Among the cases, an index of free $25(OH)_2$ vitamin D and free testosterone were significantly related to both urinary markers suggesting a combined effect of androgen deficiency and vitamin D deficiency on bone resorption among men.

3. Diet

A case-control study from the United Kingdom reported that men with daily intakes of calcium above 1 g had a lower risk of hip fracture (Cooper *et al.*, 1988). Several prospective studies have examined the relationship between nutrient intake and risk of hip fracture. In the Rancho Bernardo Study, a wide spectrum of dietary data was measured (Table I) (Holbrook *et al.*, 1988). The only variable that was statistically significant was calcium intake estimated from a 24-hour recall. The mean intake of calcium per day was 634 mg/day in the men who experienced a hip fracture compared to 787 mg/day in men who did not fracture ($p = 0.03$). The relative risk of hip fracture was 0.3 in men with the highest tertile of calcium intake compared with the lower 2 tertiles. This study was limited in its small number of hip fractures in men ($n = 15$).

In the middle-aged cohort from Norway, men who reported four or more glasses of milk per day had about a 50% reduced risk of hip fracture ($RR = 0.46$; 0.22 to 0.98) (Meyer *et al.*, 1997). Men with the highest intake of total calcium had a reduced risk of hip fracture, but confidence intervals were wide and included 1.0. There was little association between nondairy animal protein or coffee consumption and hip fracture in this study.

In the NHANES I Epidemiologic Follow-up study, there was a trend of decreasing risk of hip fracture with increasing intake of calcium and protein but neither association was statistically significant (Mussolino *et al.*, 1998). No association between dietary calcium, calcium supplement use, or total calcium intake was found in the Leisure World cohort (Paganini-Hill *et al.*, 1991).

Among Chinese men, a very low intake of calcium (< 75 mg/day) was associated with a twofold increased risk of hip fracture (Lau *et al.*, 1988).

The magnitude of the association between calcium and hip fracture risk was similar in Chinese men and Chinese women. Chinese diets are characteristically low in calcium: the mean intake in Hong Kong was 171 mg/day compared to U.S. populations (mean ≈ 700 mg/day). These data suggest a lower threshold among populations with traditionally low calcium intakes.

4. Alcohol

Increased alcohol consumption was associated with an increased risk of hip fracture among men in the Framingham cohort (Felson *et al.*, 1988). A history of alcoholism or problem drinking was also associated with an increased risk of hip fracture (Grisso *et al.*, 1991). In contrast, most other studies have not found an association between moderate alcohol consumption and hip fracture in men (Hemenway *et al.*, 1994b; Paganini-Hill *et al.*, 1991; Langlois *et al.*, 1998; Mussolini *et al.*, 1998; Grisso *et al.*, 1991). There is a well-established relationship between alcohol abuse and lower BMD (Bikle *et al.*, 1985). Moderate alcohol consumption on the other hand, may be more common among healthier individuals. For example, the percent of men who reported drinking alcohol in the past year was actually higher among the controls than cases in one study (Langlois *et al.*, 1998).

5. Smoking

Current cigarette smoking was significantly associated with the risk of hip fracture (Grisso *et al.*, 1991, 1997; Forsen *et al.*, 1994; Paganini-Hill *et al.*, 1991). The relative risk of hip fracture among male smokers versus nonsmokers ranged from 1.8 (Forsen *et al.*, 1994) to 2.23 (Paganini-Hill *et al.*, 1991). This association was independent of other risk factors for hip fracture. Pipe smoking was also associated with an increased relative risk of hip fracture: $RR = 2.6$ (1.0 to 6.8) (Grisso *et al.*, 1997). In one prospective study, the risk of hip fracture associated with smoking was elevated, but confidence intervals included 1.0 (Mussolino *et al.*, 1998). There was no association between smoking and hip fracture in the Established Populations for the Epidemiologic Study of the Elderly (EPESE) (Table I) study (Langlois *et al.*, 1998). Failure to detect an association between smoking and hip fracture in the Health Professionals Follow-up Study may have reflected limited power because fewer than 3% of the cohort reported smoking more than 25 cigarettes per day (Hemenway *et al.*, 1994b). There was no association with former smoking and hip fracture in several studies (Grisso *et al.*, 1997; Hemenway *et al.*, 1994b; Paganini-Hill *et al.*, 1991).

6. Physical Activity

Among Chinese men, daily walking was associated with a reduced risk of hip fracture, but confidence intervals included 1.0 (Lau *et al.*, 1988). In a large case-control study of 356 men with a first hip fracture, the physical activity index included the number of hours in the year before their hip fracture that was spent not only in sports or recreational activity but also in heavy outdoor/indoor work, household repairs, or car repairs (Grisso *et al.*, 1997). High activity corresponded to one hour per day or more of heavy physical activity, whereas moderate activity had a wide range with as little as 15 minutes per day up to an hour per day. The odds ratio (95% confidence interval (CI)) of experiencing a hip fracture was significantly reduced for men reporting moderate (0.3; 0.2 to 0.5) or high (0.2; 0.1 to 0.3) levels of activity compared to men with low activity (Grisso *et al.*, 1997).

Prospectively, one or more hours of exercise per day was associated with a 40% reduction in the risk of hip fracture (Paganini-Hill *et al.*, 1991). This association was independent of smoking and body mass index and was similar to that observed among women in the same cohort. Similarly in a cohort from Norway, the rate of hip fracture was higher among men reporting no exercise compared to exercisers (Forsen *et al.*, 1994). The incidence rate of hip fracture increase with age in both the inactive men and the exercisers, but the rate of increase was much greater in the inactive men (Figure 2). The incidence of hip fracture among men ⩾ age 75 who exercised was similar to the rate among men 10 years younger who did not exercise. In this study, the effect of physical activity on hip fracture was independent of age, BMI, smoking, and ill health.

Few studies have attempted to separate occupational physical activity from leisure-time activity. This issue may be more important for men than women because occupational activity levels for men may be more heterogeneous. Occupational activity, but not leisure activity, was associated with a reduced risk of hip fracture in one study (Meyer *et al.*, 1993). However, this association was limited to "intensive" activity and was not significant in

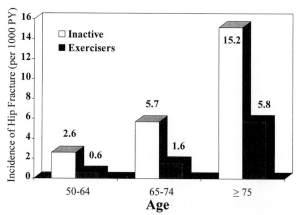

FIGURE 2   Incidence rate of hip fracture in older men by physical activity per 1000 person years (PY). Data from Forsen *et al.* (1994).

multivariate models. In Canada, incidence rates of hip fracture in men were lowest in rural areas (< 100 persons) and villages (100 to 500 persons) compared to cities (Ray *et al.*, 1990). This may reflect greater physical activity, in particular, occupational activity in the rural areas.

Higher levels of physical activity during childhood and young adulthood could reduce the risk of hip fracture by maximizing peak skeletal mass. In one study of Chinese men, higher levels of activity at age 35 were associated with a reduced risk of hip fracture (Lau *et al.*, 1988).

7. Anthropometry

In case-control (Grisso *et al.*, 1991, 1997; Karlsson *et al.*, 1993) and prospective studies (Meyer *et al.*, 1995; Paganini-Hill *et al.*, 1991; Forsen *et al.*, 1994; Meyer *et al.*, 1993), body mass index was inversely related to the risk of hip fracture in men. Men with a BMI < 25 kg/m^2 had an increased incidence of hip fracture at every age (50–64, 65–74, ≥75), but the effect of BMI appeared actually greatest in younger men (Forsen *et al.*, 1994). Body mass index was also related to the risk of fatal hip fracture (Meyer *et al.*, 1995): the age-adjusted relative risk in the three highest versus the lowest quartiles of BMI was 0.57 (0.52 to 0.62). A decrease of 1 SD in skinfold thickness was associated with a twofold excess risk of hip fracture, a finding which is consistent with the results of studies using BMI (Nyquist *et al.*, 1998).

The Health Professionals Follow-up Study did not report a significant association between BMI and hip fracture, but this may have reflected a narrow range of BMI among these health professionals and low power (Hemenway *et al.*, 1994b).

Because obese individuals tend to be less active, Forsen *et al.* (1994) tested for an interaction between BMI and level of physical activity. Among women with low BMI but the highest level of physical activity, there was no increase in hip fracture risk. This observation was, however, not observed in men.

The effect of BMI on fatal hip fracture tended to wane over the 14-year follow-up period. This may reflect changes in body weight during follow-up (Meyer *et al.*, 1997). In the NHANES I Epidemiologic Follow-up, BMI was not significantly related to hip fracture. Of importance, however, a 10% weight loss from maximum was associated with a 2.27 (1.13 to 4.59) relative risk of hip fracture which was independent of smoking, physical activity, age, alcohol consumption, number of chronic conditions, and dietary intake (Mussolini *et al.*, 1998). Similarly, a 10% weight loss since age 50 was associated with an increased risk of hip fracture, whereas a 10% gain was associated with a reduced risk of hip fracture in the EPESE study (Langlois *et al.*, 1998) (Figure 3). This association was independent of BMI and a number of other important risk factors for hip fracture. The observation that weight loss may be more strongly related to hip fracture than current BMI or body weight is similar to what has been observed among women (Cummings

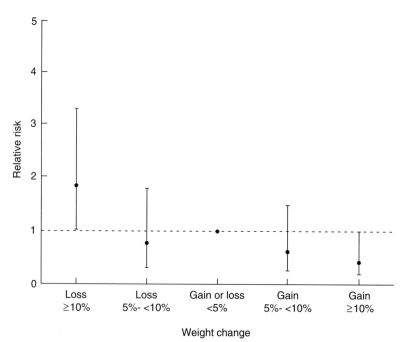

FIGURE 3   Association between change in body weight after the age of 50 years and the risk of hip fracture. The relative risks are adjusted for age at baseline, body mass index (a measure of weight in kilograms divided by the square of the height in meters) at age 50 years, cigarette smoking, alcohol consumption in the past year, number of medical conditions, impaired mobility and disability in activities of daily living, use of thiazide diuretics, physical activity level, and mental status score. Men with a weight loss or gain of less than 5% served as the reference group. The T bars indicate the upper and lower 95% confidence intervals. From Langlois *et al.* (1998). *Arch. Int. Med.* **158**, 990–996.

et al., 1995). However, none of these studies controlled for BMD. Because weight loss is associated with increased bone loss in men (Glynn *et al.*, 1996), it will be important to test whether this association is independent of BMD.

Taller men had an increased risk of hip fracture in some studies (Hemenway *et al.*, 1994b; Grisso *et al.*, 1997; Paganini-Hill *et al.*, 1991; Meyer *et al.*, 1993). Height was not related to fatal hip fracture (Meyer *et al.*, 1995). A 3.2-cm loss of height was associated with a 2.5-fold increase in hip fracture risk among men (Center *et al.*, 1998). These findings are consistent with what has been observed among older women (Cummings *et al.*, 1995).

8. Medications

Thiazide diuretic use was associated with a 33% reduction in the risk of hip fracture in men and women combined (LaCroix *et al.*, 1990). In this study, about one third of the hip fractures occurred in men, but results are not presented separately for the men. In a follow-up report of men from the same cohort, the prevalence of use of thiazide diuretics did not differ in men who had a subsequent hip fracture compared to those who did not (Langlois *et al.*, 1998). Use of nonreserpine antihypertensive medications was not associated with the risk of hip fracture in the Leisure World cohort, but the prevalence of use of these medications was relatively low (Paganini-Hill *et al.*, 1991). Five or more years of use of thiazide diuretics was associated with a lower risk of hip fracture, but this was not statistically significant (Grisso *et al.*, 1997; Poor *et al.*, 1995b).

Corticosteroid use was not associated with an increased risk of hip fracture (Poor *et al.*, 1995b; Grisso *et al.*, 1997), but this may have reflected low statistical power. Use of anticonvulsants was associated with a threefold increased risk of hip fracture which approached statistical significance (Poor *et al.*, 1995b). Use of psychotropic drugs was associated with a twofold increased risk of hip fracture (Grisso *et al.*, 1997). This study did not stratify by long or short half-life which may be important since, in women, the long-acting benzodiazepines were associated with an increased risk of hip fractures (Cummings *et al.*, 1995). Calcium channel blockers were associated with a reduced risk of hip fracture, but the underlying mechanism is unknown (Langlois *et al.*, 1997).

Finally, a history of cimetidine use was associated with a relative risk (95% CI) of 2.5 (1.4 to 4.6) for hip fracture (Grisso *et al.*, 1997). The authors speculated that chronic cimetidine use may block androgen receptors or inhibit estradiol hydroxylation, but further studies are needed.

9. Institutionalism

Men living in institutions were 13.3 (95% CI: 11.3 to 15.5) times more likely to experience a hip fracture than those living in private homes (Butler *et al.*, 1996). The difference in hip fracture rates by place of residence were greatest among younger men (age 60 to 64) but persisted through age 90.

10. Fracture History

A previous hip fracture occurred in 13% of women and 7% of men who presented with a new incident hip fracture (Falch *et al.*, 1985). History of any fracture after age 40 was also found to be more common among men who experience a hip fracture up to age 80 for men and 70 for women (Finsen and Benum, 1986).

Two studies specifically focused on whether a distal forearm fracture predicted the risk of hip fracture in men. A previous Colles' fracture was associated with a relative risk of 6.4 (2.6 to 13.1) for a hip fracture (Owen *et al.*, 1982). This association was substantially stronger in men than women. Similar findings were reported by Mallmin *et al.* (1993), although the magnitude of the association was smaller.

I I. Fluoride

Water fluoride concentration at the optimal level (1 ppm) has been associated with a slight increased risk of hip fracture in men (Jacobsen *et al.*, 1992b), a decreased risk (Lehmann *et al.*, 1998), or no association (Cooper *et al.*, 1990; Karagas *et al.*, 1996a).

12. Falls

Most hip fractures occur because of a fall, and many risk factors for falls are important risk factors for hip fractures in women (Cummings *et al.*, 1995). Men who reported falling two or more times in the past year were at a substantially increased risk of hip fracture (Cumming and Klineberg, 1994). This association was much stronger among men than women: the odds ratio (95% CI) for a hip fracture associated with four or more falls in the past year was 20.5 (3.3 to 125.1) in men and 4.38 (1.93 to 9.93) in women. Most of the falls which led to hip fractures in men occurred indoors with little seasonality (Poor *et al.*, 1995a).

The incidence of falls increases markedly with age in men: the percent of men age 60 to 64 who fell two or more times was 4% compared to about 9% among men age $\geqslant$80 (Nguyen *et al.*, 1996), although the overall rate of falling in men may be less than that observed among women (Sattin *et al.*, 1990).

Few studies have assessed the relationship between fall risk factors and subsequent hip fractures. Impaired vision was related to hip fractures in women but not men, but the number of hip fractures in men was very small ($n = 16$) (Felson *et al.*, 1989). Blindness was associated with an increased risk of hip fracture in one study (Poor *et al.*, 1995b). Greater upper body strength may improve one's ability to break the impact of a fall. Men with a grip strength $<$28.0 kg were at a higher risk of hip fracture than men with greater grip strength (Coupland *et al.*, 1993). A 10 kg greater quadricep strength was associated with about 50% decrease in hip fracture risk in Australian men (Nguyen *et al.*, 1996). Increased body sway was also associated with an increased risk of hip fracture (Nguyen *et al.*, 1996). Finally, medical conditions linked with falling, such as movement or balance disorders, were associated with almost a sevenfold increase in risk of hip fracture (OR = 6.9; 95% CI 3.3 to 14.8) (Poor *et al.*, 1995b). Similarly, lower limb dysfunction or ambulation problems were associated with an increased risk of hip fracture (Grisso *et al.*, 1991, 1997).

The characteristics of the fall has been shown to influence the risk of hip fractures in older men (Schwartz *et al.*, 1998). Men who reported hitting the hip/thigh in a fall had a substantially elevated risk of hip fracture: OR = 97.8; 95% CI 31.7 to 302. Falling sideways was associated with an increased risk of hip fracture, whereas falling forward or backward, a reduced risk. These case-control data support observations in women that characteristics of the falls are important determinants of whether or not a hip fracture occurs.

13. Medical Conditions

The number of chronic conditions or self-report of ill-health may identify men at high risk of hip fractures. In the largest case-control study of hip fracture, two or more chronic diseases were associated with an increased risk of hip fracture, but confidence intervals included one. Prospectively, self-report of bronchitis, thyroid disease, diabetes, kidney disease, heart disease, or stroke was associated with RR of 1.91 (1.19 to 3.06) (Mussolini et al., 1998). Finally, there was about a twofold increased risk of hip fracture among men who reported ill-health (Forsen et al., 1994).

In terms of specific medical conditions leading to hip fractures in men, the most comprehensive study was carried out by Poor et al. (1995b) using case control data from the Mayo Clinic. In general, medical conditions associated with secondary osteoporosis were associated with a twofold increased risk of hip fracture, whereas conditions associated with falling, a sevenfold increased risk.

Specific conditions associated with hip fracture in men include thyroidectomy (Poor et al., 1995b; Nguyen et al., 1997), hyperparathyroidism (Larsson et al., 1993), hypogonadism (Stanley et al., 1991; Jackson et al., 1992), gastric resection (Poor et al., 1995b), chronic bronchitis (Poor et al., 1995b), stroke (Grisso et al., 1997; Meyer et al., 1993), Parkinsonism (Poor et al., 1995b), dementia (Poor et al., 1995b) and alcoholism (Poor et al., 1995b). Osteoarthritis was reported to be protective for hip fractures (Dequeker et al., 1993), whereas rheumatoid arthritis was associated with an increased risk (Paganini-Hill et al., 1991). An association between diabetes was reported in one study (Meyer et al., 1993) but not in others (Poor et al., 1995b; Grisso et al., 1997). Urolithiasis was associated with a reduced risk of hip fracture in one study (Poor et al., 1995b) but not in a later study (Melton et al., 1998). An increased risk of fractures has been reported following either surgical (Daniell, 1997) or medical treatment (Townsend et al., 1997) for prostate cancer.

14. Biochemical Differences

In a case-control study, male hip fracture patients had significantly lower albumin, lower $25(OH)_2$ vitamin D and insulin-like growth factor-binding protein 3 (IGFBP3) levels than hospital and community controls (Thiebaud et al., 1997). These data may reflect an overall poor nutritional state among the men who sustained a hip fracture.

Similarly, Boonen et al. (1997) reported lower $1,25(OH)_2$ vitamin D levels in male hip fracture patients and controls. The differences were quite large, corresponding to about 1 SD difference. Parathyroid hormone (PTH) levels were also significantly higher among the cases. These data are consistent with secondary hyperparathyroidism as an important risk factor for hip fractures in men.

Male hip fracture patients were also found to have significantly lower total testosterone, free testosterone index, and dehydroepiandrosterone sulfate (DHEAS) than controls suggesting androgen deficiency as a major cause of hip fractures (Boonen et al., 1997). In this study, there was no difference in total estradiol levels between cases and controls, although the free estradiol index was higher among the controls. The hip fracture cases in this study had on average about 6 kg lower body weight than the controls, and none of these findings were adjusted for differences in body weight.

15. Family History and Genetics

Adult men with a family history of osteoporosis have lower BMD compared to men without a history of osteoporosis (Soroko et al., 1994). A son is almost four times more likely to have low BMD if his father also has low BMD, and nearly eight times more likely if both parents have low BMD (Jouanny et al., 1995). Men with a parental history of hip fracture have 30% greater risk of prevalent vertebral deformity (95% CI: 1.0, 1.7) compared to men without a parental history of such fractures (Diaz et al., 1997a). Polymorphisms in genes that encode the vitamin D and estrogen receptors, and type IαI collagen, transforming growth factor-β, α_2HS-glycoprotein, apolipoprotein E, and interleukin 6 have been associated with modest differences in BMD in some studies of pre- and postmenopausal women (Zmuda et al., 1998). Although gender plays an important role in the development of osteoporosis, genetic studies have almost exclusively focused on women. Future candidate gene association studies will need to include large numbers of men to test whether gender modifies the effects of genetic polymorphisms on BMD and the risk of fracture.

C. Risk Factors for Vertebral Fracture

1. Age and Race

The risk of symptomatic vertebral fracture increases rapidly with age in both men and women. For instance, incidence rates of symptomatic vertebral fractures increased from 18/100,000 PY among men ages 55 to 64 years to 1244/100,000 PY among those aged 85 years and older in a study of Rochester, Minnesota, residents (Cooper et al., 1992). Corresponding rates were 241/100,000 and 1167/100,000 among women of ages 55 to 64 and >85 years, respectively. Similar age-related trends have been observed in other studies (Nguyen et al., 1996; Jacobsen et al., 1992a; Hu et al., 1996).

Many vertebral fractures are asymptomatic, however, with only about one third coming to medical attention (Cooper et al., 1992). Recent population-based reports using vertebral morphometry suggest a high overall prevalence of vertebral deformity and rapid rise with age. For example, the prevalence of vertebral deformity defined by the Eastell method increased from 16.5%

to 29.1% among men of ages 50 to 54 and 75 to 79 years, respectively, in the European Vertebral Osteoporosis Study (EVOS) (O'Neill *et al.*, 1996). Corresponding prevalence estimates increased from 11.5% to 34.8% among 50- to 54- and 75- to 79-year-old women. These prevalence estimates are completely dependent on the criteria used for diagnosis. Using the McCloskey-Kanis method of diagnosis, for example, the prevalence of vertebral deformity increased from 9.9% to 18.1% among 50- to 54- and 75- to 79-year-old men, respectively, in EVOS (O'Neill *et al.*, 1996). Corresponding prevalence estimates increased from 5.0% to 24.7% among 50- to 54- and 75- to 79-year-old women. Similar findings across age groups were reported among Australian (Jones *et al.*, 1996) and Asian (Tsai *et al.*, 1996) men.

There is little information on racial differences in vertebral fracture prevalence or incidence diagnosed clinically or using vertebral morphometry. In one study, hospital discharge data for vertebral fractures were greatest in white women (17.1/10,000 per year) followed by white men (9.9/10,000 per year), black women (3.7/10,000 per year), and black men (2.5/10,000 per year) (Jacobson *et al.*, 1992a).

2. Skeletal Fragility

Bone mineral density is a major determinant of vertebral body strength (Myers and Wilson, 1997), and low BMD is strongly associated with increased risk of vertebral fracture in case-control and prospective studies in women (Ross *et al.*, 1990). There are limited prospective data in men, but most cross-sectional studies indicate that vertebral fractures are also associated with significantly reduced BMD in men measured at both axial and appendicular skeletal sites and by several techniques (Table III).

Similar associations between BMD and prevalent vertebral deformities in men and women have been documented in two recent studies (Jones *et al.*, 1996; Lunt *et al.*, 1997). The risk of prevalent vertebral deformity (4-SD criteria) associated with 1-SD decrement in femoral neck BMD measured by DXA was 1.97 in men (95% CI: 1.12, 3.45) and 1.99 in women (95% CI: 1.20, 2.38) (Jones *et al.*, 1996). Corresponding risk estimates for each SD reduction in lumbar spine BMD were 2.10 in men (95% CI: 1.15, 3.52) and 1.49 in women (95% CI: 0.96, 2.39). The risk of deformity (McCloskey-Kanis method) involving the midheight only or mid and anterior heights was significantly and similarly (OR = 1.73 to 2.55 in men and 1.78 to 3.35 in women) associated with reduced spine and femoral neck BMD measured by DXA in a second study (Lunt *et al.*, 1997). Lumbar spine BMD was a significantly better predictor of these deformities than femoral neck BMD in men, whereas there was no difference between skeletal sites in women.

At least two prospective studies have also demonstrated that low BMD is associated with vertebral fracture risk in men (Nguyen *et al.*, 1996; Ross *et al.*, 1996). A 1-SD decrement in femoral neck BMD was associated with a nearly twofold (*RR:* 1.92; 95% CI: 1.45, 2.56) greater risk of symptomatic

TABLE III Selected Cross-Sectional Studies Comparing BMD in Male Vertebral Fracture Patients and Controls

Author	Cases	Controls	Diagnostic method	Measurement of BMD	Skeletal site	Results Cases	Results Controls	Comments
Mann et al. (1992)	14	130	≥ 3 SD reduction in H_a/H_p or H_m/H_p	DPA (Lunar DP4)	Spine (g/cm^2)[a] Femoral neck (g/cm^2)[a]	0.98 0.74	1.19** 0.87**	Similar results obtained using 2 SD criteria and H_a/H_p, H_m/H_p ratio <0.80 No adjustments for age or weight
Resch et al. (1992)	27	19	2 or more atraumatic crush fractures	SPA (Novo-Osteodensiometer) QCT (Toshiba TCT 400)	Distal forearm (units) Spine (mg/ml)	42.4 80.6	50.8** 130.4***	Age-matched controls
Ito et al. (1993)	6 6	19 (50–59 yr) 9 (60–69 yr)	H_a/H_p, H_m/H_p, $H_p/H_{p\pm1}$, $H_a/H_{a\pm1}$, or $H_m/H_{m\pm1} \leq 0.85$	DXA (Hologic 1000) QCT (Siemens)	Spine (g/cm^2) 50–59 yr 60–69 yr Spine (mg/cm^3) Trabecular 50–59 yr 60–69 yr Cortical 50–59 yr 60–69 yr	0.85 0.74 78.1 64.4 209.1 258.5	0.93 0.89** 109.3* 97.6* 313.3*** 281.3	Age did not differ between cases and controls Results are for men with large osteophytes
Johansson et al. (1994)	15	124	$H_a/H_p \leq 0.66$	DPA	Calcaneus (g/cm^2)	0.38	0.43	Age, weight, and height similar in cases and controls
Resch et al. (1995)	71	130	>15% decrease in H_a/H_p or 15% in both relative to intact adjacent vertebrae	QCT (Toshiba TCT 400)	Spine (mg/ml)	75	132***	BMD-fracture relation independent of age
Stewart et al. (1995)	38	209	>25% decrease in H_a, and/or H_m relative to H_p or in H_p relative to 2 adjacent vertebrae	DXA (Norland XR-26)	Spine (g/cm^2) Femoral neck (g/cm^2) Trochanter (g/cm^2)	1.02 0.81 0.79	1.07 0.83 0.80	Cases and controls had similar age, weight, and height
Need et al. (1998)	42	92	$H_a/H_p \leq 0.80$ $H_p \leq 0.80$	Molgaard bone mineral analyzer	Forearm (g/ml)	0.38	0.44***	Cases were older and weighed less than controls, but no adjustments were made
Vega et al. (1998)	30	26	≥ 1 atraumatic wedge or compression fracture	DXA (Lunar DPX-L)	Spine (g/cm^2)	0.84	1.21***	Age-matched controls had similar weight and height

[a]BMD values estimated from bar graph; H_a indicates anterior height; H_p, posterior height; H_m, middle height.
$* p < 0.05$; $** p < 0.01$; $*** p < 0.001$.

vertebral fractures over 5-years in the Dubbo cohort (Nguyen *et al.*, 1996). A second study followed 996 men and 911 women for 6 to 8 years and identified a total of 144 women and 42 men with new vertebral fractures defined as a decrease in vertebral height of more than 15% on serial radiographs (Ross *et al.*, 1996). The risk (95% CI) of vertebral deformity in men increased with each SD decrement in BMD at the ultradistal radius (1.63; 1.16, 2.29), proximal radius (1.64; 1.16, 2.32), and calcaneus (2.02; 1.49, 2.72), and an interaction term for gender and BMD was not statistically significant. Thus, both cross-sectional and prospective studies suggest that the ability of BMD measurements to predict vertebral fracture risk may be similar between men and women.

Quantitative ultrasound parameters may predict vertebral fracture risk in men. A 1-SD decrease in patellar ultrasound velocity was associated with a 28% increase in the risk of prevalent vertebral deformity (95% CI: 1.06, 1.54) independent of radial bone mass in 182 men ages 50 years and older (Stegman *et al.*, 1996). However, Stewart *et al.* (1995) were unable to demonstrate differences in calcaneal ultrasound attenuation between 38 male vertebral fracture patients and 209 controls of similar age, body weight, and height (96.1 ± 25.3 versus 95.7 ± 24.9 db/MHz, respectively).

The overall size of vertebral bodies also contribute to bone strength (Myers and Wilson, 1997). Women with vertebral fractures have 5–12% smaller cross-sectional area of unfractured vertebrae compared to age, height, and BMD matched controls (Gilsanz *et al.*, 1995). Other prospective studies demonstrate that vertebral dimensions predict vertebral fracture incidence in older women, and that the combination of bone mass and vertebral area predicts fracture risk better than BMD alone (Ross *et al.*, 1995). Thus, measures of vertebral bone mass and size may provide unique information about bone strength and vertebral fracture risk. One cross-sectional study found 11–15% smaller vertebral area and width in 30 men with vertebral fractures compared with 26 age-matched controls (Vega *et al.*, 1998), suggesting that smaller vertebral size may also contribute to increased vertebral fracture risk in men. Furthermore, men have 30–40% larger cross-sectional area and volume of vertebrae compared with women (Gilsanz *et al.*, 1994), and vertebral area increases by 25–30% between the ages of 20 to 80 years in men, but not in women (Mosekilde and Mosekilde, 1990). Thus, greater vertebral size during skeletal development or continuous periosteal growth with aging in men may confer a biomechanical advantage and contribute to lower vertebral fracture risk in men compared with women.

3. Alcohol

Alcohol abuse has been documented in about 7% of men presenting with clinical vertebral fractures (Table IV). A clinic-based, case-control study found twofold greater risk of clinical vertebral fracture among men who reported drinking any alcohol compared those who did not drink (Seeman *et al.*,

TABLE IV Summary of Characteristics of
Men Aged 21 to 90 Years Presenting with
Symptomatic Vertebral Fractures in Selected
Case-Series[a]

	Number (%)
Secondary osteoporosis	228 (57.7)
Steroid therapy	59 (14.9)
Hypogonadism	41 (10.4)
Alcohol abuse	26 (6.6)
Neoplastic disease	14 (3.5)
Gastric or intestinal surgery	14 (3.5)
Nephrolithiasis	7 (1.8)
Anticonvulsant therapy	6 (1.5)
Osteogenesis imperfecta	6 (1.5)
Malabsorption	4 (1.0)
Hyperthyroidism	3 (0.8)
Hemochromatosis	3 (0.8)
Cushings Disease	3 (0.8)
ACTH tumor	2 (0.5)
Addisons Disease	2 (0.5)
Homocystinuria	2 (0.5)
Hyperparathyroidism	2 (0.5)
Neurologic disorders	2 (0.5)
Immobilization	1 (0.3)
Acromegaly	1 (0.3)
Panhypopituitarism	1 (0.3)
Hematologic disorder	1 (0.3)
Childhood rickets	1 (0.3)
Multiple causes	27 (6.8)
Primary osteoporosis	167 (42.3)
Total	395 (100)

[a]Summarized from the following case-series: Seeman *et al.*, 1983; Francis *et al.*, 1989; Baillie *et al.*,
1992; Peris *et al.*, 1995; Kelepouris *et al.*, 1995;
Delichatsio *et al.*, 1995.

1983). In contrast, Diaz *et al.* (1997b) were unable to link the frequency
of alcohol intake to prevalent vertebral deformity risk in a large population-
based study of older European men.

4. Smoking

Cigarette smoking has been associated with an increased risk of clinical
vertebral fractures in two cross-sectional studies. The risk of prevalent thoracic spine fracture was 50% greater among current compared with nonsmokers independent of age and obesity in a study of men aged 15 years and
older (Santavirta *et al.*, 1992). Seeman *et al.* (1983) found twofold greater
risk of clinical vertebral fractures among current smokers compared with

nonsmokers in a clinic-based, case-control study. The risk associated with smoking tended to increase with age and was greatest among the oldest men who both smoked and drank alcohol.

5. Physical Activity

A history of very heavy levels of physical activity (e.g., continuous agricultural and construction work) has been associated with a 50–70% increase in the risk of prevalent vertebral deformity among older men (Silman *et al.*, 1997). Current walking or cycling for a half-hour or more per day was associated with a 20% reduction in the risk of prevalent vertebral deformities in older women, but not among older men (Silman *et al.*, 1997). Others have also found a 50–70% increase in the risk of prevalent thoracic spine fractures associated with agricultural or industrial work (Santavirta *et al.*, 1992), suggesting that vertebral fractures among some older men may be related to trauma earlier in life.

A limited number of cross-sectional (Johansson *et al.*, 1994) and prospective (Nguyen *et al.*, 1996) studies have found that lower muscular strength is also associated with increased vertebral fracture risk in older men. The relative risk (95% CI) of incident clinical vertebral fracture per 10 kg decrease in quadriceps strength was 1.89 (95% CI: 1.33, 2.63) over 5 years in the Dubbo cohort (Nguyen *et al.*, 1996).

6. Anthropometry

Johnell *et al.* (1997) investigated the association between anthropometric measurements and prevalent vertebral deformities in a cross-sectional study of 7454 men ages 50 years and older. Current and self-reported height at age 25 years were not associated with vertebral deformity. Men with the greatest weight gain since age 25 years (>13 kg) had a 20–30% reduction in the risk of vertebral deformities. Heavier current weight was also associated with a 25–37% lower risk of vertebral deformity. The mechanisms linking body weight and weight change to vertebral deformity risk among older men are not clear, but low body mass in later years may be a marker of overall frailty and poor health.

7. Medications

Chronic corticosteroid use is the most common characteristic of men presenting with symptomatic vertebral fractures (Table IV). Systemic steroid use was associated with a twofold (OR: 2.16; 95% CI: 1.14, 4.11) and inhaled steroid use a 38% (95% CI: 0.71, 2.69) greater risk of vertebral fractures compared with never users in a study of male patients with chronic obstructive pulmonary disease (COPD) (McEvoy *et al.*, 1998). Moreover, systemic steroid users were more likely to have multiple and more severe vertebral fractures compared with never users and inhaled steroid users.

Thiazide diuretic use has been associated with greater BMD in men (Wasnich *et al.*, 1983; Morton *et al.*, 1994; Glynn *et al.*, 1995), and a lower prevalence of vertebral compression fractures determined radiographically was found among thiazide users compared with nonusers (3.5% versus 6.3%, respectively) in a study of 1368 older men (Wasnich et al., 1983). However, the number of cases in that study was small, and the difference in prevalence did not achieve statistical significance.

8. Medical Conditions

Hypogonadism is an established cause of osteoporosis in men (Orwoll and Klein, 1995) and has been documented in about 10% of men presenting with clinical vertebral fractures in case series (Table IV). Neoplastic disease is also a common secondary cause of spinal osteoporosis and vertebral fractures in men (Francis et al., 1989; Baillie et al., 1992). A history of peptic ulcer disease (Santavirta et al., 1992) and partial gastrectomy (Mellstrom et al., 1993) may also be important causes of secondary osteoporosis and have been associated with three- to fourfold increases in vertebral fracture risk in men. Men with kidney stones were four times more likely to suffer a clinical vertebral fracture compared to men without stones in a population-based retrospective cohort study (Melton et al., 1998). A history of tuberculosis was associated with a threefold greater risk of prevalent thoracic spine fractures among men but not among women (Santavirta et al., 1992). A number of other endocrinopathies and hereditary disorders have been documented in men with symptomatic vertebral fractures in case-series of men presenting to metabolic bone disease clinics, but current evidence suggests that these other factors make only a minor contribution (Table IV).

9. Primary Osteoporosis

About 40% of men presenting with symptomatic vertebral fractures may have no identifiable secondary cause of osteoporosis (Table IV). We know very little about the pathophysiology of primary osteoporosis in men. In some studies, men with vertebral fractures had about 18–30% lower fractional calcium absorption and $1,25(OH)_2$ vitamin D concentrations compared with controls (Francis et al., 1989; Need et al., 1998). About 40% of men with vertebral fractures and primary osteoporosis had hypercalciuria in one study (Peris et al., 1995). Urinary hydroxyproline excretion may be elevated in some (Resch et al., 1992; Need et al., 1998) but not all (Francis et al., 1989) men with vertebral fractures. Other recent reports have found lower insulin-like growth factor (IGF) I or IGF binding protein 3 levels in men with idiopathic osteoporosis and vertebral fractures (Johansson et al., 1997; Kurland et al., 1997; Ljunghall et al., 1992).

D. Risk Factors for Osteoporotic Fracture

The incidence of all fractures in men increased with age (Nguyen et al., 1996): the incidence (per 10,000 PY) was 177 among men of age 60 to 64;

172, age 65 to 69; 169, age 70 to 74; 343, age 75 to 79; and 811, age ≥80. In a cohort study from Norway, an age-related increase in fracture risk was observed for the weight-bearing skeleton but not for the non-weight-bearing skeleton (Joakimsen *et al.*, 1998). High rates of all fractures were reported among men in the United States living in nursing homes (Rudman and Rudman, 1989).

Radial bone mineral content was associated with fragility fractures (vertebrae, hip, distal forearm, and pelvis) below ages 70 to 80 (Gardsell *et al.*, 1990). A decrease of 1 SD in femoral neck BMD was associated with a relative risk of 1.47 (1.25 to 1.73) (Nguyen *et al.*, 1996). Melton *et al.* (1997) reported that wrist BMD was the best predictor of osteoporotic fracture risk in men, whereas total hip BMD was the strongest predictor of osteoporotic fractures among women. Low patella ultrasound measurements were related to increased risk of self-reported low trauma fractures (Travers-Gustafson *et al.*, 1995). A decrease of 1 SD in the apparent velocity of ultrasound was associated with an odds ratio of 1.69 (1.24 to 2.32).

In multivariate models, age, BMD, quadriceps strength, and body sway were independent predictors of osteoporotic fractures in men (Nguyen *et al.*, 1996). Fractures also tended to occur in men with lower body weight and a previous history of fracture, falls in past 12 months, and shorter current height. Moderate alcohol use and physical activity were associated with a reduced risk of fracture, but neither association was statistically significant. Among Swedish men, a history of falls, vertebral fractures, cerebral disorders, lower grip strength, and weight were all predictive of fragility fractures (Gardsell *et al.*, 1990). The relative risk of osteoporotic fractures was reduced among men with osteoarthritis, but confidence intervals included one (Jones *et al.*, 1995). Finally, hypogonadal men had a greater incidence of fracture (22%) than eugonadal men (4.5%; $p < 0.05$) (Swartz and Young, 1988).

Among the large cohort of men from Sweden, high levels of total physical activity among men age 45 years or older was associated with a 70% decreased risk of fractures at weight bearing sites ($RR = 0.30$; 0.1 to 0.8) but not at non-weight-bearing sites ($RR = 1.0$; 0.6 to 1.7) (Joakimsen *et al.*, 1998). Both leisure time physical activity and physical activity at work were associated with a reduced risk of fractures at weight-bearing sites. There was little difference in the effect of either type of activity on fracture risk (Joakimsen *et al.*, 1998).

E. Risk Factors for Wrist Fractures

Male incidence rates of wrist fracture show little variability with age from age 40 to 70 (Hemenway *et al.*, 1994a; Joakimsen *et al.*, 1998) but appear to increase after age 80 in men: the incidence of distal forearm fracture was 1.21 per 1000 PY among men age of 80 to 84 and 2.64 among men of age 95 to 99 (Baron *et al.*, 1994). There was no association with smoking, alcohol, height, or relative weight and wrist fractures in men (Hemenway *et al.*, 1994a). The only significant risk factor identified was left handedness or being forced to change from left-handed to right-handed.

II. Summary and Future Directions

There have been few prospective studies of risk factors for fracture in men. The cohort studies that have been completed were not specifically designed to answer questions about osteoporotic fractures in older men; hence, many important risk factors were not measured. The number of hip fractures in many studies was small, thereby limiting their statistical power. Few of these studies included men who are at the greatest risk of hip fracture (i.e., those of age ≥ 80 years). Hip fractures in younger men may have a different etiology than osteoporosis.

The most common risk factors examined in these studies were age, anthropometry, smoking, alcohol consumption, and physical activity. In general, the direction of these relationships is similar to that observed among women. Older men have higher fracture rates than younger men. Lower BMI is associated with an increased risk of fractures, but this association may not be independent of weight loss. Aging is accompanied by marked changes in body composition including an increase in fat mass and loss of lean mass. These changes appear to occur in both men and women and could contribute to the increase risk of hip fracture with age. However, nothing is known about whether changes in body composition predict the risk of hip fracture in men.

Men who smoke cigarettes have higher rates of fracture in most studies. In the past, the prevalence of cigarette smoking was greater in men than women in cohort studies of older men (Fingerhut and Warner, 1997). Hence, the attributable risk of fractures associated with cigarette smoking may actually be higher in men than women. However, the prevalence of smoking has been declining in men so there may be a cohort effect with respect to smoking. Little is known about cigar, pipe, smokeless tobacco, or passive smoking and the risk of fracture in men.

Heavy alcohol use or alcohol abuse may increase the risk of fractures. Moderate intakes appear to have little effect on fractures. Higher levels of leisure time physical activity have been associated with reduced hip fracture risk, but essentially nothing is known about historical physical activity. Occupational activity may also be an important risk factor for fractures in men, and this effect may differ by fracture site. For example, certain types of occupational activity may actually increase the risk of vertebral fractures but decrease the risk of hip fractures.

There is a paucity of research on skeletal determinants of fracture in men. In particular, more prospective data are needed on which skeletal sites are the best predictors of fractures. Clinically, DXA is most widely used. Studies need to incorporate these clinical measures for evaluation of their sensitivity and specificity in men as well as use other skeletal determinants of fractures including quantitative ultrasound, geometric measures, and biochemical markers. The high rate of hip fractures among the very old reflects not only skeletal fragility but also an increased risk of falling. No comprehensive prospective study of hip fracture in men which includes both detailed assessment of skeletal status as well as risk of falling has been carried out. Finally, most of the data on fracture risk is limited to white men.

In conclusion, much progress has been made in improving our understanding of the risk factors for fractures in older women. This knowledge has primarily come from large prospective cohort studies such as the Study of Osteoporotic Fractures (Cummings *et al.*, 1995). Similar efforts are needed for men. Large, longitudinal studies with fracture as the outcome, in particular, hip fracture, should be completed. These studies should include a number of skeletal determinants and life-style and environmental risk factors for fractures and falls as well as genetic markers of susceptibility. There is limited information on the association between genetic variation and fracture risk in men. Improving our understanding of the genetics of osteoporosis could help to identify men at greatest risk of fracture. There may also be important interactions between genetic polymorphisms and environmental risk factors. There is an urgent need to complete these studies so that the risks and benefits of certain preventive measures (e.g., calcium and exercise) can be understood. For example, Dawson-Hughes *et al.* (1997) recently showed a reduction in fractures and bone loss in a 3-year clinical trial of calcium and vitamin D supplementation. About half of these subjects were men. Thus, calcium supplementation may be warranted among men considered at high risk of osteoporotic fracture. Finally, several pharmacologic therapies have recently been approved for the prevention and treatment of osteoporosis in women such as the new bisphosphonates. Identification of men at highest risk of fracture because of their risk factors could help to identify men who may be in need of these pharmacologic therapies.

References

Baillie, S. P., Davison, C. E., Johnson, F. J., and Francis, R. M. (1992). Pathogenesis of vertebral crush fractures in men. *Age Ageing* **21**, 139–141.

Baron, J. A., Barrett, J., Malenka, D., Fisher, E., Kniffin, W., Bubolz, T., and Tosteson, T. (1994). Racial differences in fracture risk. *Epidemiology* **5**, 42–47.

Bauer, D. C., Gluer, C. C., Cauley, J. A., Vogt, M., Ensrud, K. E., Genant, H. K., and Black, D. M.: For the Study of the Osteoporotic Fractures Research Group (1997). Broadband ultrasound attenuation predicts fractures strongly and independently of densitometry in older women. *Arch. Intern. Med.* **157**, 629–634.

Bauer, R. L. (1988). Ethnic differences in hip fracture: A reduced incidence in Mexican Americans. *Am. J. Epidemiol.* **127**, 145–149.

Beck, T. J., Ruff, C. B., Scott, W. W., Plato, C. C., Tobin, J. D., and Quan, C. A. (1992). Sex differences in geometry of the femoral neck with aging: A structural analysis of bone mineral data. *Calcif. Tissue Int.* 50, 24–29.

Bikle, D. D., Genant, H. K., Cann, C., Recker, R. R., Halloran, B. P., and Strewler, G. J. (1985). Bone disease in alcohol abuse. *Ann. Intern. Med.* 103, 42–48.

Boonen, S., Vanderschueren, D., Cheng, X. G., Verbeke, G., Dequeker, J., Geusens, P., Broos, P., and Bouillon, R. (1997). Age-related (Type II) femoral neck osteoporosis in men: Biochemical evidence for both hypovitaminosis D- and androgen deficiency-induced bone resorption. *J. Bone Miner. Res.* 12, 2119–2126.

Boyce, W. J., and Vessey, M. P. (1985). Rising incidence of fracture of the proximal femur. *Lancet* 1, 150–151.

Brandenburger, G. H. (1993). Clinical determination of bone quality: Is ultrasound an answer? *Calcif. Tissue Int.* 53, S151–S156.

Burger, H., Van Daele, P. L. A., Grashuis, K., Hofman, A., Grobbee, D. E., Schutte, H. E., Birkenhager, J. C., and Pols, H. A. P. (1997). Vertebral deformities and functional impairment in men and women. *J. Bone Miner. Res.* 12, 152–157.

Butler, M., Norton, R., Lee-Joe, T., Cheng, A., and Campbell, J. A. (1996). The risks of hip fracture in older people from private homes and institutions. *Age Ageing* 25, 381–385.

Center, J. R., Nguyen, T. V., Pocock, N. A., Noakes, K. A., Kelly, P. J., Eisman, J. A., and Sambrook, P. N. (1998). Femoral neck axis length, height loss and risk of hip fracture in males and females. *Osteoporos. Int.* 8, 75–81.

Cooper, C., Barker, D. J. P., and Wickham, C. (1988). Physical activity, muscle strength and calcium intake in fracture of the proximal femur in Britain. *Br. Med. J.* 297, 1443–1446.

Cooper, C., Wickham, C., Lacey, R. F., and Parker, D. J. (1990). Water fluoride concentration and fracture of the proximal femur. *J. Epidemiol. Commun. Health* 44, 17–19.

Cooper, C., Atkinson, E. J., O'Fallon, W. M., and Melton, L. J. III (1992). Incidence of clinically diagnosed vertebral fractures: A population-based study in Rochester, Minnesota, 1985–1989. *J. Bone Miner. Res.* 7, 221–227.

Coupland, C., Wood, D., and Cooper, C. (1993). Physical inactivity is an independent risk factor for hip fracture in the elderly. *J. Epidemiol. Commun. Health* 47, 441–443.

Cumming, R. G., and Klineberg, R. J. (1994). Fall frequency and characteristics and the risk of hip fractures. *J. Am. Geriatr. Soc.* 42, 774–778.

Cummings, S. R., Nevitt, M. C., Browner, W. S., Stone, K., Fox, K. M., Ensrud, K. E., Cauley, J. A., Black, D., and Vogt, T. M.: For The Study Of Osteoporotic Fractures Research Group (1995). Risk factors for hip fracture in white women. Study of osteoporotic fractures research group. *N. Engl. J. Med.* 332, 767–773.

Daniell, H. W. (1997). Osteoporosis after orchiectomy for prostate cancer. *J. Urol.* 157, 439–444.

Dawson-Hughes, B., Harris, S. S., Krall, E. A., and Dallal, G. E. (1997). Effect of calcium and vitamin D supplementation on bone density in men and women 65 years of age or older. *N. Engl. J. Med.* 337, 670–667.

De Laet, C. E. D. H., van Hout, B. A., Burger, H., Hofman, A., and Pols, H. A. P. (1997). Bone density and risk of hip fracture in men and women: Cross sectional analysis. *Br. Med. J.* 315, 221–225.

Delichatsios, H. K., Lane, J. M., and Rivlia, R. S. (1995). Bone histomorphometry in men with spinal osteoporosis. *Calcif. Tissue Int.* 56, 359–363.

Dequeker, J., Johnell, O., and The MEDOS Study Group (1993). Osteoarthritis protects against femoral neck fracture: The MEDOS Study Experience. *Bone* 14, S51–S56.

Diaz, M. N., O'Neill, T. W., and Silman, A. J. (1997a). The influence of family history of hip fracture on the risk of vertebral deformity in men and women: The European Vertebral Osteoporosis Study. *Bone* 20, 145–149.

Diaz, M. N., O'Neill, T. W., and Silman, A. J. (1997b). The influence of alcohol consumption on the risk of vertebral deformity. *Osteoporos. Int.* 7, 65–71.

Falch, J. A., Ilebekk, A., and Slungaard, U. (1985). Epidemiology of hip fractures in Norway. *Acta Orthop. Scand.* **56,** 12–16.

Faulkner, K. G., Cummings, S. R., Black, D., Palermo, L., Gluër, C., and Genant, H. K. (1993). Simple measurement of femoral geometry predicts hip fracture: The Study of Osteoporotic Fractures. *J. Bone Miner. Res.* **9,** 1065–1070.

Felson, D. T., Kiel, D. P., Anderson, J. J., and Kanel, W. B. (1988). Alcohol consumption and hip fractures: The Framingham Study. *Am. J. Epidemiol.* **128,** 1102–1110.

Felson, D. T., Anderson, J. J., Hannan, M. T., Milton, R. C., Wilson, P. W. F., and Kiel, D. P. (1989). Impaired vision and hip fracture: The Farmington Study. *J. Am. Geriatr. Soc.* **37,** 495–500.

Fingerhut, L. A., and Warner, M. (1997). "Injury Chartbook: Health, United States 1996–1997." National Center for Health Statistics, Hyattsville, MD.

Finsen, V., and Benum, P. (1986). Past fractures indicate increased risk of hip fracture. *Acta. Orthop. Scand.* **57,** 337–339.

Forsen, L., Bjorndal, A., Bjarveit, K., Edna, T., Holmen, J., Jessen, V., and Westberg, G. (1994). Interaction between current smoking, leanness, and physical inactivity in the prediction of hip fracture. *J. Bone Miner. Res.* **9,** 1671–1678.

Francis, R. M., Peacock, M., Marshall, D. H., Horsman, A., and Aaron, J. E. (1989). Spinal osteoporosis in men. *Bone Miner.* **5,** 347–357.

Gardsell, P., Johnell, O., and Nilsson, B. E. (1990). The predictive value of forearm bone mineral content measurements in men. *Bone* **11,** 229–232.

Gilsanz, V., Boechat, M. I., Gilsanz, R., Loro, M. L., Roe, T. F., and Goodman, W. (1994). Gender differences in vertebral sizes in adults: Biomechanical implications. *Radiology* **190,** 678–682.

Gilsanz, V., Loro, M. L., Roe, T. F., Sayre, J., Gilsanz, R., and Schulz, E. E. (1995). Vertebral size in elderly women with osteoporosis: Mechanical implications and relationship to fractures. *J. Clin. Invest.* **95,** 2332–2337.

Glynn, N. W., Meilahn, E. N., Charron, M., Anderson, S. T., Kuller, L. H., and Cauley, J. A. (1995). Determinants of bone mineral density in older men. *J. Bone Miner. Res.* **10,** 1769–1777.

Glynn, N. W., Zmuda, J. M., and Cauley, J. A. (1996). Weight change and bone mineral in older men: A longitudinal study. *J. Bone Miner. Res.* **11,** S155.

Grisso, J. A., Chiu, G. Y., Maislin, G., Steinmann, W. C., and Portale, J. (1991). Risk factors for hip fractures in men: A preliminary study. *J. Bone Miner. Res.* **6,** 865–868.

Grisso, J. A., Kelsey, J. L., O'Brien, L. A., Miles, C. G., Sidney, S., Maislin, G., LaPann, K., Moritz, D., and Peters, B., and the Hip Fracture Study Group (1997). Risk factors for hip fracture in men. *Am. J. Epidemiol.* **145,** 786–793.

Heaney, R. P., Barger-Lux, M. J., Davies, K. M., Ryan, R. A., Johnson, M. I., and Gong, G. (1997). Bone dimensional change with age: Interactions of genetic, hormonal, and body size variables. *Osteoporosis Int.* **7,** 426–431.

Hemenway, D., Azrael, D. R., Rimm, E. B., Feskanich, D., and Willet, W. C. (1994a). Risk factors for wrist fracture: Effect of age, cigarettes, alcohol, body height, relative weight, and handedness on the risk for distal forearm fractures in men. *Am. J. Epidemiol.* **140,** 361–367.

Hemenway, D., Azrael, D. R., Rimm, E. B., Feskanich, D., and Willett, W. C. (1994b). Risk factors for hip fracture in US men aged 40 through 75 years. *Am. J. Public Health* **84,** 1843–1845.

Holbrook, T. L., Barrett-Connor, E., and Wingard, D. (1988). Dietary calcium and risk of hip fracture: 14-year prospective population study. *Lancet* **2,** pp. 1046–1049.

Hu, R., Mustard, C. A., and Burns, C. (1996). Epidemiology of incident spinal fracture in a complete population. *Spine* **21,** 492–499.

Ito, M., Hayashi, K., Yamada, M., Uetani, M., and Nakamura, T. (1993). Relationship of osteophytes to bone mineral density and spinal fracture in men. *Radiology* **189,** 497–502.

Jackson, J. A., Riggs, M. W., and Spiekerman, A. M. (1992). Testosterone deficiency as a risk factor for hip fractures in men: A Case-Control Study. *Am. J. Med. Sci.* **304,** 4–8.

Jacobsen, S. J., Goldberg, J., Miles, T. P., Brody, J. A., Stiers, W., and Rimm, A. A. (1990). Hip fracture incidence among the old and very old: A population-based study of 745,435 cases. *Am. J. Public Health* **80,** 871–873.

Jacobsen, S. J., Cooper, C., Gottlieb, M. S., Goldberg, J., Yahnke, D. P., and Melton, L. J., III. (1992a). Hospitalization with vertebral fracture among the aged: A National Population-Based Study, 1986–1989. *Epidemiology* **3,** 515–518.

Jacobsen, S. J., Goldberg, J., Cooper, C., and Lockwood, S. A. (1992b). The association between water fluoridation and hip fracture among white women and men aged 65 years and older. *Ann. Epidemiol.* **2,** 617–626.

Joakimsen, R. M., Fønnebø, V., Magnus, J. H., Størmer, J., Tollan, A., and Søgaard, J. (1998). The Tromsø Study: Physical activity and the incidence of fractures in a middle-aged population. *J. Bone Miner. Res.* **13,** 1149–1157.

Johansson, A. G., Eriksen, E. F., Lindh, E., Langdahl, B., Blum, W. F., Lindahl, A., Ljunggren, O., and Ljunghall, S. (1997). Reduced serum levels of the growth hormone-dependent insulin-like growth factor binding protein and a negative bone balance at the level of individual remodeling units in idiopathic osteoporosis in men. *J. Clin. Endocrinol. Metab.* **82,** 2795–2798.

Johansson, C., Mellstrom, D., Rosengren, K., and Rundgren, A. (1994). A community-based population study of vertebral fractures in 85-year-old men and women. *Age Ageing* **114,** 388–392.

Johnell, O., O'Neill, T., Felsenberg, D., Kanis, J., Cooper, C., and Silman, A. J. (1997). Anthropometric measurements and vertebral deformities. *Am. J. Epidemiol.* **146,** 287–293.

Jones, G., Nguyen, T., Sambrook, P. N., Lord, S. R., Kelly, P. J., and Eisman, J. A. (1995). Osteoarthritis, bone density, postural stability, and osteoporotic fractures: A population based study. *J. Rheumatol.* **22,** 921–925.

Jones, G., White, C., Nguyen, T., Sambrook, P. N., and Kelly, P. J., and Eisman, J. A. (1996). Prevalent vertebral deformities: Relationship to bone mineral density and spinal osteophytosis in elderly men and women. *Osteoporosis Int.* **6,** 233–239.

Jouanny, P., Guillemin, F., Kuntz, C., Jeandel, C., and Pourel, J. (1995). Environmental and genetic factors affecting bone mass: Similarity of bone density among members of healthy families. *Arthritis Rheum.* **38,** 61–67.

Karagas, M. R., Baron, J. A., Barrett, J. A., and Jacobsen, S. J. (1996a). Patterns of fracture among the United States elderly: Geographic and fluoride effects. *Ann. Epidemiol.* **6,** 209–216.

Karagas, M. R., Lu-Yao, G. L., Barrett, J. A., Beach, M. L., and Baron, J. A. (1996b). Heterogeneity of hip fracture: Age, race, sex, and geographic patterns of femoral neck and trochanteric fractures among the US elderly. *Am. J. Epidemiol.* **143,** 677–682.

Karlsson, M. K., Johnell, O., Nihlsson, B. E., Sernbo, I., and Obrant, K. J. (1993). Bone mineral mass in hip fracture patients. *Bone* **14,** 161–165.

Karlsson, K. M., Sernbo, I., Obrant, K. J., Redlund-Johnell, I., and Johnell, O. (1996). Femoral neck geometry and radiographic signs of osteoporosis as predictors of hip fracture. *Bone* **18,** 327–330.

Kelepouris, N., Harper, K. D., Gannon, F., Kaplan, F. S., and Haddad, J. G. (1995). Severe osteoporosis in men. *Ann. Intern. Med.* **123,** 452–460.

Kurland, E. S., Rosen, C. J., Cosman, F., McMahon, D., Chan, F., Shane, E., Lindsay, R., Dempster, D., and Bilezikian, J. P. (1997). Insulin-like growth factor-I in Idiopathic osteoporosis. *J. Clin. Endocrinol. Metab.* **82,** 2799–2805.

LaCroix, A. Z., Weinpahl, J., White, L. R., Wallace, R. B., Scherr, P. A., George, L. K., Cornoni-Huntley, J., and Ostfield, A. M. (1990). Thiazide diuretic agents and the incidence of hip fracture. *N. Engl. J. Med.* **322,** 286–290.

Langlois, J. A., Pahor, M., Bauer, D., and Havlik, R. (1997). Calcium channel blocker use and risk of hip fracture in old age. *J. Bone Miner. Res.* **12,** S359 (abstract).

Langlois, J. A., Visser, M., Davidovic, L. S., Maggi, S., Li, G., and Harris, T. (1998). Hip fracture risk in older white men is associated with change in body weight from age 50 years to old age. *Arch. Intern. Med.* **158**, 990–996.

Larsson, K., Ljunghall, S., Krusemo, U. B., Naessen, T., Lindh, E., and Persson, I. (1993). The risk of hip fractures in patients with primary hyperparathyroidism: A population-based cohort study with a follow-up of 19 years. *J. Intern. Med.* **234**, 585–593.

Lau, E., Donnan, S., Barker, D. J. P., and Cooper, C. (1988). Physical activity and calcium intake in fracture of the proximal femur in Hong Kong. *Br. Med. J.* **297**, 1441–1443.

Lehmann, R., Wapniarz, M., Hofman, B., Pieper, B., Haubitz, I., and Allolio, B. (1998). Drinking water fluoridation: Bone mineral density and hip fracture incidence. *Bone* **22**, 273–278.

Ling, X., Aimin, L., Xihe, Z., Xiaoshu, C., and Cummings, S. R. (1996). Very low rates of hip fracture in Beijing, People's Republic of China. *Am. J. Epidemiol.* **144**, 901–907.

Ljunghall, S., Johansson, A. G., Burman, P., Kampeo, L. E., and Karlsson, F. A. (1992). Low plasma levels of insulin-loke growth factor 1 (IGF-1) in male patients with idiopathic osteoporosis. *J. Intern. Med.* **232**, 59–64.

Lunt, M., Felsenberg, D., Reeve, J., Benevolenskaya, L., Cannata, J., Dequeker, J., Dodenhof, C., Falch, J. A., Masaryk, P., Pols, H. A. P., Poor, G., Reid, D. M., Scheidt-Nave, C., Weber, K., Verlow, J., Kanis, J. A., O'Neill, T. W., and Silman, A. J. (1997). Bone density variation and its its effects on risk of vertebral deformity in men and women studied in thirteen European centers: The EVOS Study. *J. Bone Miner. Res.* **12**, 1883–1894.

Mallmin, H., Ljunghall, S., Persson, I., Naessen, T., Krusemo, U., and Bergstrom, R. (1993). Fracture of the distal forearm as a forecaster of subsequent hip fracture: A population-based cohort study with 24 years of follow-up. *Calcif. Tissue Int.* **52**, 269–272.

Mann, T., Oviatt, S. K., Wilson, D., Nelson, D., and Orwoll, E. S. (1992). Vertebral deformity in men. *J. Bone Miner. Res.* **7**, 1259–1265.

Marshall, D., Johnell, O., and Wedel, H. (1996). Meta-analysis of how well measures of bone mineral density predict occurrence of osteoporosis fractures. *Br. Med. J.* **312**, 1254–1259.

McEvoy, C. E., Ensrud, K. E., Bender, E., Genant, H. K., Yu, W., Griffith, J. M., and Niewhoehner, D. E. (1998). Association between corticosteroid use and vertebral fractures in older men with chronic obstructive pulmonary disease. *Am. J. Respir. Crit. Care Med.* **157**, 704–709.

Mellstrom, D., Johansson, C., Johnell, O., Linstedt, G., Lundberg, P.-A., Obrant, K., Schoon, I.-M., Toss, G., and Ytterberg, B.-O. (1993). Osteoporosis, metabolic aberrations, and increased risk for vertebral fractures after partial gastrectomy. *Calcif. Tissue Int.* **53**, 370–377.

Melton, L. J., III, O'Fallon, W. M., and Riggs, B. L. (1987). Secular trends in the incidence of hip fractures. *Calcif. Tissue Int.* **41**, 57–64.

Melton, L. J., III, Atkinson, E. J., O'Connor, M. K., O'Fallon, W. M., and Riggs, B. L. (1997). Fracture prediction by BMD in men versus women. *J. Bone Miner. Res.* **12**, F543.

Melton, L. J., III, Crowson, C. S., Khosla, S., Wilson, D. M., and O'Fallon, W. M. (1998). Fracture risk among patients with urolithiasis—a population-based cohort study. *Kidney Int.* **53**, 459–464.

Meyer, H. E., Tverdal, A., and Falch, J. A. (1993). Risk factors for hip fractures in middle-aged Norwegian women and men. *Am. J. Epidemiol.* **137**, 1203–1211.

Meyer, H. E., Tverdal, A., and Falch, J. A. (1995). Body height, body mass index, and fatal hip fractures: 16 years' follow-up of 674,000 Norwegian women and men. *Epidemiology* **6**, 299–305.

Meyer, H. E., Pederson, J. I., Loken, E. B., and Tverdal, A. (1997). Dietary factors and the incidence of hip fracture in middle-aged Norwegians. *Am. J. Epidemiol.* **145**, 117–123.

Morton, D. J., Barrett-Connor, E. L., and Edelstein, S. L. (1994). Thiazides and bone mineral density in elderly men and women. *Am. J. Epidemiol.* **139**, 1107–1115.

Mosekilde, L., and Mosekilde, L. (1990). Sex differences in age-related changes in vertebral body size, density and biomechanical competence in normal individuals. *Bone* **11**, 67–73.

Mussolino, M. E., Looker, A. C., Madans, J. H., Langlois, J. A., and Orwoll, E. S. (1998). Risk factors for hip fracture in white men: The NHANES I Epidemiologic Follow-up Study. *J. Bone Miner. Res.* **13**, 918–924.

Myers, E. R., and Wilson, S. E. (1997). Biomechanics of osteoporosis and vertebral fracture. *Spine* **22**, 25S–31S.

Naessen, T., Parker, R., Persson, I., Zack, M., and Adami, H.-O. (1989). Time trends in incidence rates of first hip fracture in the Uppsala health care region, Sweden, 1965–1983. *Am. J. Epidemiol.* **130**, 289–299.

Need, A. G., Morris, H. A., Horowitz, M., Scopacasa, F., and Nordin, B. E. C. (1998). Intestinal calcium absorption in men with spinal osteoporosis. *Clin. Endocrinol.* **48**, 163–168.

Nguyen, T. V., Eisman, J. A., Kelly, P. J., and Sambrook, P. N. (1996). Risk factors for osteoporotic fractures in elderly men. *Am. J. Epidemiol.* **144**, 255–263.

Nguyen, T. V., Heath, H., Bryant, S. C., O'Fallon, W. M., and Melton, L. J. (1997). Fractures after thyroidectomy in men: A population-based cohort study. *J. Bone Miner. Res.* **12**, 1092–1099.

Nyquist, F., Gardsell, P., Sernbo, I., Jeppsson, J. O., and Johnell, O. (1998). Assessment of sex hormones and bone mineral density in relation to occurrence of fracture in men: A prospective population-based study. *Bone* **22**, 147–151.

Obrant, K. J., Bengner, U., Johnell, O., Nilsson, B. E., and Sernbo, I. (1989). Increasing age-adjusted risk of fragility fractures: A sign of increasing osteoporosis in successive generations? *Calcif. Tissue Int.* **44**, 157–167.

O'Neill, T. W., Felsenberg, D., Varlow, J., Cooper, C., Kanis, J. A., and Silman, A. J. (1996). The prevalence of vertebral deformity in European men and women: The European Vertebral Osteoporosis Study. *J. Bone Miner. Res.* **11**, 1010–1018.

Orwoll, E. S., and Klein, R. F. (1995). Osteoporosis in men. *Endocr. Rev.* **16**, 87–116.

Owen, R. A., Melton, L. J., Ilstrup, D. M., Johnson, K. A., and Riggs, B. L. (1982). Colles' fracture and subsequent hip fracture risk. *Clin. Orthop.* **171**, 37–43.

Paganini-Hill, A., Chao, A., Ross, R. K., and Henderson, B. E. (1991). Exercise and other factors in the prevention of hip fracture: The Leisure World Study. *Epidemiology* **2**, 16–25.

Peris, P., Guanabens, N., Monegal, A., Suris, X., Alvarez, L., Desoba, M. J. M., Hernandez, M., and Gomez, J. M. (1995). Aetiology and presenting symptoms in male osteoporosis. *Br. J. Rheumatol.* **34**, 936–941.

Poor, G., Atkinson, E. J., Lewallen, D. G., O'Fallon, W. M., and Melton, L. J., III. (1995a). Age-related hip fractures in men: Clinical spectrum and short-term outcomes. *Osteoporosis Int.* **5**, 419–426.

Poor, G., Atkinson, E. J., O'Fallon, W. M., and Melton, L. J., III. (1995b). Predictors of hip fractures in elderly men. *J. Bone Miner. Res.* **10**, 1900–1907.

Ray, N. F., Chan, J. K., Thaner, M., and Melton, L. J., III. (1997). Medical expenditures for the treatment of osteoporotic fractures in the United States in 1995: Report from the National Osteoporosis Foundation. *J. Bone Miner. Res.* **12**, 24–35.

Ray, W. A., Griffin, M. R., West, R., Strand, L., and Melton, L. J., III. (1990). Incidence of hip fracture in Saskatchewan, Canada, 1976–1985. *Am. J. Epidemiol.* **131**, 502–509.

Resch, A., Schneider, B., Bernecker, P., *et al.* (1995). Risk of vertebral fractures in men: Relationship to mineral density of the vertebral body. *AJR Am. J. Roentgenol.* **164**, 1447–1450.

Resch, H., Pietschmann, P., Woloszczuk, W., Krexner, E., Bernecker, P., and Willvonseder, R. (1992). Bone mass and biochemical parameters of bone metabolism in men with spinal osteoporosis. *Eur. J. Clin. Invest.* **22**, 542–545.

Ross, P. D., Davis, J. W., Vogel, J. M., and Wasnich, R. D. (1990). A critical review of bone mass and the risk of fractures in osteoporosis. *Calcif. Tissue Int.* **46**, 149–161.

Ross, P. D., Norimatsu, H., Davis, J. W., Yano, K., Wasnich, R. D., Fujiwara, S., Hosoda, Y., and Melton, L. J. (1991). A comparison of hip fracture incidence among native Japanese, Japanese Americans, and American Caucasians. *Am. J. Epidemiol.* **133**, 801–809.

Ross, P. D., Huang, C., Davis, J. W., and Wasnich, R. D. (1995). Vertebral dimension measurements improve prediction of vertebral fracture incidence. *Bone* **16**, 257S–262S.

Ross, P. D., Kim, S., and Wasnich, R. D. (1996). Bone density predicts vertebral fracture risk in both men and women. *J. Bone Miner. Res.* **11**, 132 (abstr.).

Rudman, I. W., and Rudman, D. (1989). High rate of fractures for men in nursing homes. *Am. J. Phys. Med. Rehabil.* **68**, 2–5.

Santavirta, S., Konttinen, Y. T., Heliovaara, M., Knekt, P., Luthje, P., and Aromaa, A. (1992). Determinants of osteoporotic thoracic vertebral fracture. Screening of 57,000 Finnish women and men. *Acta Orthop. Scand.* **63**, 198–202.

Sattin, R. W., Lambert Huber, D. A., DeVito, C. A., Rodriguez, J. G., Ros, A., Bacchelli, S., Stevens, J. A., and Waxweiler, R. J. (1990). The incidence of fall injury events among the elderly in a defined population. *Am. J. Epidemiol.* **131**, 1028–1037.

Schwartz, A. V., Kelsey, J. L., Sidney, S., and Grisso, J. A. (1998). Characteristics of falls and risk of hip fracture in elderly men. *Osteoporosis Int.* **8**, 240–246.

Seeman, E., Melton, L. J., III, O'Fallon, W. M., and Riggs, B. L. (1983). Risk factors for spinal osteoporosis in men. *Am. J. Med.* **75**, 977–983.

Silman, A. J., O'Neill, T. W., Cooper, C., Kanis, J., and Felsenberg, D. (1997). Influence of physical activity on vertebral deformity in men and women: Results from the European Vertebral Osteoporosis Study. *J. Bone Miner. Res.* **12**, 813–819.

Silverman, S. L., and Madison, R. E. (1988). Decreased incidence of hip fracture in Hispanics, Asians, and Blacks: California Hospital Discharge Data. *Am. J. Public Health* **78**, 1482–1483.

Soroko, S. B., Barrett-Connor, E., Edelstein, S. L., and Kritz-Silverstein, D. (1994). Family history of osteoporosis and bone mineral density at the axial skeleton: the Rancho Bernardo study. *J. Bone Miner. Res.* **9**, 761–769.

Stanley, H. L., Schmitt, B. P., Poses, R. M., and Deiss, W. P. (1991). Does hypogonadism contribute to the occurrence of a minimal trauma hip fracture in elderly men? *J. Am. Geriatr. Soc.* **39**, 766–771.

Stegman, M. R., Davies, K. M., Heaney, R. P., Recker, R. R., and Lappe, J. M. (1996). The association of patellar ultrasound transmissions and forearm densitometry with vertebral fracture, number and severity: The Saunders County Bone Quality Study. *Osteoporosis Int.* **6**, 130–135.

Stewart, A., Felsenberg, D., Kalidis, L., and Reid, D. M. (1995). Vertebral fractures in men and women: How discriminative are bone mass measurements? *Br. J. Radiol.* **68**, 614–620.

Swartz, C. M., and Young, M. A. (1988). Male hypogonadism and bone fracture. *N. Engl. J. Med.* Letter to Editor, p. 996.

Thiebaud, D., Burckhardt, P., Costanza, M., Sloutskis, D., Gilliard, D., Quinodoz, F., Jacquet, A. F., and Burnand, B. (1997). Importance of albumin, 25(OH)-vitamin D and IGFBP-3 as risk factors in elderly women and men with hip fracture. *Osteoporosis Int.* **7**, 457–462.

Townsend, M. F., Sanders, W. H., Northway, R. O., and Graham, S. D. (1997). Bone fractures associated with lutenizing hormone-releasing hormone agonists used in the treatment of prostate carcinoma. *Cancer (Philadelphia)* **79**, 45–50.

Travers-Gustafson, D., Stegman, M. R., Heaney, R. P., and Recker, R. R. (1995). Ultrasound, densitometry, and extraskeletal appendicular fracture risk factors: A cross-sectional report on the Saunders County Bone Quality Study. *Calcif. Tissue Int.* **57**, 267–271.

Tsai, K., Twu, S., Chieng, P., Yang, R., and Lee, T. (1996). Prevalence of vertebral fractures in Chinese men and women in urban Taiwanese communities. *Calcif. Tissue Int.* **59**, 249–253.

Vega, E., Ghiringhelli, G., Mautalen, C., Valzacchi, G. R., Scaglia, H., and Zylberstein, C. (1998). Bone mineral density and bone size in men with primary osteoporosis and vertebral fractures. *Calcif. Tissue Int.* **52**, 465–469.

Wasnich, R. D., Benfante, R. J., Yano, K., Heilbrun, L., and Vogel, J. M. (1983). Thiazide effect on the mineral content of bone. *N. Engl. J. Med.* **309**, 344–347.

Zmuda, J. M., Cauley, J. A., Ferrell, R. E. (1999). Recent progress in understanding the genetic susceptibility to osteoporosis. *Genet. Epidemiol.* (in press).

Chapter 19

John P. Bilezikian[*,†]
Etah S. Kurland[*]
Clifford J. Rosen[‡]

Departments of *Medicine and †Pharmacology
College of Physicians and Surgeons
Columbia University
New York, New York
‡St. Joseph Hospital
Bangor, Maine

Idiopathic Osteoporosis in Men

I. Introduction

Only in the past decade has attention been focused upon the increasingly important problem of osteoporosis in men. In a biomedical world that has invested its investigative resources in the gender affected most by osteoporosis, progress has previously been limited to insights gained about women. We have not learned much about how the same disorder may affect men. The mind set of studying osteoporosis in women rather exclusively, because women are most often affected by osteoporosis, has led not only to a paucity of information about osteoporosis in men but also to a tendency to assume that what is the case for women is necessarily also the case for men. In addition, the rather exclusive focus on women has undoubtedly led to an underreporting of the problem in men. Despite the dearth of information about osteoporosis in men, a cohort has emerged in whom no clear-cut etiologies are evident. Osteoporosis in such men is termed "idiopathic." In this chapter, we will describe this interesting group of individuals with respect to risk factors, clinical characteristics, possible etiologies, therapeutic approaches, and directions for needed research.

II. Definition

If one surveys a typical population of men with osteoporosis, several etiologies will surface frequently. They are alcohol abuse, glucocorticoid excess (either endogenous-Cushing's syndrome or, more commonly, chronic glucocorticoid therapy), and hypogonadism (Orwoll and Klein, 1995; Klein and Orwoll, 1994). In addition, other etiologies are important to consider, including primary hyperparathyroidism, excessive thyroid hormone exposure (hyperthyroidism or overtreatment with thyroid hormone), multiple myeloma and other malignancies, anticonvulsant use, gastrointestinal disorders, and high dose chemotherapeutics (Scane *et al.*, 1993; Seeman, 1993; Scane and Francis, 1993). A listing of etiologies of osteoporosis in men is found in Table I. Idiopathic osteoporosis can be defined simply as osteoporosis that occurs without any known cause.

In most series that have been reported, the number of men whose osteoporosis remains unexplained after a routine evaluation is approximately 50% (Parfitt and Duncan, 1982; Seeman *et al.*, 1983; Francis *et al.*, 1989; Baillie *et al.*, 1992; Resch *et al.*, 1992). It is difficult to be sure of the "real" incidence of idiopathic osteoporosis because many series come from referral centers that tend to attract small numbers of more unusual patients. Such series might therefore overestimate the proportion of men with unexplained disease. With modern diagnostic tools and greater insight into the mechanisms of bone loss in this population, the number of men whose osteoporosis cannot be explained will inevitably tend to decline. Nevertheless, in the broadest terms, a reasonable estimate is between 40 and 60% of the known osteoporotic male population (Parfitt and Duncan, 1982; Seeman *et al.*, 1983; Francis *et al.*, 1989; Baillie *et al.*, 1992; Resch *et al.*, 1992).

We also suggest that the diagnosis of idiopathic osteoporosis be applied only to men under the age of 70 years. By that stage of life it is to be expected that the poorly understood process of age-related bone loss has inevitably occurred, a phenomenon quite distinct from the unexpected appearance of osteoporosis in a younger man. Moreover, in older men with osteoporosis, it is more likely that the disease is at least in part the result of the cumulative effects of factors that affected skeletal health earlier in life (e.g., failure to achieve adequate peak bone mass, calcium undernutrition, inadequate exercise, and declines in gonadal hormones) (Finkelstein *et al.*, 1987, 1992, 1996; Bendavid *et al.*, 1996; Mussolino *et al.*, 1998; Stepan *et al.*, 1989; Francis

TABLE I   Secondary Causes of Osteoporosis in Men

I. Hormonal
  Hypogonadism
  Cushing's syndrome
  Hyperthyroidism
  Hyperparathyroidism (1° or 2°)

II. Medication/drug-related
  Glucocorticoids
  Anticonvulsants
  Thyroid hormone
  Alcohol
  High-dose or long-term chemotherapeutics (methotrexate)

III. Genetic
  Osteogenesis imperfecta (adult form)
  Homocystinuria

IV. Gastrointestinal
  Malabsorption syndromes
  Primary biliary cirrhosis
  Postgastrectomy

V. Systemic illnesses
  Mastocytosis
  Rheumatoid arthritis
  Multiple myeloma
  Other malignancies

VI. Other
  Hypercalciuria

---

et al., 1986; Garn *et al.*, 1992; Hannan *et al.*, 1992; Comston *et al.*, 1989; Smith and Walker, 1964; Brockstedt *et al.*, 1993; Nicolas *et al.*, 1994) but are not now identifiable. Again, this situation should be considered pathophysiologically different from that affecting younger men with osteoporosis of uncertain cause.

III. Characteristics of Idiopathic Osteoporosis in Men

Fracture or symptomatic back pain is the most characteristic presenting feature of idiopathic male osteoporosis. This feature is quite different from the typical postmenopausal woman with osteoporosis in whom the diagnosis is more likely made by bone mass measurement. Selective screening of the female population at risk for osteoporosis more often leads to the recognition of osteoporosis well before clinical sequellae (height loss, back pain, or overt fractures) have developed (Epstein and Miller, 1997). In men, it is still uncommon for bone mass measurement to be obtained, even in the presence of clear-cut risk factors for the disease. In virtually all series that have been published on this subject (Francis et al., 1989; Jackson et al., 1987; Khosla et al., 1994; Kelepouris et al., 1995; Jackson and Kleerekoper, 1990; Ljung-hall et al., 1992; Reed et al., 1995; Pacifici, 1997; Kurland et al., 1997), the initial presentation has been fracture or back pain.

Kurland and her associates have recently reported 24 men who appear to be quite representative of the syndrome. All patients were under 70 years of age (mean 50.5 ± 1.9 yr, range 29–67). Seventeen men (71%) came to medical attention because of fracture. Thirteen had experienced vertebral fractures; 3 had sustained stress fractures of the lower extremities; and 1 broke his hip. The remaining seven patients were evaluated for unexplained back pain. Although routine x-rays of the spine did not reveal fracture, osteopenia was apparent. Subsequently, osteoporosis was established by dual energy x-ray absorptiometry (DEXA). None of the men were alcohol abusers, but 38% did have a history of prior smoking. All men enjoyed an active life-style with many involved in a formal daily exercise program. Average daily calcium intake was over 1400 mg calcium. Gonadal, hepatic, and adrenal functions were normal. Other characteristics of the group are illustrated in Tables II and III. Serum calcium, phosphorus, 25-hydroxyvitamin D, 1,25-dihydroxyvitamin D, and TSH were all normal. Although the mean parathyroid hormone (PTH) concentration was also normal (25 ± 2.2 pg/ml-nl, 10–65), this is somewhat lower than one might expect for a group of 50-year-old men. Moreover, five patients had PTH values no greater than 15 pg/ml. Typical of most modern series of men with idiopathic osteoporosis (Kelepouris et al., 1995; Reed et al., 1995), hypercalciuria was not present. The average urinary calcium concentration was 158 ± 15 mg/g Cr (Table III). Serum and urinary markers of bone turnover were all normal albeit in the lower end of the normal range. In general, markers of bone

TABLE II   Markers of Bone Turnover

Parameter	Mean ± SEM	Normal range
Urinary calcium excretion (mg/g creatinine)	158 ± 15	150–300
Free pyridinoline (nmol/mmol creatinine)	19.5 ± 1.4	8–71
N-Telopeptide (nmol BCE/mmol creatinine)	26.0 ± 3.1	12–105
Osteocalcin (ng/mL)	5.67 ± .39	2.4–11.7
Bone-specific alkaline phosphatase (BASP, ng/mL)	11.6 ± 1.1	2.9–20.1
Procollagen (PICP, ng/mL)	96.8 ± 5.7	50–170

Reprinted with permission from Kurland et al., Insulin-like growth factor-1 in men with idiopathic osteoporosis, J. Clin. Endocrinol. Metab. **82**, 2799–2805, 1997, © The Endocrine Society.

TABLE III   Relationship among Serum IGF-I, Osteocalcin, and Bone Density
at the Spine, Hip, and Radius

	IGF-I		*Osteocalcin*	
	Correlation coefficient	*p value*	*Correlation coefficient*	*p value*
Lumbar spine BMD	+0.39	<0.001	+0.2	0.29
Femoral neck BMD	+0.05	0.61	+0.1	0.58
1/3 site distal radius BMD	+0.04	0.69	+0.44	<0.002

Reprinted with permission from Kurland *et al.*, Insulin-like growth-factor 1 in men with idiopathic osteoporosis, *J. Clin. Endocrinol. Metab.* **82,** 2799–2805, 1997, © The Endocrine Society.

resorption correlated well with markers of bone formation, suggesting that there was no obvious disturbance of the coupling between bone formation and bone resorption. Bone mass measurement by DEXA revealed marked reductions at the lumbar spine, hip, and forearm (Figure 1). T-scores were -3.50 ± 0.15 at the lumbar spine; -3.03 ± 0.15 at the femoral neck; and -2.12 ± 0.26 at the distal radius (1/3 site).

Eighteen men underwent percutaneous bone biopsy (Table IV). To quantify dynamic indices, they were prepared with two time-spaced doses of tetracycline. Bone volume was reduced by 31% ($p < 0.001$). Cortical width

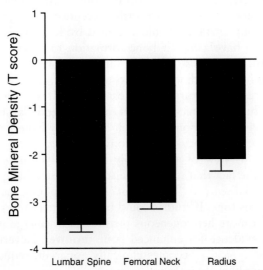

FIGURE 1   Bone density in men with idiopathic osteoporosis. T-scores for three sites are shown ± SEM. Marked reductions are seen at all sites. Reprinted with permission from E. S. Kurland *et al.* (1997). Insulin-like growth factor-I in men with idiopathic osteoporosis. *J. Clin. Endocrinol. Metab.* **82,** 2799–2806, © The Endocrine Society.

TABLE IV   Bone Histomorphometry

Parameter	Osteoporotic	Normal	p value
Bone volume (%)	13.3 ± 4.7	19.3 ± 3.1	0.001
Cortical width (μm)	776.6 ± 317.2	1081 ± 331	0.05
Eroded surface (%)	3.8 ± 1.3	3.5 ± 1.6	NS
Osteoid surface (%)	9.6 ± 4.5	14.4 ± 5.9	0.01
Mineralizing surface (%)	7.6 ± 4.7	18.3 ± 7.5	0.001
Mineral apposition rate (μm/day)	0.7 ± 0.07	0.68 ± 0.16	NS
Bone formation rate (μm³/μm²/day)	0.06 ± 0.03	0.13 ± 0.07	0.01
Adjusted apposition rate (μm/day)	0.56 ± 0.25	0.58 ± 0.22	NS

Reprinted with permission from Kurland *et al.*, Insulin-like growth factor-1 in men with idiopathic osteoporosis, *J. Clin. Endocrinol. Metab.* **82**, 2799–2805, 1997, © The Endocrine Society.

was reduced by 28% ($p < 0.05$); osteoid surface, by 33% ($p < 0.01$), and bone formation rate, by an impressive 54% ($p < 0.04$. Mineralizing surface was reduced by 42% ($p < 0.001$). Eroded surface was not increased. This profile suggests a low turnover state. Similar results were obtained in men studied by Jackson *et al.* (1987), Jackson and Kleerekoper (1990), Kelepouris *et al.* (1995), and Reed *et al.* (1995). In addition, DeVernejoul *et al.* (1983), Khosla *et al.* (1994), and Darby and Meunier (1981) and Johansson *et al.* (1997) reported reduction in mean wall thickness, the amount of bone deposited by the osteoblast in each remodeling unit. Jackson *et al.* (1987; Jackson and Kleerekoper, 1990), also demonstrated significantly reduced osteoblastic surface. The only noteworthy exception among these studies is the youngest group (<44 years old), studied by Kelepouris *et al.* (1995), who appeared to have a higher bone formation rate than the older men (>44 years old). From these results a rather uniform histomorphometric picture emerges in men with idiopathic osteoporosis. It is characterized best by reduced indices of bone turnover (Khosla, 1997). It is much different from the active bone turnover typically seen in early hypogonadal states and other disorders associated with bone loss such as primary hyperparathyroidism, hyperthyroidism, malignancy, and anticonvulsant use.

Tempering this view of a uniformly low turnover state in idiopathic osteoporosis is the fact that most of the series reported have involved men with far advanced disease. A "burned out" histomorphometric picture might be expected at this time. If studies could be conducted earlier in the course of the disease, a more heterogeneous picture might emerge with some patients showing evidence for enhanced bone turnover. Nevertheless, at the time the disease typically becomes clinically apparent, reduced indices of bone turnover are likely to be found.

There is a subset of men with osteoporosis characterized by hypercalciuria (Jackson *et al.*, 1987; Reed *et al.*, 1995; Perry *et al.*, 1982) and biochemical indices that suggest high bone turnover (Resch *et al.*, 1992). Although osteoporotic men with hypercalciuria may represent a subset of idiopathic osteoporosis, or in fact a phenotype that surfaces earlier in the course of the disease, they appear to be different from the group under discussion. In the study of Reed *et al.* (1995), low turnover was seen along with hypercalciuria in some patients. Although, in these cases, one could point to hypercalciuria, with or without accelerated bone resorption, as being "etiological," and therefore not part of the syndrome of idiopathic osteoporosis, the mechanisms of bone loss in men with hypercalciuria are still not clear (Ghazalie *et al.*, 1997; Pacifici, 1997). It remains to be seen how this subgroup of men with osteoporosis will relate to the larger group being discussed in this chapter.

IV. Etiological Considerations

This section considers possible etiologies for the syndrome of idiopathic osteoporosis in men. Obviously, the topics considered in this section are discussed as hypotheses. By no means have they been established as causes. We have been necessarily selective because data are in general sparse, and it is not useful to consider all conceivable etiologies for this syndrome. A review of information for which data have recently become available exemplifies the kinds of research directions being taken by investigators in the field.

A. Insulin-like Growth Factor-I

Growth factors for bone are being increasingly recognized for their pivotal role in establishing and maintaining skeletal mass (Canalis, 1995; Canalis *et al.*, 1993). Insulin-like growth factor-I (IGF-I) has received attention because it appears to be one of the most abundant skeletal growth factors, and it is essential for osteoblast function (Jones and Clemmons, 1995; Rajaram *et al.*, 1997; Canalis, 1997). Studies by Rosen and his colleagues have provided intriguing evidence for the possibility that the genetic regulation of IGF-I might be determinant of peak bone mass in the mouse (Beamer *et al.*, 1996; Rosen *et al.*, 1997). In human subjects, too, evidence is accumulating that IGF-I might play an important role (Romagnoli *et al.*, 1994; Boonen *et al.*, 1996; Fall *et al.*, 1998). The first reports of low IGF-I levels in men with idiopathic osteoporosis came from Ljunghall *et al.* (1992). In their study of 12 middle-aged men, a significant reduction in IGF-I values was noted and shown to be correlated with bone density of the spine and forearm. Similarly, in a group of 18 men with osteoporosis, Reed and her colleagues (1995) showed that IGF-I levels were reduced.

The patients reported by Kurland *et al.* (1997) support a potential role for deficient IGF-I in this syndrome. The mean IGF-I concentration was reduced in men with idiopathic osteoporosis when compared to that of a group of normal men (157 ± 8.6 ng/ml versus 197 ± 14 ng/ml, $p < 0.04$).

IGF-I levels declined, as expected, as a function of age, but even when the data are expressed as a function of age (Figure 2A) or as a distribution of Z-scores (Figure 2B), it is apparent that these men have low IGF-I levels. IGF-I levels were inversely correlated with percent eroded surface by histo-

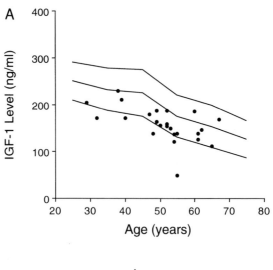

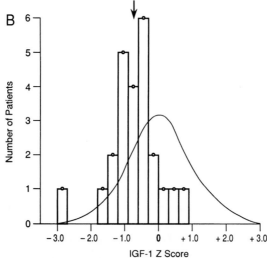

FIGURE 2   (A) IGF-I levels in men with idiopathic osteoporosis. Serum IGF–1 levels declined significantly with age ($r = 0.49$; $p < 0.02$). The data points are shown in relationship to the age-specific mean ± 1 SD. (B) Distribution of IGF-I Z-scores in men with idiopathic osteoporosis. The graph shows the mean Z-score, -0.75, is significantly lower ($p = 0.0002$) than the theoretical Gaussian distribution of the normal population, where $Z = 0$. Reprinted with permission from E. S. Kurland *et al.* (1997). Insulin-like growth factor-I in men with idiopathic osteoporosis. *J. Clin. Endocrinol. Metab.* **82**, 2799–2806, © The Endocrine Society.

morphometry, potentially as a result of a reduction in the stimulus to bone formation (i.e., reduced IGF-I levels), with a consequent increase in the relative extent of bone surface occupied by the resorptive process. By multiple regression analysis, IGF-I was shown to explain 15% of the variance in bone mineral density at the lumbar spine. The major circulating binding protein for IGF-I, IGFBP3, was also in the lower end of the normal range (2616 ± 101 ng/ml; nl, 2100–5000).

B. Growth Hormone

It is attractive to consider the possibility that men with idiopathic osteoporosis and reduced IGF-I levels have a deficiency in growth hormone. Skeletal and other actions of growth hormone are mediated by IGF-I. In fact, IGF-I levels are used as a reflection of growth hormone levels (Blum *et al.*, 1993), and, in states of growth hormone deficiency bone density, can be reduced (Rosen *et al.*, 1993) with low IGF-I levels (Hoffman *et al.*, 1994). In the patients we have reported with reduced concentrations of IGF-I, all other indices of anterior pituitary function were normal. Thus, if growth hormone deficiency is present it represents an isolated pituitary abnormality, a rather uncommon finding in adults who have no previous history of anterior pituitary disease (Hoffman *et al.*, 1994). In the Ljunghall report (Ljunghall *et al.*, 1992), growth hormone secretion appeared to be normal despite low IGF-I levels.

To test the hypothesis that abnormalities in growth hormone regulation may be responsible for the low IGF-I levels, growth hormone secretory reserve was evaluated in 14 men (Kurland *et al.*, 1998a). Growth hormone secretion was stimulated by two agonists: arginine infusion (which inhibits somatostatin) and L-dopa (which directly stimulates GHRH release). The protocol consisted of a 30-g intravenous arginine infusion over 30 min followed 1 h later by the oral administration of L-dopa (500 mg). Twelve of 14 patients responded maximally to arginine with mean peak values of 14.0 ± 2.8 ng/ml, representing a mean 17.7-fold increase over baseline. Only two patients responded with less than a threefold increase to arginine, but these two patients clearly responded satisfactorily to L-dopa (Figure 3). There was no relationship between growth hormone secretory capacity and IGF-I levels. The growth hormone responses in this study are similar in magnitude to those noted by others (Baum *et al.*, 1996; Rahim *et al.*, 1996).

The diagnostic criteria needed to establish normalcy of growth hormone secretory reserve are less well established for adults than they are for children. Furthermore, it is not clear that arginine can be used as informatively as insulin tolerance testing as an adequate stimulus to growth hormone secretion (Rahim *et al.*, 1996; de Boer *et al.*, 1995; Thorner *et al.*, 1995; Hoffman *et al.*, 1994; de Boer and van der Veen, 1997). Nevertheless,

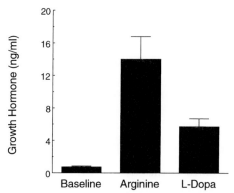

FIGURE 3   Peak responsiveness of growth hormone to stimulation by arginine or *L*-dopa. Data are shown as peak response to arginine (45–60 min) or to *L*-dopa (120–180 minutes) in relationship to baseline. Fold increase for arginine was 17.7 ± 2.8; for *L*-dopa, it was 9.2 ± 2.2. From Kurland *et al.* (1998a), with permission.

provocative testing with insulin and arginine have both been shown to reflect 24-h quantititive and qualitative secretory growth hormone dynamics (Baum *et al.*, 1996; Reutens *et al.*, 1996; Toogood *et al.*, 1996). Therefore, growth hormone secretory reserve in these men with idiopathic osteoporosis and reduced IGF-I levels appears to be normal.

C. Other Factors That Could Account for Reduced IGF-I Levels

Reduced IGF-I levels in men with idiopathic osteoporosis are difficult to explain by abnormalities of growth hormone secretory reserve or in growth hormone secretory dynamics. Thus, there is a dissociation between growth hormone and IGF-I in this syndrome. A similar dissociation between IGF-I and growth hormone has been demonstrated in other situations such as malnutrition (Rosen and Conover, 1997; Estivarez and Ziegler, 1997; Grinspoon *et al.*, 1995) and in genetic mouse models (Rosen *et al.*, 1997).

Regulators of skeletal IGF-I production might be an attractive focus for inquiry because, after the liver, the skeleton is the largest source of circulating IGF-I (Rosen *et al.*, 1994). Reduced skeletal levels of IGF-I could be responsible both for reduced bone turnover and for low circulating levels. In this regard, PTH is a regulator of IGF-I production in bone, and a reduction in PTH-mediated IGF-I production could be an important mechanism. The fact that circulating PTH levels in the cohort studied by Kurland *et al.* (1997) were lower than expected adds support for this possibility. Moreover, in postmenopausal osteoporotic women, there is some evidence for deficient secretory dynamics of parathyroid hormone (Silverberg *et al.*, 1989). It is also possible that other regulators of local IGF-I production such as gonadal steroids, dihydroepiandrosterone, interleukin–1, and PDGF could be involved.

D. Genetics of IGF–I in Men with Idiopathic Osteoporosis

There is strong hereditability of IGF-I in healthy, free-living adults (Grogean et al., 1997; Comuzzie et al., 1996). There is also a strong association between IGF-I and bone density among inbred strains of mice (Beamer et al., 1996; Rosen et al., 1997). It is therefore possible that the low IGF-I levels in men with idiopathic osteoporosis are genetically determined, a hypotheses we have recently tested (Rosen et al., 1998). We examined a highly polymorphic microsatellite region of the IGF-I gene composed of variable cytosine-adenosine (CA) which repeats 1 kb upstream from the transcription start site (Rotwein et al., 1986; Weber and May, 1989). The most frequent allele in our population sample is 192 base pairs in length, corresponding to the observations of Weber and May (1989). The frequency of homozygosity for the 192 allele in the men with idiopathic osteoporosis was compared to three other groups who did not have osteoporosis: 30 healthy men of similar age; 37 healthy postmenopausal women; and 79 men and women some of whom had coronary artery disease but none of whom had osteoporosis. The men with osteoporosis had a frequency of homozygosity of the 192/192 polymorphism of 64% (16 of 25), twice as high as the frequency of homozygosity (32%) in the groups without osteoporosis. It was also possible to compare this polymorphism with circulating IGF-I levels, across all groups. The mean IGF-I level in those with the 192/192 genotype was significantly lower than in subjects with any other genotype (129 ± 7 ng/ml versus 154 ± 9 ng/ml, p 0.03). When this group was divided by gender, it was also evident that normal men with the 192/192 genotype had lower IGF–1 levels (158.6 ± 9 versus 188.8 ± 8.6 ng/ml, p 0.02). In the 12 normal men who demonstrated homozygosity for 192/192, the mean T-score for bone mass at the spine and the hip was lower than 18 men who displayed other genotypes.

The data suggest that there is an association between low levels of IGF-I, low bone density, and a 192/192 polymorphism of the IGF-I gene, but the cause of this association is not yet clear. How IGF-I may be altered in its synthesis, regulation, translation, or stability in the presence of the 192/192 polymorphism is not known. It is intriguing to note that a promoter region containing a cyclic AMP response element possibly inducible by PTH is located very near this microsatellite region (McCarthy et al., 1989). In addition, estrogen interacts with a cyclic AMP inducible protein which, in turn, helps to regulate IGF. This observation may be relevant in view of the relationship between estrogen and IGF-I (McCarthy et al., 1997). Obviously, much more work is needed to establish a *bona fide* interaction among this polymorphism of the IGF-I gene, the clinical IGF-I phenotype, and osteoporosis. Different groups of subjects as well as more definitive linkage studies are clearly needed.

E. Sex Steroids

It may seem puzzling to include a discussion of sex steroids in men with idiopathic osteoporosis because the syndrome excludes abnormalities of gonadal function. Men with hypogonadism have a ready explanation for reduced bone mass, much in the way that postmenopausal women typically become osteoporotic because of estrogen deficiency. However, recent studies have called attention to a possible role for estrogens in the skeletal health of men.

Two genetic paradigms of estrogen action in the male have dramatically highlighted this possibility. In 1994, Smith *et al.* described a 28-year old man with a disruptive mutation of the estrogen receptor alpha gene associated with resistance to the action of estrogen. When discovered, the man was tall (204 cm) and still growing. He was well-masculinized with normal levels of testosterone and dihydrotestosterone. Estradiol and estrone levels were elevated 2 to 2.5 times greater than the upper limits for a male. Indices of bone formation and bone resorption were all elevated. Bone mineral density was more than 2 standard deviations (SD) below the mean for 15-year old boys (the patient's bone age). Not unexpectedly, administration of estrogen to this patient did not result in any improvement.

In addition, Morishima *et al.* (1995) described a 24-year-old man with a mutation in the aromatase gene responsible for conversion of androgens to estrogens. The genetic defect was shown to be a point mutation in exon IX of the gene at position 1123, yielding a gene product completely devoid of aromatase activity. This man, like the patient reported by Smith *et al.* (1994), was 204 cm tall and still growing. Androgen levels were elevated (androstenedione, testosterone, and dihydrotestosterone), and estradiol and estrone levels were undetectable. Of interest, the gonadotropins (LH, FSH) were mildly increased. Bone mass was reduced at all sites. If one corrects for the size of the bones (Carter *et al.*, 1992), it is apparent that volumetric density was reduced even further than that depicted by the areal density provided by DEXA. With this correction, *T*-scores were −1.99, −2.12, and −7.75 at the lumbar spine, femoral neck, and distal radius (1/3 site), respectively. In contrast to the individual reported by Smith *et al.*, this patient responded to therapy with conjugated estrogens (Bilezikian *et al.*, 1998). He quickly stopped growing and experienced closure of the epiphyses and a maturation of bone age. Over a period of 3 years, estrone and estradiol levels increased to normal and elevated gonadotropins and indices of bone turnover decreased to normal (Figure 4). He experienced a dramatic increase in bone mass at all sites (20.7% in the lumbar spine, 15.7% in the femoral neck, and 12.9% in the forearm) (Figure 5). Another male reported with aromatase deficiency

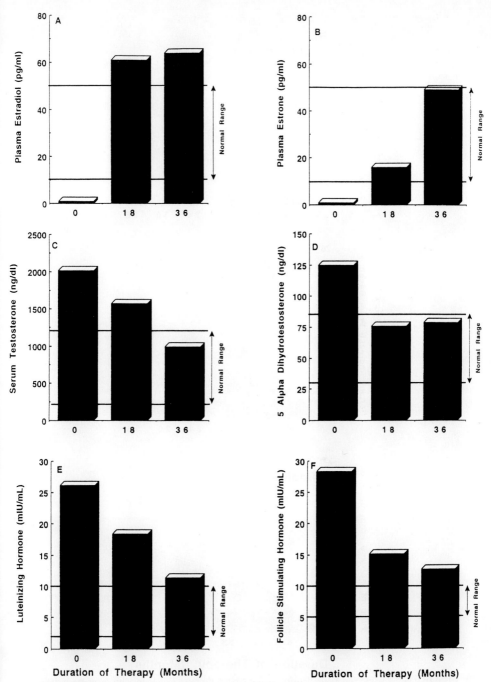

FIGURE 4 Changes in sex steroids and gonadotropins with estrogen therapy. The data are shown at baseline, 18 months, and 36 months after conjugated estrogen therapy was provided for a man with aromatase deficiency (see text). Estradiol (A), estrone (B), testosterone (C), 5-alpha dihydrotestosterone (D), luteinizing hormone (E), and follicle-stimulating hormone (F). The normal range for each index is given by the horizontal bars.

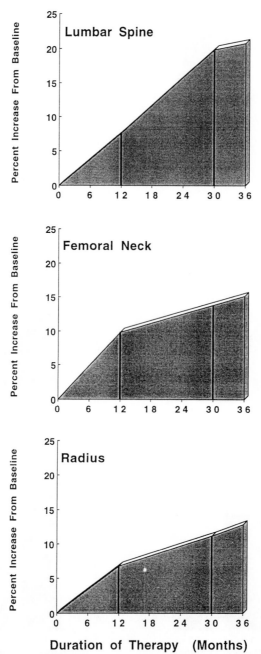

FIGURE 5 Changes in bone density with estrogen therapy in a man with aromatase deficiency. The percentage increases from baseline values are depicted for each site. After baseline determination, specific measurements were made at 12, 30, and 36 months after therapy (vertical bars) for each site. Increases are 20.7% (lumbar spine); 15.7% (femoral neck) and 12.9% (distal radius). From Bilezikian *et al.* (1998), with permission. Copyright © 1998 Massachusetts Medical Society. All rights reserved.

also experienced an improvement in bone mass after a shorter, 6-month course of therapy with estrogen (Carani *et al.*, 1997). These cases illustrate the importance of estrogen in establishing bone mass in the male, as well as the remarkable therapeutic potential of estrogen in this setting.

Obviously, mutations in the estrogen receptor or in the aromatase gene are unlikely to explain male osteoporosis, as such mutations are rare. But these experiments of nature point out the potential importance of estrogen in the male skeleton. Experimental studies in male rats also support the concept that estrogens are important in establishing peak bone mass (Vanderschueren *et al.*, 1997.

In 1997, Slemenda *et al.* reported a group of older men, in whom sex steroid and bone mass measurements were made over a period of 2 years. Bone mass was positively associated with estradiol concentrations ($r = +0.21 \pm 0.35$; p 0.01–0.05) at all skeletal sites. Surprisingly, weak negative correlations were observed between serum testosterone and bone density ($r = -0.20$ to -0.28; $p = 0.03$–0.10). Similarly, Khosla *et al.* (1998) have studied an age-stratified sample of 346 men, 23–90 years old. In a multivariate analysis, bioavailable serum estrogen was a consistent independent predictor of bone density. Anderson *et al.* (1997) have treated eugonadal, osteoporotic men with testosterone. They were able to correlate the increase in bone mass with an increase in estradiol levels, but not with the rise in testosterone levels. These observations suggest that in men with idiopathic osteoporosis, estrogen levels could contribute to bone loss and to therapeutic bone gain with androgens.

V. Clinical Approach and Management

The evaluation of the male patient with osteoporosis assumes that the diagnosis has been confirmed by densitometry and that a complete history and physical examination have been performed. The next step is to consider potential secondary causes of bone loss (Table I). Routine measurements of calcium, phosphorus, alkaline phosphatase, and serum proteins, as well as liver, renal, adrenal, pituitary, and thyroid function tests are appropriate. Sex steroid measurements should include total testosterone, estrone, estradiol, and sex hormone binding globulin. Tests of the calciotropic axis should include parathyroid hormone, 25-hydroxyvitamin D and 1,25 dihydroxyvitamin D levels. Specific markers of bone formation (serum bone-specific alkaline phosphatase activity or osteocalcin) and of bone resorption (urinary calcium, collagen, N-telopepetide, or deoxypyridinoline) may be useful. A percutaneous bone biopsy may be helpful to ascertain more definitively the histomorphometric indices of the disorder. The bone biopsy may also help identify potentially occult causes such as osteomalacia, osteogenesis imperfecta, mastocytosis and malignancy (Table V).

TABLE V   Diagnostic Evaluation for Osteoporosis in Men

The protocol herein considers diagnostic measures for all definable causes for osteoporosis in men. Depending upon the information provided by the patient, some or all of the following are indicated.

1. Routine measurements: serum calcium, phosphorus, alkaline phosphatase, albumin, protein electrophoresis; urinary calcium; immunoelectrophosphoresis
2. Tests of organ systems: liver, renal, adrenal, pituitary, thyroid function tests
3. Hormonal: sex steroid measurements—total testosterone, estrone, estradiol, sex hormone binding globulin
4. Calciotropic axis:
   a. serum: parathyroid hormone, 25-hydroxyvitamin D, 1,25 dihydroxyvitamin D
   b. specific markers of bone formation: serum bone-specific alkaline phosphatase activity or osteocalcin
   c. specific markers of bone resorption: urinary collagen crosslinks-*N*-telopeptide or deoxypyridinoline
   d. percutaneous bone biopsy: if potential causes not readily apparent are still possible: occult forms of osteomalacia, osteogenesis imperfecta, mastocytosis, malignancy

Initial therapeutic approaches are similar to those considered in osteoporotic women. Dietary calcium intake should be 1500 mg, consistent with the National Institute of Health (NIH) guidelines for optimal calcium intake (Bilezikian and Panel Members, 1994) and the new Food and Nutrition Board (FNB) (1998) recommendation. Although 1200 mg is recommended by the FNB for men older than 50, it seems prudent to ensure adequacy in osteoporosis by aiming for 1500 mg. Given the pervasive nature of vitamin D deficiency in this country (Thomas *et al.*, 1998), adequate vitamin D nutrition should be ensured. Even if vitamin D deficiency is not present (i.e., 25-hydroxyvitamin D > 20 ng/ml), individuals should receive 600–800 IU/day. This is somewhat higher than the current RDA for vitamin D but consistent with the newer FNB guidelines.

Adequate exercise is strongly recommended (see Chapter 8). In individuals who have sustained vertebral fractures or other complications, exercise should be appropriate to the setting. The nature of the exercise and its extent are issues that sometimes may require the services of a physical therapist. Weight training that provides a mechanical stimulus to selected sites may also have a role. Smoking should be avoided and excessive alcohol intake eliminated. In general, androgen therapy is not recommended in individuals with normal gonadal function.

There are inadequate data concerning more specific therapies. There is no information yet about bisphosphonate therapy in men with idiopathic osteoporosis. Typical of the gender bias alluded to earlier, excellent data are available on the efficacy of alendronate in postmenopausal women (Liberman *et al.*, 1995; Black *et al.*, 1996; Hosking *et al.*, 1998), but evaluations of the use of alendronate in men are still ongoing. One might consider it reasonable to prescribe alendronate in men with idiopathic osteoporosis, assuming that the results will be similar to those of women. Although this assumption is not unfounded, supporting data are not yet available.

In view of the fact that bone dynamics appear to be suppressed in many men with idiopathic osteoporosis, an attractive therapeutic approach is the use of an anabolic agent. It has been known for years that intermittent, low-dose administration of parathyroid hormone can be associated with anabolic effects at cancellous sites (Slovik *et al.*, 1986; Dempster *et al.*, 1993; Rosen and Donahue, 1996; Morley *et al.*, 1997). Slovik *et al.* (1986) showed that intermittent parathyroid hormone administered to four men with idiopathic osteoporosis was associated with a remarkable 198% increase in lumbar spine bone density within 12 months (by CAT scan densitometry). Cortical bone (distal radius) did not change, but overall calcium retention improved. More recently, Kurland *et al.* (1998b) have gained experience in using parathyroid hormone (1–34) in men with idiopathic osteoporosis. The study involved 23 men and was randomized, double-blinded, and placebo-controlled. After 18 months, the ten patients who received parathyroid hormone (400 IU daily) demonstrated a 13.5% increase in bone mass in the lumbar spine ($p < 0.03$), and no change in the forearm. Such impressive gains are promising and encourage further development of parathyroid hormone as a therapeutic agent in states of low turnover osteoporosis.

VI. Future Directions

As we become more aware of the problem of osteoporosis in men, the diagnosis will be made with increasing frequency. Many of these men can be expected to present without known cause. Similarly, an increasingly large group of premenopausal women who are osteoporotic without overt explanation may be uncovered (Kulak *et al.*, 1998). For both groups, a concerted, systematic inquiry is needed to elucidate the underlying causes. It is likely that a number of different etiologies will be established. To gain greatest insight into the basic and clinical factors that lead to bone loss and eventual complications in this syndrome, the investigative approach needs to consider both genetic and physiological mechanisms.

Acknowledgments

Some of the work cited in this chapter was supported by Grants FD-R 001024 from the Food and Drug Administration and AR 39191 and RR-MO1–000645 from the National Institutes of Health.

References

Anderson, F. H., Francis, R. M., Peaston, R. T., and Wastell, H. J. (1997). Androgen supplementation in eugonadal men with osteoporosis: Effects of six months' treatment on markers of bone formation and resorption. *J. Bone Miner. Res.* **12**, 472–478.

Baillie, S. P., Davison, C. E., Johnson, F. J., and Francis, R. M. (1992). Pathogenesis of vertebral crush fractures in men. *Age Ageing* **21**, 139–141.

Baum, H. B. A., Biller, B. M. K., Katznelson, L., Oppenheim, D. S., Clemmons, D. R., Cannistraro, K. B., Schoenfeld, D. A., Best, S. A., and Klibanski, A. (1996). Assessment of growth hormone (GH) secretion in men with adult-onset GH deficiency compared with that in normal men: A Clinical Research Center Study. *J. Clin. Endocrinol. Metab.* **81**, 84–92.

Beamer, W. G., Donahue, L. R., Rosen, C. J., and Baylink, D. J. (1996). Genetic variability in adult bone density among inbred strains of mice. *Bone* **18**, 397–403.

Bendavid, E. J., Shan, J., and Barrett-Connor, E. (1996). Factors associated with bone mineral density in middle-aged men. *J. Bone Miner. Res.* **11**, 1185–1190.

Bilezikian, J. P., and Panel Members (1994) Optimal calcium intake: Statement of the consensus development panel on optimal calcium intake. *J. Am. Med. Assoc.* **272**, 1942–1948.

Bilezikian, J. P., Morishima, A., Bell, J., and Grumbach, M. M. (1998). A marked effect of estrogens to enhance peak bone mass in a man with aromatase deficiency. *N. Engl. J. Med.* **339**, 599–603.

Black, D. M., Cummings, S. R., Karpf, D. B., Cauley, J. A., Thompson, D. E., Nevitt, M. C., Bauer, D. C., Genant, H. K., Haskell, W. L., Marcus, R., Ott, S. M., Torner, J. C., Quandt, S. A., Reiss, T. F., and Ensrud, K. E. (1996). Randomised trial of effect of alendronate on risk of fracture in women with existing vertebral fractures *Lancet* **348**, 1535–1541.

Blum, W. F., Albertsson, K., Roseberg, D., and Ranke, M. B. (1993). Serum levels of IGF-I and IGFBP-3 reflect spontaneous growth hormone secretion. *J. Clin. Endocrinol. Metab.* **76**, 1610–1630.

Boonen, S., Lesaffre, E., Dequeker, J., Aerssens, J., Nijs, J., Pelemans, W., and Bouillon, R. (1996). Relationship between baseline IGF-I and femoral neck bone density in women aged over 70 years. *J. Am. Geriatr. Soc.* **44** 1301–1306.

Brockstedt, H., Kassem, M., Eriksen E. F., Mosekilde, L., and Melsen, F. (1993). Age- and sex-related changes in iliac cortical bone mass and remodeling. *Bone* **14**, 681–691.

Canalis, E. (1995). Growth hormone skeletal growth factors and osteoporosis. *Endocr. Pract.* **1**, 39–43.

Canalis, E. (1997). Insulin-like growth factors and osteoporosis. *Bone* **21**, 215–216.

Canalis, E., Pash, J. M., and Varghese, S. (1993). Skeletal growth factors. *Crit. Rev. Eukaryoic Gene Expression.* **3**, 155–166.

Carani, C., Qin, K., Simoni, M., Faustini-Fustini, M., Serpente, S., Boyd, J., Korach, K. S., and Simpson, E. R. (1997). Effect of testosterone and estradiol in a man with aromatase deficiency. *N. Engl. J. Med.* **337**, 91–95.

Carter, D.R., Bouxsein, M. L., and Marcus, R. (1992). New approaches for interpreting projected bone densitometry data. *J. Bone Miner. Res.* **7**, 137–145.

Compston, J. E., Mellish, R. W. E., Croucher, P., Newcombe, R., and Garrahan, N. J. (1989). Structural mechanisms of trabecular bone loss in man. *Bone Miner.* **6**, 339–350.

Commuzie, A. G., Biangero, J., Mahaney, M. C., *et al.* (1996). Genetic and environmental correlations among hormone levels and measures of body fat accumulation and topography. *J. Clin. Endocrinol. Metab.* **81**, 597–600.

Darby, A. J., and Meunier, P. J. (1981). Mean wall thickness and formation periods of trabecular bone packets in idiopathic osteoporosis. *Calcif. Tissue Int.* **33**, 199–204.

de Boer, H., and van der Veen, E. A. (1997). Editorial: Why retest young adults with childhood-onset growth hormone deficiency? *J. Clin. Endocrinol. Metab.* **82**, 2032–2036.

de Boer, H., Blok, G. J., and van der Veen, E. A. (1995). Clinical aspects of growth hormone deficiency in adults. *Endocr. Rev.* **16**, 63–86.

Dempster, D. W., Cosman, G., Parisien, M., Shen, V., and Lindsay, R. (1993). Anabolic action of parathyroid hormone on bone. *Endocr. Rev.* **14**, 690–709.

DeVernejoul, M. C., Bielkoff, J., Herve, M., Gueris, J., Hott, M., Modrowski, D., Kuntz, D., Miravet, L., and Ryckewaert, A. (1983). Evidence for defective osteoblastic function: A role for alcohol and tobacco consumption in osteoporosis in middle-aged men. *Clin. Othop. Relat. Res.* **179**, 107–115.

Epstein, S., and Miller, P. (1997). Bone mass measurements: The case for selected screening? *Trends Endocrinol. Metab.* **8**, 157–160.

Estivarez, C. E., and Ziegler, T. R. (1997). Nutrition and the IGF system. *Endocrine*, **4**, 65–71.

Fall, C., Hindmarsh, P., Dennison, E., Kellingray, S., Barker, D., and Cooper, C. (1998). Programming of growth hormone secretion and bone mineral density in elderly men: A hypothesis. *J. Clin. Endocrinol. Metab.* **83**, 135–139.

Finkelstein, J. S., Klibanski, A., Neer, R. M., Greenspan, S. L., Rosenthal D. I., and Crowley, W. F. (1987). Osteoporosis in men with idiopathic hypogonadotropic hypogonadism. *Ann. Intern. Med.* **106**, 354–361.

Finkelstein, J. S., Neer, R. M., Biller, B. M. K., Crawford, J. D., and Klibanski, A. (1992). Osteopenia in men with a history of delayed puberty. *N. Engl. J. Med.* **326**, 600–604.

Finkelstein, J. S., Klibanski, A., and Neer, R. M. (1996). A longitudinal evaluation of bone mineral density in adult men with histories of delayed puberty. *J. Clin. Endocrinol. Metab.* **81**, 1152–1155.

Food and Nutrition Board, Institute of Medicine, National Research Council (1998). "Dietary Reference Intakes." National Academy Press, Washington, D C.

Francis, R. M., Peacock, M., Aaron, J. E., Selby, P. L., Taylor, G. A., Thompson, J., Marshall, D. H., and Horsman, A. (1986). Osteoporosis in hypogonadal men: Role of decreased plasma 1,25-dihydroxyvitamin D, calcium malabsorption, and low bone formation. *Bone* **7**, 261–268.

Francis, R. M., Peacock, M., Marshall, D. H., Horsman, A., and Aaron, J. E. (1989). Spinal osteoporosis in men. *Bone Miner.* **5**, 347–357.

Garn, S. M., Sullivan, T. V., Decker, S. A., Larkin, F. A., and Hawthorne, V. M. (1992). Continuing bone expansion and increasing bone loss over a two-decade period in men and women from a total community sample. *Am. J. Hum. Biol.* **4**, 57–67.

Ghazalie, A., Fuentes, V., Desaint, C., Bataille, P., Westeel, A., Brazier, M., Prin, L., and Fournier, A. (1997). Low bone mineral density and peripheral blood monocyte activation profile in calcium stone formers with idiopathic hypercalciuria. *J. Clin. Endocrino. Metab.* **82**, 32–38.

Grinspoon, S. K., Baum, H. B. A., Peterson, S., and Klibanski, A. (1995). Effects of rhIGF–1 administration on bone turnover during short-term fasting. *J. Clin. Invest.* **96**, 900–905.

Grogean, T., Vereault, D., Millard, P. S., *et al.* (1997). A comparative analysis of methods to measurement IGF–1 in human serum. *Endocr. Metab.* **4**, 109–114.

Hannan, M. T., Felson, D. T., and Anderson, J. J. (1992). Bone mineral density in elderly men and women: Results from the Framingham osteoporosis study. *J. Bone Miner. Res.* **7**, 547–553.

Hoffman, D. M., O'Sullivan, A. J., Baxter, R. C., and Ho, K. K. Y. (1994). Diagnosis of growth-hormone deficiency in adults. *Lancet* **343**, 1064–1068.

Hosking, D., Chilvers, C. E. D., Christiansen, C., Ravn, P., Wasnich, R., Ross, P., McClung, M., Balske, A., Thompson, D., Daley, M., and Yates, A. J. (1998). Prevention of bone loss with alendronate in postmenopausal women under 60 years of age. *N. Engl. J. Med.* **338**, 485–492.

Jackson, J. A., and Kleerekoper, M. (1990). Osteoporosis in men: Diagnosis, pathophysiology, and prevention. *Medicine* **69**, 137–152.

414   Bilezikian *et al.*

Jackson, J. A., Kleerekoper, M., Parfitt, A. M., Rao, D. S., Villanueva, A. R., and Frame, B. (1987). Bone histomorphometry in hypogonadal and eugonadal men with spinal osteoporosis. *J. Clin. Endocrinol. Metab.* **65**, 53–58.

Johansson, A. G., Eriksen, E. F., and Lindh, E., *et al.* (1997). Reduced serum levels of the growth hormone-dependent IGF binding protein and a negative bone balance at the level of individual remodeling units in idiopathic osteoporosis in men. *J. Clin. Endocrinol. Metab.* **82**, 2795–2798.

Jones, J. I., and Clemmons, D. R. (1995). Insulin-like growth factors and their binding proteins: Biomedical actions. *Endocr. Rev.* **16**, 3–34.

Kelepouris, N., Harper, K. D., Gannon, F., Kaplan, F. S., and Haddad, J. G. (1995). Severe osteoporosis in men. *Ann. Intern. Med.* **123**, 452–460.

Khosla, S. (1997). Editorial: Idiopathic osteoporosis—is the osteoblast to blame? *J. Clin. Endocrinol. Metab.* **82**, 2792–2794.

Khosla, S., Lufkin, E. G., Hodgson, S. F., Fitzpatrick, L. A., and Melton, L. J., III (1994). Epidemiology and clinical features of osteoporosis in young individuals. *Bone* **15**, 551–555.

Khosla, S., Melton, L. J., III, Atkinson, E. J., O'Fallon, W. M., Klee, G. G., and Riggs, B. L. (1998). Relationship of serum sex steroid levels and bone turnover markers with bone mineral density in men and women: A key role for bioavailable estrogen. *J. Clin. Endocrinol. Metab.* **83**, 2266–2274.

Klein, R. F., and Orwoll, E. S. (1994). Bone loss in men: Pathogenesis and therapeutic considerations. *Endocrinologist* **4**, 252–269.

Kulak, C. A. M., Schussheim, D. H., McMahon, D., Silverberg, S. J., Bilezikian, J. P., and Shane, E. (1998). Low bone mass in premenopausal women. *Endo. Soc. 80th Annu. Meet.* pp. 3–87.

Kurland, E. S., Rosen, C. J., Cosman, F., McMahon, D., Chan, F., Shane, E., Lindsay, R., Dempster, D., and Bilezikian, J. P. (1997). Insulin-like growth factor-1 in men with idiopathic osteoporosis. *J. Clin. Endocrinol. Metab.* **82**, 2799–2805.

Kurland, E. S., Chan, F. K. W., Rosen, C. J., and Bilezikian, J. P. (1998a). Normal growth hormone secretory reserve in men with idiopathic osteoporosis and reduced circulating levels of insulin-like growth factor–1. *J. Clin. Endocrinol. Metab.* **83**, 1–4.

Kurland, E. S., Cosman, F., McMahon, D. J., Rosen, C. J., Lindsay, R., and Bilezikian, J. P. (1998b). Parathyroid hormone (PTH1–34) increases cancellous bone mass markedly in men with idiopathic osteoporosis. *Bone* **1039** (suppl. 5), abstract.

Liberman, U. A., Weiss, S. R., Broll, J., Minne, H. W., Quan, H., Bell, N. H., Rodriquez-Portales, J., Downs, R. W., Dequeker, J., Favus, M., Seeman, E., Recker, R. R., Capizzi, T., Santora, A. C., II, Lombardi, A., Shah, R. V., Hirsch, L. J., and Karpf, D. B. (1995). Effect of oral alendronate on bone mineral density and the incidence of fractures in postmenopausal osteoporosis. *N. Engl. J. Med.* **333**, 1437–1443.

Ljunghall, S., Johansson, A. G., Burman, P., Kampe, O., Lindh, E., and Karlson, R. A. (1992). Low plasma levels of insulin-like growth factor 1 (IGF–1) in male patients with idiopathic osteoporosis. *J. Intern. Med.* **232**, 59–64.

McCarthy, T. L., Centrella, M., and Canalis, E. (1989). PTH enhances the transcript and polypeptide levels of IGF–1 in osteoblast enriched cultures from fetal rate calvariae. *Endocrinology (Baltimore)* **124**, 1247–1253.

McCarthy, T. L., Ji, C., Shu, H., *et al.* (1997). 17β-estradiol potentially suppresses cAMP-induced IGF–1 gene activation in primary rat osteoblast cultures. *J. Biol. Chem.* **272** 18132–18139.

Morishima, A., Grumbach, M. M., Simpson, E. R., Fisher, C., and Qin, K. (1995). Aromatase deficiency in male and female siblings caused by a novel mutation and the physiological role of estrogens. *J. Clin. Endocrinol. Metab.* **80**, 3689–3698.

Morley, P., Whitfield, J. F., and Willick, G. E. (1997). Anabolic effects of parathyroid hormone on bone. *Trends Endocrinol. Metab.* **8**, 225–231.

Mussolino, M. E., Looker, A. C., Madans, J. H., Langlois, J. A., and Orwoll, E. S. (1998). Risk factors for hip fracture in white men: The NHANES I epidemiologic follow-up study. *J. Bone Miner. Res.* **13**, 918–924.

Nicolas, V., Prewett, A., and Bettica, P. (1994). Age-related decreases in insulin-like growth factor-1 and transforming growth factor-β in femoral cortical bone from both men and women: Implications for bone loss with aging. *J. Clin. Endocrinol. Metab.* **78**, 1011–1016.

Orwoll, E. S., and Klein, R. F. (1995). Osteoporosis in men. *Endocr. Rev.* **16**, 87–116.

Pacifici, R. (1997). Idiopathic hypercalciuria and osteoporosis-distinct clinical manifestations of increased cytokine-induced bone resorption? *J. Clin. Endocrinol. Metab.* **82**, 29–31.

Parfitt, A. M., and Duncan, H. (1982). Metabolic bone disease affecting the spine. *In* "The Spine" (R. Rothman, ed.), 2nd ed., pp. 775–905. Saunders, Philadelphia.

Perry, H. M., III, Fallon, M. D., Bergfeld, M., Teitelbaum, S. L., and Avioli, L. V. (1982). Osteoporosis in young men. *Arch. Intern. Med.* **142**, 1295–1298.

Rahim, A., Toogood, A. A., and Shalet, S. M. (1996). The assessment of growth hormone status in normal young adult males using a variety of provocative agents. *Clin. Endocrinol. (Oxford)* **45**, 557–562.

Rajaram, S., Baylink, D. J., and Mohan, S. (1997). Insulin-like growth factor-binding proteins in serum and other biological fluids: Regulation and functions. *Endocr. Rev.* **18**, 801–831.

Reed, B. Y., Zwerwekh, J. E., Sakhaee, K., Breslau, N. A., Gottschalk, F., and Pak, C. Y. C. (1995). Serum IGF 1 is low and correlated with osteoblastic surface in idiopathic osteoporosis. *J. Bone Miner. Res.* **10**, 1218–1224.

Resch, H., Pietschmann, P., Woloszczuk, W., Krexner, E., Bernecker, P., and Willvonseder, R. (1992). Bone mass and biochemical parameters of bone metabolism in men with spinal osteoporosis. *Eur. J. Clin. Invest.* **22**, 542–545.

Reutens, A. T., Veldhuis, J. D., Hoffman, D. M., Leung, K. C., and Ho, K. K. Y. (1996). A highly sensitive growth hormone (GH) enzyme-liked immunoabsorbent assay uncovers increased contribution of a tonic mode of GH secretion in adults with organic GH deficiency. *J. Clin. Endocrinol. Metab.* **81**, 1591–1597.

Romagnoli, E., Minisola, S., Carnevale, V., Rosso, R., Pacitti, M. T., Scarda, A,. Scarnecchia, L., and Mazzuoli, G. (1994). Circulating levels of IGFBP–3 and IGF–1 in perimenopausal women. *Osteoporosis Int.* **4**, 305–308.

Rosen, C. J., and Conover, C. (1997). Growth insulin like growth factor–1 axis in aging: a summary of an NIA sponsored symposium. *J. Clin. Endocrinol. Metab.* **82**, 3919–3922.

Rosen, C. J., and Donahue, L. R. (1996). Parathyroid hormone and osteoporosis. *Cur. Opin. Endocrinol. Diabetes.* **3**, 532–539.

Rosen, C. J., Donahue, L. R., and Hunter, S. J. (1994). Insulin-like growth factors and bone: The osteoporosis connection. *Proc. Soc. Exp. Biol. Med.* **206**, 83–102.

Rosen, C. J., Dimai, H. P., Vereault, D., Donahue, L. R., Beamer, W. G., Farley, J., Linkhart, S., Linkhart, T., Mohan, S., and Baylink, D. J. (1997). Circulating and skeletal insulin-like growth factor–1 (IGF–1) concentrations in two inbred strains of mice with different bone mineral densities. *Bone* **21**, 217–223.

Rosen, C. J., Kurland, E. S., Vereault, D., Adler, R. A., Rackoff, P. J., Craig, W. Y., Witte, S., Rogers, J., and Bilezikian, J. P. (1998). An association between serum IGF–1 and a simple sequence repeat in the IGF–1 gene: implications for genetic studies of bone mineral density. *J. Clin. Endocrinol. Metab.* **83**, 2286–2290.

Rosen, T., Hansson, T., Granhed, H., Szucs, J., and Bengtsson, B. A. (1993). Reduced bone mineral content in adult patients with growth hormone deficiency. *Acta Endocrinol. (Copenhagen)* **129**, 201–206.

Rotwein, P., Pollock, K. M., Didler, D. K., and Krivi, G. G. (1986). Organization and sequence of the human IGF–1 gene. *J. Biol. Chem.* **26**, 4828–4832.

Scane, A. C., and Francis, R. M. (1993). Risk factors for osteoporosis in men. *Clin. Endocrinol.* **38**, 15–16.

Scane, A. C., Sutcliffe, A. M., and Francis, R. M. (1993). Osteoporosis in men. *Bailliere's Clin. Rheumatol.* 7, 589–601.

Seeman, E. (1993). Osteoporosis in men: Epidemiology, pathophysiology, and treatment possibilities. *Am. J. Med.* 95, 5S–28S.

Seeman, E., Melton, L. J., III, O'Fallon, W. M., and Riggs, B. L. (1983). Risk factors for spinal osteoporosis in men. *Am. J. Med.* 75, 977–983.

Silverberg, S. J., Shane, E., de la Cruz, L., Segre, G. V., Clemens, T. L., and Bilezikian, J. P. (1989). Abnormalities in parathyroid hormone secretion and 1,25-dihydroxyvitamin D3 formation in osteoporosis. *N. Engl. J. Med.* 320, 277–281.

Slemenda, C. W., Longcope, C., Zhou, L., Hui, S. L., Peacock, M., and Johnston, C. C. (1997). Sex steroids and bone mass in older men. *J. Clin. Invest.* 100, 1755–1759.

Slovik, D. M., Rosenthal, D. I., Doppelt, S. H., Potts, J. T., Jr, Daly, M. A., Campbell, J. A., and Neer, R. M. (1986). Restoration of spinal bone in osteoporosis men by treatment with human parathyroid hormone (1–34) and 1,25 dihydroxyvitamin D. *J. Bone Miner. Res.* 1, 377–381.

Smith, E. P., Boyd, J., Frank, G. R., Takahashi, H., Cohen, R. M., Specker, B., Williams, T. C., Lubahn, D. B., and Korach, K. S. (1994). Estrogen resistance caused by a mutation in the estrogen-receptor gene in a man. *N. Engl. J. Med.* 331, 1056–1061.

Smith, R. W. J., and Walker, R. R. (1964). Femoral expansion in aging women: Implications for osteoporosis and fractures. *Science* 145, 156–157.

Stepan, J. J., Lachman, M., Zverina, J., Pacovsky, V., and Baylink, D. J. (1989). Castrated men exhibit bone loss: Effect of calcitonin treatment on biochemical indices of bone remodeling. *J. Clin. Endocrinol. Metab.* 69, 523–527.

Thomas, M. K., Lloyd-Jones, D. M., Thadhani, R. I., Shaw, A. C., Deraska, D. J., Kitch. B. T., Vamvakas, E. C., Dick, I. M., Prince, R. L., and Finkelstein, J. S. (1998). Hypovitaminosis D in medical inpatients *N. Engl. J. Med.* 338, 777–783.

Thorner, M. O., Bengtsson, B. A., Ho, K. Y., *et al.* (1995). The diagnosis of growth hormone deficiency in adults. *J. Clin. Endocrinol. Metab.* 80, 3097–3098.

Toogood, A. A., O'Neill, P. A., and Shalet, S. M. (1996). Beyond the somatopause: Growth hormone deficiency in adults over the age of 60 years. *J. Clin. Endocrinol. Metab.* 81, 460–465.

Vanderschueren, D., Van Herck, E., Nijs, J., Ederveen, A. G. H., De Coster, R., and Bouillon. R. (1997). Aromatase inhibition impairs skeletal modeling and decreases bone mineral density in growing male rats. *Endocrinology (Baltimore)* 138, 2301–2307.

Weber, J. L., and May, P. E. (1989). Abundant class of human DNA polymorphisms which can be typed using the polymerase chain reaction. *Am. J. Hum. Genet.* 44, 188–196.

Chapter 20

Ian R. Reid

Department of Medicine
University of Auckland
Private Bag 92019
Auckland, New Zealand

Glucocorticoids and Osteoporosis

I. Introduction

Glucocorticoid excess occurs in two clinical contexts. Endogenous hypercortisolism is the cause of Cushing's syndrome, where spontaneous fractures, particularly of the vertebrae, were noted in the first descriptions of this condition almost 70 years ago. The therapeutic use of glucocorticoid drugs is a much more common cause of glucocorticoid excess, and fractures were also reported to occur in this context within a few years of the introduction of these agents. Even though these drugs substantially reduce the morbidity and mortality of many inflammatory conditions, some of their side effects, particularly the development of osteoporosis, substantially curtail their use. Therefore, the assessment of osteopenia and, where appropriate, its treatment have become an integral part of the management of patients requiring these medications.

II. Clinical Presentation

A. Effects on Bone Mass

Bone mass decreases rapidly after the initiation of steroid therapy (Lo Cascio *et al.*, 1990), and with continued use of these agents there is an ongoing loss of bone (Saito *et al.*, 1995). A prospective study has shown an 8% decrease in trabecular bone density at the lumbar spine after 20 weeks of treatment with prednisone in a mean dose of 7.5 mg/day (Laan *et al.*, 1993). Cross-sectionally, reductions in bone density of the lumbar spine and proximal femur of about 20% are demonstrable after several years of treatment (Reid *et al.*, 1992b). However, the rate of loss is greater in trabecular bone (probably because of its greater surface to volume ratio), and cross-sectional studies commonly show a bone mass reduction of the order of 40% in this bone compartment (Reid and Heap, 1990; Reid *et al.*, 1992a). The degree of bone loss is related to the average glucocorticoid dose and to its duration (Reid and Heap, 1990; Buckley *et al.*, 1995). Despite occasional anecdotal comments in the literature to the contrary, there is no clear evidence that the effect of glucocorticoids on bone loss is significantly different between the sexes (Reid and Heap, 1990). In their prospective study, Laan *et al.* (1993) found no impact of sex on bone loss, and the same was true in the longitudinal study of Saito *et al.* (1995). Similarly, in patients with Addison's disease, there is no consistent evidence of a difference between the sexes in the incidence of osteopenia (Florkowski *et al.*, 1994; Zelissen *et al.*, 1994).

Bone loss appears to occur in virtually everyone who takes supraphysiological doses of glucocorticoids (Laan *et al.*, 1993; Rizzato and Montemurro, 1993). As a result, bone density remains normally distributed in steroid-treated patients studied cross-sectionally, where the mean is displaced below the normal value, but the standard deviation is little changed. Therefore, there is a substantial overlap in bone density values between those receiving steroids and normal subjects. This does not imply that individuals are resistant to the effects of steroids, merely that some started at the upper end of the normal range and have therefore ended up at the upper end of the steroid-treated range. Such individuals are likely to have a lesser fracture risk and, therefore, are less in need of osteoporotic therapies. For this reason, the measurement of bone density is important to determine which steroid-treated patients require interventions to increase bone mass.

It is also important to note that the osteopenia produced by glucocorticoids is almost completely reversible when the glucocorticoid excess is no longer present. This has been demonstrated in prospective studies of glucocorticoid drug use, which have demonstrated a regaining of bone density over the same time span as its loss occurred (Laan *et al.*, 1993; Rizzato and Montemurro, 1993). Similarly, substantial increases in bone density have been observed following cure of Cushing's syndrome (Lufkin *et al.*, 1988; Hermus *et al.*, 1994) such that subjects with a history of cured Cushing's syndrome a decade previously have normal bone density (Manning *et al.*, 1992).

One strategy for reducing the systemic dose of glucocorticoids is to administer them locally (e.g., by inhalation in patients with pulmonary diseases such as asthma). While this approach often produces good disease control there is still significant systemic absorption of the glucocorticoid, resulting in adrenal suppression in 15% of patients (Grebe *et al.*, 1997), reduction in markers of osteoblast activity (Struijs and Mulder, 1997), modest reductions in bone density (Struijs and Mulder, 1997) and increases in other side effects such as cataract formation (Cumming *et al.*, 1997) and growth retardation (Doull *et al.*, 1996). Thus, while local administration of steroids probably has a better risk-benefit profile than systemic use, caution is still required. In contrast, the use of alternate day administration of glucocorticoids appears to confer no benefit from the point of view of bone loss.

B. Fractures

Because glucocorticoids have their greatest effect on trabecular bone, fractures are most common in regions of the skeleton which are predominantly trabecular, such as the vertebral bodies and ribs. Approximately one third of patients have evidence of vertebral fractures after 5–10 years of glucocorticoid treatment (Adinoff and Hollister, 1983; Luengo *et al.*, 1991; Michel *et al.*, 1991; Laan *et al.*, 1992; Spector *et al.*, 1993; Lems *et al.*, 1995). The risk of hip fracture is also increased nearly threefold in patients taking glucocorticoids (Cooper *et al.*, 1995). Fracture risk is related to the duration of glucocorticoid use, age, and body weight (inversely) and to female sex (Michel *et al.*, 1993).

In a recent prospective study of patients treated with glucocorticoids plus a placebo, Adachi *et al.* (1997b) observed new vertebral fractures in 3 out of 25 men, 0 out of 8 premenopausal women, and 7 out of 32 postmenopausal women over a period of 12 months. The differences in fracture rates between the postmenopausal women and the men can probably be accounted for by differences in their baseline bone density. The small number of premenopausal women make it unwise to comment on their relative fracture rate. It should be noted, however, that the premenopausal women in this study showed substantial losses of bone density during the study (e.g., -4.6% in the lumbar spine, -6.0% in the femoral trochanter) arguing against any suggestion that they may be less at risk of steroid-induced bone loss. Adinoff and Hollister (1983) studied two cohorts of patients receiving steroids. In one, fractures tended to be more common in men, but in the other the reverse was seen. In a group of 100 subjects on steroids reported by Luengo *et al.* (1991), the prevalence of fractures was approximately equal between the sexes. Both these studies are complicated by the fact that data for pre- and postmenopausal women are not analyzed separately. At the present time, the data indicate that all individuals lose bone when treated with supraphysiological doses of glucocorticoids, and whether fracture results is determined by the baseline bone density, the dose of glucocorticoid used, and the period of its use.

III. Pathophysiology

Because of the widespread distribution of the glucocorticoid receptor, these agents are able to have an impact on bone and calcium metabolism at many levels. Other than the changes in sex hormone levels, there is no clear evidence that these effects are gender-specific, although this has not been addressed in any detail. The various sites of action of glucocorticoids will now be reviewed.

A. Osteoblasts

The most consistently demonstrated effects of glucocorticoids on bone are in the osteoblast, whether studied *in vivo* or *in vitro*. Both animal and human studies of bone histomorphometry demonstrate impaired bone formation. Both the rate of bone production within each bone modeling unit and the duration of activity of each unit are reduced (Dempster, 1989). *In vitro*, glucocorticoids can be characterized as increasing osteoblast differentiation and decreasing osteoblast proliferation. The former effect may be partly attributable to increased production of bone morphogenic protein-6 (Boden *et al.*, 1997) and the latter to reduced expression of cyclin-dependent kinases and cyclin-D3 together with enhanced transcription of inhibitors of cyclin-dependent kinases (Rogatsky *et al.*, 1997). There is also evidence for glucocorticoid regulation of a number of important osteoblastic genes including those for type I collagen, osteocalcin, osteopontin, fibronectin, β-1 integrin, bone sialoprotein, alkaline phosphatase, collagenase, and the nuclear proto-oncogenes, c-myc, c-fos, and c-jun. In osteoblast precursor cells, gene expression is modulated to produce a more differentiated osteoblastic phenotype, whereas in the mature osteoblast, cell proliferation and matrix synthesis are reduced by glucocorticoids. These effects may be biphasic with respect to both dose and time, inhibition of osteoblast proliferation, and activity being evident at high hormone concentrations and with long exposure periods (Dietrich *et al.*, 1979; Gallagher *et al.*, 1984).

Osteoblasts produce factors which act in an autocrine manner to regulate their own activity. Insulin-like growth factors (IGF)-1 and -2 act in this way, and their local synthesis is inhibited by glucocorticoids. Their local activity is modulated by the interplay of specific binding proteins and there is now evidence for a reduction in the levels of the stimulatory binding proteins, IGFBP-3 and IGFBP-5 (Okazaki *et al.*, 1994; Chevalley *et al.*, 1996; Gabbitas *et al.*, 1996) and for increased production of IGFBP-6, an inhibitor of IGF-2 activity (Gabbitas and Canalis, 1996). However, blocking the effects of endogenous IGFs does not abrogate the effect of glucocorticoids on osteoblast proliferation and collagen synthesis. Transforming growth factor-β is a further important autocrine factor modulated by glucocorticoids (Centrella *et al.*, 1991; Oursler *et al.*, 1993).

B. Osteoclasts

The effects of glucocorticoids on osteoclasts are contradictory. There is evidence that glucocorticoids increase osteoclast formation from precursor cells in bone marrow (Shuto *et al.*, 1994; Kaji *et al.*, 1997) but also that they lead to apoptosis of mature osteoclasts (Tobias and Chambers, 1989; Dempster *et al.*, 1997). These opposing effects may account for the findings in organ culture that glucorticoids can either increase or decrease bone resorption, depending on the culture conditions (Caputo *et al.*, 1976; Gronowicz *et al.*, 1990; Lowe *et al.*, 1992). In organ culture, glucocorticoid effects may be contributed to by their inhibition of the local production of osteolytic cytokines such as interleukin-1 and the tumor necrosis factors.

Animal and human studies are also difficult to interpret. In sheep (Chavassieux *et al.*, 1997), the eroded perimeter is increased, but the number of osteoclasts is diminished, consistent with findings in human studies. These findings could be accounted for by a reduced rate of recruitment of osteoblasts to the previously resorbed bone, leaving eroded surfaces unfilled for a greater time than normal. Thus, they do not necessarily imply increased rates of bone resorption. Most of the human studies of biochemical markers of bone resorption would be consistent with this conclusion.

C. Intestinal and Renal Handling of Calcium and Phosphate

Studies have consistently demonstrated an inhibition of calcium absorption associated with glucocorticoid treatment. This is not mediated by changes in vitamin D metabolites and is therefore likely to represent a direct effect on the calcium transport system in the small intestine.

Within weeks of glucocorticoid treatment, there is a substantial rise in urine calcium excretion (Gray *et al.*, 1991; Welten *et al.*, 1994) which is not accounted for by changes in the serum-ionized calcium or the glomerular filtration rate. These changes persist in patients receiving long-term therapy, in whom bone resorption rates are normal (Reid and Ibberston, 1987). This suggests that glucocorticoids directly regulate tubular resorption of calcium. There is also evidence for malabsorption of phosphate in both the gut and renal tubule associated with glucocorticoid use (Cosman *et al.*, 1994).

D. Vitamin D and Parathyroid Hormone

There is no consistent evidence suggesting that changes in vitamin D metabolism mediate the osteopenic effects of glucocorticoids. *In vitro*, glucocorticoids increase parathyroid hormone (PTH) release from cultured parathyroid glands, but hyperparathyroidism is only inconsistently demonstrated in human studies.

E. Sex Hormones

Both Cushing's syndrome (Smals *et al.*, 1977) and the administration of glucocorticoids are associated with reduced serum testosterone levels in men. Hypogonadism in Cushing's syndrome is not surprising because many of these patients have pituitary tumors that might directly interfere with gonadotropin production. However, hypogonadism in steroid-treated men has only been more recently recognized. Reid *et al.* reported a nearly 50% reduction in both total and free testosterone concentrations in asthmatic men receiving glucocorticoids, in comparison with age-matched asthmatic control subjects not receiving such treatment (Reid *et al.*, 1985). This has now been confirmed by a number of other groups (MacAdams *et al.*, 1986; Morrison *et al.*, 1994; Fitzgerald *et al.*, 1997) and in a further cohort that Reid *et al.* have reported (Figure 1) (Reid *et al.*, 1994).

It has become apparent that estrogen is also important to the development and maintenance of normal bone mass in men. The recent observation

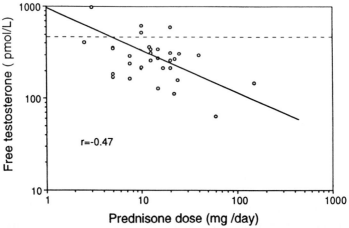

FIGURE I Relationship between circulating free testosterone concentrations and prednisone dose in 32 male asthmatic patients. The reference range for free testosterone in our laboratory is 380–1200 pmol/L, and the lower end of this range is indicated in the figure by the broken line. The inverse correlation between these variables is significant ($p = 0.007$). Reprinted from Reid *et al.* (1994), pp. 7–18, by courtesy of Marcel Dekker, Inc.

of Pearce *et al.* (1998), that there is a reduction in serum estradiol concentrations of nearly one half in men treated with prednisone 50 mg/day for 2 months, is therefore likely to be relevant to the mechanism of steroid-induced bone loss.

In early studies, reduced testosterone levels were associated with elevations of follicle stimulating hormone (FSH) and luteinizing hormone (LH), indicating a direct testicular effect of glucocorticoids. In subsequent studies (MacAdams *et al.*, 1986; Morrison *et al.*, 1994), gonadotropins were not elevated, suggesting that glucocorticoids were acting centrally to suppress the pituitary–gonadal axis. Pearce *et al.* (1998) have shown there to be transient elevations of FSH but a decrease in LH. Thus, there is some conflict in the clinical data as to whether this is a central or peripheral effect. However, there is evidence from other studies suggesting that glucocorticoids may act at both sites. Thus, corticotrophin-releasing factor, ACTH, and cortisol have all been shown to diminish either basal or GnRH-stimulated release of LH in rats (Mann *et al.*, 1982; Ringstom and Schwartz, 1985; Rivier and Vale, 1985), and prednisolone reduces stimulated LH levels in women (Sakakura *et al.*, 1975). On the other hand, adrenocorticotrophic hormone (ACTH) has been shown to reduce plasma testosterone in rats even when human chorionic gonadotropin (HCG) is co-administered (Saez *et al.*, 1977), and acute administration of cortisol to men has been shown to reduce testosterone and increase gonadotropin levels (Doerr and Pirke, 1976). Administration of dexamethasone for 3 days to normal men depresses the testosterone response to HCG (Schaison *et al.*, 1978). The mechanism of the peripheral effect of glucocorticoids may be to decrease the number of LH receptors on the Leydig cells since reduced numbers of binding sites for HCG have been reported in the testes of steroid-treated rats (Saez *et al.*, 1977). The effect of glucocorticoids to reduce adrenal production of dehydroepiandrosterone sulfate (DHEAs) is not thought to be relevant because ACTH administration, which will increase production of DHEAS, also decreases circulating testosterone concentrations (Irvine *et al.*, 1974). Thus, the action of glucocorticoids on the pituitary–gonadal axis is probably both central and peripheral, the balance of these effects varying between clinical studies. This heterogeneity among clinical studies may also be contributed to by the fact that many of the conditions for which glucocorticoids are prescribed can themselves lead to hypogonadism (Turner and Wass, 1997).

IV. Patient Evaluation

As discussed earlier, many subjects taking glucocorticoids have bone density levels within the normal range. Therefore, the universal use of antiosteoporotic therapies in steroid-treated subjects is not appropriate, and patients should be evaluated to determine their fracture risk. To some extent, fracture risk can be assessed clinically based on past fracture history, sex, weight, cigarette smoking, the frequency of falls, and the like. However, much more reliable fracture prediction is possible with bone densitometry, and this should ideally be undertaken in all subjects receiving long-term glucocorticoid therapy. Bone loss is initially most marked in the spine, and assessment of spinal bone mass by quantitative computed tomography or dual-energy x-ray absorptiometry (DXA) is appropriate. DXA should preferably be undertaken in the lateral projection since this avoids measurement of the cortical bone of the posterior processes (Reid et al., 1992a), though the antero-posterior projection is frequently used. There is preliminary evidence that ultrasound assessment of bone is as satisfactory as conventional bone densitometry (Blanckaert et al., 1997).

Of the various biochemical markers of bone turnover, the one most consistently influenced by glucocorticoids is osteocalcin, which is decreased in a dose-dependent fashion (Reid et al., 1986). However, there is no evidence that measuring this or other markers of turnover permits a more accurate prediction of bone loss than would be possible from knowledge of the glucocorticoid dose alone (Reid and Heap, 1990). Other biochemical indices of calcium metabolism have not been shown to have a specific role in predicting rates of bone loss.

As discussed earlier, hypogonadism is common in glucocorticoid-treated men. This is frequently asymptomatic, and the presence of normal libido and potency does not rule out the finding of reduced serum testosterone. It is therefore wise to assess this hormone in steroid-treated men because its replacement is an option for therapy.

The decision to recommend the use of specific antiosteoporotic therapies in steroid-treated subjects is based largely on their fracture history and bone density findings, together with their expected steroid dose in the immediate future. A history of fractures after minimal trauma is clearly an indication for treatment. If a patient's bone density is toward the lower part of the young normal range, their fracture risk is already increased above average. If the subject is only just commencing glucocorticoid therapy, then a further 10–20% decline in bone density can be expected over the following years, placing their bone density in the clearly osteoporotic range. For this reason, such individuals would usually be offered treatment. On the other hand, subjects with a bone density in the upper part of the young normal range can be monitored without intervention initially. A flowchart for making these decisions in a glucocorticoid-treated man is provided in Figure 2.

It is my own practice to vary the intensity of intervention according to the degree of osteopenia and severity of past fracture history. Thus if a patient has already had multiple fractures after minor trauma and/or has a bone density markedly below the normal range, then intervention with multiple agents (e.g., testosterone replacement and a bisphosphonate) may be

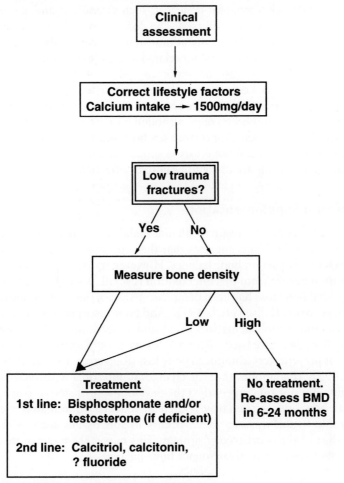

FIGURE 2   Flowchart for the evaluation and treatment of men receiving glucocorticoid therapy. Copyright © 1998 I. R. Reid, used with permission.

indicated. In a fracture-free individual with a bone density toward the lower end of the young normal range, then intervention with a single agent may be adequate initial management.

V. Management

In managing the osteoporosis of a steroid-treated patient, the intention is either to increase bone density (in established osteoporosis) or to prevent bone loss (in the patient just beginning steroid therapy) with a view to preventing fractures. Other risk factors for bone loss, such as smoking and maintenance of body weight, should be addressed. The dose of systemic steroid should be minimized and, if possible, locally administered steroids substituted for systemic medication. Other factors not related to bone mass optimization, such as falls prevention, may also be important. Most of the studies of specific interventions in steroid osteoporosis have been carried out in both men and women. In many, it is not possible to assess the outcomes in the two sexes separately from the published data; although where this information is available, it will be mentioned. Apart from sex hormone effects, the pathogenesis of glucocorticoid-induced bone loss is similar in men and women, and the available interventions are likely to be equally effective.

A. Calcium Supplementation

The occurrence of intestinal calcium malabsorption and hypercalciuria in steroid-treated patients suggests that the provision of extra calcium may have a positive impact on bone balance. However, most evidence suggests that the potential benefit from this intervention is small. A slight reduction in the rate of radial bone loss has been demonstrated with the daily administration of hydroxyapatite (Nilsen et al., 1978), and bone resorption is suppressed by simple calcium supplementation (Reid and Ibbertson, 1986). However, a number of studies have used calcium alone as a comparator and shown that it does not prevent steroid-induced bone loss (Reid et al., 1988a,b; Sambrook et al., 1993). This implies that the changes in intestinal and renal handling of calcium are not fundamental to the development of steroid osteoporosis and that bone loss is primarily related to reduced bone matrix synthesis, comparable to the wasting which occurs in soft tissues such as skin and muscle during glucocorticoid treatment. This moves the focus of therapy to attempting to more directly influence bone balance.

B. Bisphosphonates

Bisphosphonates bind directly to bone mineral and inhibit osteoclastic bone resorption. An increasing number of agents of this class are entering clinical trials or coming into routine clinical use, the individual members of the class differing in their antiresorptive potency and, in some cases, in their side effects. There is increasing evidence of their efficacy in steroid osteoporosis. Oral pamidronate substantially increases the bone density of steroid-treated patients (Reid et al., 1988a,b) and the same medication given by 3-monthly infusions has been shown to completely prevent bone loss in patients being started on prednisolone (Boutsen et al., 1997). There is a steadily increasing number of studies demonstrating the efficacy of oral etidronate, and this treatment has high patient acceptability because medication is taken for only 2 weeks every 3 months. The largest of these studies is the multicenter Canadian study of patients beginning steroid therapy (Adachi *et al.*, 1997b). Bone loss was prevented in the lumbar spine and femur, although the between-groups differences were not as substantial as in the pamidronate studies. This study demonstrated a reduction in height loss, and the overall incidence of vertebral fractures was reduced 40% with etidronate treatment, although this was only statistically significant amongst postmenopausal women. However, this study does suggest that, as in postmenopausal osteoporosis, the beneficial effects on bone mass produced by bisphosphonates translate into a reduced incidence of fractures in steroid-treated subjects.

Most of the bisphosphonate trials have assessed efficacy in the total patient population without a separate analysis by sex. However, the Canadian etidronate study did provide this, demonstrating efficacy in men as well as in women. In a study of pamidronate by Reid *et al.*, all 11 male patients who received active therapy showed increases in bone density at 12 months (Reid *et al.*, 1988b).

All bisphosphonates are very insoluble and therefore have low oral bioavailability. They must, therefore, be taken fasting with water at least 30 minutes before food. Etidronate occasionally causes diarrhea. The aminobisphosphonates, such as pamidronate and alendronate, may cause upper gastrointestinal irritation, particularly in patients with gastroesophageal reflux.

C. Vitamin D and Its Metabolites

This group of compounds has been evaluated as a therapy for steroid osteoporosis over several decades, but the inconsistencies in the outcomes of the various studies mean that their place is still uncertain. Much of the early work in humans was carried out by Hahn and co-workers. They demonstrated significant increases in forearm bone density from the use of calciferol 50,000 units three times per week plus calcium 500 mg/day (Hahn and Hahn, 1976). In a subsequent study using 25-hydroxyvitamin D (40 μg/day) similar beneficial effects on bone density were found (Hahn *et al.*, 1979), but in a third trial of calcitriol (0.4 μg/day), they found it to be no different from calcium in its effect on forearm density (Dykman *et al.*, 1984). Subsequently, Braun *et al.* (1983) demonstrated a beneficial effect of alphacalcidol (2 μg/day) on trabecular bone volume over a 6-month period but Bijlsma *et al.* (1988) failed to show any benefit from the use of dihydrotachysterol in a 2-year study. In 1989, Di Munno *et al.* reported a substantial gain in radial bone mineral content in patients starting glucocorticoids who were also given 25-hydroxyvitamin D (35 μg/day), in comparison with substantial losses in those given placebo.

Sambrook *et al.* (1993) have reported a large study in which patients beginning glucocorticoid therapy were randomly assigned to receive calcium, calcium plus calcitriol (mean dose 0.6 μg/day) or these two agents combined with calcitonin, over a 12-month period. Bone loss from the lumbar spine was 4.3, 1.3, and 0.2% in the respective groups. There was a similar but nonsignificant trend in distal radial bone loss but no evidence whatsoever of reduced bone loss in the proximal femur (3% in all groups). Although there was clearly a benefit from the use of calcitriol, it was less than that seen in a comparable trial in which etidronate was administered from the time of introduction of steroid therapy (Mulder and Struys, 1994). Furthermore, several groups have documented that etidronate also prevents femoral bone loss (Diamond *et al.*, 1995; Struys *et al.*, 1995). In contrast, one recent study of bone loss after cardiac transplantation compared the effects of alphacalcidol and etidronate (Van Cleemput *et al.*, 1996). Neither therapy completely prevented bone loss, but the vitamin D metabolite was superior to the bisphosphonate. It should be noted, however, that many of the patients in this study were vitamin D deficient. Adachi *et al.* (1996) have recently reexamined the effect of calciferol (50,000 units/week) plus calcium (1000 mg/day) in a randomized controlled trial. At the end of 3 years, they found no suggestion of any beneficial effect from the use of this intervention. This contrasts with the findings of Buckley *et al.* (1996) who showed prevention of bone loss with calcium (1000 mg/day) and calciferol (500 units/day) in patients who were, for the most part, already established on steroid therapy. It is unclear whether the different outcomes of these studies relate to the dose of vitamin D used, to the initial vitamin D status of the patients, or to different effects of these interventions in subjects initiating or continuing steroid treatment.

The relatively small number of studies with each agent and the variability of their outcomes make it difficult to determine the optimal course with respect to vitamin D and its metabolites in the prevention of steroid osteoporosis. Many suggest their use as adjunctive therapy to either sex hormone replacement or bisphosphonates in patients with severe steroid osteoporosis or as a second-line therapy in patients for whom these other agents are not acceptable. Calciferol is always indicated to treat proven vitamin D deficiency (i.e., subnormal circulating concentrations of 25-hydroxyvitamin D).

D. Fluoride

Fluoride ion is a potent osteoblast mitogen which has been demonstrated to produce substantial and cumulative increases in bone density with prolonged therapy. However, at only slightly higher doses than those necessary to increase bone density, it interferes with bone mineralization, and this is thought to account for the inconsistent data regarding its antifracture efficacy in postmenopausal osteoporosis, the condition in which it has been most extensively studied. There is clear evidence of its capacity to increase bone mass in steroid-treated subjects, but its antifracture efficacy in this context has not been adequately assessed. It is attractive as an adjunctuve agent in patients with severe steroid osteoporosis. For instance, Lems *et al.* (1997) have recently demonstrated increases in lumbar spine bone density of almost 5% per annum above those achieved with cyclical etidronate therapy alone. The absence of definitive efficacy data suggests that it should not be used as a first line agent in steroid osteoporosis at present.

E. Calcitonin

Calcitonin directly inhibits bone resorption via specific receptors on osteoclasts. It has been used in some countries for the management of postmenopausal osteoporosis, even though its effectiveness is generally less than that of hormone replacement therapy or the bisphosphonates. There have now been several controlled trials in steroid-treated subjects suggesting that it slows bone loss. Rizzato *et al.* (1988) found that injections of salmon calcitonin (100 IU every 1–2 days) prevented bone loss over a 15-month period, whereas vertebral bone mass declined 14% in the control group. Using a similar regimen, Luengo *et al.* (1990) found an increase in spinal bone density of 4% in those receiving calcitonin, whereas there was a 2.5% decrease in the density in the control group over a 12-month period. Similar results using intranasal calcitonin have been reported by Montemurro *et al.* (1991) and by Adachi *et al.* (1997a), the latter group finding a 3.7% between-groups difference in lumbar spine bone density after 12 months therapy with calcitonin or placebo. Thus, calcitonin is likely to be effective, but its side effects and cost make it less attractive than sex hormone therapy or the bisphosphonates.

F. Testosterone Supplementation

The frequent occurrence of hypogonadism in steroid-treated men and the knowledge that hypogonadism in other contexts is associated with reversible bone loss suggest that testosterone supplementation should be of benefit. Reid *et al.* have recently reported increases in lumbar spine bone density of 5% in steroid-treated subjects given monthly injections of testosterone esters (250 mg) (Figure 3) (Reid *et al.*, 1996). Circulating testosterone levels returned to baseline between each injection, suggesting that reduction in the interval between injections might increase efficacy. Testosterone was also found to reverse glucocorticoid effects on soft tissue composition, increasing lean mass and reducing fat mass (Figure 4). Some men experienced significant increases in energy and well-being, and the intervention was generally well tolerated, even though there were reductions in serum HDL cholesterol concentrations. Biochemical markers of bone turnover were reduced following testosterone therapy suggesting that the intervention primarily had an antiresorptive effect. This could be mediated directly by androgen receptors, but circulating estradiol levels were doubled following testosterone administration, and this could account for much of the antiresorptive effect seen.

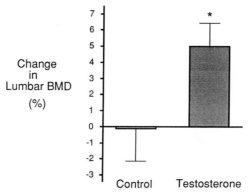

FIGURE 3   Rate of change of lumbar spine bone mineral density during control or testosterone treatment periods, each of 12 months duration. Data are mean ± SEM. There was a significant difference between groups ($p = 0.05$). Reproduced with permission from Reid *et al.*, *Arch. Int. Med.*, June 10, 1996, **156**, 1173–1177. Copyright 1996, American Medical Association.

The relative merits of testosterone supplementation in comparison with other therapeutic options require further exploration. In the available studies, testosterone was given by intramuscular injection which is associated by some discomfort, and many patients would prefer oral bisphosphonates or bisphosphonates by three monthly intravenous infusions. There is concern regarding androgen effects on the cardiovascular system, on the prostate, and on hematocrit, but how these considerations should be weighed against

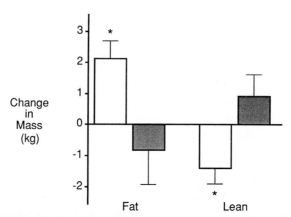

FIGURE 4   Changes in fat and lean body masses during the control period (open bars) and during treatment with testosterone (shaded bars). There were significant between-groups differences for both fat ($p = 0.03$) and lean ($p = 0.02$) masses. Reproduced with permission from Reid *et al.*, *Arch. Int. Med.*, June 10, 1996, **156**, 1173–1177. Copyright 1996, American Medical Association.

the potential increase in well-being is unclear. At the present time, testosterone clearly provides a further therapeutic option, one which can be combined with other interventions in the patient with severe osteoporosis.

VI. Research Directions

Steroid osteoporosis is a less prevalent problem than postmenopausal osteoporosis, so pharmaceutical companies tend to accord it a secondary priority. Thus, much of the clinical research at the present time is directed toward assessing the efficacy of agents already established in the management of postmenopausal osteoporosis. This is particularly true of the third generation bisphosphonates, and preliminary reports indicate that both alendronate and risedronate prevent bone loss in steroid-treated subjects of either sex. The analogs of parathyroid hormone should also be assessed in steroid osteoporosis.

For more than a decade the possibility of developing bone-sparing glucocorticoids was explored. While early results with deflazacort were encouraging, more recent data suggest that those studies were based on incorrect assumptions regarding the dose-equivalence of deflazacort, and that when it is used in doses of comparable therapeutic efficacy, it has no advantage over conventional glucocorticoids (Weisman, 1993; Di Munno *et al.*, 1995; Krogsgaard *et al.*, 1996).

There is clearly also a need for research on fracture prediction in steroid-treated subjects, both male and female. Data on fracture prediction based on bone density have all been acquired in the context of postmenopausal osteoporosis. There are suggestions that the "fracture threshold" is different in steroid-treated subjects (Luengo *et al.*, 1991) or that bone mass and fracture risk are unrelated in these individuals (Peel *et al.*, 1995). Because most decisions regarding the need for therapy are made on the basis of bone density measurements, resolution of these questions is important.

References

Adachi, J. D., Bensen, W. G., Bianchi, F., Cividino, A., Pillersdorf, S., Sebaldt, R. J., Tugwell, P., Gordon, M., Steele, M., Webber, C., and Goldsmith, C. H. (1996). Vitamin D and calcium in the prevention of corticosteroid induced osteoporosis—a 3 year followup. *J. Rheumatol.* **23,** 995–1000.

Adachi, J. D., Bensen, W. G., Bell, M. J., Bianchi, F. A., Cividino, A. A., Craig, G. L., Sturtridge, W. C., Sebaldt, R. J., Steele, M., Gordon, M., Themeles, E., Tugwell, P., Roberts, R., and Gent, M. (1997a). Salmon calcitonin nasal spray in the prevention of corticosteroid-induced osteoporosis. *Br. J. Rheumatol.* **36,** 255–259.

Adachi, J. D., Bensen, W. G., Brown, J., Hanley, D., Hodsman, A., Josse, R., Kendler, D. L., Lentle, B., Olszynski, W., Stemarie, L. G., Tenenhouse, A., and Chines, A. A. (1997b).

Intermittent etidronate therapy to prevent corticosteroid-induced osteoporosis. *N. Engl. J. Med.* **337**, 382–387.

Adinoff, A. D., and Hollister, J. R. (1983). Steroid-induced fractures and bone loss in patients with asthma. *N. Engl. J. Med.* **309**, 265–268.

Bijlsma, J. W., Raymakers, J. A., Mosch, C., Hoekstra, A., Derksen, R. H., Baart de la Faille, H., and Duursma, S. A. (1988). Effect of oral calcium and vitamin D on glucocorticoid-induced osteopenia. *Clin. Exp. Rheumatol.* **6**, 113–119.

Blanckaert, F., Cortet, B., Coquerelle, P., Flipo, R. M., Duquesnoy, B., Marchandise, X., and Delcambre, B. (1997). Contribution of calcaneal ultrasonic assessment to the evaluation of postmenopausal and glucocorticoid-induced osteoporosis. *Rev. Rhum. Mal. Osteo-Articulaires* **64**, 305–313.

Boden, S. D., Hair, G., Titus, L., Racine, M., McCuaig, K., Wozney, J. M., and Nanes, M. S. (1997). Glucocorticoid-induced differentiation of fetal rat calvarial osteoblasts is mediated by bone morphogenetic protein-6. *Endocrinology (Baltimore)* **138**, 2820–2828.

Boutsen, Y., Jamart, J., Esselinckx, W., Stoffel, M., and Devogelaer, J. P. (1997). Primary prevention of glucocorticoid-induced osteoporosis with intermittent intravenous pamidronate—a randomized trial. *Calcif. Tissue Int.* **61**, 266–271.

Braun, J. J., Birkenhager-Frenkel, D. H., Rietveld, A. H., Jr., Visser, J. T. J., and Birkenhager, J. C. (1983). Influence of 1α(OH)D3 administration on bone and bone mineral metabolism in patients on chronic glucocorticoid treatment; a double-blind controlled study. *Clin. Endocrinol. (Oxford)* **18**, 265–273.

Buckley, L. M., Leib, E. S., Cartularo, K. S., Vacek, P. M., and Cooper, S. M. (1995). Effects of low dose corticosteroids on the bone mineral density of patients with rheumatoid arthritis. *J. Rheumatol.* **22**, 1055–1059.

Buckley, L. M., Leib, E. S., Cartularo, K. S., Vacek, P. M., and Cooper, S. M. (1996). Calcium and vitamin D-3 supplementation prevents bone loss in the spine secondary to low-dose corticosteroids in patients with rheumatoid arthritis—a randomized, double-blind, placebo-controlled trial. *Ann. Intern. Med.* **125**, 961–968.

Caputo, C. B., Meadows, D., and Raisz, L. G. (1976). Failure of estrogens and androgens to inhibit bone resorption in tissue culture. *Endocrinology (Baltimore)* **98**, 1065–1068.

Centrella, M., McCarthy, T. L., and Canalis, E. (1991). Glucocorticoid regulation of transforming growth factor beta 1 activity and binding in osteoblast-enriched cultures from fetal rat bone. *Mol. Cell. Biol.* **11**, 3390–3396.

Chavassieux, P., Buffet, A., Vergnaud, P., Garnero, P., and Meunier, P. J. (1997). Short-term effects of corticosteroids on trabecular bone remodeling in old ewes. *Bone* **20**, 451–455.

Chevalley, T., Strong, D. D., Mohan, S., Baylink, D. J., and Linkhart, T. A. (1996). Evidence for a role for insulin-like growth factor binding proteins in glucocorticoid inhibition of normal human osteoblast-like cell proliferation. *Eur. J. Endocrinol.* **134**, 591–601.

Cooper, C., Coupland, C., and Mitchell, M. (1995). Rheumatoid arthritis, corticosteroid therapy and hip fracture. *Ann. Rheum. Dis.* **54**, 49–52.

Cosman, F., Nieves, J., Herbert, J., Shen, V., and Lindsay, R. (1994). High-dose glucocorticoids in multiple sclerosis patients exert direct effects on the kidney and skeleton. *J. Bone Miner. Res.* **9**, 1097–1105.

Cumming, R. G., Mitchell, P., and Leeder, S. R. (1997). Use of inhaled corticosteroids and the risk of cataracts. *N. Engl. J. Med.* **337**, 8–14.

Dempster, D. W. (1989). Bone histomorphometry in glucocorticoid-induced osteoporosis. *J. Bone Miner. Res.* **4**, 137–141.

Dempster, D. W., Moonga, B. S., Stein, L. S., Horbert, W. R., and Antakly, T. (1997). Glucocorticoids inhibit bone resorption by isolated rat osteoclasts by enhancing apoptosis. *J. Endocrinol.* **154**, 397–406.

Diamond, T., McGuigan, L., Barbagallo, S., and Bryant, C. (1995). Cyclical etidronate plus ergocalciferol prevents glucocorticoid-induced bone loss in postmenopausal women. *Am. J. Med.* **98**, 459–463.

Dietrich, J. W., Canalis, E. M., Maina, D. M., and Raisz, G. (1979). Effects of glucocorticoids on fetal rat bone collagen synthesis in vitro. *Endocrinology (Baltimore)* **104**, 715–721.

Di Munno, O., Beghe, F., Favini, P., Di Giuseppe, P., Pontrandolfo, A., Occhipinti, G., and Pasero, G. (1989). Prevention of glucocorticoid-induced osteopenia: Effect of oral 25-hydroxyvitamin D and calcium. *Clin. Rheumatol.* **8**, 202–207.

Di Munno, O., Imbimbo, B., Mazzantini, M., Milani, S., Occhipinti, G., and Pasero, G. (1995). Deflazacort versus methylprednisolone in polymyalgia rheumatica: Clinical equivalence and relative antiinflammatory potency of different treatment regimens. *J. Rheumatol.* **22**, 1492–1498.

Doerr, P., and Pirke, K. M. (1976). Cortisol-induced suppression of plasma testosterone in normal adult males. *J. Clin. Endocrinol. Metab.* **43**, 622–629.

Doull, I., Freezer, N., and Holgate, S. (1996). Osteocalcin, growth, and inhaled corticosteroids—a prospective study. *Arch. Dis. Child.* **74**, 497–501.

Dykman, T. R., Haralson, K. M., Gluck, O. S., Murphy, W. A., Teitelbaum, S. L., Hahn, T. J., and Hahn, B. H. (1984). Effect of oral 1,25-dihydroxy-vitamin D and calcium on glucocorticoid-induced osteopenia in patients with rheumatic diseases. *Arthritis Rheum.* **27**, 1336–1343.

Fitzgerald, R. C., Skingle, S. J., and Crisp, A. J. (1997). Testosterone concentrations in men on chronic glucocorticosteroid therapy. *J. R. Coll. Physicians London* **31**, 168–170.

Florkowski, C. M., Holmes, S. J., Elliot, J. R., Donald, R. A., and Espiner, E. A. (1994). Bone mineral density is reduced in female but not male subjects with Addison's disease. *N.Z. Med. J.* **107**, 52–53.

Gabbitas, B., and Canalis, E. (1996). Cortisol enhances the transcription of insulin-like growth factor-binding protein-6 in cultured osteoblasts. *Endocrinology (Baltimore)* **137**, 1687–1692.

Gabbitas, B., Pash, J. M., Delany, A. M., and Canalis, E. (1996). Cortisol inhibits the synthesis of insulin-like growth factor-binding protein-5 in bone cell cultures by transcriptional mechanisms. *J. Biol. Chem.* **271**, 9033–9038.

Gallagher, J. A., Beresford, J. N., MacDonald, B. R., and Russell, R. G. G. (1984). Hormone target cell interactions in human bone. *In* "Osteoporosis" (C. Christiansen, ed.), pp. 431–439. Copenhagen.

Gray, R. E., Doherty, S. M., Galloway, J., Coulton, L., de Broe, M., and Kanis, J. A. (1991). A double-blind study of deflazacort and prednisone in patients with chronic inflammatory disorders. *Arthritis Rheum.* **34**, 287–295.

Grebe, S. K. G., Feek, C. M., Durham, J. A., Kljakovic, M., and Cooke, R. R. (1997). Inhaled beclomethasone dipropionate suppresses the hypothalamo-pituitary-adrenal axis in a dose dependent manner. *Clin. Endocrinol. (Oxford)* **47**, 297–304.

Gronowicz, G., McCarthy, M. B., and Raisz, L. G. (1990). Glucocorticoids stimulate resorption in fetal rat parietal bones in vitro. *J. Bone Miner. Res.* **5**, 1223–1230.

Hahn, T. J., and Hahn, B. H. (1976). Osteopenia in patients with rheumatic diseases: Principles of diagnosis and therapy. *Semin. Arthritis Rheum.* **6**, 165–188.

Hahn, T. J., Halstead, L. R., Teitelbaum, S. L., and Hahn, B. H. (1979). Altered mineral metabolism in glucocorticoid-induced osteopenia. *J. Clin. Invest.* **64**, 655–665.

Hermus, A. R., Huysmans, D. A., Smals, A. G., Corstens, F. H., and Kloppenborg, P. W. (1994). Remarkable improvement of osteopenia after cure of Cushings syndrome. *Horm. Metab. Res.* **26**, 209–210.

Irvine, W. J., Toft, A. D., and Wilson, K. S. (1974). The effect of synthetic corticotropin analogues on adrenocortical, anterior pituitary and testicular function. *J. Clin. Endocrinol. Metab.* **39**, 522–529.

Kaji, H., Sugimoto, T., Kanatani, M., Nishiyama, K., and Chihara, K. (1997). Dexamethasone stimulates osteoclast-like cell formation by directly acting on hemopoietic blast cells and enhances osteoclast-like cell formation stimulated by parathyroid hormone and prostaglandin e-2. *J. Bone Miner. Res.* **12**, 734–741.

Krogsgaard, M. R., Thamsborg, G., and Lund, B. (1996). Changes in bone mass during low dose corticosteroid treatment in patients with polymalgia rheumatica—a double blind, prospective comparison between prednisolone and deflazacort. *Ann. Rheum. Dis.* **55**, 143–146.

Laan, R. F. J. M., van Riel, P. L. C. M., van Erning, L. J. T., Lemmens, J. A. M., Ruijs, S. H. J., et al. (1992). Vertebral osteoporosis in rheumatoid arthritis patients: Effect of low dose prednisone therapy. *Br. J. Rheumatol.* **31**, 91–96.

Laan, R. F. J. M., Vanriel, P. L. C. M., Vandeputte, L. B. A., Vanerning, L. J. T. O., Vanthof, M. A., and Lemmens, J. A. M. (1993). Low-dose prednisone induces rapid reversible axial bone loss in patients with rheumatoid arthritis—a randomized, controlled study. *Ann. Intern. Med.* **119**, 963–968.

Lems, W. F., Jahangier, Z. N., Jacobs, J. W. G., and Bijlsma, J. W. J. (1995). Vertebral fractures in patients with rheumatoid arthritis treated with corticosteroids. *Clin. Exp. Rheumatol.* **13**, 293–297.

Lems, W. F., Jacobs, J. W. G., Bijlsma, J. W. J., Vanveen, G. J. M., Houben, H. M. L., Haanen, H. C. M., Gerrits, M. I., and Vanrijn, H. J. M. (1997). Is addition of sodium fluoride to cyclical etidronate beneficial in the treatment of corticosteroid induced osteoporosis. *Ann. Rheum. Dis.* **56**, 357–363.

Lo Cascio, V., Bonucci, E., Imbimbo, B., Ballanti, P., Adami, S., Milani, S., Tartarotti, D., and DellaRoca, C. (1990). Bone loss in response to long-term glucocorticoid therapy. *Bone Miner.* **8**, 39–51.

Lowe, C., Gray, D. H., and Reid, I. R. (1992). Serum blocks the osteolytic effect of cortisol in neonatal mouse calvaria. *Calcif. Tissue Int.* **50**, 189–192.

Luengo, M., Picado, C., Del Rio, L., Guanabens, N., Montserrat, J. M., and Setoain, J. (1990). Treatment of steroid-induced osteopenia with calcitonin in corticosteroid-dependent asthma. A one-year follow-up study. *Am. Rev. Respir. Dis.* **142**, 104–107.

Luengo, M., Picado, C., Del Rio, L., Guanabens, N., Montserrat, J. M., and Setoain, J. (1991). Vertebral fractures in steroid dependent asthma and involutional osteoporosis: A comparative study. *Thorax* **46**, 803–806.

Lufkin, E. G., Wahner, H. W., and Bergstralh, E. J. (1988). Reversibility of steroid-induced osteoporosis. *Am. J. Med.* **85**, 887–888.

MacAdams, M. R., White, R. H., and Cipps, B. E. (1986). Reduction of serum testosterone levels during chronic glucocorticoid therapy. *Ann. Intern. Med.* **104**, 648–651.

Mann, D. R., Jackson, G. C., and Blank, M. S. (1982). Influence of adrenocorticotropin and adrenalectomy on gonadotropin secretion in immature rats. *Neuroendicronology* **34**, 20–26.

Manning, P. J., Evans, M. C., and Reid, I. R. (1992). Normal bone mineral density following cure of Cushing's syndrome. *Clin. Endocrinol. (Oxford)* **36**, 229–234.

Michel, B. A., Bloch, D. A., and Fries, J. F. (1991). Predictors of fractures in early rheumatoid arthritis. *J. Rheumatol.* **18**, 804–808.

Michel, B. A., Bloch, D. A., Wolfe, F., and Fries, J. F. (1993). Fractures in rheumatoid arthritis—an evaluation of associated risk factors. *J. Rheumatol.* **20**, 1666–1669.

Montemurro, L., Schiraldi, G., Fraioli, P., Tosi, G., Riboldi, A., and Rizzato, G. (1991). Prevention of corticosteroid-induced osteoporosis with salmon calcitonin in sarcoid patients. *Calcif. Tissue Int.* **49**, 71–76.

Morrison, D., Capewell, S., Reynolds, S. P., Thomas, J., Ali, N. J., Read, G. F., Henley, R., and Riadfahmy, D. (1994). Testosterone levels during systemic and inhaled corticosteroid therapy. *Respir. Med.* **88**, 659–663.

Mulder, H., and Struys, A. (1994). Intermittent cyclical etidronate in the prevention of corticosteroid-induced bone loss. *Br. J. Rheumatol.* **33**, 348–350.

Nilsen, K. H., Jayson, M. I. V., and Dixon, A. StJ. (1978). Microcrystalline calcium hydroxyapatite compound in corticosteroid-treated rheumatoid patients: A controlled study. *Br. Med. J.* **2**, 1124.

Okazaki, R., Riggs, B. L., and Conover, C. A. (1994). Glucocorticoid regulation of insulin-like growth factor-binding protein expression in normal human osteoblast-like cells. *Endocrinology (Baltimore)* **134**, 126–132.

Oursler, M. J., Riggs, B. L., and Spelsberg, T. C. (1993). Glucocorticoid-induced activation of latent transforming growth factor-beta by normal human osteoblast-like cells. *Endocrinology (Baltimore)* **133**, 2187–2196.

Pearce, G., Tabensky, D. A., Delmas, P. D., Baker, H. W. G., and Seeman, E. (1998). Corticosteroid-induced bone loss in men. *J. Clin. Endocrinol. Metab.* **83**, 801–806.

Peel, N. F. A., Moore, D. J., Barrington, N. A., Bax, D. E., and Eastell, R. (1995). Risk of vertebral fracture and relationship to bone mineral density in steroid treated rheumatoid arthritis. *Ann. Rheum. Dis.* **54**, 801–806.

Reid, I. R., and Heap, S. W. (1990). Determinants of vertebral mineral density in patients receiving chronic glucocorticoid therapy. *Arch. Intern. Med.* **150**, 2545–2548.

Reid, I. R., and Ibbertson, H. K. (1986). Calcium supplements in the prevention of steroid-induced osteoporosis. *Am. J. Clin. Nutr.* **44**, 287–290.

Reid, I. R., and Ibberston, H. K. (1987). Evidence for decreased tubular reabsorption of calcium in glucorticoid-treated asthmatics. *Horm. Res.* **27**, 200–204.

Reid, I. R., France, J. T., Pybus, J., and Ibbertson, H. K. (1985). Low plasma testosterone levels in glucocorticoid-treated male asthmatics. *Br. Med. J.* **291**, 574.

Reid, I. R., Chapman, G. E., Fraser, T. R. C., Davies, A. D., Surus, A. S., Meyer, J., Huq, N. L., and Ibbertson, H. J. (1986). Low serum osteocalcin levels in glucocorticoid-treated asthmatics. *J. Clin. Endocrinol. Metab.* **62**, 379–383.

Reid, I. R., King, A. R., Alexander, C. J., and Ibbertson, H. K. (1988a). Prevention of steroid-induced osteoporosis with (3-amino-1-hydroxypropylidene)-1,1-bisphosphonate (APD). *Lancet* **1**, 143–146.

Reid, I. R., Heap, S. W., King, A. R., and Ibbertson, H. K. (1988b). Two-year follow-up of bisphosphonate (APD) treatment in steroid osteoporosis. *Lancet* **2**, 1144.

Reid, I. R., Evans, M. C., and Stapleton, J. (1992a). Lateral spine densitometry is a more sensitive indicator of glucocorticoid-induced bone loss. *J. Bone Miner. Res.* **7**, 1221–1225.

Reid, I. R., Evans, M. C., Wattie, D. J., Ames, R., and Cundy, T. F. (1992b). Bone mineral density of the proximal femur and lumbar spine in glucocorticoid-treated asthamtic patients. *Osteoporosis Int.* **2**, 103–105.

Reid, I. R., Veale, A. G., and France, J. T. (1994). Glucocorticoid osteoporosis. *J. Asthma* **31**, 7–18.

Reid, I. R., Wattie, D. J., Evans, M. C., and Stapleton, J. P. (1996). Testosterone therapy in glucocorticoid-treated men. *Arch. Intern. Med.* **156**, 1173–1177.

Ringstom, S. J,, and Schwartz, N. Z. (1985). Cortisol suppresses the LH, but not the FSH, response to gonadotropin-releasing hormone after orchidectomy. *Endocrinology (Baltimore)* **116**, 472–474.

Rivier, C., and Vale, W. (1985). Effects of long-term administration of corticotropin-releasing factor on the pituitary-adrenal and pituitary-gonadal axis in the male rat. *J. Clin. Invest.* **75**, 689–694.

Rizzato, G., and Montemurro, L. (1993). Reversibility of exogenous corticosteroid-induced bone loss. *Eur. Respir. J.* **6**, 116–119.

Rizzato, G., Tosi, G., Schiraldi, G., Montemurro, L., Zanni, D., and Sisti, S. (1988). Bone protection with salmon calcitonin (sCT) in the long-term steroid therapy of chronic sarcoidosis. *Sarcoidosis* **5**, 99–103.

Rogatsky, I., Trowbridge, J. M., and Garabedian, M. J. (1997). Glucocorticoid receptor-mediated cell cycle arrest is achieved through distinct cell-specific transcriptional regulatory mechanisms. *Mol. Cell. Biol.* **17**, 3181–3193.

Saez, J. M., Morera, A. M., Haour, F., and Evain, D. (1977). Effects of in vivo administration of dexamethasone, corticotropin and human chorionic gonadotropin on steroidogenesis and protein and DNA synthesis of testicular interstitial cells in prepubertal rats. *Endocrinology (Baltimore)* **101**, 1256–1263.

Saito, J. K., Davis, J. W., Wasnich, R. D., and Ross, P. D. (1995). Users of low-dose glucocorticoids have increased bone loss rates: A longitudinal study. *Calcif. Tissue Int.* **57**, 115–119.

Sakakura, M., Takebe, K., and Nakagawa, S. (1975). Inhibition of luteinizing hormone secretion induced by synthetic LRH by long-term treatment with glucocorticoids in human subjects. *J. Clin. Endocrinol. Metab.* **40**, 774–779.

Sambrook, P., Birmingham, J., Kelly, P., Kempler, S., Nguyen, T., Pocock, N., and Eisman, J. (1993). Prevention of corticosteroid osteoporosis—a comparison of calcium, calcitriol, and calcitonin. *N. Engl. J. Med.* **328**, 1747–1752.

Schaison, G., Durand, F., and Mowszowicz, I. (1978). Effect of glucocorticoids on plasma testosterone in men. *Acta Endocrinol. (Copenhagen)* **89**, 126–131.

Shuto, T., Kukita, T., Hirata, M., Jimi, E., and Koga, T. (1994). Dexamethasone stimulates osteoclast-like cell formation by inhibiting granulocyte-macrophage colony-stimulating factor production in mouse bone marrow cultures. *Endocrinology (Baltimore)* **134**, 1121–1126.

Smals, A. G. H., Kloppenborg, P. W. C., and Benraad, T. J. (1977). Plasma testosterone profiles in Cushing's syndrome. *J. Clin. Endocrinol. Metab.* **45**, 240–245.

Spector, T. D., Hall, G. M., McCloskey, E. V., and Kanis, J. A. (1993). Risk of vertebral fracture in women with rheumatoid arthritis. *Br. Med. J.* **306**, 558.

Struijs, A., and Mulder, H. (1997). The effects of inhaled glucocorticoids on bone mass and biochemical markers of bone homeostasis—a 1-year study of beclomethasone versus budesonide. *Neth. J. Med.* **50**, 233–237.

Struys, A., Snelder, A. A., and Mulder, H. (1995). Cyclical etidronate reverses bone loss of the spine and proximal femur in patients with established corticosteroid-induced osteoporosis. *Am. J. Med.* **99**, 235–242.

Tobias, J., and Chambers, T. J. (1989). Glucocorticoids impair bone resorptive activity and viability of osteoclasts disaggregated from neonatal rat long bones. *Endocrinology (Baltimore)* **125**, 1290–1295.

Turner, H. E., and Wass, J. A. H. (1997). Gonadal function in men with chronic illness. *Clin. Endocrinol. (Oxford)* **47**, 379–403.

Van Cleemput, J., Daenen, W., Geusens, P., Dequeker, J., Van de Werf, F., and Vanhaecke, J. (1996). Prevention of bone loss in cardiac transplant recipients—a comparison of bisphosphonates and vitamin D. *Transplantation* **61**, 1495–1499.

Weisman, M. H. (1993). Dose equivalency of deflazacort and prednisone in the treatment of steroid dependent rheumatoid arthritis. *Proc. Int. Symp. Osteoporosis, 4th,* Copenhagen, p. 515.

Welten, D. C., Kemper, H. C. G., Post, G. B., Vanmechelen, W., Twisk, J., Lips, P., and Teule, G. J. (1994). Weight-bearing activity during youth is a more important factor for peak bone mass than calcium intake. *J. Bone Miner. Res.* **9**, 1089–1096.

Zelissen, P. M. J., Croughs, R. J. M., Vanrijk, P. P., and Raymakers, J. A. (1994). Effects of glucocorticoid replacement therapy on bone mineral density in patients with Addison disease. *Ann. Intern. Med.* **120**, 207–210.

Chapter 21

Robert F. Klein

Bone and Mineral Unit
Oregon Health Sciences University
and the Portland VA Medical Center
Portland, Oregon

Alcohol

I. Introduction

Prolonged alcohol abuse results in a host of abnormal clinical, biochemical, and physiologic findings that stem from the toxic effects of ethanol on the liver (e.g., cirrhosis), bone marrow (e.g., anemia), and brain (e.g., addiction, dementia). It therefore is not surprising that long-term alcohol abuse has been shown to be detrimental to skeletal integrity (reduced bone mass and increased fracture incidence). However, some studies of subjects with more moderate intake suggest a potentially beneficial effect of alcohol to slow the normal decline in bone mass that accompanies aging. This section reviews significant research findings describing the skeletal consequences of alcohol consumption. The specific topics addressed include epidemiological studies of the effect of alcohol intake on bone mass and fracture incidence; clinical investigations into the nutritional and hormonal consequences of alcohol intake on skeletal integrity; basic science studies on the effect of alcohol on bone cell biology; and appropriate therapeutic modalities.

II. Alcohol-Induced Osteoporotic Fractures _____

Since the time of the ancient Egyptians, alcohol abuse has been known to confer a high risk for skeletal fracture (Conn, 1985; Seller, 1985; Mathew, 1992). However, recent scientific studies of fracture prevalence in alcoholic subjects are, for the most part, based on small, inadequately controlled series. Of 19 alcoholic subjects (15 men and 4 women) examined by Schnitzler and Solomon (1984), 8 were found to have severe osteoporosis with a total of 52 fractured bones—19 vertebral compression fractures, 6 rib fractures, and 10 hip fractures! Lindsell et al. (1982) compared chest x-rays of 72 subjects with alcoholic cirrhosis to those of 149 controls. Rib fractures were four times more common in the alcoholic population (28% versus 7%). Similarly, Israel and colleagues (1980) found 29% of 198 male alcoholics had rib or vertebral fractures on x-ray compared to 2% of nonalcoholic control males. Finally, Crilly et al. (1988) evaluated 50 male alcoholics and found that 25 exhibited roentgenologic evidence of at least two atraumatic spinal crush fractures. These observations have prompted some investigators to suggest that the presence of fractures on chest x-ray films may serve as a useful indicator of occult alcoholism in men (Israel et al., 1980; Lindsell et al., 1982). In contrast, only a small proportion of fractures in women are attributable to alcohol abuse. Johnell et al. (1985) found a history of alcohol abuse in 25% of all men but only 4% of women hospitalized for lower limb fractures.

Even though men hospitalized for alcohol-related problems are much more likely to have experienced an osteoporotic fracture, the effect of moderate alcohol consumption on the bones of healthy subjects has not been well explored. Evidence from population studies is inconsistent, with some reporting a positive association between alcohol intake and fracture occurrence, and others detecting no such association. In a study of 105 men with vertebral compression fractures secondary to osteoporosis (Seeman and Melton, 1983), alcohol consumption was found to be a highly significant risk factor (relative risk = 2.4 overall). The risk of osteoporosis increased by 0.7% for each ounce-year of cumulative exposure ($p = 0.01$). The risk further increased with age (relative risk = 20.2 for individuals 70 years and over). The Framingham Observational Study also has examined the association between alcohol consumption and hip fracture (Felson et al., 1988). During 117,224 person-years of follow-up, 217 hip fractures occurred (174 in women and 43 in men) and the relative risk increased by 28% for every 7 drinks per week consumption. However, other studies of similar size and design have not identified any significant association between alcohol intake and fracture risk. Hemenway and colleagues (1994) recorded 271 wrist fractures in a prospective study of 51,529 men aged 50 to 75 years during 271,522 person-years of observation. Risk of wrist fracture was unrelated to alcohol consumption. Similarly, no association was detected between frequency of alcohol intake and either vertebral deformity (Naves Diaz *et al.*, 1997) or distal forearm fracture (O'Neill *et al.*, 1996). However, it is possible that preferential mortality and an unequal reporting of abstention between the fracture cases and controls may have limited the ability of these epidemiological surveys to demonstrate a significant risk of alcohol consumption.

Thus, accumulating evidence suggests that excessive alcohol intake increases the risk of fracture. However, the skeletal consequences of smaller amounts of alcohol consumption are less clear. Because of the much larger number of people at risk from moderate alcohol consumption, it is crucial that the impact of social drinking on skeletal integrity be better assessed. Unfortunately, the majority of available data on this issue comes from case-control and cohort studies designed to identify general risk factors for osteoporotic fractures, not to specifically explore the impact of alcohol consumption on fracture incidence. A study of the relationship between alcohol intake and fracture risk would be a formidable undertaking, but likely to have important public health implications, considering the prevalence of osteoporosis and prominence of drinking in American society.

III. Alcohol-Induced Osteopenia

Although the relationship between excessive alcohol ingestion and bone disease has been established, the mechanisms by which alcohol induces osteoporotic fractures remain unclear. An association between alcoholism and accidental injury is well recognized (Lucas, 1987). Alcohol intoxication creates conditions that favor accidents and falls, facilitating bone fractures (Lucas, 1987). In a study comparing the blood alcohol level (BAL) of fall subjects with non-fall controls, relative risks were 1 (BAL 0–0.1%), 3 (BAL 0.1–0.15%), and 60 (BAL $\geq$ 0.16%) (Honkanen *et al.*, 1983) (Figure 1). In addition to the direct effects of intoxication, the impaired muscle control that can accompany alcohol-associated neuromuscular disabilities, withdrawal fits and hypoglycemic attacks probably also contribute to the increased fall frequency. However, emerging evidence suggests that alcoholics may also suffer from a generalized skeletal fragility that makes their bones more liable to fracture.

Bone density is an important determinant of bone strength and is a predictor of fractures. Saville (1965) was the first to demonstrate the association of reduced bone mineral density (osteopenia) with alcohol abuse. Using postmortem material from 198 cadavers, he observed that fat-free bone mass was markedly reduced in the 39 samples from individuals with a history of

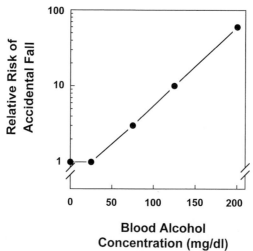

FIGURE I   Relative risk of injury from accidental fall related to blood alcohol concentration. Data from Honkanen *et al.* (1983).

alcoholism. He noted that the bone mass of young alcoholic males was comparable to that of elderly postmenopausal females. Subsequent studies over the past quarter century have clearly demonstrated clinically relevant reductions in bone mass in alcoholics, especially in the iliac crest, calcaneus, vertebral column, and hip (Spencer *et al.,* 1986; Diamond *et al.,* 1989; Peris *et al.,* 1995). In a recent prospective case-control analysis of risk factors for the development of osteoporosis, average alcohol consumption was two to three times higher in both osteoporotic males ($p = 0.001$) and osteoporotic females ($p = 0.01$) than that of age-matched controls (Blaauw *et al.,* 1994). Slemenda and colleagues (Slemenda *et al.,* 1992) found in a 16-year follow-up study of 111 men that those who drank more than 1.5 drinks per day experienced more rapid bone loss than those who did not imbibe. Spencer and colleagues (1986) reviewed thoraco-lumbar spine x-rays of 96 ambulatory men with chronic alcoholism and noted osteopenia in 47%. One-half of those affected were under the age of 50. Diamond *et al.* (1989) found that 38% of ambulatory patients with alcoholic liver disease had reduced bone mineral density of the spine, forearm, or both. Chon examined 32 nonhospitalized, Caucasian alcoholic men and found the subjects' average femoral neck and lumbar spine bone mineral density values were, respectively, 0.56 and 0.57 standard deviations below the age-matched normative values (Chon *et al.,* 1992). Finally, Peris and colleagues (1995) reported that 29% of chronic alcoholic male subjects exhibited lumbar spine bone mineral density values below the fracture threshold as compared to only 8% of the age-matched control population.

Still, reduced bone density is not universally reported. In one prospective epidemiological study of 142 men and 220 women, bone density was measured 12 years after documentation of alcohol intake by questionnaire (Holbrook and Barrett-Connor, 1993). Increasing alcohol consumption was associated with higher bone density at the hip in men and spine in women (Figure 2). The Study of Osteoporotic Fractures (7963 ambulatory, Caucasian women, 65 years or older) has also found that moderate alcohol intake is associated with higher bone density (Orwoll *et al.*, 1996). A small study of 19 premenopausal alcoholic women found no difference in spine, hip or forearm bone density (Laitinen *et al.*, 1993), but a larger cross-sectional study of postmenopausal women by this research group observed a positive

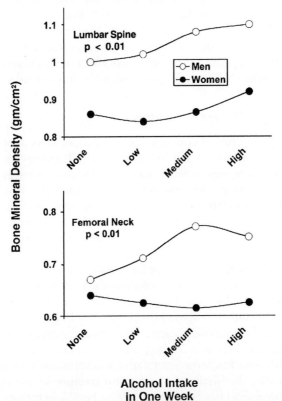

**Alcohol Intake
in One Week**

FIGURE 2   Adjusted mean bone mineral density of femoral neck and lumbar spine in relation to alcohol intake in one week. In this study, low alcohol intake = 0.1 − 19.1 g for men and 0.1 − 14.3 g for women; medium intake = 19.2 − 41.1 g for men, 14.4 − 28.8 g for women: high intake = ⩾ 41.2 g for men, ⩾ 28.9 g for women. This figure was first published in the BMJ [Holbrook, T. L., and Barrett-Connor, E., A prospective study of alcohol consumption and bone mineral density, *Br. Med. J.* 1993; **306**:1506–1509] and is reproduced by permission of the BMJ.

correlation between alcohol intake and bone density (Laitinen *et al.*, 1991c). May and colleagues (1995) examined 458 men over the age of 60. Mean bone density at the proximal femur was significantly higher in the drinkers ($n = 335$) as compared with the non-drinkers ($n = 123$), but after adjusting for smoking, caffeine intake and physical activity, the difference remained significant at the trochanter only. Lastly, a community-based sample of ambulatory men over the age of 50 found no association between bone density and alcohol consumption (Glynn *et al.*, 1995). Of note, only 26% of this cohort consumed more than one standard drink per day.

Hence, the excessive consumption of alcoholic beverages is recognized as a significant determinant of reduced bone mass and increased fracture rates in epidemiological surveys of both men and women. The degree to which alcohol contributes to osteopenia in the entire population is not yet known. There are intriguing new data suggesting that more modest alcohol consumption is less likely to be associated with low bone density and may even be associated with higher bone density. Moderate alcohol intake may affect endogenous hormone levels (*vide infra*) to indirectly augment skeletal mass. However, the evidence for a protective effect of moderate alcohol consumption is not entirely compelling and should be interpreted with caution.

A. Limitations of Current Studies

To evaluate the clinical consequences of alcohol consumption successfully, a number of obstacles must be recognized and circumvented (Seeman, 1996). First, it is extremely difficult to define, let alone accurately quantify lifetime alcohol exposure, and this issue is compounded further when studying elderly individuals with impaired recall. Second, most studies treat alcohol consumption as a continuous variable. Biphasic effects of alcohol (protective at one level of consumption and harmful at another) would likely be obscured in such analyses. Third, individuals rarely, if ever, vary in their exposure to only one factor. Confounding by known and unknown factors must be assessed and taken into account in analyses. Finally, small sample sizes, preferential mortality, biological variation, and measurement error can reduce the power of studies to detect effects that may be small at the individual level but are of considerable societal importance. Any association (either positive or negative) between drinking and fracture rates will be difficult to demonstrate because fractures are relatively uncommon events, especially in men. Currently, the lifetime risk of a hip fracture in the United States (Rochester, Minnesota) has been calculated to be 6% in men and 17.5% in women from age 50 onward (Melton and Chrischilles, 1992). Attention to these serious methodological issues (e.g., adequate sample size, accurate assessment of "lifetime" alcohol exposure, proper accounting for relevant covariates such as tobacco exposure, appropriate representation of all levels of alcohol intake, etc.) are lacking from most published studies and may result in a distorted estimation of the true consequences of alcohol on the skeleton. Even when they are accounted for, current studies document associations but do not prove causality. Despite adjusting for known covariates, the association between social drinking and increased bone density found in some studies may not be causal. Moderate alcohol intake may merely be a marker for relative affluence (resulting in better nutrition and a healther life-style during peak bone mass acquisition earlier in life). A randomized intervention study will likely be required to ultimately prove the existence of a cause-and-effect relationship.

IV. Potential Mechanisms of Alcohol-Induced Bone Disease

A. Effect of Alcohol on Adult Bone

Microscopic examination of bone (bone histomorphometry) from alcoholic subjects has provided important insight into the specific nature of the skeletal disorder induced by ethanol. Adult bone mass is regulated by a remodeling cycle that is composed of an initial period of resorption by osteoclasts followed by a balanced amount of new bone formation by osteoblasts. Skeletal remodeling is a continuous process with approximately 10% of bone undergoing the process at any given time. Bone formation and bone resorption rates are tightly coupled, allowing for large amounts of bone to be replaced throughout adult life without significant alterations in total bone mass.

Baran and co-workers (1980) found that chronic (8 weeks) exposure of rats to alcohol resulted in diminished trabecular bone volume and enhanced bone resorption. Using scanning electron microscopy, Peng and colleagues (1988) found that the trabeculae of femurs from ethanol-fed rats were thinner than those from control rats. These ultrastructural changes in bone morphology were accompanied by a substantial compromise in the overall mechanical strength of the bone. Turner *et al.* (1987) observed significant reductions in bone matrix synthesis and mineralization rates in rats receiving intoxicating amounts of ethanol for 3 weeks.

Similar alcohol-induced histomorphometric abnormalities have been found in humans. Schnitzler and Solomon (1984) found a reduction in bone formation parameters and an increase in bone resorption parameters in alcoholic patients, leading them to conclude that alcohol uncouples the normal association between bone formation and resorption. Diamond and co-workers (1989) examined 28 alcoholic subjects and found markedly diminished bone formation rates in the alcoholics as compared to 36 nonalcoholic control subjects (0.1 $\mu m^3/\mu m^2$/day versus 0.06 $\mu m^3/\mu m^2$/day, respectively). However, bone resorption was relatively active because no significant differences in osteoclast parameters (number, resorption surface area, etc.) were found between these two groups. Crilly *et al.* (1988) compared 16 actively imbibing alcoholic subjects with 9 chronic alcoholics who had been abstinent for at least 3 months prior to study. The actively drinking subjects were found to have 60% fewer osteoblasts and a 50% lower mineralization rate. Resorption parameters were not different (Table I). Similarly, in a study of 20 alcoholic men, Chappard *et al.* (1991) noted significant defects in osteoblastic function with reduced osteoid parameters associated with decreased mineralization rates and reduced mineralized surfaces. As a consequence, bone formation rate and trabecular thickness were significantly reduced; conversely, osteoclast number was not significantly different from normal. The overall impression from these studies seems to be that alcoholic bone disease is characterized by considerable suppression of bone formation, whereas indices of bone resorption, for the most part, do not differ substantially from that observed in control subjects.

Studies on alcohol abstainers have demonstrated a rapid recovery of osteoblast function (as assessed histomorphometrically and by biochemical parameters of bone remodeling) within as little as 2 weeks after cessation of drinking (Feitelberg *et al.*, 1987; Diamond *et al.*, 1989; Laitinen *et al.*, 1992a). Moreover, a recent report suggests that bone, once lost, can be at least partially restored when alcohol abuse is discontinued (Peris *et al.*, 1994). Hence, the bone loss in alcoholism appears to be a consequence of an imbalance in the normal tight coupling of resorption and formation, with normal resorption activity outstripping a repressed formation process. To date, no histomorphometric analyses have been performed on moderate

TABLE I Comparison of Bone Histomorphometric Parameters in Abstainers and Current Drinkers

Parameters	Abstainers (n = 9)	Drinkers (n = 16)	Significance (p value)
Bone formation			
Osteoid volume (%)	0.68 ± 0.17	0.38 ± 0.08	NS
Osteoid seam width (μm)	11.4 ± 0.68	7.95 ± 0.48	0.001
Osteoid surface with osteoblasts (%)	20.1 ± 4.3	5.5 ± 1.7	0.01
Ostoeblasts/10 cm surface	143.5 ± 18.3	51.5 ± 18	0.003
Bone resorption			
Extent of surface with lacunae (%)	6.9 ± 1.03	5.5 ± 0.07	NS
Extent of surface with osteoclasts (5)	0.76 ± 0.24	1.11 ± 0.22	NS
Osteoclasts/10 surface	17.1 ± 3.4	21.3 ± 5.1	NS
Mineralization			
Mineralization rate (μm/day)	0.52 ± 0.1	0.26 ± 0.07	0.04
Mineralization lag time (days)	28 ± 4	61 ± 10	0.006
Osteon remodeling time (days)	140 ± 20	423 ± 78	0.003

Adapted from Orwoll and Klein (1996). Data from Crilly *et al.* (1988).

drinkers. Such studies would be important to confirm and possibly extend the previous reports of increased bone density. The microscopic examination of skeletal tissue has the added benefit of identifying possible cellular mechanisms by which moderate alcohol intake effects skeletal physiology.

B. Effect of Alcohol on Growing Bone

Conservative estimates based on nutritional studies indicate that at least 15% of adult women and 25% of adult men consume on average two or more drinks per day (Flegal, 1990; O'Hare, 1991; Simon et al., 1991). The problem of adolescent drinking may be even more significant. Over 90% of teenagers are "drinkers" (Smart et al., 1985; Arria et al., 1991), and 10% of these young individuals drink daily (Schuckit, 1989). The skeletal consequences of alcohol intake during adolescence, when the rapid skeletal growth ultimately responsible for achieving peak bone mass is occurring, may be especially harmful. In a recent series of experiments, Sampson and colleagues (1996, 1997; Hogan et al., 1997) have examined the effect of alcohol on the early phases of skeletal development in a growing animal model. Rats were chronically exposed to alcohol from the age of 1 to 3 months (a developmental period comparable to that of human adolescence and young adulthood). Reduced caloric intake associated with alcohol consumption was accounted for with a pair-fed group and permitted the isolation of alcohol-specific effects. Gross skeletal morphology was not affected by alcohol, but bone density (determined by tibial calcium content) was 25% lower in the alcohol-exposed animals, and whole bone strength was 40% lower. These studies indicate that the adolescent skeleton is especially sensitive to the adverse effects of alcohol on bone formation. By limiting peak bone mass attainment, the development of osteoporosis later in life may be increased and its onset hastened. Adolescent alcohol consumption is frequently heavy and episodic ("binge drinking") (Wechsler et al., 1994). No animal studies have, as of yet, examined the impact of episodic alcohol intake and compared it to continuous alcohol exposure. Furthermore, studies are needed to determine if alcohol consumption during adolescence has a lasting effect on age-related osteopenia and subsequent fracture risk.

C. Alcohol and Nutrition

Normal bone formation depends on adequate nutrition and the presence of appropriate levels of a variety of endocrine, paracrine, and autocrine factors. The effect of ethanol on the skeleton could therefore be mediated directly through a toxic effect on bone or indirectly through an effect on nutritional status or hormonal regulation of bone metabolism. Disturbances in mineral homeostasis are an obvious mechanism for bone disease in alcoholics. Mild hypocalcemia, hypophosphatemia, and hypomagnesemia are frequently present in ambulatory alcoholics because of poor dietary intake, malabsorption, and increased renal excretion (Kalbfleisch *et al.*, 1963; Territo and Tanaka, 1974; Bikle *et al.*, 1985; Laitinen *et al.*, 1992a). Yet, no histomorphometric study has demonstrated any evidence of nutritional deficiency, except in patients with fat malabsorption resulting from alcohol-induced pancreatic or liver disease or those who have previously undergone gastric surgery (Johnell *et al.*, 1982b).

Vitamin D is a fat-soluble vitamin that stimulates intestinal absorption of calcium and is necessary for mineralization of new skeletal tissue. The circulating levels of 25-hydroxyvitamin D (25-OHD) generally provide a reliable assessment of vitamin D status because, unlike vitamin D itself, most of 25OHD circulated in blood where it is bound to vitamin D-binding protein and albumin. Both of these proteins are synthesized in the liver, and their levels are reduced in liver disease (Bikle *et al.*, 1986) which can complicate the assessment of vitamin D status in such individuals. Early studies found circulating levels of the vitamin D metabolites to be low (Verbanck *et al.*, 1977; DeVernejoul *et al.*, 1983; Mobarhan *et al.*, 1984; Lalor *et al.*, 1986), but subsequent investigation has excluded vitamin D deficiency as a major cause of alcohol-induced bone disease by demonstrating normal vitamin D absorption (Scott *et al.*, 1965; Sorensen *et al.*, 1977) and conversion to active metabolites (Posner *et al.*, 1978) in most alcoholic individuals and, more directly, by the measurement of normal free concentrations of $1,25(OH)_2D$ (the biologically active metabolite of vitamin D) in patients with alcoholic cirrhosis and alcoholic bone disease (Bikle *et al.*, 1984, 1985). These findings do not exclude the possibility of an alcohol-induced vitamin D-resistant state, but the lack of histomorphometric evidence of osteomalacia in vitamin D-replete osteopenic alcoholic subjects (Bikle *et al.*, 1985; Diamond *et al.*, 1989) argues strongly against such a possibility.

D. Alcohol and Calciotropic Hormones

Calcitonin is a peptide produced by the thyroid C cells that functions as an inhibitor of bone resorption. Williams and colleagues administered 0.8 g/kg of ethanol to normal nonalcoholic men and noted a 38% increase in plasma calcitonin levels 3 hours later (Williams *et al.*, 1978). In view of the fact that calcitonin exerts a protective effect on bone, alcohol-induced hypercalcitoninemia might explain the observation that a moderate intake of alcohol is associated with higher bone density. However, no data exist about the duration of this induction in chronic alcoholism.

Parathyroid hormone (PTH) is the principal regulator of blood calcium levels. The production of calcium is stimulated by a decrease in blood calcium and its major actions are to increase the release of calcium from bone and reduce kidney excretion of calcium. An elevated PTH level would be a sensitive indicator of reduced circulating calcium but most studies have failed to demonstrate this. PTH levels may be normal, reduced or elevated in alcoholic subjects (Johnell *et al.*, 1982a; Bjorneboe *et al.*, 1988; Bikle *et al.*, 1993). A likely explanation for the discrepant reports of PTH values is the molecular heterogeneity of PTH fragments in the circulation and the immunoheterogeneity of the radioimmunoassays employed in the various studies. PTH is metabolized in the liver, which is frequently damaged with alcohol ingestion.

Recent studies suggest that alcohol may directly interfere with PTH secretion. Laitinen and colleagues (1991a) administered alcohol to normal volunteers over a 3-hour period and observed a marked decrease in intact PTH levels. PTH levels then rebounded to above baseline levels after 8 hours and remained elevated for the remainder of the study (16 hours). The fall in PTH was accompanied by a fall in blood calcium and a dramatic increase in urinary calcium excretion. These findings suggest that the response of the parathyroid gland is impaired even in the presence of hypocalcemia. It is possible that alcohol-induced changes in intracellular calcium, especially within the parathyroid gland, may explain the reduced PTH levels (Brown *et al.*, 1995). Subsequently, Laitinen examined the effects of more prolonged alcohol consumption and observed an increase in PTH levels accompanied by a rise in serum-ionized calcium after 3 weeks (Laitinen *et al.*, 1991b). Thus, alcohol appears to have both acute and chronic effects on PTH secretion with the net result that immunoreactive levels of PTH are slightly increased. There are no reports on PTH bioactivity in the serum of alcoholic subjects to give a definitive account. However, the classic signs of hyperparathyroidism such as osteitis fibrosa cystica and accelerated bone remodeling are not seen on bone biopsies of affected patients (Bikle *et al.*, 1985; Crilly *et al.*, 1988; Diamond *et al.*, 1989; Lindholm *et al.*, 1991). Thus, no convincing evidence can be marshaled to support a major role for an indirect effect of ethanol on bone via alterations in nutritional status or calciotropic hormone levels.

E. Alcohol and Sex Steroid Hormones

Hypogonadism is a well-described risk factor for osteoporosis. Alcohol abuse has been associated with sexual dysfunction in both men and women (Van Thiel, 1983; Gavaler, 1991; Wright *et al.*, 1991). Men who have a long-term history of alcohol abuse often suffer from impotence, sterility, and testicular atrophy (Valimaki *et al.*, 1982) and have reduced concentrations of plasma testosterone (Van Thiel *et al.*, 1974, 1975; Boydon and Parmenter, 1983). Although most studies of alcoholic men with bone disease report normal androgen levels (Bikle *et al.*, 1985; Laitinen *et al.*, 1992b; Gonzalez-Calvin *et al.*, 1993), reduced serum-free testosterone concentrations in alcoholic subjects with osteoporosis were reported by Diamond (Diamond *et al.*, 1989). The testosterone levels were on average lower than those of the male control subjects but still fell within the normal range for the general male population overall.

In contrast, moderate alcohol consumption has been shown to increase estradiol levels in both premenopausal (Reichman *et al.*, 1993) and postmenopausal women (Gavaler *et al.*, 1993; Gavaler, 1995; Ginsburg *et al.*, 1995, 1996) as well as in men (Anderson *et al.*, 1986) (Figure 3). Animal studies indicate that moderate alcohol levels increase the production of estradiol through peripheral conversion (aromatization) of testosterone (Chung, 1990). Relative to the skeleton, studies have shown that osteoblasts possess aromatase activity (Purohit *et al.*, 1992), thus providing a potential source for

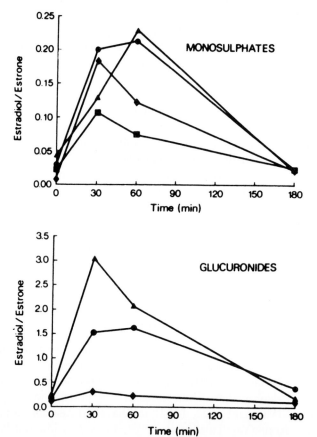

FIGURE 3   Effect of ethanol on the levels of estrogen conjugates. Ratios between estradiol and estrone in the monosulphate and glucuronide fractions from four men given 0.3 g ethanol/ kg body weight at time 0 are depicted in the right and left panels, respectively. Reprinted from *J. Steroid Biochem.*, **24**, Anderson, S. H. G., Cronholm, T., and Sjövall, J., Effects of ethanol on the levels of unconjugated and conjugated androgens and estrogens in plasma of men, 1193–1198, 1986, with permission from Elsevier Science.

estradiol in the bone microenvironment. In addition to increasing endogenous estrogen levels, certain alcoholic beverages contain isoflavanoid compounds known as phytoestrogens (Gavaler *et al.*, 1995). These nonsteroidal substances of plant origin are capable of binding to the estrogen receptor (Gavaler *et al.*, 1987) and eliciting relevant estrogenic responses in both ovariectomized animals (Gavaler *et al.*, 1987) and postmenopausal women (Gavaler *et al.*, 1991; Van Thiel *et al.*, 1991).

Estrogen receptors are present in the bone of both men and women, and it is clear that inadequate exposure to endogenous estrogens in young men can have serious skeletal consequences (Smith *et al.*, 1994; Morishima *et al.*, 1995). Recently, Slemenda *et al.* (1997) identified a significant positive association between bone density and serum estradiol concentrations in healthy older men that was of similar strength to that observed in women (Slemenda *et al.*, 1996). These observations suggest that estrogens are involved in the development and/or maintenance of the male skeleton, just as they are in the female. Elevated circulating levels of estrogens (both endogenous hormone and ingested phytoestrogen) in response to alcohol intake may be a possible explanation for the observations in certain epidemiological studies that moderate drinking is associated with increased bone density. However, the level of alcohol consumption is likely to be an important factor relative to bone metabolism because consumption of more than one standard drink per day confers no additional benefit on estradiol levels in postmenopausal women (Gavaler *et al.*, 1993), and chronic alcohol abuse is clearly responsible for bone disease. Further investigation will be required to identify potential associations between alcohol, alterations in sex steroid levels, and osteoporosis.

F. Alcohol and Bone Cells

Alcoholism is associated with profound alterations in the growth and proliferation of a wide variety of cell types. Biochemical and histomorphometric evaluation of alcoholic subjects reveal a marked impairment in osteoblastic activity with normal osteoclastic activity. These findings argue strongly that a primary target of ethanol's adverse effects on the skeleton is the osteoblast. Because bone remodeling and mineralization are dependent upon osteoblasts, it follows that a deleterious effect of alcohol on these cells will ultimately lead to reduced bone mass and fractures. Friday and Howard (1991) examined the effects of ethanol on the proliferation and function of cultured normal human osteoblastic cells. Ethanol induced a dose-dependent reduction in cell protein and DNA synthesis as assessed by incorporation of [^{3}H]-proline and [^{3}H]-thymidine, respectively. The antiproliferative effects of ethanol on normal human osteoblastic cells were reconfirmed in a subsequent report by Chavassieux *et al.* (1993). In similar studies on chick calvarial cells, Farley and co-workers (1985) also observed an inhibition of osteoblastic cell proliferation by ethanol (0.3%). Moreover, ethanol prevented the normal mitogenic effects of sodium fluoride and insulin-like growth factor-II (IGF-II) on these cell cultures. In addition, ethanol also suppressed bone formation in chick calvariae *in vitro*, as measured by the incorporation of [³H]-proline into collagen, the major protein in bone.

Ethanol-associated reductions in cell number must stem from either overt toxicity or inhibition of intracellular signaling processes that regulate cell replication. Recently, ethanol-enhanced apoptosis has been described in both thymocytes (Ewald and Shao, 1993) and in hypothalamic β-endorphin neurons (De *et al.*, 1994). In many other cell types, however, ethanol-induced reductions in cell division are reversible and associated with depletion of cellular polyamine levels (Shibley *et al.*, 1995). Polyamines are naturally oc-curring aliphatic amines that have been implicated as regulators of both DNA (Janne *et al.*, 1978) and protein synthesis (Jacob *et al.*, 1981) and may also affect the expression of genes that regulate cell division (Luscher and Eisenman, 1988). Chronic exposure to ethanol results in alterations in poly-amine metabolism that may contribute to the pathogenesis and/or progres-sion of liver disease in alcoholic individuals (Diehl *et al.*, 1988, 1990a,b). In a series of experiments on osteoblast-like osteosarcoma cell cultures, Klein and Carlos (1995) observed that the induction of cellular ODC activity (the ini-tial and often rate-limiting step in polyamine biosynthesis) was impaired by ethanol in a dose-dependent fashion that directly paralleled its antiprolifer-ative effects (Figure 4). Addition of polyamines restored the rate of cell pro-liferation in the ethanol-exposed cell cultures to that observed in the control cultures. Additional studies failed to find any evidence for induction of apop-

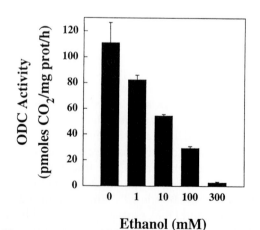

Ethanol (mM)

FIGURE 4   Concentration-dependent inhibition of osteoblastic UMR 106-01 ornithine de-carboxylase (ODC) activity by ethanol (Klein and Carlos, 1995). Measurements were conducted on proliferating cell cultures treated with varying doses of ethanol for 6 hours. The ODC activity of quiescent cultures was 7.7 ± 0.9 pmol/$^{14}CO_2$/mg protein/hr. Reprinted from Klein (1997), with permission.

tosis by ethanol in these osteoblast-like cell cultures (Klein *et al.*, 1996). The half-maximally effective concentration of ethanol to inhibit osteoblast proliferation *in vitro* was ∼50 mM, a level well within the physiologic range observed in actively imbibing alcoholic subjects. The 10-mM dose (equivalent to a "legal" blood alcohol level of 0.044%) also resulted in a substantial (20%) decline. These findings of a direct inhibitory effect of clinically relevant concentrations of ethanol on proliferation of these osteoblast-like osteosarcoma cells support the histomorphometric observations of a reduced number of osteoblasts and impaired bone formation activity in humans consuming excessive amounts of ethanol (DeVernejoul *et al.*, 1983; Bikle *et al.*, 1985; Crilly *et al.*, 1988; Diamond *et al.*, 1989; Bikle, 1993). Furthermore, these studies indicate that impairment of cellular polyamine synthesis plays a critical role in mediating the antiproliferative effects of ethanol because the administration of exogenous polyamines overcame the inhibitory effect of ethanol on cell proliferation. Moreover, these studies suggest that ethanol must perturb some intracellular process that normally results in stimulation of the polyamine biosynthetic pathway, a vital step in osteoblast proliferation.

Further evidence implicating a direct effect of ethanol on osteoblast activity comes from studies examining the effects of ethanol on circulating osteocalcin levels. Osteocalcin is a small peptide synthesized by active osteoblasts, a portion of which is released into the circulation. Levels of osteocalcin are positively correlated with histomorphometric parameters of bone formation in healthy individuals (Garcia-Carrasco *et al.*, 1988) and patients with metabolic bone disease (Delmas *et al.*, 1985). Chronic alcoholic patients exhibit significantly lower osteocalcin levels than age-matched controls (Labib *et al.*, 1989). Moreover, alcohol exerts a dose-dependent suppressive effect on circulating osteocalcin levels (Rico *et al.*, 1987; Nielsen *et al.*, 1990; Laitinen *et al.*, 1991b) (Figure 5). The consumption of 50 g of ethanol (equivalent to four "shots" of scotch whisky) over 45 min resulted in a 30% decrease in serum osteocalcin levels detectable 2 hours later (Nielsen *et al.*, 1990). Beyond these fragmentary attempts at characterization, however, little further is known about the mechanisms whereby ethanol impairs osteoblast proliferation and growth.

G. Alcohol and Intracellular Signaling Processes

The specific subcellular mechanism(s) whereby ethanol inflicts damage on any part of the body is currently not known. It has been proposed that ethanol may become incorporated into biologic membranes and disrupt, or disorder, hydrophobic interactions between phosopholipid acyl chains. The effects of ethanol on membrane lipids may, in turn, influence the function of proteins residing within the lipid environment of the cell membrane. Specifically, there is increasing evidence that ethanol may exert significant effects on transmembrane signal transduction processes that constitute major branches

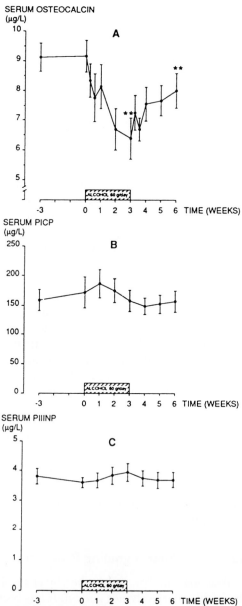

FIGURE 5 Effect of moderate alcohol ingestion on circulating osteocalcin levels (Laitinen *et al.*, 1991b). Ethanol (60 g/day) was administered to 10 healthy male volunteers for 3 weeks (shown in the hatched bar). The drinking period was preceded and followed by an abstinence period of 3 weeks. The values are expressed as means ± SEM. ** $p < 0.01$ for differences from the last preceding sober or drinking value.

of cellular control mechanisms (Hoek and Rubin, 1990; Hoffman and Tabakoff, 1990; Taylor, 1997).

Recent studies indicate that ethanol directly interferes with the functioning of the Type 1 insulin-like growth factor receptor (IGF-IR). Resnicoff *et al.* found that inhibition of both fibroblast (Resnicoff *et al.*, 1993) and neural cell (Resnicoff *et al.*, 1994) proliferation by ethanol correlated with an impairment of IGF-IR tyrosine autophosphorylation, an intracellular reaction necessary for IGF-dependent growth (Figure 6). This effect was observed in both intact cells and immunopurified IGF-IR preparations of cell lysates, suggesting that ethanol directly inhibits the receptor kinase rather than stimulates a tyrosine phosphatase. The inhibition of IGF-I signaling by ethanol was confirmed by a decrease in proto-oncogene expression that occurs distal to the receptor. In related work, Sasaki and Wands (1994) reported that chronic ethanol exposure severely diminished tyrosyl phosphorylation of IRS-1, a known substrate of the tyrosine kinase activity of the IGF-IR. The IGFs are considered to be the most important local regulators of bone remodeling. Both IGF-I and IGF-II are produced by cultures of osteoblastic cells under serum-free conditions (Canalis *et al.*, 1991), and osteoblasts are dependent on signaling through the IGF-IR for *in vitro* survival and proliferation

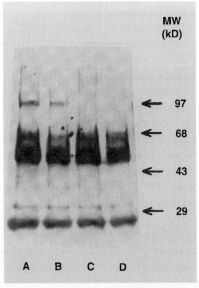

FIGURE 6   Effect of ethanol on autophosphorylation of the type 1 insulin-like growth factor (IGF-1) receptor. Tyrosine phosphorylation of the subunit of the IGF-1 receptor was visualized by Western immunoblotting. (A) No addition; (B) IGF-1 (10 ng/ml); (C) ethanol alone (100 mM), 10 minutes; (D) IGF-1 plus ethanol, 10 minutes. Reprinted from Resnicoff *et al.* (1994), with permission.

(Kappel *et al.*, 1994). The IGFs increase a preosteoblastic cell population that eventually differentiates into mature osteoblasts. And, independent of their effects on cell replication, IGFs increase collagen synthesis and matrix apposition. Through these actions, it is apparent that the IGFs play a fundamental role in the maintenance of bone mass. Based on the findings of Resnicoff *et al.* (1993, 1994), it is interesting to speculate that the reduced osteoblast number and bone formation that characterized alcoholic bone disease may stem entirely from a single defect in intracellular signaling by the IGF receptor induced by ethanol.

V. Therapy of Alcohol-Induced Bone Disease _____

Not only is our understanding of the cellular mechanisms for alcohol-induced skeletal damage incomplete but, sadly, so too is our ability to treat the clinical bone disease effectively. Patients with "idiopathic" osteoporosis should be routinely and thoroughly questioned about drinking habits, and osteoporosis should be suspected in every chronic alcohol abuser. In one study of men with vertebral fracture, alcohol abuse was identified as an underlying cause in 11% of subjects (Kanis, 1994). Alcoholism is a subtle disease in most patients, and the diagnosis may be missed unless the patient is specifically questioned. A history of sporadic alcohol ingestion should arouse suspicion. Symptoms such as low back pain, which can indicate the presence of osteoporosis, may be minimized or overlooked in these patients because of the more obvious acute and chronic complications of alcoholism.

Once the diagnosis of alcohol-induced bone disease has been established, a number of measures are recommended. Aggressive medical and psychiatric treatment should be pursued in the hopes of interrupting the cycle of chronic alcohol ingestion thereby diminishing the risk of further skeletal deterioration. Unfortunately, the personality disturbances and low compliance of most alcohol abusers reduces the long-term success of such therapeutic interventions (Mossberg *et al.*, 1985). The cessation of alcohol intake will, presumably, stop further progression of bone loss, but data are scant. Moreover, no evidence has been reported that bone, once lost, will be restored when alcohol abuse is discontinued. Studies on alcohol abstainers have demonstrated a rapid recovery of osteoblast function (as assessed histomorphometrically and by biochemical parameters of bone remodeling) within as little as 2 weeks after cessation of drinking, but no significant differences in bone mineral content were observed between abstainers and actively drinking men (Feitelberg *et al.*, 1987; Diamond *et al.*, 1989; Laitinen *et al.*, 1992a). The relatively short period of abstinence, however, makes these results inconclusive. On a positive note, Peris *et al.* found evidence for an increase in bone mass after discontinuation of ethanol (Peris *et al.*, 1994), a finding that suggests there is an opportunity to reduce fracture risk in former drinkers.

Most alcoholics have low turnover osteoporosis. The challenge in this disorder is to stimulate bone formation. Current osteoporosis therapies (sex steroids, selective estrogen receptor modulators, calcitonin, bisphosphonates) work primarily by inhibiting bone resorption. Histomorphometric studies indicate that by the time an alcoholic subject comes to medical attention, bone resorption is normal or reduced. Certainly all subjects, especially those adolescents who imbibe, will benefit from steps to ensure calcium sufficiency (1000–1500 mg of elemental calcium per day). Evidence that calcium supplementation will correct the bone disease of alcoholics has not been reported, but it is reasonable to minimize the impact of this potential risk factor for reduced bone mass. Tobacco use and excessive consumption of phosphate-binding antacids should be discouraged. Adequate vitamin D nutrition and physical exercise should be encouraged. Patients who present with very low serum 25-hydroxyvitamin D levels that cannot be explained by comparably reduced vitamin D-binding protein and albumin levels should be considered for aggressive vitamin D supplementation (ergocalciferol 50–150,000 IU/week). Calcifediol is somewhat better absorbed than ergocalciferol in patients with steatorrhea so that if treatment with ergocalciferol fails to increase circulating levels of 25-hydroxyvitamin D, calcifediol (50 μg three times per week) is an effective alternative. Agents such as fluoride, parathyroid hormone, or growth hormone may stimulate bone formation, but such regimens remain investigational, and no therapeutic trials in alcoholic men have been reported. The toxic effects of alcohol and fluoride on the gastrointestinal tract may likely preclude its use in the individual who continues to drink. Thus, the appropriate management of alcohol-induced bone disease remains uncertain, and prevention rather that correction should be the goal.

VI. Conclusion

Recent studies suggest a dose-dependent relationship between alcohol consumption and fracture risk in both women and men. This increased risk may be, at least in part, attributable to a reduction in bone density in those with excessive alcohol intake. Alcoholic bone disease is characterized by impaired bone formation in the face of relatively normal bone resorption. The uncoupling of these two physiologic processes results in defective remodeling of skeletal tissue and, in turn, reduced bone mass and increased fracture risk. The growing skeleton may be especially sensitive to the adverse effects of alcohol. Experiments using well-defined osteoblastic model systems indicate that the observed reductions in bone formation result from a direct, antiproliferative effect of ethanol on the osteoblast itself. Further studies are necessary to establish the underlying mechanisms by which ethanol exerts its antiproliferative effects on the osteoblast. At present, sustained reduction in alcohol intake is the only effective therapy for alcohol-induced bone disease. Unfortunately, the long-term success of such therapy is poor. An improved understanding of the pathogenesis of alcohol-induced bone disease may lead to alternative therapeutic avenues.

Of considerable interest, because of the large proportion of our society that is affected, is the provocative finding of increased bone density in social drinkers with more moderate alcohol consumption. Whether this increase in bone density can be ascribed to direct stimulatory effects of ethanol on estrogen and/or calcitonin levels or to concomitant life-style and/or socioeconomic factors has yet to be adequately explored. Specific studies are needed to address the question of whether moderate alcohol consumption is a protective factor against fracture, and if so, at what level the skeletal advantages of alcohol intake are obviated by the increased risks from alcohol excess.

References

Anderson, S. H. G., Cronholm, T., and Sjövall, J. (1986). Effects of ethanol on the levels of unconjugated and conjugated androgens and estrogens in plasma of men. *J. Steroid Biochem.* **24**, 1193–1198.

Arria, A. M., Targer, R. E., and van Thiel, D. H. (1991). The effects of alcohol abuse on the health of adolescents. *Alcohol Abuse Adolesc. Health* **15**, 52–57.

Baran, D. T., Teitelbaum, S. L., Bergfeld, M. A., Parker, G., Cruvant, E. M., and Avioli, L. V. (1980). Effect of alcohol ingestion on bone and mineral metabolism in rats. *Am. J. Physiol.* **238**, E507–E510.

Bikle, D. D. (1993). Alcohol-induced bone disease. In "Osteoporosis: Nutritional Aspects" (A. P. Simopoulos and C. Galli, eds.), pp. 53–79. Karger, Basel.

Bikle, D. D., Gee, E., Halloran, B., and Haddad, J. G. (1984). Free 1,25-dihydroxyvitamin D levels in serum from normal subjects, pregnant subjects and subjects with liver disease. *J. Clin. Invest.* **74**, 1966–1971.

Bikle, D. D., Genant, H. K., Cann, C. E., Recker, R. R., Halloran, B. P., and Strewler, G. J. (1985). Bone disease in alcohol abuse. *Ann. Intern. Med.* **103**, 42–48.

Bikle, D. D., Gee, E., Halloran, B., Kowalski, M. A., Ryzen, E., and Haddad, J. G. (1986). Assessment of the free fraction of 25-hydroxyvitamin D in serum: Its regulation by albumin and the vitamin D-binding protein. *J. Clin. Endocrinol. Metab.* **63**, 954–959.

Bikle, D. D., Stesin, A., Halloran, B., Steinbach, L., and Recker, R. (1993). Alcohol-induced bone disease: Relationship to age and parathyroid hormone levels. *Alcohol: Clin. Exp. Res.* **17**, 690–695.

Bjorneboe, G.-E. A., Bjorneboe, A., Johnson, J., Skylv, N., Oftebro, H., Gautvik, K. M., Hoiseth, A., Mørland, J., and Drevon, C. A. (1988). Calcium status and calcium-regulating hormones in alcoholics. *Alcohol: Clin. Exp. Res.* **12**, 229–232.

Blaauw, R., Albertse, E. C., Beneke, T., Lombard, C. J., Laubscher, R., and Hough, F. S. (1994). Risk factors for the development of osteoporosis in a South African population. *S. Afr. Med. J.* **84**, 328–332.

Boydon, T. W., and Parmenter, R. W. (1983). Effects of ethanol on the male hypothalamic-pituitary-gonadal axis. *Endocr. Rev.* **4**, 389–395.

Brown, E. M., Pollak, M., Chou, Y. H., Seidman, C. E., Seidman, J. G., and Herbert, S. C. (1995). Cloning and functional characterization of extracellular Ca2+-sensing receptors from parathyroid and kidney. *Bone* **17**(2 Suppl.), S7–S11.

Canalis, E., Centrella, M., and McCarthy, T. L. (1991). Regulation of insulin-like growth factor-II production in bone cultures. *Endocrinology (Baltimore)* **129**(5), 2457–2462.

Chappard, D., Plantard, B., Petitjean, M., Alexandre, C., and Riffat, G. (1991). Alcoholic cirrhosis and osteoporosis in men: A light and scanning electron microscopy study. *J. Stud. Alcohol* **52**(3), 269–274.

Chavassieux, P., Serre, C. M., Vernaud, P., Delmas, P. D., and Meunier, P. J. (1993). *In vitro* evaluation of dose-effects of ethanol on human osteoblastic cells. *Bone Miner.* **22**, 95–103.

Chon, K. S., Sartoris, D. J., Brown, S. A., and Clopton, P. (1992). Alcoholism-associated spinal and femoral bone loss in abstinent male alcoholics, as measured by dual X-ray absorptiometry. *Skeletal Radiol.* **21**, 431–436.

Chung, K. W. (1990). Effects of chronic ethanol intake on aromatization of androgens and concentration of estrogen and androgen receptors in rat liver. *Toxicology* **62**, 285–295.

Conn, H. O. (1985). Natural history of complications of alcoholic liver disease. *Acta Med. Scand.* **703** (Suppl.), 127–134.

Crilly, R. G., Anderson, C., Hogan, D., and Delaquerrière-Richardson, L. (1988). Bone histomorphometry, bone mass, and related parameters in alcoholic males. *Calcif. Tissue Int.* **43**, 269–276.

De, A., Boyadjieva, N. I., Pastorcic, M., Reddy, B. V., and Sarkar, D. K. (1994). Cyclic AMP and ethanol interact to control apoptosis and differentiation in hypothalamic β-endorphin neurons. *J. Biol. Chem.* **269**, 26697–26705.

Delmas, P. D., Malaval, L., Arlot, M. E., and Meunier, P. J. (1985). Serum bone Gla-protein compared to bone histomorphometry in endocrine diseases. *Bone* **6**, 339–341.

DeVernejoul, M. C., Bielakoff, J., Herve, M., Gueris, J., Hott, M., Modrowski, D., Kuntz, D., Miravet, L., and Ryckewaert, A. (1983). Evidence for defective osteoblastic function. A role for alcohol and tobacco consumption in osteoporosis in middle-aged men. *Clin. Orthop.* **179**, 107–115.

Diamond, T., Stiel, D., Luzner, M., Wilkinson, M., and Posen, S. (1989). Ethanol reduces bone formation and may cause osteoporosis. *Am. J. Med.* **86**, 282–288.

Diehl, A. M., Chacon, M., and Wagner, P. (1988). The effect of chronic ethanol feeding on ornithine decarboxylase activity and liver regeneration. *Hepatology* **8**, 237–242.

Diehl, A. M., Abdo, S., and Brown, N. (1990a). Supplemental putrescine reverses ethanol-associated inhibition of liver regeneration. *Hepatology* **12**, 633–637.

Diehl, A. M., Wells, M., Brown, N. D., Thorgeirsson, S. S., and Steer, C. J. (1990b). Effect of ethanol on polyamine synthesis during liver regeneration in rats. *J. Clin. Invest.* **85**, 385–390.

Ewald, S. J., and Shao, H. (1993). Ethanol increases apoptotic cell death of thymocytes in vitro. *Alcohol: Clin. Exp. Res.* **17**, 359–365.

Farley, J. R., Fitzsimmons, R., Taylor, A. K., Jorch, U. M., and Lau, K. H. (1985). Direct effects of ethanol on bone resorption and bone formation *in vitro*. *Arch. Biochem. Biophys* **238**, 305–314.

Feitelberg, S., Epstein, S., Ismail, F., and D'Amanda, C. (1987). Deranged bone mineral metabolism in chronic alcoholism. *Metab. Clin. Exp.* **36**, 322–326.

Felson, D. T., Kiel, D. P., and Anderson, J. J. (1988). Alcohol consumption and hip fractures: The Framingham Study. *Am. J. Epidemiol.* **128**, 1102–1110.

Flegal, K. M. (1990). Agreement between two dietary methods in the measurement of alcohol consumption. *J. Stud. Alcohol.* **51**, 408–414.

Friday, K., and Howard, G. A. (1991). Ethanol inhibits human bone cell proliferation and function *in vitro*. *Metab., Clin. Exp.* **40**, 562–565.

Garcia-Carrasco, M., Gruson, M., and DeVernejoul, C. (1988). Osteocalcin and bone histomorphometric parameters in adults without bone disease. *Calcif. Tissue Int.* **42**, 13–17.

Gavaler, J. S., (1991). Effects of alcohol on female endocrine function. *Alcohol Health Res. World* **15**, 104–109.

Gavaler, J. S. (1995). Alcohol effects on hormone levels in normal postmenopausal women with alcohol-induced cirrhosis. *Recent Dev. Alcohol.* **12**, 199–208.

Gavaler, J. S., Rosenblum, E. R., Van Thiel, D. H., Eagon, D. K., Pohl, C. R., Campbell, I. M., Imhoff, A. F., and Gavaler, J. (1987). Biologically active phyto-estrogens are present in bourbon. *Alcohol: Clin. Exp. Res.* **11**, 399–406.

Gavaler, J. S., Galvao-Teles, A., Monteiro, E., Van Thiel, D. H., and Rosenblum, E. R. (1991). Clinical responses to the administration of bourbon phytoestrogens to normal postmenopausal women. *Hepatology* **14**, 193.

Gavaler, J. S., Deal, S. R., Vanthiel, D. H., Arria, A., and Allan, M. J. (1993). Alcohol and estrogen levels in postmenopausal women—The spectrum of effect. *Alcohol: Clin. Exp. Res.* **17**, 786–790.

Gavaler, J. S., Rosenblum, E. R., Deal, S. R., and Bowie, B. T. (1995). The phytoestrogen congeners of alcoholic beverages: Current status. *Proc. Soc. Exp. Biol. Med.* **208**, 98–102.

Ginsburg, E. S., Walsh, B. W., Shea, B. F., Gao, X., Gleason, R. E., and Barbieri, R. L. (1995). The effects of ethanol on the clearance of estradiol in postmenopausal women. *Fertil. Steril.* **63**, 1227–1230.

Ginsburg, E. S., Mello, N. K., Mendelson, J. H., Barbieri, R. L., Teoh, S. K., Rothman, M., Gao, X., and Sholar, J. W. (1996). Effects of alcohol ingestion on estrogens in postmenopausal women. *JAMA, J. Am. Med. Assoc.* **276**, 1747–1751.

Glynn, N. W., Meilahn, E. N., Charron, M., Anderson, S. J., Kuller, L. H., and Cauley, J. A. (1995). Determinants of bone mineral density in older men. *J. Bone Miner. Res.* **10**, 1769–1777.

Gonzalez-Calvin, J. L., Garcia-Sanchez, A., Bellot, V., Munoz-Torres, M., Raya-Alvarez, E., and Salvatierra-Rios, D. (1993). Mineral metabolism, osteoblastic function and bone mass in chronic alcoholism. *Alcohol Alcohol.* **28**, 571–579.

Hemenway, D., Azrael, D. R., Rimm, E. B., Feskanich, D., and Willett, W. C. (1994). Risk factors for wrist fracture: Effect of age, cigarettes, alcohol, body height, relative weight, and handedness on the risk for distal forearm fractures in men. *Am. J. Epidemiol.* **140**, 361–367.

Hoek, J. B., and Rubin, E. (1990). Alcohol and membrane-associated signal transduction. *Alcohol Alcohol.* **25**, 143–156.

Hoffman, P. L., and Tabakoff, B. (1990). Ethanol and guanine nucleotide binding proteins: A selective interaction. *FASEB J.* **4**, 2612–2622.

Hogan, H. A., Sampson, H. W., Cashier, E., and Ledoux, N. (1997). Alcohol consumption by young actively growing rats: A study of cortical bone histomorphometry and mechanical properties. *Alcohol: Clin. Exp. Res.* **21**, 809–816.

Holbrook, T. L., and Barrett-Connor, E. (1993). A prospective study of alcohol consumption and bone mineral density. *Br. Med. J.* **306**, 1506–1509.

Honkanen, R., Ertama, L., Kuosmanen, P., Linniola, M., Alha, A., and Visuri, T. (1983). The role of alcohol in accidental falls. *J. Stud. Alcohol* **44**, 231–245.

Israel, Y., Orrego, H., Holt, S., Macdonald, D. W., and Meema, H. E. (1980). Identification of alcohol abuse: Thoracic fractures on routine chest x-rays as indicators of alcoholism. *Alcoholism* **4**, 420–422.

Jacob, S. T., Duceman, B. W., and Rose, K. M. (1981). Spermine mediated phosphorylation of RNA polymerase I and its effect on transcription. *Med. Biol.* **59**, 381–388.

Janne, J., Poso, H., and Raina, A. (1978). Polyamines in rapid growth and cancer. *Biochim. Biophys. Acta* **473**, 241–293.

Johnell, O., Kristensson, H., and Nilsson, B. E. (1982a). Parathyroid activity in alcoholics. *Br. J. Addict.* **77**, 93–95.

Johnell, O., Nilsson, B. E., and Wikluind, P. E. (1982b). Bone morphometry in alcoholics. *Clin. Orthop.* **165**, 253–258.

Johnell, O., Kristenson, H., and Redlund-Johnell, I. (1985). Lower limb fractures and registration for alcoholism. *Scand. J. Soc. Med.* **13**, 95–97.

Kalbfleisch, J. M., Lindeman, R. D., Ginn, H. E., and Smith, W. O. (1963). Effects of ethanol administration on urinary excretion of magnesium and other electrolytes in alcoholic and normal subjects. *J. Clin. Invest.* **42**, 1471–1475.

Kanis, J. A. (1994). Assessment of bone mass and osteoporosis. *In* "Osteoporosis" (R. Marcus, ed.), p. 144. Blackwell Scientific Publications, Oxford.

Kappel, C. G., Velez-Yanguas, M. C., Hirschfeld, S., and Helman, L. J. (1994). Human osteosarcoma cell lines are dependent on insulin-like growth factor I for *in vitro* growth. *Cancer Res.* **54**, 2803–2807.

Klein, R. F., and Carlos, A. S. (1995). Inhibition of osteoblastic cell proliferation and ornithine decarboxylase activity by ethanol. *Endocrinology (Baltimore)* **136**, 3406–3411.

Klein, R. F., Fausti, K. A., and Carlos, A. S. (1996). Ethanol inhibits human osteoblastic cell proliferation. *Alcohol: Clin. Exp. Res.* **20**, 572–578.

Labib, M., Abdel-Kader, M., Ranganath, L., Teale, D., and Marks, V. (1989). Bone disease in chronic alcoholism: The value of plasma osteocalcin measurement. *Alcohol Alcohol.* **24**, 141–144.

Laitinen, K., Lamberg-Allardt, C., Tunninen, R., Karonen, S.-L., Tahtela, T., Ylikahri, R. and Valimaki, M. (1991a). Transient hypoparathyroidism during acute alcohol intoxication. *N. Engl. J. Med.* **324**, 721–727.

Laitinen, K., Lamberg-Allardt, C., Tunninen, R., Karonen, S. L., Ylikhari, R., and Valimaki, M. (1991b). Effects of 3 weeks moderate alcohol intake on bone and mineral metabolism in normal men. *Bone Miner.* **13**, 139–151.

Laitinen, K., Valimaki, M., and Keto, P. (1991c). Bone mineral density measured by dual-energy X-ray absorptiometry in healthy Finnish women. *Calcif. Tissue Int.* **48**, 224–231.

Laitinen, K., Lamberg-Allardt, C., Tunninen, R., Harkonen, M., and Valimaki, M. (1992a). Bone mineral density and abstention-induced changes in bone and mineral metabolism in noncirrhotic male alcoholics. *Am. J. Med.* **93**, 642–650.

Laitinen, K., Tahtela, R., and Valimaki, M. (1992b). The dose-dependency of alcohol-induced hypoparathyroidism, hypercalciuria, and hypermagnesuria. *Bone Miner.* **19**(1), 75–83.

Laitinen, K., Karkkainen, M., Lalla, M., Lambergallardt, C., Tunninen, R., Tahtela, R., and Valimaki, M. (1993). Is alcohol an osteoporosis-inducing agent for young and middle-aged women? *Metab., Clin. Exp.* **42**(7), 875–881.

Lalor, B. C., France, M. W., Powell, D., Adams, P. H., and Counihan, T. B. (1986). Bone and mineral metabolism and chronic alcohol abuse. *Q. J. Med.* **59**, 497–511.

Lindholm, J., Steiniche, T., Rasmussen, E., Thamsborg, G., Nielsen, I. O., Brockstedt-Rasmussen, H., Storm, T., Hyldstrup, L., and Schou, C. (1991). Bone disorder in men with chronic alcoholism: A reversible disease? *J. Clin. Endocrinol. Metab.* **73**, 118–124.

Lindsell, D. R., Wilson, A. G., and Maxwell, J. D. (1982). Fractures on the chest radiograph in detection of alcoholic liver disease. *Br. Med. J.* **285**, 597–599.

Lucas, E. G. (1987). Alcohol in industry. *Br. Med. J.* **291**, 460–461.

Luscher, B., and Eisenman, R. N. (1988). *c*-Myc and *c*-myb protein degradation: Effect of metabolic inhibitors and heat shock. *Mol. Cell. Biol.* **8**, 2504–2512.

Mathew, V. M. (1992). Alcoholism in biblical prophecy. *Alcohol Alcohol.* **27**, 89–90.

May, H., Murphy, S., and Khaw, K. T. (1995). Alcohol consumption and bone mineral density in older men. *Gerontology* **41**, 152–158.

Melton, L. J., III, and Chrischille, E. A. (1992). Perspective: How many women have osteoporosis? *J. Bone Miner. Res.* **7**, 1005–1010.

Mobarhan, S. A., Russell, R. M., Recker, R. R. et al. (1984). Metabolic bone disease in alcoholic cirrhosis: A comparison of the effect of vitamin D,25-hydroxyvitamin D, or supportive treatment. *Hepatology* **4**, 266–273.

Morishima, A., Grumbach, M. M., Simpson, E. R., Fisher, C., and Qin, K. (1995). Aromatase deficiency in male and female siblings caused by a novel mutation and the physiological role of estrogens. *J. Clin. Endocrinol. Metab.* **80**, 3689–3698.

Mossberg, D., Liljeberg, P., and Borg, S. (1985). Clinical conditions in alcoholics during long term abstinence: A descriptive longitudinal study. *Alcohol* **2**, 551–553.

Naves Diaz, M., O'Neill, T. W., and Silman, A. J. (1997). The influence of alcohol consumption on the risk of vertebral deformity. *Osteoporosis Int.* **7**, 65–71.

Nielsen, H. K., Lundby, L., and Rasmussen, K. (1990). Alcohol decreases serum osteocalcin in a dose-dependent way in normal subjects. *Calcif. Tissue Int.* **46**, 173–178.

O'Hare, T. (1991). Measuring alcohol consumption: A comparison of the retrospective diary and the quantity-frequency method in a college drinking survey. *J. Stud. Alcohol* **52**, 500–502.

O'Neill, T. W., Marsden, D., Adams, J. E., and Silman, A. J. (1996). Risk factors, falls, and fracture of the distal forearm in Manchester, UK. *J. Epidemiol. Commun. Health* **50**, 288–292.

Orwoll, E. S., Bauer, D. C., Vogt, T. M., and Fox, K. M. (1996). Axial bone mass in older women. *Ann. Intern. Med.* **124**, 187–196.

Peng, T.-C., Kusy, R. P., Hirsch, P. F., and Hagaman, J. R. (1988). Ethanol-induced changes in the morphology and strength of femurs of rats. *Alcohol: Clin. Exp. Res.* **12**, 655–659.

Peris, P., Pares, A., Guanabens, N., Delrio, L., Pons, F., Deosaba, M. J. M., Monegal, A., Caballeria, J., Rodes, J., and Munozgomez, J. (1994). Bone mass improves in alcoholics after 2 years of abstinence. *J. Bone Miner. Res.* **9**(10), 1607–1612.

Peris, P., Guañabens, N., Parés, A., Pons, F., del Rio, L., Monegal, A., Suris, X., Caballería, J., Rodés, J., and Muñoz-Gómez, J. (1995). Vertebral fractures and osteopenia in chronic alcoholic patients. *Calcif. Tissue Int.* **57**, 111–114.

Posner, D. B., Russell, R. M., and Ansood, S. (1978). Effective 25-hydroxylation of vitamin D in alcoholic cirrhosis. *Gastroenterology* **74**, 866–870.

Purohit, A., Flanagan, A. M., and Reed, M. J. (1992). Estrogen synthesis by osteoblast cell lines. *Endocrinology (Baltimore)* **131**, 2027–2029.

Reichman, M. E., Judd, J. T., Longcope, C., Schatzkin, A., Clevidence, B. A., Nair, P. P., Campbell, W. S., and Taylor, P. R. (1993). Effects of alcohol consumption on plasma and urinary hormone concentrations in premenopausal women. *J. Natl. Canc. Inst.* **85**, 722–727.

Resnicoff, M., Sell, C., Ambrose, D., Baserga, R., and Rubin, R. (1993). Ethanol inhibits the autophosphorylation of the insulin-like growth factor 1 (IGF-1) receptor and IGF-1-mediated proliferation of 3T3 cells. *J. Biol. Chem.* **268**(29), 21777–21782.

Resnicoff, M., Rubini, M., Baserga, R., and Rubin, R. (1994). Ethanol inhibits insulin-like growth factor-I mediated signalling and proliferation of C6 rat glioblastoma cells. *Lab. Invest.* **71**, 657–662.

Rico, H., Cabranes, J. A., Cabello, J., Gomez-Castresana, F., and Hernandez, E. R. (1987). Low serum osteocalcin in acute alcohol intoxication: A direct effect of alcohol on osteoblasts. *Bone Miner.* **2**, 221–225.

Sampson, H. W., Perks, N., Champney, T. H., and DeFee, B. (1996). Alcohol consumption inhibits bone growth and development in young actively growing rats. *Alcohol: Clin. Exp. Res.* **20**, 1375–1384.

Sampson, H. W., Chaffin, C., Lange, J., and DeFee, B. (1997). Alcohol consumption by young actively growing rats: A histomorphometric study of cancellous bone. *Alcohol: Clin. Exp. Res.* **21**, 352–359.

Sasaki, Y., and Wand, J. R. (1994). Ethanol impairs insulin receptor substrate-1 mediated signal transduction during rat liver regeneration. *Biochem. Biophys. Res. Comm.* **199**, 403–409.

Saville, P. D. (1965). Changes in bone mass with age and alcoholism. *J. Bone Jt. Surg., Am. Vol.* **47A**, 492–499.

Schnitzler, C. M., and Solomon, L. (1984). Bone changes after alcohol abuse. *S. Afr. Med. J.* **66**, 730–734.

Schukit, M. A. (1989). Alcoholism: An introduction. *In* "Drug and Alcohol Abuse: A Clinical Guide to Diagnosis and Treatment" (M. A. Schuckit, ed.), pp. 45–76. Plenum Medical Book Company, New York.

Scott, K. G., Smyth, F. S., Peng, C. T. *et al.* (1965). Measurements of the plasma levels of tritiated labelled vitamin D in control and rachitic, cirrhotic and osteoporotic patients. *Strahlentherapie* **60** (suppl.), 317.

Seeman, E. (1996). The effects of tobacco and alcohol use on bone. *In* "Osteoporosis" (R. Marcus, D. Feldman, and J. Kelsey, eds.), pp. 577–598. Academic Press, San Diego, CA.

Seeman, E., and Melton, L. J., III (1983). Risk factors for spinal osteoporosis in men. *Am. J. Med.* **75**, 977–983.

Seller, S. C. (1985). Alcohol abuse in the old testament. *Alcohol Alcohol.* **20**, 69–76.

Shibley, I. A. J., Gavigan, M. D., and Pennington, S. N. (1995). Ethanol's effect on tissue poly-amines and ornithine decarboxylase activity: A concise review. *Alcohol: Clin. Exp. Res.* **19**, 209–215.

Simon, D. G., Eley, J. W., Greenberg, R. S., Newman, N., Gillespie, T., and Moore, M. (1991). A survey of alcohol use in an inner-city ambulatory care setting. *J. Gen. Intern. Med.* **6**, 295–298.

Slemenda, C. W., Christian, J. C., Reed, T., Reister, T. K., Williams, C. J., and Johnston, C. C., Jr. (1992). Long-term bone loss in men: Effects of genetic and environmental factors. *Ann. Intern. Med.* **117**(4), 286–291.

Slemenda, C. W., Longcope, C., Peacock, M. P., Hui, S. L., and Johnston, C. C. (1996). Sex steroids, bone mass and bone loss. A prospective study of pre-, peri- and postmenopausal women. *J. Clin. Invest.* **97**, 14–21.

Slemenda, C. W., Longcope, C., Zhou, L., Hsui, S. L., Peacock, M., and Johnston, C. C. (1997). Sex steroids and bone mass in older men. Positive associations with serum estrogens and negative associations with androgens. *J. Clin. Invest.* **100**, 1755–1759.

Smart, R. G., Goodstadt, M. S., and Adlaf, E. M. (1985). Trends in the prevalence of alcohol and other drug use among Ontario students. *Can. J. Public Health* **76**, 157–161.

Smith, E. P., Body, J., Frank, G. R., Takahashi, H., Cohen, R. M., Specker, B., and Williams, T. C. (1994). Estrogen resistance caused by a mutation in the estrogen receptor gene in a man. *N. Engl. J. Med.* **331**, 1056–1061.

Sorensen, O. H., Lund, B., Hilden, M., and Lund, B. (1977). 25-Hydroxylation in chronic alcoholic liver disease. *In* "Vitamin D: Biochemical, Chemical and Clinical Aspects Related to Calcium Metabolism" (A. W. Norman, K. Schaefer, and J. W. Coburn, eds.), pp. 843–845. de Guyter, Hawthorne, NY.

Spencer, H., Rubio, N., Rubio, E., Indreika, M., and Seitam, A. (1986). Chronic alcoholism. Frequently overlooked cause of osteoporosis in men. *Am. J. Med.* **80**, 393–397.

Taylor, R. (1997). Anesthesiologists wake up to the biochemical mechanisms of their tools. *J. NIH Res.* **9**, 37–41.

Territo, M. C., and Tanaka, K. R. (1974). Hypophosphatemia in chronic alcoholism. *Arch. Intern. Med.* **134**, 445–447.

Turner, R. T., Greene, V. S., and Bell, N. H. (1987). Demonstration that ethanol inhibits bone matrix synthesis and mineralization in the rat. *J. Bone Miner. Res.* **2**, 61–66.

Valimaki, M., Salaspuro, M., and Ylikahri, R. (1982). Liver damage and sex hormones in chronic male alcoholics. *Clin. Endocrinol. (Oxford)* **17**, 469–477.

Van Thiel, D. H. (1983). Ethanol: Its adverse effects upon the hypothalamic-pituitary-gonadal axis. *J. Lab. Clin. Med.* **101**, 21–33.

Van Thiel, D. H., Lester, R., and Sherins, R. J. (1974). Hypogonadism in alcoholic liver disease: Evidence for a double defect. *Gastroenterology* **67**, 1188–1199.

Van Thiel, D. H., Gavaler, J. S., Lester, R., and Goodman, M. D. (1975). Alcohol-induced testicular atrophy. An experimental model for hypogonadism occurring in chronic alcoholic men. *Gastroenterology* **69**, 326–332.

Van Thiel, D. H., Galvao-Teles, A., Monteiro, E., Rosenblum, E. R., and Gavaler, J. S. (1991). The phytoestrogens present in de-ethanolized bourbon are biologically active: A preliminary study in a postmenopausal women. *Alcohol: Clin. Exp. Res.* **15**, 822–823.

Verbanck, M. Z., Verbanck, J., Brauman, J., and Mullier, J. T. (1977). Bone histology and 25OH-vitamin D plasma levels in alcoholics without cirrhosis. *Calcif. Tissue Res.* **22**, 538–541.

Wechsler, H., Davenport, A., Dowdall, G., Moeykens, B., and Castillo, S. (1994). Health and behavioral consequences of binge drinking in college. *JAMA, J. Am. Med. Assoc.* **272**, 1672–1677.

Williams, G. A., Bowser, E. N., Hargis, G. K., Kukreja, S. C., Shah, J. H., Vora, N. M., and Henderson, W. J. (1978). Effect of ethanol on parathyroid hormone and calcitonin secretion in man. *Proc. Soc. Exp. Biol. Med.* **159**, 187–191.

Wright, H. I., Gavaler, J. S., and van Thiel, D. H. (1991). Effects of alcohol on the male reproductive system. *Alcohol Health Res. World* **15**, 110–114.

Chapter 22

Joseph E. Zerwekh

Center for Mineral Metabolism and Clinical Research
University of Texas Southwestern Medical Center
Dallas, Texas

Hypercalciuria and Bone Disease

I. Introduction

Hypercalciuria has long been a consistent finding in the majority of patients with nephrolithiasis. The advent of bone densitometric measurements has also linked hypercalciuria (Seeman *et al.*, 1983; Bordier *et al.*, 1977; Pietschmann *et al.*, 1992; Sakhaee *et al.*, 1985a) with reductions in bone mineral density (BMD). More attention has been focused on the association of hypercalciuria and osteopenia in men, but this bias may reflect the greater prevalence of hypercalciuria in men than women. Moreover, in contrast to women in whom the cessation of menses is such a dominant factor in the pathophysiology of osteoporosis, in male osteoporosis without clear secondary causes, underlying metabolic abnormalities such as hypercalciuria assume greater prominence. This chapter will focus on five specific areas regarding hypercalciuria and osteoporosis in men: (1) a review of the primary mechanisms for hypercalciuria as gleaned from studies in patients with idiopathic hypercalciuria and renal stone disease, (2) a review of the prevalence and nature of the hypercalciuria observed in osteoporotic men, (3) a consideration of possible pathophysiological mechanisms contributing to the hypercalciuria in osteoporotic men, (4) a discussion of the appropriate diagnostic evaluation for determining the mechanism of hypercalciuria in male osteoporotic patients, and (5) a consideration of potential therapeutic modalities.

II. Primary Mechanisms of Hypercalciuria

The term "idiopathic hypercalciuria" was introduced by Albright *et al.* in 1953. Although several mechanisms were considered to explain the cause of the hypercalciuria, none proved to be entirely correct. Today, idiopathic hypercalciuria denotes an increased urinary excretion of calcium for which there is no readily apparent cause (hypercalcemia, sarcoidosis, excessive vitamin D ingestion, glucocorticoid excess, thyrotoxicosis, immobilization, etc.). Reasonable upper limits for 24-hr urinary calcium excretion in outpatients on a free diet are 250 mg (6.2 mmol) per day in women, 300 mg (7.5 mmol) per day in men, or 4 mg (0.1 mmol) per kilogram of body weight per day in patients of either sex (Coe *et al.*, 1992). A more rigid definition of hypercalciuria is a urinary calcium excretion of more than 200 mg/day after 1 week on a diet restricted in calcium and salt (400 mg calcium and 100 mEq sodium daily) (Pak *et al.*, 1974, 1975). With either of these definitions, more subtle forms of hypercalciuria might be missed unless it is ensured that at least one 24-hr urine specimen is collected while the patient is on a 1000-mg calcium diet or an oral 1000-mg oral calcium load test is performed.

Hypercalciuria can result from three different mechanisms individually or in some combination: (a) increased intestinal calcium absorption, (b) increased bone resorption, and (c) defective renal tubular calcium reabsorption. Regardless of the cause, calcium excreted in the urine must ultimately be derived from dietary calcium, bone mineral, or both. There appear to be subsets of patients with idiopathic hypercalciuria in whom each of these mechanisms predominates.

A. Absorptive Hypercalciuria

The primary abnormality in absorptive hypercalciuria (AH) is the intestinal hyperabsorption of calcium. The consequent increase in serum calcium (within the normal range) both increases the renal filtered load of calcium and suppresses parathyroid function. The resulting enhancement of calcium excretion contributes to the maintenance of normal serum calcium levels.

Although AH is the single most common cause of kidney stones, accounting for up to nearly 45% of patients with nephrolithiasis (Pak *et al.*, 1980), the cause of the intestinal hyperabsorption of calcium has not been clearly delineated. Evidence is mounting that AH itself may be a heteroge-neous condition. Increased serum 1,25-dihydroxyvitamin D [1,25(OH)$_2$D] levels were found in 30–80% of patients (Kaplan *et al.*, 1977; Broadus *et al.*, 1984), and Insogna *et al.* (1985) reported, using the infusion equilibrium technique, that patients with severe AH have increased 1,25(OH)$_2$D synthe-sis. The cause of increased 1,25(OH)$_2$D levels remains unclear because serum immunoreactive parathyroid hormone (iPTH) and phosphorus levels are generally normal. Other causes of AH may be an increased sensitivity to 1,25(OH)$_2$D or vitamin D independent mechanisms.

There is mounting evidence that patients with AH tend to have reduced spinal bone density. Spinal bone density was observed to be 10% below age- and sex-adjusted normal values as assessed by dual energy x-ray absorptiom-etry (Pietschmann *et al.*, 1992). Seventy-five percent of hypercalciuric pa-tients had bone mineral density values below the normal mean. Others also noted diminished spinal bone density in AH (Barkin *et al.*, 1985; Bataille *et al.*, 1991; Pacifici *et al.*, 1990). The cause of reduced bone mineral density is not clear but may result from (1) large urinary calcium losses exceed-ing intake and leading to a net negative calcium balance, (2) increased 1,25(OH)$_2$D-mediated bone resorption or diminished bone formation, or (3) in the case of stone-formers, the result of chronic adherence to a calcium-restricted diet.

B. Resorptive Hypercalciuria

In resorptive hypercalciuria, the primary disorder is an increased rate of bone resorption. Skeletal calcium mobilization increases the ambient concentration of calcium in serum, thus suppressing parathyroid function, 1,25(OH)$_2$D synthesis, and intestinal calcium absorption, as well as increasing the filtered load of calcium. Examples of resorptive hypercalciuria include the immobilization syndrome, cancer-associate osteolysis, and hyperthyroid-ism. Hypercalciuria observed in patients with primary hyperparathyroidism, distal renal tubular acidosis (RTA), glucocorticoid excess, and sarcoidosis may have a resorptive component.

If these well-known causes of bone resorption are excluded, there is a subset of patients with idiopathic hypercalciuria that have normal serum calcium, fasting hypercalciuria, and normal or suppressed iPTH values. This presentation, sometimes referred to as "unclassified hypercalciuria," is com-patible with neither classic AH nor renal hypercalciuria (see next section). Although this pattern may result from delayed clearance of absorbed cal-cium in patients with AH, in some patients it persists even after a prolonged fast or after treatment with sodium cellulose phosphate (an agent which binds intestinal calcium and lowers urinary calcium excretion). This constellation of findings occurs in approximately 18% of stone-formers (Levy *et al.*, 1995) and is most likely derived from increased skeletal resorption. Postulated causes include a primary enhancement of $1,25(OH)_2D$ production or increased vitamin D receptor concentrations in bone, prostaglandin excess, or overproduction of cytokines (such as IL-1) by bone marrow macrophages. Stone patients in this category, with persistent fasting and 24-hr hypercalciuria despite a low-calcium diet, appear to have the most severe and prevalent bone loss.

C. Renal Hypercalciuria

In renal hypercalciuria (RH) the primary abnormality is thought to be an impairment in the renal tubular reabsorption of calcium (Coe *et al.*, 1973; Pak, 1979). The consequent reduction in serum calcium concentration (within the normal range) stimulates parathyroid function, with a secondary increase in the renal synthesis of $1,25(OH)_2D$. Increased parathyroid hormone and $1,25(OH)_2D$ levels then stimulate, respectively, mobilization of calcium from bone and intestinal absorption of calcium. These effects restore serum calcium toward baseline. The observed restoration of normal serum iPTH, $1,25(OH)_2D$, and intestinal calcium absorption by correction of the renal calcium leak with thiazide diuretics lends further support to this pathogenetic scheme (Zerwekh and Pak, 1980). Using a rigid definition of renal hypercalciuria (normocalcemia with fasting hypercalciuria in the presence of secondary hyperparathyroidism), the frequency of this hypercalciuric variant is currently much less than that of AH, and it is believed to be less than 2% of all stone formers (Levy *et al.*, 1995).

The cause of the primary renal calcium leak is not known. There may be a more generalized disturbance in renal tubular function in RH, as shown by the exaggerated natriuretic response to thiazide (Sakhaee *et al.*, 1985b) and an exaggerated calciuric response to a carbohydrate load (Barilla *et al.*, 1978). Although some suggest that the renal leak of calcium is the result of an excessive dietary sodium intake, when a limited number of RH patients were placed on a very low sodium intake (9 meq/day) for a week, fasting hypercalciuria and secondary hyperparathyroidism were still evident (unpublished observations).

There is limited information on bone density in patients with RH. In a group of renal hypercalciuric patients, bone density at the distal radius was 7.5% below that of age- and sex-matched control subjects (Lawoyin *et al.*, 1979). These limited results would be consistent with cortical bone loss due to secondary hyperparathyroidism. More significant bone loss in RH may be averted by a compensatory intestinal hyperabsorption of calcium that results from the PTH-induced renal synthesis of $1,25(OH)_2D$.

D. Mixed Causes of Hypercalciuria

It is clear that hypercalciuria may be based on a single dominant mechanism. However, it is also apparent that there is a degree of overlap among the various classifications. For example, patients with AH driven by calcitriol excess or sensitivity may also have increased bone resorption. Moreover, if PTH is suppressed in these patients, they may have reduced tubular reabsorption of calcium. Those classified as renal hypercalciurics have secondary hyperparathyroidism, which may increase intestinal calcium absorption via calcitriol synthesis and enhance bone resorption. Although there are simple tests for discriminating these mechanisms of hypercalciuria from one another (Pak *et al.*, 1975), there has been limited application of such tests in hypercalciuric osteoporotic men. These tests are considered in more detail in Section V.

There are some dietary habits that can contribute to hypercalciuria, probably by mixed mechanisms. For example, excessive intake of dietary calcium would be expected to suppress PTH and promote losses at the kidney due to the lack of PTH-mediated increases in renal tubular calcium reabsorption. Other nutritional factors also need to be considered when interpreting both 24 hr and fasting urinary calcium excretion on a random diet. Excessive animal protein intake can contribute to hypercalciuria. The protein-mediated increase in urinary calcium has been speculated to be of skeletal origin, and protein excess has been reported to lead to osteoporosis (Wachman and Bernstein, 1968) and hypercalciuria (Breslau *et al.*, 1988; Jaeger *et al.*, 1987). In fact, when consumed in isolation, animal protein can induce a metabolic acidosis from the increased dietary sulfate, and acidosis can increase the release of bone calcium salts that act to buffer the proton load (Lemann *et al.*, 1966). Even though intestinal calcium absorption may be decreased slightly by acidosis, the filtered load is nevertheless increased and contributes to hypercalciuria. Tubular reabsorption of calcium is also decreased, either because of a direct effect of acidosis or by sulfate complexation of calcium (Lemann, 1980). Despite this effect of animal protein ingestion on renal calcium handling, its impact on mineral and skeletal metabolism is uncertain. The consumption of animal protein as part of a mixed meal essentially eliminates the hypercalciuric effect, and the degree of negative calcium balance induced by dietary protein intake in free-living adults is very small.

There is also evidence that dietary sodium inhibits tubular reabsorption of calcium, thereby promoting an excess calcium excretion (Lemann, 1992; Breslau *et al.*, 1982). Therefore, it is important to bear in mind that certain dietary indiscretions may lead to hypercalciuria and, if of sufficient magnitude and length, may ultimately lead to bone loss and osteoporosis.

III. Potential Mechanisms for the Findings of Concomitant Hypercalciuria and Osteoporosis in Men

Based on the previous discussion, it is apparent that hypercalciuria in osteoporotic men could be explained by several mechanisms. Conceptually, mostsimple is the case of increased bone resorption, in which the hypercalciuria reflects an increased filtered load of calcium derived from the skeleton. Greater difficulty is encountered in attempting to explain the association of absorptive hypercalciuria and osteoporosis in men. Nevertheless, a comparison of clinical, biochemical, and histological findings among patients with idiopathic hypercalciuria and those with idiopathic osteoporosis demonstrate a number of similarities between the two diseases as summarized in Table 1. The following consideration will explore each of these mechanisms for hypercalciuria in men with idiopathic osteoporotic in light of the similarities between this disease and the observed osteopenia in hypercalciuric stone-formers.

A. Resorptive Hypercalciuria

Because the vast majority of the body calcium is contained within bone mineral, increased bone resorption would be expected to decrease bone mass and increase urinary calcium excretion. Indeed, several studies in calcium stone formers with idiopathic hypercalciuria have documented decreased bone mineral density (Lawoyin *et al.*, 1979; Fuss *et al.*, 1983; Pacifici *et al.*, 1990; Pietschmann *et al.*, 1992). When performed, histological or biochemical studies have also provided evidence of increased bone resorption or a high turnover state of bone remodeling in some patients (Steiniche *et al.*,

TABLE I Comparison of Selected Clinical, Biochemical, and Histological Findings in Patients with Idiopathic Hypercalciuria (IH) and Those with Idiopathic Osteoporosis (IO)

Parameter	IH	IO
Male/female	2/1	1/1
24-hr urinary Ca (800 mg/day intake)	Invariable ↑	Frequently ↑ (8–100% of cases)
Fasting urinary Ca	Rarely ↑ in AH variant (By definition always ↑ in fasting hypercalciuria)	Frequently ↑
Intestinal Ca absorption	Invariably ↑ in AH	Frequently ↑
Serum iPTH	Normal or ↓	Normal or ↓
Serum 1,25(OH)₂D	↑ in 30–35% of patients	↑ in up to 25% of IO patients
Vertebral BMD	↓ modestly in 75% of AH patients	↓ markedly in all patients
Bone histology		
Formation indices	↓ in majority of patients	↓ or normal
Resorption indices	↑ in 80% of patients	↑ in 30–50% of all IO patients
Mode of inheritance	Autosomal dominant	?

Abbreviations: ↑, increased; ↓, decreased.

1989; Da Silva *et al.*, 1993; Heilberg *et al.*, 1994; Bataille *et al.*, 1995). Thus, in stone-forming patients with fasting hypercalciuria the decrease in BMD is greater or more frequent (Lawoyin *et al.*, 1979; Lindergard *et al.*, 1983; Pacifici *et al.*, 1990; Heilberg *et al.*, 1994; Pietschmann *et al.*, 1992) than when the hypercalciuria is of the absorptive type. The lack of more significant bone loss in patients with absorptive hypercalciuria may be the result of increased intestinal calcium absorption which would help to attenuate the negative calcium balance resulting from increased bone resorption. Two exceptions to this general observation are the series by Bataille *et al.* (1991) and Fuss *et al.* (1983) that reported no difference in bone loss between patients with absorptive hypercalciuria and those with fasting hypercalciuria. Thus, a majority of patients with fasting hypercalciuria and nephrolithiasis demonstrate reduced BMD as a result of increased bone resorption.

The critical question that remains to be answered is what physiological derangement is promoting increased bone resorption and the attendant hypercalciuria. In the face of normal or suppressed parathyroid hormone and normal $1,25(OH)_2D$ observed in the majority of patients with fasting hypercalciuria, the cause of increased bone resorption remains unknown. One possible explanation may come from the studies of Pacifici *et al.* (1990) that demonstrated that monocytes from patients with fasting hypercalciuria overproduced interleukin-1 (IL-1), a cytokine that is a potent stimulator of bone resorption both *in vitro* and *in vivo* (Gowen and Mundy, 1986). Interestingly, high IL-1 production was not found in patients classified as having absorptive hypercalciuria (Pacifici *et al.*, 1990). Comparable findings were recently reported by Weisinger *et al.* (1996), who suggested that IL-1α was responsible for the increased bone resorption because *in vitro* production of IL-1α (and not IL-1β, IL-6, or TNFα) in unstimulated cultures of peripheral blood mononuclear cells was inversely correlated with the Z score of the lumbar spine mineral density. More recently, Weisinger (1996) reported that the expression of IL-1α mRNA is increased in unstimulated blood monocytes from hypercalciuric patients when compared to normocalciuric stone formers or healthy controls. Still to be resolved is whether the increased IL-1α production is caused by augmented transcription of the IL-1α gene or to stabilization of the IL-1α mRNA. These results were confirmed in a more recent investigation (Ghazali *et al.*, 1997) and extended to include increased monocyte production of TNFα and granulocyte macrophage-colony stimulating factor (GM-CSF) in unstimulated peripheral blood monocytes from stone formers with idiopathic hypercalciuria and fasting hypercalciuria. Interestingly, these findings were not observed in patients having dietary hypercalciuria. Ghazali and colleagues also reported that bone density was significantly lower in idiopathic hypercalciuric patients than in age-matched controls. However, unlike Weisinger *et al.* (1996), Ghazali's study failed to find a correlation between cytokine production and bone density but did report a positive correlation between bone density and lipopolysaccharide induced GM-CSF levels. It should also be borne in mind that cytokine levels reflect the rate of bone remodeling at the time of sample procurement, whereas bone density measurements reflect all past and current events capable of influencing skeleton development and maturation. Although these studies in hypercalciuric calcium stone formers provide evidence that increased bone resorption is the result of a cytokine-mediated process, similar findings in patients with idiopathic osteoporosis subsequently found to have hypercalciuria have not been reported. Thus, none of these studies demonstrate the existence of a cause-effect relationship between increased production of cytokines, bone loss, and hypercalciuria. However, they do provide an avenue of investigation into the pathogenesis of increased bone resorption and hypercalciuria in men with idiopathic osteoporosis.

B. Renal Hypercalciuria

Renal hypercalciuria, while not as prevalent as resorptive or absorptive hypercalciuria, has been associated with reduced radial bone mineral density in a limited number of stone-forming patients (Lawoyin *et al.*, 1979) and more recently with reduced lumbar spine density (Heilberg *et al.*, 1994). The loss of bone mineral at the radius, a site rich in cortical bone, is consistent with the bone-resorbing action of parathyroid hormone and suggests the secondary hyperparathyroidism that results from the renal leak of calcium is responsible for the skeletal changes. Limited bone biopsy data in renal hypercalciuric stone formers (Heilberg *et al.*, 1994) and in a small population of postmenopausal women with renal hypercalciuria (Sakhaee *et al.*, 1985a) corroborate the notion of increased osteoclastic bone resorption in this hypercalciuric variant. That these abnormalities may reflect parathyroid hormone-dependent osteoclastic resorption and bone turnover is supported by the reduction of indices of resorption after correction of secondary hyperparathyroidism with hydrochlorothiazide therapy. Although intestinal calcium absorption may also be increased via a parathyroid hormone-mediated increase in $1,25(OH)_2D$, the magnitude of this increase does not appear to be sufficient enough to prevent the osteoclastic resorption of bone. Overall, there are limited references to this type of osteoporosis in women, and no reports to date in osteoporotic men. Nevertheless, it is conceivable that a subset of men with renal hypercalciuria and osteoporosis does exist.

C. Absorptive Hypercalciuria

Absorptive hypercalciuria is often reported in male osteoporotic hypercalciuric patients. In its purest form, fasting calcium excretion is not increased, thus negating increased bone resorption as a potential mechanism. However, there also appears to be a subset of male osteoporotic patients with absorptive hypercalciuria who may also have a component of resorptive hypercalciuria as suggested by histological analysis (Perry *et al.*, 1982; Steiniche *et al.*, 1989; Da Silva *et al.*, 1993) or modest elevations in fasting urinary calcium (Zerwekh *et al.*, 1992).

In the investigation by Zerwekh *et al.* (1992), a careful evaluation of intestinal calcium absorption, urinary calcium (fasting and post calcium load), PTH, and vitamin D metabolites supported an absorptive type of hypercalciuria in nine men with idiopathic osteoporosis and hypercalciuria. Although mean fasting urinary calcium was at the upper limit of normal for the group, there was no histological evidence of increased bone resorption as compared to the nonhypercalciuric group of osteoporotic men. On the contrary, bone formation rate was significantly decreased for the entire group of osteoporotic men as compared to normal men. More interestingly, bone formation rate was significantly decreased in the hypercalciuric group as compared to the normocalciuric osteoporotic men. Biopsy analysis of the nine men also demonstrated normal mean resorption parameters. However, adjusted apposition rate was significantly less in the hypercalciuric, osteoporotic men as compared to seven osteoporotic men without hypercalciuria. This reduction in bone formation was associated with significant increases in the mineralization lag time and formation period. This observation of low bone formation in the presence of absorptive hypercalciuria was previously suggested by Malluche *et al.* (1980), who presented static and dynamic histology data in 15 hypercalciuric calcium stone formers on a free diet. The hypercalciuria was believed to be of the absorptive type because oral administration of cellulose phosphate (which complexes calcium in the gut) reduced urinary calcium excretion by 40% or more in all patients. Bone histomorphometry disclosed a picture best described as reduced bone formation in the presence of normal bone resorption. Osteoblastic surface was decreased as was mineral apposition rate and double labeled surfaces. Similar findings were also reported by Bataille *et al.* (1995), although, in that series only one patient was reported to have pure absorptive hypercalciuria, limiting the value of the observation. The cause of reduced bone formation in men with osteoporosis is not known. Recently, there has been increasing attention directed at a possible defect in insulin-like growth factor-1 (IGF-1) synthesis or action (Ljunghall *et al.*, 1992; Reed *et al.*, 1995; Dempster *et al.*, 1996).

Another question that needs to be addressed is the cause of intestinal hyperabsorption of calcium. Like their hypercalciuric stone-forming counterparts, the majority of the hypercalciuric osteoporotic men have relatively normal concentrations of calcitriol, the principal modulator of intestinal calcium absorption. In a minority of these men, elevations in serum calcitriol are found, which may explain the absorptive hypercalciuria, and may suggest a component of increased vitamin D-mediated bone resorption. In the remaining patients with normal $1,25(OH)_2D$ concentrations, there may be increased sensitivity of target organs to the action of this vitamin D metabolite.

This mechanism could also explain the similarities between hypercalciuric osteoporotic men and hypercalciuric calcium stone formers with reduced bone mass. If the skeleton were to display more sensitivity than the intestine, osteoporosis would be expected to result. Increased skeletal sensitivity to $1,25(OH)_2D$ would be expected to increase bone resorption and possibly reduce bone formation through the inhibitory actions of $1,25(OH)_2D$ on collagen synthesis as observed *in vitro* (Rowe and Kream, 1982). On the contrary, if the intestine were more sensitive, then AH would be present with only modest reductions in skeletal bone mass. Whether any of these potential mechanisms will prove to be correct must await more detailed investigations in hypercalciuric osteoporotic men.

IV. Prevalence and Forms of Hypercalciuria in Men with Osteoporosis

Although hypercalciuria can be a finding in men with secondary osteoporosis due to various causes (endocrinopathies, neoplastic diseases, immobilization, or drug-induced) interest in its occurrence has been directed mainly at men with primary (idiopathic) osteoporosis. Investigations in osteoporotic men in which the presence or lack of hypercalciuria was noted are summarized in Table II. It should be pointed out that, in most of these studies, patients were evaluated while consuming a random diet of undefined composition. Although a majority of the studies have used the definitions of hypercalciuria described earlier (Section II) during a random diet, there have been few attempts to determine whether hypercalciuria is still prevalent on a standard or calcium-restricted diet. This is of central importance in ascertaining whether the hypercalciuria is due to a primary mechanism or whether it is the result of nutritional habits.

Despite the lack of such dietary considerations in the majority of studies summarized in Table II, several interesting observations emerge. Hypercalciuria has been noted in a majority of these investigations. In only two studies was hypercalciuria not observed. The investigations by Jackson *et al.* (1987) and Francis *et al.* (1989) failed to find that hypercalciuria was a feature of their male idiopathic osteoporotic populations when mean urinary calcium excretion was compared to that in a group of normal men. Because individual data were not addressed in these two studies, it is not possible to determine if the prevalence of hypercalciuria was increased. For the remaining investigations summarized in Table II, the prevalence of hypercalciuria varied from 8 to 100% of the studied patients. This large range may be the result of failure to control the diet during study, inclusion of women in some studies, and possible referral bias. Nevertheless, hypercalciuria does appear to be a frequent finding in men with idiopathic osteoporosis, with a mean prevalence of about 30%.

TABLE II Summary of Studies That Have Assessed Urinary Calcium Excretion in Male Osteoporotic Subjects

Study	Patient population	Percent with hypercalciuria	Mechanism of hypercalciuria	Bone Bx findings	Notes
Jackson (1958)	27 men 11 women	7/27 men (26%) 3/11 women (27%)	Not examined	Not performed	Stated that hypercalciuria present in 16/27 men (59%) on initial exam
Hioco et al. (1964)	42 men	Very common	—	Not performed	↑resorption/↓formation by ^{45}Ca kinetic analysis
Bordier et al. (1973)	10 men 1 women	4/11 (30%)	Probably resorptive	↓resorption ↓formation	Hypercalciuria result of ↓skeletal accretion
Perry et al. (1982)	5 men	5/5 (100%)	Absorptive component in all; 4/5 with resorptive component	↑resorption ↑formation	—
De Vernejoul et al. (1983)	11 men	2/11 (18%)	Absorptive	Nl resorption ↓formation	Study complicated by excessive alcohol and tobacco consumption in patients
Jackson et al. (1987)	8 men	0/8 (0%)	—	↓formation	—
Francis et al. (1989)	40 men	Mean value in 34 patients not different from control	—	↓formation	Low intestinal calcium absorption
Resch et al. (1992)	27 men	Group mean significantly greater than control mean	Not examined	Not performed but ↑OHPro and alk. phos.; implied ↑turnover	—
Zerwekh et al. (1992)	16 men	9/16 (56%)	Absorptive	↓formation but ES > in presence of hypercalciuria	—
Khosla et al. (1994)	26 men 30 women	5/56 (8%)	Not examined	Heterogeneous picture ↑resorption ↓formation	Biopsy data in 18 patients only
Delichatsios et al. (1995)	7 men	3/7 (43%)	Not assessed	↑resorption Nl formation	Hypercalciuric patients had greater resorption indices
Peris et al. (1995)	18 men	8/18 (44%)	Not determined	Not performed but OHPro↓ in 2 hypercalciuric patients	↓Tm PO$_4$/GFR in hypercalciuric patients

Abbreviations: ↑, increased; ↓, decreased; OHPro, hydroxyproline.

Only three studies directly examined the mechanism of hypercalciuria found in osteoporotic men. Interestingly, all three of these studies (Perry *et al.,* 1982; De Vernejoul *et al.,* 1983; Zerwekh *et al.,* 1992) demonstrated that the hypercalciuria was of the absorptive type as determined from normal fasting calcium/creatinine (De Vernejoul *et al.,* 1983), increased fractional intestinal calcium absorption as measured isotopically and by the calciuric response to a 1 g calcium load (Zerwekh *et al.,* 1992), and from decreases in urinary calcium excretion following reduction of dietary calcium (Perry *et al.,* 1982). Another study (De Vernejoul *et al.,* 1983) was complicated by the high prevalence of excessive smoking and alcohol use in their patient population, both of which have been established as risk factors for osteoporosis and probably contributed to the low bone formation rates seen in their patients. Despite drawbacks and limitations in some studies, there appears to be a frequent association of intestinal hyperabsorption of calcium in the face of reduced bone formation in many hypercalciuric osteoporotic men.

More than one mechanism may be operative in contributing to hypercalciuria in some osteoporotic men. For example, four of five men in Perry's study probably had both resorptive and absorptive components, because 24-hr urinary calcium did not completely return to normal values after calcium restriction. In addition, all of Perry's patients demonstrated high bone turnover when bone biopsies were examined, consistent with increased bone resorption. Similarly, Bordier *et al.* (1973) found decreased bone mineral accretion (i.e., decreased bone formation) in four hypercalciuric osteoporotics, but also noted that increased bone resorption may have contributed to hypercalciuria.

Although $1,25(OH)_2D$ is a potent stimulator of intestinal calcium absorption, the serum concentration of this vitamin D metabolite was normal in all of Perry's subjects. In Zerwekh's study, the mean serum $1,25(OH)_2D$ concentration was not significantly different from the normal control value. However, four of the nine hypercalciuric patients demonstrated frank increases in the circulating concentration of this vitamin D metabolite despite normal serum iPTH and phosphorus concentrations. This finding may be the result of disordered regulation of the renal 25-hydroxyvitamin D_3-1α-hydroxylase as has been proposed for patients with absorptive hypercalciuria and nephrolithiasis (Broadus *et al.,* 1984; Insogna *et al.,* 1985). An increase in serum $1,25(OH)_2D$ would also be expected to promote increased bone resorption and might explain why some patients demonstrate a component of resorptive hypercalciuria (Perry *et al.,* 1982). For those idiopathic osteoporotic men with normal serum calcitriol concentration, increased intestinal calcium absorption may be the result of a primary defect at the intestine.

For the remaining studies listed in Table II, a resorptive mechanism of hypercalciuria was suggested by either increased bone resorption and/or increased urinary hydroxyproline excretion. Unfortunately, there was no assessment of fasting urinary calcium excretion in the majority of these studies.

Thus, the available data don't strongly support the common existence of a primary renal calcium leak in male idiopathic osteoporotic patients, as has been reported for postmenopausal osteoporotic women (Morris *et al.*, 1991; Nordin *et al.*, 1994). Although a renal leak of calcium would be expected to cause secondary hyperparathyroidism, increased serum $1,25(OH)_2D$ levels, and increased intestinal calcium absorption, serum iPTH concentrations have not been elevated in male idiopathic osteoporotic men (Perry *et al.*, 1982; De Vernejoul *et al.*, 1983; Jackson *et al.*, 1987; Francis *et al.*, 1989; Resch *et al.*, 1992; Zerwekh *et al.*, 1992; Delichatsios *et al.*, 1995; Peris *et al.*, 1995).

Taken together, the available literature documents the presence of hypercalciuria in a large fraction of men with idiopathic osteoporosis. It is evident that a proportion of hypercalciuric osteoporotic men demonstrate absorptive hypercalciuria, independent of increased bone resorption. Whether the coexistence of intestinal hyperabsorption of calcium and osteoporosis in men are related or represent two separate disease processes remains to be established. Additional studies are also needed to delineate fully the true prevalence of renal hypercalciuria in this group of male osteoporotic patients. It may be that renal hypercalciuria has the same prevalence in male osteoporotics as in patients with nephrolithiasis (i.e., approximately 2%). If true, then many additional osteoporotic, hypercalciuric patients will be needed to obtain meaningful data on the prevalence and skeletal effects of renal hypercalciuria.

V. Clinical Evaluation

In light of the frequent association of low bone mass with hypercalciuria, bone mineral density should be assessed in all patients who are evaluated for hypercalciuria and nephrolithiasis. In this way, patients with low bone mass who are at increased risk for an osteoporotic fracture can be identified and appropriate preventive or treatment strategies instigated. The measurement can also serve as a baseline by which to gauge future changes in bone mass. Similarly, in men with osteoporosis consideration should routinely be given to the possibility that a primary hypercalciuric disorder may be contributing to the skeletal disorder. An evaluation should rely on a testing regimen described briefly by Pak *et al.* (1980). This approach can be used to exclude secondary causes of osteoporosis and to identify and characterize hypercalciuria.

Although the work-up for stone-forming patients utilizes three different urine collections, in the evaluation of patients presenting with osteoporosis sufficient information can be initially obtained with one 24-hr urine collection. The patient is advised to discontinue any medications that might influence calcium homeostasis such as calcium and vitamin D supplements, thiazide diuretics, and bisphosphonates (female patients currently taking estrogen are allowed to continue on this therapy). If hypercalciuria is found to be present, further evaluation is warranted for classification. After 2–3 weeks the patient returns to the clinic (after another 24-hr urine collection the day before) for a 12-hr fast performed while maintaining high intake of distilled water to ensure adequate urine flow during the testing period. On the morning of the test, the patient empties the bladder, consumes 300 ml of distilled water, and begins a 2-hr fasting urine collection. At the end of the 2-hr period, the urine is collected, the volume is measured, and an aliquot is removed for testing. Fasting blood is drawn for routine serum chemistries, complete blood count, osteocalcin, bone-specific alkaline phosphatase, type I procollagen extension peptide, vitamin D metabolites, iPTH, cortisol, total and free testosterone, LH, and serum protein electrophoresis. Urine tests include calcium, phosphorus, sodium, cortisol, protein electrophoresis, pH, deoxypyridinoline, and creatinine. After the fasting blood collection, a 1-g elemental calcium load is given, and urine is collected during the ensuing 4 hr with continued hydration. The fasting urine calcium excretion is expressed as milligrams of calcium per deciliter of glomerular filtrate (as determined by clearance of creatinine), normal being less than 0.11. Urinary calcium excretion after calcium loading is expressed as milligrams of calcium per milligram of creatinine, the normal ratio being less than 0.2.

Hypercalciuria is diagnosed when the 24-hr urinary excretion of calcium is greater than 4 mg/kg on a random diet. The serum calcium, phosphorus, PTH level, and urinary excretion of calcium in response to the fast and calcium loading identify the pathophysiology of the hypercalciuria. Assuming that the fast was adequate, fasting hypercalciuria indicates either an excessive filtered load of calcium, or reduced renal reabsorption. The finding of fasting hypercalciuria in the face of normal iPTH and normal bone resorption may signify improper preparation by the patient for the fast and load test. Under such conditions, the test should be repeated after administration of sodium cellulose phosphate (Calcibind), a nonabsorbable binder of dietary calcium. If increased skeletal resorption is contributing to an increased filtered load and fasting hypercalciuria, then urinary markers of bone resorption should also be elevated. Patients with elevated 24-hr urine calcium excretion and a normal fasting urinary calcium excretion but exaggerated calciuric response to the calcium load have absorptive hypercalciuria. An algorithm for delineating the hypercalciuric mechanism as well as suggested therapeutic modalities for each hypercalciuric variant is depicted in Figure 1.

VI. Therapeutic Considerations in the Hypercalciuric Osteoporotic Male

Treatment of the hypercalciuric osteoporotic man should initially be directed at correcting any underlying defect in bone remodeling. For example, the use of bisphosphonates in those patients with histological or bio-

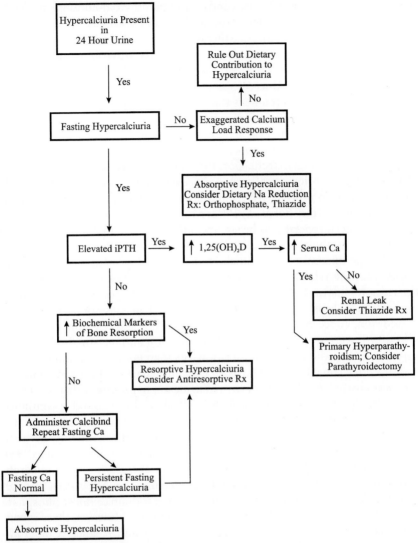

FIGURE I   Flow diagram of the diagnostic and potential therapeutic approach to the hypercalciuric male osteoporotic patient.

chemical evidence of increased bone resorption will, in most cases, also correct resultant resorptive hypercalciuria.

In some osteoporotic men, particularly in those with a history of nephrolithiasis, hypercalciuria may be the result of a primary renal calcium leak. Although hypercalciuria in these men may be exacerbated by increased bone resorption secondary to an increase in parathyroid hormone, and an increase in intestinal calcium absorption secondary to a parathyroid-hormone-mediated increase in circulating calcitriol, the underlying hypercalciuric defect is of renal origin. In such cases, thiazide therapy is indicated. By correcting the renal calcium leak, thiazide reverses secondary hyperparathyroidism and restores a normal serum calcitriol level and intestinal calcium absorption. Thiazide has been shown to produce a sustained correction of hypercalciuria in stone-forming patients commensurate with a restoration of normal serum $1,25(OH)_2D$ levels and intestinal calcium absorption during up to 10 years of therapy (Preminger and Pak, 1986). Furthermore, thiazide therapy in such renal hypercalciuric patients appears to stabilize bone density. Previous studies have also suggested that thiazide, through its hypercalciuric action, might cause skeletal retention of calcium in those without hypercalciuria. Thiazide has been found to prevent age-related decline in bone density of the appendicular skeleton (Transbol et al., 1982; Morton et al., 1994). Moreover, bone density has been reported to be significantly increased in hypertensive male patients taking thiazide (Wasnich et al., 1983) through a reduction of the rate of bone mineral loss (Wasnich et al., 1990). Ray et al. (1989) also reported that the relative risk of hip fracture was halved by an exposure to thiazides for more than 6 years. Unfortunately, the specific use of thiazide diuretics in male osteoporotic hypercalciuric patients has not been reported. In addition, concern has been expressed regarding the potential deleterious effects of lowering serum calcitriol concentration and intestinal calcium absorption during thiazide administration. Such an effect might minimize the positive effect thiazides may have on calcium balance. However, concomitant administration of calcitriol with thiazide might improve calcium balance substantially through the hypocalciuric effect of thiazide and a continued calcitriol-mediated increase in intestinal calcium absorption. This regimen has been used in postmenopausal osteoporotic women with an improvement in calcium balance and attenuation of further bone loss (Sakhaee et al., 1993).

In patients with absorbtive hypercalciuria, correction of the hyperabsorption of calcium and the ensuing hypercalciuria can be effected through dietary calcium restriction and administration of sodium cellulose phosphate (a nonabsorbable calcium-binding resin) with meals. However, there is concern that this approach may induce negative calcium balance (Coe et al., 1982), and it is probably in the best interest of the patient with reduced bone mass or established osteoporosis to avoid the tendency to correct the hyperabsorption of calcium. It may be preferable to use such agents as thiazides or orthophosphates, which decrease urinary calcium excretion more than they decrease intestinal calcium absorption (Coe et al., 1988).

VII. Summary

Although several secondary causes of osteoporosis in men can promote hypercalciuria, there is an increasing awareness that a significant proportion of men with primary osteoporosis also demonstrate primary hypercalciuria. The prevalence of hypercalciuria in men with idiopathic osteoporosis has been shown to range from 8 to 100%, but studies that suggest an exceptionally high prevalence of hypercalciuria may suffer from a lack of consideration of dietary habits, which may have contributed to the hypercalciuria. In light of the limited data available, the overall prevalence of hypercalciuria is estimated to be on the order of 30%. Additional studies of osteoporotic men in controlled study environments are needed to ascertain the true prevalence of hypercalciuria.

Hypercalciuria in osteoporosis may simply represent a manifestation of increased bone resorption, but few studies have confidently identified the nature of the hypercalciuria as resorptive, renal leak, or absorptive. It has been proposed that hypercalciuria with increased bone resorption may be the result of osteoclastic activation by cytokines, a condition also reported in women. A limited number of studies have documented hypercalciuria in the face of normal bone resorption, suppressed bone formation, and augmented intestinal calcium absorption, but neither the stimulus for increased intestinal calcium absorption nor for suppressed bone formation has been elucidated to date.

Defining the hypercalciuric variant in osteoporotic men is a relatively simple task and, in men with osteoporosis, can aid in the selection of the appropriate pharmacologic agent. Ideally, such an agent should reduce urinary calcium excretion, promote positive calcium balance, and at the same time halt or reverse the osteoporotic process.

References

Albright, F., Henneman, P., Benedict, P. H., and Forbes, A. P. (1953). Idiopathic hypercalciuria: A preliminary report. *Proc. R. Soc. Med.* **46**, 1077–1081.

Barilla, D. E., Townsend, J., and Pak, C. Y. C. (1978). An exaggerated augmentation of renal calcium excretion following oral glucose ingestion in patients with renal hypercalciuria. *Ivest.Urol.* **15**, 486–488.

Barkin, J., Wilson, D. R., Manuel, A., Bayley, A., Murray, T., and Harrison, J. (1985). Bone mineral content in idiopathic calcium nephrolithiasis. *Miner. Electrolyte Metab.* **11**, 19–24.

Bataille, P., Achard, J. M., Fournier, A., Boudailliez, B., Westeel, P. F., el Esper, N., Bergot, C., Jans, I., Lalau, J. D., Petit, J., Henon, G., Jeantet, M. A. L., Bouillon, R., and Sebert, J. L. (1991). Diet, vitamin D and vertebral mineral density in hypercalciuric calcium stone formers. *Kidney Int.* **39**, 1193–1205.

Bataille, P., Hardy, P., Marie, A., Steinche, I., Cohen Solal, M. E., Brazier, M., Werteel, A., and Fournier, A. (1995). Decreased bone formation in idiopathic hypercalciuric calcium stone formers explains reduced bone density. *J. Bone Min. Res.* **10**(Suppl.), 395–401.

Bordier, P. J., Miravet, L., and Hioco, D. (1973). Young adult osteoporosis. *Clin. Endocrinol. Metab.* **2**, 277–292.

Bordier, P. J., Ryckewart, A., Gueris, J., and Rasmussen, H. (1977). On the pathogenesis of so-called idiopathic hypercalciuria. *Am. J. Med.* **63**, 398–409.

Breslau, N. A., McGuire, J. L., Zerwek, J. E., and Pak, C. Y. C. (1982). The role of dietary sodium on renal excretion and intestinal absorption of calcium and on vitamin D metabolism. *J. Clin. Endocrinol. Metab.* **55**, 369–373.

Breslau, N. A., Brinkley, L., Hill, K. D., and Pak, C. Y. C. (1988). Relationship of animal protein-rich diet to kidney stone formation and calcium metabolism. *J. Clin. Endocrinol. Metab.* **66,** 140–146.

Broadus, A. E., Insogna, K. L., Lang, R., Ellison, A. F., and Dreyer, B. E. (1984). Evidence for disordered control of 1,25-dihydroxy-vitamin D production in absorptive hypercalciuria. *N. Engl. J. Med.* **311,** 73–80.

Coe, F. L., Canterbury, J. M., Firpo, J. J., and Reiss, E. (1973). Evidence for secondary hyperparathyroidism in idiopathic hypercalciuria. *J. Clin. Invest.* **52,** 134–142.

Coe, F. L., Favus, M. J., and Crockett, T. (1982). Effects of low-calcium diet on urine calcium excretion, parathyroid function and serum $1,25(OH)_2D_3$ levels in patients with idiopathic hypercalciuria and in normal subjects. *Am. J. Med.* **72,** 25–32.

Coe, F. L., Parks, J. H., Bushinsky, D. A., Langman, C. B., and Favus, M. J. (1988). Chlorthalidone promotes mineral retention in patients with idiopathic hypercalciuria. *Kidney Int.* **33,** 1140–1146.

Coe, F. L., Parks, J. H., and Asplin, J. R. (1992). The pathogenesis and treatment of kidney stones. *N. Engl. J. Med.* **327,** 1141–1152.

Da Silva, A. M. M., Dos Reis, L. M., and Pereira, R. C. (1993). Bone histomorphometric and bone mineral content in idiopathic hypercalciuria patients. *Int. Congr. Nephrol., 12th,* Jerusalem, Israel, Abstr., p. 620.

Delichatsios, H. K., lane, J. M., and Rivlin, R. S. (1995). Bone histomorphometry in men with spinal osteoporosis. *Calcif. Tissue Int.* **56,** 359–363.

Dempster, D. W., Kurland, E., Cosman, F., Schnitzer, M., Parisien, M., Chan, F., Shane, E., Rosen, C., Lindsay, R., and Bilezikien, J. P. (1996). Bone histomorphometry in osteoporotic men with low circulating levels of insulin-like growth factor-1 (IGF-1). *J. Bone Miner. Res.* **11,** (Suppl. 1), Abstract S327.

De Vernejoul, M. C., Bielakoff, J., Herve, M., Gueris, J., Hott, M., Modrowski, D., Kuntz, D., Miravet, L., and Ryckewart, A. (1983). Evidence for defective osteoblastic function; a role for alcohol and tobacco consumption in osteoporosis in middle-aged men. *Clin. Orthop. Relat. Res.* **179,** 107–115.

Francis, R. M., Peacock, M., Marshall, D. H., Horsman, A., and Aaron, J. E. (1989). Spinal osteoporosis in men. *Bone Miner.* **5,** 347–357.

Fuss, M., Gillet, C., Simon, J, Vandewalle, J. C., Schoutens, A., and Bergmann, P. (1983). Bone mineral content in idiopathic renal stone disease and in primary hyperparathyroidism. *Eur. Urol.* **9,** 32–34.

Ghazali, A., Fuentes, V., Desaint, C., Bataille, P., Westeel, A., Brazier, M., Prin, L., and Fournier, A. (1997). Low bone mineral density and peripheral blood monocyte activation profile in calcium stone formers with idiopathic hypercalciuria. *J. Clin. Endocrinol. Metab.* **82,** 32–38.

Gowen, M., and Mundy, G. R. (1986). Actions of interleukin-1, interleukin-2, and interferon γ on bone resorption *in vitro. J. Immunol.* **136,** 2478–2482.

Heilberg, I. P., Martini, L. A., Szejnfeld, V. L., Carvalho, A. B., Draibe, S. A., Ajzen, H., Ramos, O. L., and Schor, N. (1994). Bone disease in calcium stone forming patients. *Clin. Nephrol.* **42,** 175–182.

Insogna, K. L., Broadus, A. E., Dreyer, B. E., Ellison, A. F., and Gertner, J. M. (1985). Elevated production rate of 1,25-dihydroxy-vitamin D in patients with absorptive hypercalciuria. *J. Clin. Endocrinol. Metab.* **61,** 490–495.

Jackson, J. A., Kleerekoper, M., Parfitt, A. M., Rao, D. S., Villanueva, A. R., and Frame, B. (1987). Bone histomorphometry in hypogonadal and eugonadal men with spinal osteoporosis. *J. Clin. Endocrinol. Metab.* **65,** 53–58.

Jackson, W. P. U. (1958). Osteoporosis of unknown cause in younger people. *J. Bone Jt. Surg., Br. Vol.* **40B,** 420–441.

Jaeger, P., Portmann, L., Ginalski, J. M., Campiche, M., and Burckhardt, P. (1987). Dietary factors and medullary sponge kidneys as causes of the so-called idiopathic renal leak of calcium. *Am. J. Nephrol.* **7,** 257–263.

Kaplan, R. A., Haussler, M. R., Deftos, L. J., Bone, H., and Pak, C. Y. C. (1977). The role of 1α,25-dihydroxyvitamin D in the mediation of intestinal hyperabsorption of calcium in primary hyperparathyroidism and absorptive hypercalciuria. *J. Clin. Invest.* 59, 756–760.

Khosla, S., Lufkin, E. G., Hodgson, S. F., Fitzpatrick, L. A., and Melton, L. J., III (1994). Epidemiology and clinical features of osteoporosis in young individuals. *Bone* 15, 551–555.

Lawoyin, S., Sismilich, S., Browne, R., and Pak, C. Y. C. (1979). Bone mineral content in patients with calcium urolithiasis. *Metab., Clin. Exp.* 28, 1250–1254.

Lemann, J., Jr. (1980). Idiopathic hypercalciuria in nephrolithiasis. In "Contemporary Issues in Nephrology" (F. L. Coe, B. M., Brenner, and J. H. Stein, eds.), pp. 86–135. Churchill-Livingstone, New York.

Lemann, J., Jr. (1992). Pathogenesis of idiopathic hypercalciuria and nephrolithiasis. In "Disorders of Bone and Mineral Metabolism" (F. L. Coe and M. J. Favus, eds.), pp. 685–706. Raven Press, NewYork.

Lemann, J., Jr., Litzow, J. R., and Lennon, E. J. (1966). The effects of chronic acid loads in normal man: Further evidence for the participation of bone mineral in the defense against chronic metabolic acidosis. *J. Clin. Invest.* 45, 1608–1614.

Levy, F. L., Adams-Huet, B., and Pak, C. Y. C. (1995). Ambulatory evaluation of nephrolithiasis: An update of a 1980 protocol. *Am. J. Med.* 98, 50–59.

Lindergard, B., Colleen, S., Mansson, W., Rademark, C., and Roglund, B. (1983). Calcium loading test and bone disease in patients with urolithiasis. *Proc. EDTA* 20, 460–465.

Ljunghall, S., Johansson, A. G., Burman, P., Kampe, O., Lindh, E., and Karlsson, F. A. (1992). Low plasma levels of insulin-like growth factor I (IGF-I) in male patients with idiopathic osteoporosis. *J. Intern. Med.* 232, 59–64.

Malluche, H. H., Tschoepe, W., Ritz, E., Meyer-Sabellek, W., and Massry, S. G. (1980). Abnormal bone histology in idiopathic hypercalciuria. *J. Clin. Endocrinol. Metab.* 50, 654–658.

Morris, H. A., Need, A. G., Horowitz, M., O'Loughlin, P. D., and Nordin, B. E. C. (1991). Calcium absorption in normal and osteoporotic post-menopausal women. *Calcif. Tissue Int.* 49, 240–243.

Morton, D. J., Barrett-Connor, E. L., and Edelstein, S. L. (1994). Thiazides and bone mineral density in elderly men and women. *Am. J. Epidemiol.* 139, 1107–1115.

Nordin, B. E. C., Horowitz, M., Need, A., and Morris, H. A. (1994). Renal leak of calcium in postmenopausal osteoporosis. *Clin. Endocrinol.* 41, 41–45.

Pacifici, R., Rothstein, M., Pifas, L., Lau, K.-H. W., Baylink, D. J., Avioli, L. V., and Hruska, K. (1990). Increased monocyte interleukin-1 activity and decreased vertebral bone density in patients with fasting idiopathic hypercalciuria. *J. Clin. Endocrinol. Metab.* 71, 138–145.

Pak, C. Y. C. (1979). Physiological basis for absorptive and renal hypercalciurias. *Am. J. Physiol.* 237, F415–F423.

Pak, C. Y. C., Ohata, M., Lawrence, E. C., and Snyder, W. (1974). The hypercalciurias. Causes, parathyroid functions and diagnostic criteria. *J. Clin. Invest.* 54, 387–400.

Pak, C. Y. C., Kaplan, R. A., Bone, H., Townsend, J., and Waters, O. (1975). A simple test for the diagnosis of absorptive, resorptive and renal hypercalciuria. *N. Engl. J. Med.* 292, 497–500.

Pak, C. Y. C., Britton, F., Peterson, R., Ward, D., Northcutt, C., Breslau, N. A., McGuire, J., Sakhaee, K., Bush, S., Nicar, M., Norman, D., and Peters, P. (1980). Ambulatory evaluation of nephrolithiasis: Classification, clinical presentation and diganostic criteria. *Am. J. Med.* 69, 19–30.

Peris, P., Guanabens, N., Monegal, A., Suris, X., Alvarez, L., Martinez de Osaba, M. J., Hernandez, M. V., and Munoz-Gomez, J. (1995). Aetiology and presenting symptoms in male osteoporosis. *Br. J. Rheum.* 34, 936–941.

Perry, H. M., III, Fallon, M. D., Bergfeld, M., Teitelbaum, S. L., and Avioli, L. V. (1982). Osteoporosis in young men; a syndrome of hypercalciuria and accelerated bone turnover. *Arch. Intern. Med.* 142, 1295–1298.

Pietschmann, F., Breslau, N. A., and Pak, C. Y. C. (1992). Reduced vertebral bone density in hypercalciuric nephrolithiasis. *J. Bone Miner. Res.* 7, 1383–1388.

Preminger, G. P., and Pak, C. Y. C. (1986). Eventual attenuation of hypocalciuric response to hydrochlorothiazide in absorptive hypercalciuria. *J. Urol.* **137**, 1104–1108.

Ray, W. A., Griffin, M. R., Downey, W., and Melton, L. J., III (1989). Long-term use of thiazide diuretics and risk of hip fracture. *Lancet* **1**, 687–690.

Reed, B. Y., Zerwekh, J. E., Sakhaee, K., Breslau, N. A., Gottschalk, F., and Pak, C. Y. C. (1995). Serum IGF-1 is low and correlated with osteoblastic surface in idiopathic osteoporosis. *J. Bone Miner. Res.* **10**, 1218–1224.

Resch, H., Pietschmann, P., Woloszczuk, W., Krexner, E., Bernecker, P., and Willvonseder, R. (1992). Bone mass and biochemical parameters of bone metabolism in men with spinal osteoporosis. *Eur. J. Clin. Invest.* **22**, 542–545.

Rowe, D. W., and Kream, B. E. (1982). Regulation of collagen synthesis in fetal rat calvaria by 1,25-dihydroxyvitamin D_3. *J. Biol. Chem.* **257**, 8009–8105.

Sakhaee, K., Nicar, M. J., Glass, K., and Pak, C. Y. C. (1985a). Postmenopausal osteoporosis as a manifestation of renal hypercalciuria with secondary hyperparathyroidism. *J. Clin. Endocrinol. Metab.* **61**, 368–373.

Sakhaee, K., Nicar, M. J., Brater, D. C., and Pak, C. Y. C. (1985b). Exaggerated natriuretic and calciuric response to hydrochlorothiazide in renal hypercalciuria but not in absorptive hypercalciuria. *J. Clin. Endocrinol. Metab.* **61**, 825–829.

Sakhaee, K., Zisman, A., Pondexter, J. R., Zerwekh, J. E., and Pak, C. Y. C. (1993). Metabolic effects of thiazide and 1,25-$(OH)_2$ Vitamin D in postmenopausal osteoporosis. *Osteoporosis Int.* **3**, 209–214.

Seeman, E., Melton, L. J., III, O'Fallon, W. M., and Riggs, B. L. (1983). Risk factors for spinal osteoporosis in men. *Am. J. Med.* **75**, 977–983.

Steiniche, T., Mosekilde, L., Christensen, M. S., and Melsen, F. (1989). A histomorphometric determination of iliac bone remodeling in patients with recurrent renal stone formation and idiopathic hypercalciuria. *Acta Pathol. Microbiol. Immunol Scand.* **97**, 309–316.

Transbol, I., Christensen, M. S., Jensen, G. F., Christiansen, C., and McNair, P. (1982). Thiazide for the postponement of postmenopausal bone loss. *Metab., Clin. Exp.* **31**, 383–386.

Wachman, A., and Bernstein, D. S. (1968). Diet and osteoporosis. *Lancet* **1**, 958–959.

Wasnich, R. D., Benfante, R. J., Yano, K., Heilbrun, L., and Vogel, J. M. (1983). Thiazide effect on the mineral content of bone. *N. Engl. J. Med.* **309**, 344–347.

Wasnich, R. D., Davis, J., Ross, P., and Vogel, J. M. (1990). Effect of thiazide on rates of bone mineral loss: A longitudinal study. *Br. Med. J.* **301**, 1303–1305.

Weisinger, J. R. (1996). New insights into the pathogenesis of idiopathic hypercalciuria: The role of bone. *Kidney Int.* **49**, 1507–1518.

Weisinger, J. R., Alonzo, E., Bellorin-Font, E., Blasini, A. M., Rodriguez, M. A., Paz-Martinez, V., and Martinis, R. (1996). Possible role of cytokines on the bone mineral loss in idiopathic hypercalciuria. *Kidney Int.* **49**, 244–250.

Zerwekh, J. E., and Pak, C. Y. C. (1980). Selective effects of thiazide therapy on serum 1,25-dihydroxyvitamin D and intestinal calcium absorption in renal and absorptive hypercalciurias. *Metab., Clin. Exp.* **29**, 13–17.

Zerwekh, J. E., Sakhaee, K., Breslau, N. A., Gottschalk, F., and Pak, C. Y. C. (1992). Impaired bone formation in male idiopathic osteoporosis: Further reduction in the presence of concomitant hypercalciuria. *Osteoporosis Int.* **2**, 128–134.

Chapter 23

Peter R. Ebeling

Bone and Mineral Service
Departments of Diabetes and Endocrinology and Medicine
The University of Melbourne
The Royal Melbourne Hospital
Victoria 3050, Australia

Secondary Causes of Osteoporosis in Men

In men with osteoporosis, it is critical to exclude underlying pathological causes as these are more likely to be present than in women (Riggs and Melton, 1986). Previous studies have shown that between 30 and 60% of men evaluated for vertebral fractures have another illness contributing to the presence of bone disease (Ebeling, 1998a; Orwoll and Klein, 1995; Francis *et al.*, 1989; Seeman and Melton, 1983; Resch *et al.*, 1992; Seeman, 1993); however, there have been fewer studies of the bone disease present in men sustaining proximal femoral (Nyquist *et al.*, 1998; Boonen *et al.*, 1997a) or other peripheral fractures. This chapter will focus on the major conditions causing osteoporosis in men which are enumerated in Table I.

I. Glucocorticoid-Induced Osteoporosis

Glucocorticoid excess (predominantly exogenous) is the most commonly identified etiological factor, accounting for 16–18% of cases (Francis *et al.*,

TABLE I   Etiology of Osteoporosis in Men

Primary	Senile
	Idiopathic
Secondary	Glucocorticoid excess (exogenous or endogenous)
	Other immunosuppressive drugs (e.g., cyclosporine A)
	Hypogonadism (including treatment for prostatic carcinoma, glucocorticoid-induced and renal insufficiency)
	Ineffective skeletal estrogen action (estrogen receptor defects, aromatase deficiency)
	Alcohol excess
	Smoking
	Chronic obstructive pulmonary disease and asthma
	Cystic fibrosis
	Gastrointestinal disease (coeliac, Crohn's diseases, short bowel syndrome, post-gastrectomy, total parenteral nutrition, lactase deficiency)
	Pernicious anemia
	Hypercalciuria
	Anticonvulsants (phenytoin, phenobarbitone)
	Thyrotoxicosis
	Hyperparathyroidism
	Immobilization
	Osteogenesis imperfecta
	Homocystinuria
	Neoplastic disease (multiple myeloma, lymphoma)
	Ankylosing spondylitis and rheumatoid arthritis
	Systemic mastocytosis

1989; Seeman and Melton, 1983). The pathophysiology of glucocorticoid-induced osteoporosis is similar in women and men, and the most important mechanism is a direct inhibition of the actions of osteoblasts, including the elaboration of growth factors promoting collagen proliferation (McCarthy *et al.*, 1990; Raisz and Simmons, 1985), and decreased osteoblast recruitment (Chuyn *et al.*, 1984). However, muscle weakness, immobility, impaired intestinal calcium absorption, hypercalciuria, and a reduction in serum total and free testosterone levels also may all contribute to glucocorticoid-associated bone loss (MacAdams *et al.*, 1986; Fitzgerald *et al.*, 1997). The cause of the reduction in serum testosterone levels of men receiving treatment with glucocorticoids is incompletely understood. The mechanisms may include central inhibition of GnRH release, suppression of pituitary sensitivity to GnRH, and a direct inhibition of testicular steroidogenesis (Veldhuis *et al.*, 1992). This common cause of osteoporosis in men is discussed in more detail in Chapter 20. Importantly, it is not uncommon for more than one risk factor to be operative in the same patient, such as long-standing tobacco and alcohol abuse in a man requiring oral glucocorticoid therapy for asthma.

II. Pulmonary Disease and Immunosuppressive Drugs _____

In men with asthma (Ebeling *et al.*, 1998b), low spinal bone density is related to both the cumulative inhaled glucocorticoid dose and the cumulative exposure to oral prednisolone. However, the cumulative exposure to oral prednisolone is a more important determinant of bone density at both the spine and the proximal femur (Fig. 1). Vertebral deformities are common in older men with chronic pulmonary disease and the likelihood of vertebral fracture is also greatest in those men using continuous systemic glucocorticoid therapy (McEvoy *et al.*, 1998). Osteoporosis is also a common accompaniment in adult male survivors with cystic fibrosis. In men with cystic fibrosis aged 25–45 years, overall fracture rates were twofold greater than

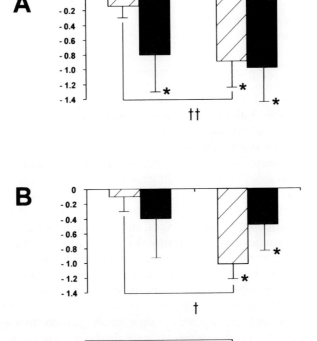

FIGURE I Effects of high-dose inhaled (IG) or prior maintenance oral (OG) glucocorticoid therapy on standardized bone mineral density in men and women. Bars indicate mean ± SEM. (A) Lumbar spine Z score. (B) Femoral neck Z score. $*p = 0.01$ compared with zero; $†p < 0.01$; $††p = 0.07$, for OG group compared with IG group. From Ebeling *et al.* (1998a), *J. Bone Miner. Res.* (in press). © American Society for Bone and Mineral Research, with permission.

in the general population, whereas vertebral compression and rib fractures were 100- and 10-fold more common, respectively, than expected in the general population (Aris *et al.*, 1998). Mean standardized bone mineral densities (BMDs) at the spine, femur, and total body were two standard deviations lower than expected. The cumulative prednisolone dose, body mass index, and age at puberty were the strongest predictors of bone density.

In animal models, cyclosporine A therapy leads to high bone turnover and rapid bone loss (Movsowitz *et al.*, 1988). In humans, immunosuppressive therapy with cyclosporine A or tacrolimus for the prevention and treatment of graft versus host disease also results in osteoporosis. The combination of glucocorticoids and cyclosporine A results in rapid bone loss following cardiac, renal, single lung and bone marrow transplantation, and vertebral fractures are not infrequent in this increasingly common clinical setting (Katz and Epstein, 1992). Following allogeneic bone marrow transplantation, bone loss at the femoral neck and lumbar spine is related to the cumulative prednisolone dose and the duration of cyclosporine A therapy used to treat graft versus host disease, as well as the pretransplantation levels of bone resorption (Ebeling *et al.*, 1999).

III. Hypogonadism

Although there is no abrupt cessation of testicular function or "andropause" comparable with the menopause in women, both total and free testosterone concentrations decline irrevocably with age in men. The decrease in free testosterone concentrations is greater than that for total testosterone because sex hormone-binding globulin levels also increase with age. Finally, age-related decreases in adrenal androgens are even greater than for testosterone and may have more impact on age-related bone loss (Clarke *et al.*, 1994). A limited correlation exists between free testosterone levels with bone density at some, but not all, skeletal sites, and these findings have been inconsistent between studies and skeletal sites (Kelly *et al.*, 1990). In a study of 90 healthy men, after controlling for age, free but not total testosterone concentrations were related to BMD at the femoral neck and Ward's triangle, but not at the lumbar spine, while an inverse relationship existed between total testosterone and fat mass (Ongphiphadhanakul *et al.*, 1995). The distribution of adipose tissue is also altered in men with postpubertal hypogonadism. Although measurements of visceral fat were similar to eugonadal men, subcutaneous and muscle fat areas were higher (Katznelson *et al.*, 1998).

In contrast to the studies of testosterone, a recent study has shown that BMD at all skeletal sites was significantly positively associated with serum estradiol concentrations in men aged over 65 years (Slemenda *et al.*, 1997). Body weight, age and serum sex steroids accounted for 30% of the variability of BMD in men with consistent positive associations between BMD and estradiol concentrations. Importantly, within the normal range, lower serum testosterone levels were not associated with low BMD. Khosla *et al.* (1998) also showed that bioavailable estradiol levels correlated positively with BMD and negatively with bone resorption in normal men aged 23–90 years. Currently, it is not therefore possible to identify a threshold serum testosterone concentration, below which bone loss will occur.

Hypogonadism is one of the most common secondary causes of osteoporosis in men, being present in up to 30% of men with osteoporotic vertebral fractures (Orwoll and Klein, 1995), and low free testosterone and 25(OH) vitamin D concentrations are common in men with hip fractures (Boonen *et al.*, 1997a). Free testosterone and 25(OH) vitamin D concentrations are both independently negatively related to deoxypyridinoline excretion in men with hip fractures, suggesting that increased bone resorption rates in these men may be important in contributing to bone loss at the femoral neck. Fragility fractures and low bone density are also common in men with prostate cancer. The cumulative incidence of osteoporotic fractures in men 7 years after orchidectomy for prostate cancer was approximately 28% (Daniell, 1997). The incidence of fragility fractures in men with prostate cancer treated with luteinizing hormone-releasing hormone agonists for 22 months, on average, was somewhat lower at 5% (Townsend *et al.*, 1997).

Androgens are important in both attainment of peak bone mass and the maintenance of bone mass in adult men. Reduced bone mass is present in men with Klinefelter's and Kallman's syndromes and also in men who have had constitutionally delayed puberty. In young men with constitutional delay of puberty (CDP), bone turnover was increased and BMD was decreased, whereas bone turnover was normal and BMD was decreased in men with idiopathic hyogonadotrophic hypogonadism (IHH). Interestingly, after testosterone therapy, BMD increased only in men with CDP and not in men with IHH, indicating that high baseline bone turnover could be a useful predictor of responses to testosterone in men with hypogonadism (Lubushutzky *et al.*, 1998).

In hypogonadism beginning in the prepubertal years, the bone deficit is more marked in cortical bone than in hypogonadism commencing after puberty. It is likely, therefore, that androgens are important in bone modeling and subperiosteal apposition. This is supported by rat studies that show an increase in subperiosteal bone formation rates after oophorectomy compared with a decrease after orchidectomy (Orwoll and Klein, 1995). By contrast, in postpubertal hypogonadism, vertebral bone loss, with reduced trabecular numbers, is greater than appendicular bone loss (Finkelstein *et al.*, 1989).

There is an interaction between testosterone concentrations and vitamin D metabolism. Francis and Peacock (1986) found that $1,25\text{-}(OH)_2D$ levels were decreased in European hypogonadal males with fragility fractures. Both bone formation parameters and plasma $1,25\text{-}(OH)_2D$ levels increased after testosterone treatment. However, in animal studies using vitamin D replete, sexually immature male chicks, circulating $1,25\text{-}(OH)_2D$ levels decreased, whereas the tissue levels of $1,25\text{-}(OH)_2D$ and the biological responses of bone and intestine to $1,25\text{-}(OH)_2D$ increased (Otremski et al., 1997). A French histomorphometric study of men with chronic hypogonadism also demonstrated low bone formation rates (Delmas and Meunier, 1981). By contrast, North American studies of men with fragility fractures have not demonstrated reduced bone formation rates, but a slight increase in mean remodeling rates comparable with postmenopausal estrogen deficiency in women (Jackson and Kleerekoper, 1987). Thus, nutritional vitamin D deficiency may have contributed to the European study findings. It is notable, however, that in all studies trabecular loss was a consistent finding.

Osteoblasts in men contain low numbers of androgen and estrogen receptors (Colvard et al., 1989; Orwoll et al., 1991; Eriksen et al., 1988). Androgens and estrogens affect bone cells by indirect and direct mechanisms secondary to changes in concentrations of both systemic and local factors. Several of these effects including proliferation, growth factor and cytokine production, and bone matrix protein production (type I collagen, osteocalcin, osteopontin) are mediated by the androgen receptor (AR). The mechanisms whereby sex hormones interact with local growth factors to exert their effects on bone cells in men needs to be further elucidated. For example, it is possible that an interaction occurs between decreasing serum concentrations of testosterone and insulin-like growth factor-1 (IGF-I) with aging resulting in reduced bone formation rates and an age-related increase in bone fragility (Boonen et al., 1997b).

Acute testosterone deficiency following orchidectomy is associated with a phase of rapid bone loss and increases in biochemical markers of bone turnover as it is in postmenopausal women (Stepan and Lachman, 1989; Goldray et al., 1993). This is followed by a phase of slower bone loss associated with low bone turnover. Histomorphometric studies have also shown that bone formation rates are reduced in chronic hypogonadism (Otremski et al., 1997; Delmas and Meunier, 1981; Jackson and Kleerekoper, 1987). In addition, it is uncertain whether testosterone therapy of eugonadal men results in significant increases in bone density. One small, nonrandomized study of parenteral testosterone therapy of eugonadal older men detected increases in spinal, but not proximal femur, bone mass (Tenover, 1992); however, a double blind, placebo-controlled trial of transdermal testosterone showed no effect (Orwoll and Oviatt, 1992). A recent open, uncontrolled study of testosterone treatment of eugonadal men with osteoporosis for 6 months showed that a 5% increase in spinal BMD was associated with large decreases in urinary excretion of deoxypyridinoline and N-telopeptide. The increase in spinal BMD was correlated with changes in estradiol but not in testosterone (Anderson et al., 1997).

This is in keeping with increasing evidence that estrogens (Vanderscheueren et al., 1996), as well as androgens, play an important role in skeletal

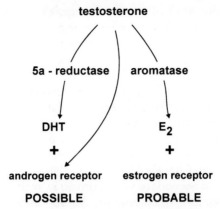

FIGURE 2   Possible modes of androgen action on bone. Testosterone may be either converted to dihyrotestosterone by 5α-reductase or converted into 17β-estradiol by aromatase. From Vanderscheueren *et al.* (1996), with permission.

maintenance in men (Fig. 2). In men peripheral aromatization of androgens to estrogens occurs, and aromatization also occurs within osteoblasts. Two human models currently exist for inefficient actions of estrogen on the male skeleton. A man with a stop mutation in the estrogen receptor gene and high circulating estradiol concentrations had failure of epiphyseal fusion, continued skeletal growth, and severe osteoporosis (Smith *et al.*, 1994). Similarly, an aromatase-deficient man developed tall stature and osteoporosis, and low-dose estrogen therapy resulted in a large increase in bone density (Ke-nan *et al.*, 1995; Morishima *et al.*, 1998).

IV. Alcohol and Osteomalacia

Alcoholic men have a high risk of osteoporotic fracture. The link between alcohol abuse and bone diseases has been well established by epidemiological studies (Seeman and Melton, 1983; Resch *et al.*, 1992). In 25–50% of men who present for medical assistance because of excessive drinking, osteopenia will be present (Orwoll and Klein, 1995). The habitual consumption of alcohol is also significantly negatively related to bone mass in men (Seeman and Melton, 1983; Resch *et al.*, 1992; Slemenda *et al.*, 1992), and in a longitudinal study, Slemenda *et al.* (1992) showed that high alcohol consumption was associated with increased rates of bone loss. However, the dose dependence of alcohol-related bone loss is unclear. For example, recent studies suggest that modest alcohol intakes may be associated with increases in bone mass. Even those men in the Framingham heart study cohort who were the heaviest drinkers (> 414 mL/week) had BMD that was, on average,

3.9% higher at all sites after adjustment for age, weight, height and smoking (Felson *et al.*, 1995). In addition, men aged 50 years and over from the European Vertebral Osteoporosis Study Group with vertebral deformities did not have a higher frequency of alcohol intake than men without vertebral deformities (Naves Diaz *et al.*, 1997). There was also a small and nonsignificant protective effect of moderately frequent alcohol intake (1–4 days per week) in men aged 65 years and older (OR = 0.81; 95% CI = 0.62, 1.08). Overall, further prospective data are required to determine at what level of alcohol ingestion the positive benefits of regular intake are overtaken by the increased risk of fragility fracture from alcohol excess. This problem is discussed in more detail in Chapter 21.

In many cases of secondary osteoporosis in men, including alcohol-related bone disease, gastrointestinal disease and anticonvulsant use, it is important to exclude vitamin D deficiency as a contributing factor. In the individual man with metabolic bone disease, the degree of vitamin D deficiency may vary from severe (osteomalacia) to mild, but the latter is also important to detect because it may lead to secondary hyperparathyroidism if it is untreated. In men with alcoholic cirrhosis and alcoholic bone disease the free concentrations of both 25(OH)D and 1,25-(OH)$_2$D are normal despite low levels of the total hormones (Bikle *et al.*, 1984, 1986). Trans-iliac bone biopsy is the definitive test to diagnose osteomalacia. Nevertheless, a measure of serum 25(OH)D concentration will provide useful information on the degree of vitamin D deficiency present (with the exception noted above).

V. Tobacco

Tobacco use is associated with decreased bone mass in women (Hopper and Seeman, 1994). In men, hip fracture rates are higher in current smokers (Paganini-Hill *et al.*, 1991) and the relative risk of vertebral fracture in smokers is 2.3 based on a previous cohort study (Seeman and Melton, 1983). This risk is independent of alcohol consumption. Both risk factors had adverse effects on BMD in men who were aged greater than 60 years and whose average duration of smoking was 36 years, indicating that prolonged exposure may be required for effects on fracture incidence. Slemenda *et al.* (1992) demonstrated in twins discordant for smoking that radial bone loss was 40% greater in the smoking twin than the nonsmoking twin (Fig. 3). The number of cigarettes smoked also correlated with the rapidity of bone loss.

A recent study (Vogel *et al.*, 1997) examined effects of smoking on bone density, and of current smoking on rates of bone loss in men. Current and past smokers had significantly lower bone density, particularly at the calcaneus (approximately 4.5%) and distal radius (approximately 2.5%). The effect was linked both to the smoking duration and to the number of ciga-

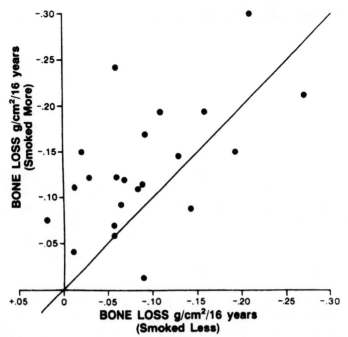

FIGURE 3   Bone loss from the distal radius in twins discordant for smoking. Points above the line indicate pairs in which the twin lost more ($p = 0.005$, two-sided exact binomial test of equal proportions). Minus values indicate bone loss. From Slemenda *et al.* (1992), with permission.

rettes smoked. The rates of bone loss measured over an average of 5 years in current smokers were 20.5, 27.2, and 9.7% greater at the calcaneus, distal, and proximal radius, respectively, than in the never smokers, but these changes did not reach significance. However, smokers of more than 20 cigarettes per day had a significantly higher rate of bone loss (by 77.6% at the distal radius), consistent with an increase in fracture risk of 10–30% per decade of smoking. This effect was similar to that demonstrated in male twins and slightly greater than the effect on spinal BMD in female twins discordant for smoking, whose BMD deficit was 9.3% for 20 pack-years (one pack-year is equivalent to 20 cigarettes per day for one year) (Hopper and Seeman, 1994).

The mechanism of the adverse effect of smoking on bone mass in men is unknown but it may be related to decreased body weight, decreased calcium absorption, and decreased estrogen levels as it is in women (Krall and Dawson-Hughes, 1991). Smoking may also have a direct toxic effect on bone metabolism. However, its effects on androgen concentrations or growth factor production in men are unknown.

VI. Gastrointestinal Disease

Several nutrients including amino acids, calcium, magnesium, and phosphorus and the fat-soluble vitamins D and K are important for the maintenance of skeletal health in normal men. Gastrointestinal disease predisposes to bone disease as a result of intestinal malabsorption of these nutrients. In men with hip fractures, a low serum albumin concentration, a nonspecific marker of nutrition, was the strongest independent variable correlated with fracture (Thiebaud *et al.*, 1997). Low femoral neck BMD was also correlated with hip fracture risk. Serum insulin-like growth factor-binding protein 3 (IGF-BP3) concentrations were lower in men with hip fractures and also correlated with BMD and albumin. Lactase deficiency can lead to low dietary calcium intakes, increased bone turnover, and osteoporotic fractures in men (Tamatani *et al.*, 1998). In addition to vitamin D deficiency, decreased vitamin K1 and K2 levels are correlated with BMD in osteopenic elderly Japanese men, suggesting that both deficiencies may cooperatively play a role in the etiology of type II osteoporosis in men (Laroche *et al.*, 1995).

In particular, gastrectomy is commonly associated with vertebral osteoporosis in men (Francis *et al.*, 1989; Seeman, 1993). Between 10 and 40% of men have low BMD following gastrectomy (Garrick *et al.*, 1971). It is not currently known whether prolonged use of powerful inhibitors of gastric acid secretion such as omeprazole may also predispose to bone loss in men, but by analogy with pernicious anemia this seems unlikely (see following discussion). Other gastrointestinal diseases, particularly small bowel disease (coeliac disease, Crohn's disease, small intestinal resection), cause bone disease equally in men and women (Orwoll and Klein, 1995). However, large bowel diseases are uncommonly associated with osteopenia.

Vitamin D deficiency and osteomalacia are associated with malabsorption. However, lesser degrees of nutrient malabsorption more commonly result in other forms of bone loss. For example, Parfitt has described focal osteomalacia (increased osteoid thickness with normal osteoid surface) or atypical osteomalacia (increased osteoid surface with normal osteoid thickness) in patients with postgastrectomy bone disease and without obvious vitamin D deficiency, secondary hyperparathyroidism, or hypophosphatemia (Parfitt and Duncan, 1982). Similar forms of bone disease are also seen in small bowel disease. All are characterized by low mineralization rates. Low turnover osteoporosis may also be seen in men with bowel disease (Rao and Honasoge, 1996). Its etiology is unknown, but in some men treatment with glucocorticoids may be partially or completely responsible.

In cholestatic or alcoholic liver disease, there is an increased incidence of metabolic bone diseases, including osteomalacia and osteoporosis. In men with cirrhosis following necrotic hepatitis, spinal BMD, serum osteocalcin and 25-(OH)D concentrations were lower than in control men. The spinal

BMD was correlated with serum 25-(OH)D concentrations or the clinical severity of cirrhosis (Chen *et al.*, 1996). It is therefore important to exclude vitamin D deficiency in men with cirrhosis of any cause or severity.

VII. Hypercalciuria

Hypercalciuria is more than twice as common in men as in women (Smith, 1989). Currently there are data that suggest a link between hypercalciuria and bone loss in some men with osteoporosis. Hypercalciuria or nephrolithiasis in men is associated with osteopenia (Pietschmann *et al.*, 1992). In men with renal hypercalciuria, this may be related to a negative calcium balance with secondary hyperparathyroidism, increased $1,25$ $(OH)_2$ vitamin D levels and increased bone turnover rates (Zerwekh *et al.*, 1992). This secondary cause of osteoporosis is more fully discussed in Chapter 22.

VIII. Anticonvulsants

Anticonvulsants (phenobarbitone, phenytoin) cause a spectrum of disorders of bone and mineral metabolism associated with hyperosteoidosis in 10–60% of men and women using these drugs (Orwoll and Klein, 1995). This is particularly important in the elderly who are at risk of epileptic seizures as a result of previous stroke or tumor (Cohen *et al.*, 1997) and in institutionalized epileptics. Nilsson *et al.* (1986) found that institutionalized epileptics had a fracture rate of 10%/year. Bone histological findings from the fracture patients revealed increased osteoid volume, increased osteoclastic resorptive activity, and reduced trabecular bone volume compared with age-matched controls. Thus, the bone disease can include a combination of osteoporosis, osteomalacia, and hyperparathyroidism. Anticonvulsants increase hepatic metabolism of vitamin D and 25-(OH)D to inactive metabolites via induction of cytochrome P_{450} enzyme activity. Circulating and tissue levels of biologically active vitamin D metabolites are decreased, and hypocalcemia, decreased intestinal calcium absorption and hypophosphatemia, secondary hyperparathyroidism, and alterations in bone remodeling result.

In epileptics receiving phenytoin, serum 25(OH)D concentrations correlate positively with serum calcium levels and BMD (Hahn *et al.*, 1972). Total body bone mineral content was 10–30% lower than age-matched normal values. The effect of anticonvulsants on BMD was related to the number of drugs used, the total daily dose, and the duration of drug therapy (Wolinsky Friedland, 1995). Phenytoin also may directly decrease intestinal calcium absorption by inhibition of cellular calcium fluxes. It inhibits PTH-induced bone resorption in a dose-dependent manner and inhibits collagen synthesis *in vitro*. In boys, sodium valproate (but not carbamazepine) therapy, resulted in significantly lower BMD by 14 and 10%, at axial and appendicular sites, respectively (Sheth *et al.*, 1995).

IX. Pernicious Anemia

In men and women with pernicious anemia, there is an increased risk of fragility fractures (Goerss *et al.*, 1992). In comparison with fracture rates from the general community, patients with pernicious anemia had a 1.9-fold increase in proximal femur fractures, a 1.8-fold increase in vertebral fractures, and a 2.9-fold increase in distal forearm fractures. The rate of proximal humerus or pelvic fractures was not increased. The mechanism of bone loss in this condition is unknown because women with pernicious anemia have normal true fractional calcium absorption and normal levels of calciotrophic hormones despite achlorhydria, indicating gastric acid is not required for absorption of dietary calcium (Eastell *et al.*, 1992).

X. Thyrotoxicosis and Thyroidectomy

Thyrotoxicosis and a past history of thyrotoxicosis are associated with osteopenia in both men and women. There are few, if any, studies of the effects of clinical or subclinical hyperthyroidism on bone in men. Studies in women suggest that thyrotoxic bone disease and osteopenia are potentially reversible disorders (Diamond *et al.*, 1994). In women with subclinical hyperthyroidism, cortical bone is adversely affected more than trabecular bone (Ross, 1994). No data exist on an increased fracture risk of subclinical hyperthyroidism in either men or women. In men with a history of thyroidectomy, the relative risk of fractures of any of the vertebrae, proximal humerus, distal radius, pelvis, or proximal femur was increased only 1.5-fold (95% confidence interval, 0.7–3.2) compared with age-matched controls (Nguyen *et al.*, 1997). This difference was entirely due to a statistically significant increase in the rate of proximal femur fractures in men who had had a thyroidectomy. Other risk factors for hip fractures included being older at the time of surgery, a greater extent of surgery, and the presence of other risk factors for osteoporosis. Thyroidectomy, performed mainly for adenoma or goiter, had little influence on the risk of fracture at other sites.

XI. Hyperparathyroidism

In the original bone densitometric studies of patients with primary hyperparathyroidism, osteopenia occurred predominantly in postmenopausal women and less commonly in premenopausal women or men (Pak *et al.*, 1975). Nevertheless, vertebral compression fractures are the mode of presentation in approximately 4% of patients with surgically proven primary hyperparathyroidism (Dauphine *et al.*, 1975). Survival in men and women following surgical treatment for primary hyperparathyroidism is usually not impaired, but the presence of osteoporosis and muscle weakness and the absence of a history of renal calculi have been associated with reductions in survival (Soreide *et al.*, 1997). In men with severe congestive heart failure, there is a high prevalence of osteoporosis and osteopenia, low vitamin D metabolite concentrations, and high bone turnover rates. Conversely, higher parathyroid hormone (PTH) concentrations were associated with better left ventricular function (Shane *et al.*, 1997). In men with chronic renal failure treated with chronic ambulatory peritoneal dialysis and 1-α-(OH)D$_3$ for 2 years, there was no change in bone mineral content of the distal radius, whereas in age-matched postmenopausal women, it decreased by 6% per year. The greater bone loss in women could therefore indicate an additive effect of hypogonadism on bone loss in secondary hyperparathyroidism in uremia, as also exists for primary hyperparathyroidism (Lyhne and Pedersen, 1995).

XII. Immobilization

Prolonged bed rest is similar to weightlessness in that it can result in bone loss. Bone lost during immobilization can be regained after weight-bearing is recommenced, but a deficit in bone mass is likely to result (Donaldson *et al.*, 1970). Osteopenia is also a rapid, constant, and permanent accompaniment of quadriplegia and paraplegia. In men with hemiplegia, the ipsilateral femoral neck BMD, measured by DXA, was lower than in the contralateral femur, but the difference was less than in women. The duration of immobilization comprised only 5% of the total variance of bone loss (del Puente *et al.*, 1996). In men with a history of a tibial fracture 9 years prior, spinal BMD measured by dual energy x-ray absorptiometry (DXA) was 12.3 or 9.5% lower in men with a history of primary nonunion and union, respectively, compared with age-, weight- and height-matched normal men (Kannus *et al.*, 1994). Therefore, bone loss due to immobilization may be long-lived.

XIII. Osteogenesis Imperfecta

Osteogenesis imperfecta in its milder forms may present as osteoporosis in either men or women (Spotila *et al.*, 1991). It is important to assess men with osteoporosis carefully for signs of osteogenesis imperfecta such as ligamentous laxity, increased elasticity of the skin, and blue sclerae. A family history of multiple and severe fragility fractures may also be present.

XIV. Homocystinuria

Osteoporosis occurs commonly in homocystinuria. By the age of 15 years, spinal osteoporosis is detected in 64% of patients with vitamin B6-unresponsive compared with 36% of vitamin B6-responsive patients (Mudd *et al.*, 1985). Deficient collagen cross-linking has been proposed as a cause of osteoporosis in homocystinuria. In ten patients with homocystinuria, concentrations of amino- and carboxy-terminal propeptides of types III and I collagen, respectively, were similar to those in healthy age-matched controls. However, the urinary excretion of the carboxy-terminal telopeptide cross-link (ICTP) was decreased consistent with normal collagen synthesis and reduced pyridinium cross-link formation in homocystinuria (Lubec *et al.*, 1996).

XV. Neoplastic Disease (Multiple Myeloma, Lymphoma)

Multiple myeloma and lymphoma are associated with bone destruction, low bone mass, and fragility fractures due to the production of cytokines. In patients with multiple myeloma, new bone formation is also inhibited. Possible mediators of this effect include lymphotoxin, interleukin-1β, parathyroid hormone-related protein (PTHrP), and interleukin-6. They can be produced by the myeloma cells or by marrow stromal cells in response to myeloma cells, and all have been implicated as possible osteoclast-activating factors (OAF) (Roodman, 1997). The cytokines were originally labeled osteoclast-activating factors because of their ability to stimulate osteoclastic bone resorption. Production of these cytokines is inhibited by glucocorticoids, and intravenous bisphosphonate therapy with monthly infusions of pamidronate for nine months reduced the skeletal morbidity associated with multiple myeloma and improved quality of life (Berenson *et al.*, 1996).

XVI. Ankylosing Spondylitis and Rheumatoid Arthritis

Cytokine production, particularly interleukin-6 (Papanicolaou *et al.*, 1998), as well as immobility and cumulative glucocorticoid therapy dose all play important roles in the etiology of osteoporosis in ankylosing spondylosis and rheumatoid arthritis. In men with ankylosing spondylitis of recent onset, spinal and femoral neck BMDs were lower than in age-matched control men, suggesting early loss of trabecular bone (Will *et al.*, 1989). Later in the disease process, spinal BMD is increased due to syndesmophyte formation. Vertebral compression fractures are present in 10–41% of patients with ankylosing spondylitis (Sivri *et al.*, 1996; Donnelly *et al.*, 1994). Patients with fractures are more likely to be male, to be older, and to have longer disease duration and more advanced spinal limitation with less mobility. There were no consistent deficits in either spinal or femoral neck BMD in fracture patients, and spinal BMD does not reliably predict the risk of vertebral fracture in men with ankylosing spondylitis.

In men with rheumatoid arthritis, osteoporosis is also more evident at the hip and radius than the spine (Dequeker *et al.*, 1995). Low-dose methotrexate therapy may increase the risk of fragility fractures and lower extremity pain syndromes in men and women with rheumatoid arthritis, but further prospective studies are required to prove this hypothesis. Few studies have addressed any problems specific to men with rheumatoid arthritis, but risk factors for osteoporosis in men are likely to be similar to those in women. In particular, consideration should be given to the treatment of underlying hypogonadism.

XVII. Systemic Mastocytosis

Mastocytosis is a spectrum of disorders in which aberrant mast cell proliferation may occur in a number of different organs (Table II). Mutations of the *c-kit* proto-oncogene, which encodes for a receptor tyrosine kinase and plays an important role in mast cell growth and differentiation during hematopoiesis, have been identified in some cases of human mastocytosis (Pignon, 1997). Mastocytosis may be indolent or aggressive, and in 75% of cases bone disease will be present (Travis *et al.*, 1988). Diffuse osteoporosis is the most common finding (28%) followed by osteosclerosis (19%); mixed sclerosis and demineralization occurs in 10% of the patients studied. The skeletal abnormalities are dependent on mast cell mediator production. Both heparin and prostaglandin D_2 may cause increased bone resorption, whereas histamine promotes bone fibrosis.

TABLE II   Classification of Mastocytosis

Indolent mastocytosis	Syncope
	Cutaneous disease
	Ulcer disease
	Malabsorption
	Bone marrow mast cell aggregates
	Skeletal disease (osteopenia, osteosclerosis, mixed)
	Hepatosplenomegaly
	Lymphadenopathy
Hematologic disorder	Myeloproliferative
	Myelodysplastic
Aggressive	Lymphadenopathic mastocytosis with eosinophilia
Mastocytic leukemia	

Recently there has been renewed interest in the prevalence of systemic mastocytosis in men with no other obvious cause of osteoporosis. In a large retrospective study by Ritzel *et al.* (1997), the prevalence of mastocytosis in patients having biopsies for osteoporosis was 1.1%, and men were equally represented with women. Osteoporosis in mastocytosis was associated with an increase in osteoid volume and osteoid surface, and an increase in eroded surface compared with the control group. Trabecular bone volume and trabecular thickness were decreased. Because osteoclast numbers were similar in both groups, these observations suggest an effect of mast cell products on osteoclasts together with an uncoupling of osteoblast and osteoclast function. It is possible the increased osteoid is due in part to calcium and/or vitamin D malabsorption caused by mastocytosis-associated gastrointestinal dysfunction.

In a smaller retrospective study of 136 bone biopsies from men with idiopathic osteoporosis, de Gennes *et al.* (1992) detected only four cases of skeletal mastocytosis, a prevalence of 3%. In a large teaching hospital in the United Kingdom, a search of all bone biopsies submitted over 5 years revealed evidence of only six cases of skeletal mastocytosis, four of whom were men (Andrew and Freemont, 1993). On the other hand, mastocytosis may present with diffuse osteopenia in up to 50% of cases (Fig. 4) with or without

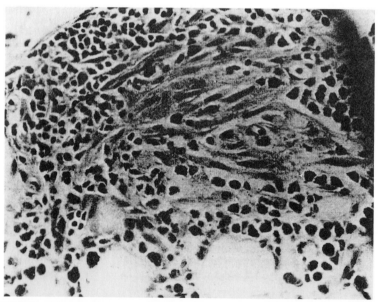

FIGURE 4   A bone marrow granuloma containing mast cells from a patient with mastocytosis. From Chines *et al. Osteoporosis Int.* (1993) S1, S148. © European Foundation for Osteoporosis, Lyons France and National Osteoporosis Foundation, Washington, D.C., U.S.A.

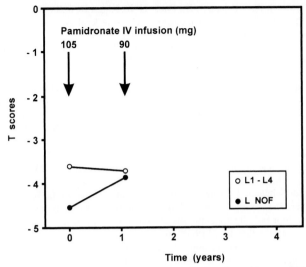

FIGURE 5   Effect of a single 105-mg intravenous infusion of pamidronate (APD) on lumbar spine and femoral neck bone mineral density in a man with osteoporosis secondary to mastocytosis. From Marshall *et al.* (1997), *Br. J. Rheumatol.* 36, 393–396, by permission of Oxford University Press.

vertebral compression fractures and in the absence of systemic symptoms or its classical cutaneous manifestation of urticaria pigmentosum (Chines *et al.*, 1993). In addition, mastocytosis may be more common as a cause of severe generalized osteopenia in younger men without clinical evidence of mast cell mediator disease (Lidor *et al.*, 1990). The treatment of men with mastocytosis has included antihistamines (H1 and H2 blockers), ketotifen, disodium chromoglycate, bisphosphonates (clodronate and pamidronate) and, most recently, interferon alpha-2b (Gruchalla, 1995). In one man with mastocytosis (Marshall *et al.*, 1997), a single infusion of 105 mg of pamidronate resulted in a 16% increase in spinal bone density over one year as measured by dual-energy x-ray absorptiometry (Fig. 5). In two small series of men treated with either daily or thrice weekly subcutaneous injections of interferon alpha-2b, trabecular BMD increased by 16%, on average, over 8 months (Lehmann *et al.*, 1996; Weide *et al.*, 1996).

References

Anderson, F. H., Francis, R. M., Peaston, R. T., and Wastell, H. J. (1997). Androgen supplementation in eugonadal men with osteoporosis: Effects of six months' treatment on markers of bone formation and resorption. *J. Bone Miner. Res.* 12, 472–478.

Andrew, S. M., and Fremont, A. J. (1993). Skeletal mastocytosis. *J. Clin. Pathol.* 46, 1033–1035.

Aris, R. M., Renner, J. B., Winders, A. D., Buell, H. E., Riggs, D. B., Lester, G. E., and Ontjes, D. A. (1998). Increased rate of fractures and severe kyphosis: Sequelae of living into adulthood with cystic fibrosis. *Ann. Intern. Med.* **128,** 186–193.

Berenson, J. R., Lichtenstein, A., Porter, L., Dimopoulos, M. A., Bordoni, R., George, S., Lipton, A., Keller, A., Ballester, O., Kovacs, M. J., Blacklock, H. A., Bell, R., Simeone, J., Reitsma, D. J., Heffernan, M., Seaman, J., and Knight, R. D. (1996). Efficacy of pamidronate in reducing skeletal events in patients with advanced multiple myeloma. Myeloma Aredia Study Group. *N. Engl. J. Med.* **334,** 488–493.

Bikle, D. D., Gee, E., and Halloran, B. (1984). Free 1,25-dihydroxyvitamin D levels in serum from normal subjects, pregnant subjects and subjects with liver disease. *J. Clin. Invest.* **78,** 748–752.

Bikle, D. D., Halloran, B. P., Gee, E., Ryzen, E., and Haddad, J. G. (1986). Free 25-hydroxyvitamin D levels are normal in subjects with liver disease and reduced total 25-hydroxyvitamin D levels. *J. Clin. Invest.* **78,** 748–752.

Boonen, S., Vanderschueren, D., Cheng, X. G., Verbeke, G., Dequeker, J., Geusens, P., Broos, P., and Bouillon, R. (1997a). Age-related (type II) femoral neck osteoporosis in men: Biochemical evidence for both hypovitaminosis D- and androgen-deficiency-induced bone resorption. *J. Bone Miner. Res.* **12,** 2119–2126.

Boonen, S., Vanderschueren, D., Geusens, P., and Bouillon, R. (1997b). Age-associated endocrine deficiencies as potential determinants of femoral neck (type II) osteoporotic fracture occurrence in elderly men. *Int. J. Androl.* **20,** 134–143.

Chen, C. C., Wang, S. S., Jeng, F. S., and Lee, S. D. (1996). Metabolic bone disease of liver cirrhosis: Is it parallel to the clinical severity of cirrhosis? *J. Gastroenterol. Hepatol.* **11,** 417–421.

Chines, A., Pacifici, R., Avioli, L. A., Korenblat, P. E., and Teitelbaum, S. L. (1993). Systemic mastocytosis and osteoporosis. *Osteoporosis Int.* **S1,** S147–S149.

Chuyn, Y. S., Kream, B. E., and Raisz, L. G. (1984). Cortisone decreases bone formation by inhibiting periosteal cell proliferation. *Endocrinology (Baltimore)* **114,** 477–480.

Clarke, B. L., Ebeling, P. R., Wahner, H. W., O'Fallon, W. M., Riggs, B. L., and Fitzpatrick, L. A. (1994). Steroid hormones influence bone histomorphometric parameters in healthy men. *Calcif. Tissue Int.* **54,** 334.

Cohen, A., Lancman, M., Mogul, H., Marks, S., and Smith, K. (1997). Strategies to protect bone mass in the older patient with epilepsy. *Geriatrics* **52,** 70.

Colvard, D. S., Eriksen, E. F., Keeting, P. E., Wilson, E. M., Lubahn, D. B., French, F. S., Riggs, B. L., and Spelsberg, T. C. (1989). Identification of androgen receptors in normal human osteoblast-like cells. *Proc. Natl. Acad. Sci. U.S.A.* **86,** 854–857.

Daniell, H. W. (1997). Osteoporosis after orchidectomy for prostate cancer. *J. Urol.* **157,** 439–444.

Dauphine, R. T., Riggs, B. L., and Scholtz, D. A. (1975). Back pain and vertebral crush fractures: an unemphasized mode of presentation of primary hyperparathyroidism. *Ann. Intern. Med.* **83,** 365–367.

de Gennes, C., Kuntz, D., and de Vernejoul, M. C. (1992). Bone mastocytosis: A report of nine cases with a bone histomorphometric study. *Clin. Orthop. Relat. Res.* **279,** 281–291.

Delmas, P., and Meunier, P. J. (1981). L'ostéoporose au cours du syndrome de Klinefelter. Donées histologiques osseuses quantitatives dans cinq cas. Relation avec la carence hormonale. *Nouv. Presse Med.* **10,** 687.

del Puente, A., Pappone, N., Mandes, M. G., Mantova, D., Scarpa, R., and Oriente, P. (1996). Determinants of bone mineral density in immobilization; a study on hemiplegic patients. *Osteoporosis Int.* **6,** 50–54.

Dequeker, J., Maenaut, K., Verwilghen, J., and Westhovens, R. (1995). Osteoporosis in rheumatoid arthritis. *Clin. Exp. Rheumatol.* **13**(S12), S21–S26.

Diamond, T., Vine, J., Smart, R., and Butler, P. (1994). Thyrotoxic bone disease in women: A potentially reversible disorder. *Ann. Intern. Med.* **120,** 8–11.

Donaldson, C. L., Hulley, S. B., and Vogel, J. M. (1970). Effect of prolonged bed rest on bone mineral. *Metab. Clin. Exp.* **19,** 1071–1084.

Donnelly, S., Doyle, D. V., Denton, A., Rolfe, I., McCloskey, E. V., and Spector, T. D. (1994). Bone mineral density and vertebral compression fracture rates in ankylosing spondylitis. *Ann. Rheum. Dis.* **53,** 117–121.

Eastell, R., Vieira, N. E., Yergey, A. L., Wahner, H. W., Silverstein, M. N., Kumar, R., and Riggs, B. L. (1992). Pernicious anemia as a risk factor for osteoporosis. *Clin. Sci.* **82,** 681–685.

Ebeling, P. R. (1998a). Osteoporosis in men. New insights into aetiology, pathogenesis, prevention and management. *Drugs Aging* **13,** 421–424.

Ebeling, P. R., Erbas, B., Hopper, J. L., Wark, J. D., and Rubinfeld, A. R. (1998b). Bone mineral density and bone turnover in asthma treated with long-term inhaled or oral glucocorticoids. *J. Bone Miner. Res.* **13,** 1283–1289.

Ebeling, P. R., Thomas, D. M., Erbas, B., Hopper, J. L., Szer, J., and Grigg, A. P. (1999). Mechanisms of bone loss in allogeneic and autologous hematopoietic stem cell transplantation. *J. Bone Miner. Res.* (in press).

Eriksen, E. F., Colvard, D. S., Berg, N. J., Graham, M. L., Mann, K. G., Spelsberg, T. C., and Riggs, B. L. (1988). Evidence of estrogen receptors in normal human osteoblast-like cells. *Science* **241,** 84–86.

Felson, D. T., Zhang, Y., Hannan, M. T., Kannel, W. B., and Kiel, D. P. (1995). Alcohol intake and bone mineral density in elderly men and women. The Framingham Study. *Am. J. Epidemiol.* **142,** 485–492.

Finkelstein, J. S., Klibanski, A., Neer, R. M., Doppelt, S. H., Rosenthal, D. I., Segré, G. V., and Crowley, W. F., Jr. (1989). Increases in bone density during treatment of men with idiopathic hypogonadotrophic hypogonadism. *J. Clin. Endocrinol. Metab.* **69,** 776–783.

Fitzgerald, R. C., Skingle, S. J., and Crisp, A. J. (1997). Testosterone concentrations in men on chronic glucocorticoid therapy. *J. R. Coll. Physicians London* **31,** 168–170.

Francis, R. M., and Peacock, M. (1986). Osteoporosis in hypogonadal men: Role of decreased plasma 1,25-dihydroxy vitamin D, calcium malabsorption and low bone formation. *Bone* **7,** 261–268.

Francis, R. M., Peacock, M., Marshall, D. H., Horsman, A., and Aaron, J. E. (1989). Spinal osteoporosis in men. *Bone Miner.* **5,** 347–357.

Garrick, R., Ireland, A. W., and Posen, S. (1971). Bone abnormalities after gastric surgery: A prospective histological study. *Ann. Intern. Med.* **75,** 221–225.

Goerss, J. B., Kim, C. H., Atkinson, E. J., Eastell, R., O'Fallon, W. M., and Melton, L. J., III (1992). Risk of fractures in patients with pernicious anemia. *J. Bone Miner. Res.* **7,** 573–579.

Goldray, D., Weisman, Y., Jaccard, N., Merdler, C., Chen, J., and Matzkin, H. (1993). Decreased bone density in elderly men treated with the gonadotrophin-releasing hormone agonist decapeptyl (D-Trp⁶-GnRH). *J. Clin. Endocrinol. Metab.* **76,** 288–290.

Gruchalla, R. S. (1995). Mastocytosis: Developments during the past decade. *Am. J. Med. Sci.* **309,** 328–338.

Hahn, T., Henden, B., and Scharp, C. (1972). Effect of chronic anticonvulsant therapy on serum 25-hydroxycalciferol levels in adults. *N. Engl. J. Med.* **287,** 900–904.

Hopper, J. L., and Seeman, E. (1994). The bone density of female twins discordant for smoking. *N. Engl. J. Med.* **330,** 387–392.

Jackson, J. A., and Kleerekoper, M. (1987). Bone histomorphometry in hypogonadal and eugonadal men with spinal osteoporosis. *J. Clin. Endocrinol. Metab.* **65,** 53–58.

Kannus, P., Jarvinen, M., Sievanen, H., Oja, P., and Vuori, I. (1994). Osteoporosis in men with a history of tibial fracture. *J. Bone Miner. Res.* **9,** 423–429.

Katz, I. A., and Epstein, S. (1992). Posttransplantation bone disease. *J. Bone Miner. Res.* **7,** 123–126.

Katznelson, L., Rosenthal, D. I., Rosol, M. S., Anderson, E. J., Hayden, D. L., Schoenfeld, D. A., and Klibanski, A. (1998). Using quantitative CT to assess adipose distribution in adult men with acquired hypogonadism. *AJR, Am. J. Roentgenol.* **170,** 423–427.

Kelly, P. J., Pocock, N. A., Sambrook, P. N., and Eisman, J. A. (1990). Dietary calcium, sex hormones and bone mineral density in men. *Br. Med. J.* **300**, 1361–1364.

Ke-nan, Q., Fisher, C. R., Grumbach, M. M., Morshina, A., and Simpson, E. R. (1995). Aromatase deficiency in a male subject: Characterization of a mutation in the CYP gene in an affected family. *Endocrinol. Soc.* **A**, pp. P3–P27.

Khosla, S., Melton, L. J. III, Atkinson, E. J., O'Fallon, W. M., Klee, G. G., and Riggs, B. L. (1998). Relationship of serum sex steroid levels and bone turnover markers with bone mineral density in men and women: A key role for bioavailable estrogen. *J. Clin. Endocrinol. Metab.* **83**, 2266–2274.

Krall, E. A., and Dawson-Hughes, B. (1991). Smoking and bone loss among postmenopausal women. *J. Bone Miner. Res.* **6**, 331–338.

Laroche, M., Bon, E., Moulinier, L., Cantagrel, A., and Mazieres, B. (1995). Lactose intolerance and osteoporosis in men. *Rev. Rheum. (Engl. Ed.)* **62**, 766–769.

Lehmann, T., Beyeler, C., Lammle, B., Hunziker, T., Vock, P., Olah, A. J., Dahinden, C., and Gerber, N. J. (1996). Severe osteoporosis due to systemic mast cell disease: Successful treatment with interferon alpha-2b. *Br. J. Rheumatol.* **35**, 898–900.

Lidor, C., Frisch, B., Gazit, D., Gepstein, R., Hallel, T., and Mekori, Y. A. (1990). Osteoporosis as the sole presentation of bone marrow mastocytosis. *J. Bone Miner. Res.* **8**, 871–876.

Lubec, B., Fang-Kircher, S., Lubec, T., Blom, H. J., and Boers, G. H. (1996). Evidence for McKusick's hypothesis of deficient collagen cross-linking in patients with homocystinuria. *Biochim. Biophys. Acta* **1315**, 159–162.

Lubushitzky, R., Front, D., Iosilevsky, G., Bettman, L., Frenkel, A., Kolodny, G. M., and Israel, O. (1998). Quantitative bone SPECT in young males with delayed puberty and hypogonadism: Implications for treatment of low bone density. *J. Nucl. Med.* **39**, 104–107.

Lyhne, N., and Pedersen, F. B. (1995). Changes in bone mineral content during long-term CAPD. Indication of a sex-dependent bone mineral loss. *Nephrol. Dial. Transplant.* **10**, 395–398.

MacAdams, M. R., White, R. H., and Chipps, B. E. (1986). Reduction of serum testosterone levels during chronic glucocorticoid therapy. *Ann. Intern. Med.* **104**, 648–651.

Marshall, A., Kavanagh, R. T., and Crisp, A. J. (1997). The effect of pamidronate on lumbar spine bone density and pain in osteoporosis secondary to systemic mastocytosis. *Br. J. Rheumatol.* **36**, 393–396.

McCarthy, T. L., Centrella, M., and Canalis, E. (1990). Cortisol inhibits the synthesis of insulin-like growth factor-I in skeletal cells. *Endocrinology (Baltimore)* **126**, 1569–1575.

McEvoy, C. E., Ensrud, K. E., Bender, E., Genant, H. K., Yu, W., Griffith, J. M., and Niewoehner, D. E. (1998). Association between corticosteroid use and vertebral fractures in older men with chronic obstructive pulmonary disease. *Am. J. Respir. Crit. Care Med.* **157**, 704–709.

Morishima, A., Grumbach, M. M., and Bilezikian, J. P. (1997). Estrogen markedly increases bone mass in an estrogen deficient young man with aromatase deficiency. *J. Bone Miner. Res.* **12**(S1), A96.

Movsowitz, C., Epstein, S., Fallon, M., Ismail, F., and Thomas, S. (1988). Cyclosporin-A *in vivo* produces severe osteopenia in the rat: Effect of dose and duration of administration. *Endocrinology (Baltimore)* **123**, 2571–2577.

Mudd, S. H., Skovby, F., Levy, H. L., Pettigrew, K. D., Wilcken, B., Pyeritz, R. E., Andria, G., Boers, G. H., Bromberg, I. L., and Cerone, R. (1985). The natural history of homocystinuria due to cystathione beta-synthase deficiency. *Am. J. Hum. Genet.* **37**, 1–31.

Naves Diaz, M., O'Neill, T. W., and Silman, A. J. (1997). The influence of alcohol consumption on the risk of vertebral deformity. European Vertebral Osteoporosis Study Group. *Osteoporosis Int.* **7**, 65–71.

Nguyen, T. T., Heath, H., III, Bryant, S. C., O'Fallon, W. M., and Melton, L. J., III (1997). Fractures after thyroidectomy in men: A population-based cohort study. *J. Bone Miner. Res.* **12**, 1092–1099.

Nilsson, O. S., Lindholm, T. S., Elmstedt, E., Lindback, A., and Lindholm, T. C. (1986). Fracture incidence and bone disease in epileptics receiving long-term anticonvulsant drug therapy. *Arch. Orthop. Trauma Surg.* **105**, 146–149.

Nyquist, F., Gardsell, P., Sernbo, I., Jeppsson, J. O., and Johnell, O. (1998). Assessment of sex hormones and bone mineral density in relation to occurrence of fracture in men: A prospective population-based study. *Bone* **22**, 147–151.

Ongphiphadhanakul, B., Rajatanavin, R., Chailurkit, L., Piaseu, N., Teearungsikul, K., Sirisriro, R., Komindr, S., and Puavilai, G. (1995). Serum testosterone and its relation to bone mineral density and body composition in normal males. *Clin. Endocrinol. (Oxford)* **43**, 727–733.

Orwoll, E. S., and Klein, R. F. (1995). Osteoporosis in men. *Endocr. Rev.* **16**, 87–116.

Orwoll, E. S., and Oviatt, S. (1992). Transdermal testosterone supplementation in normal older men. *Proc. Endocr. Soc.* A, 1071.

Orwoll, E. S., Stribska, L., Ramsey, E. E., and Keenan, E. J. (1991). Androgen receptors in osteoblast-like cell lines. *Calcif. Tissue Int.* **49**, 182–187.

Otremski, I., Lev-Ran, M., Salama, R., and Edelstein, S. (1997). The metabolism of vitamin D3 in response to testosterone. *Calcif. Tissue Int.* **60**, 485–487.

Paganini-Hill, A., Chao, A., Ross, R. K., and Henderson, B. E. (1991). Exercise and other factors in the prevention of hip fracture: The Leisure World Study. *Epidemiology* **2**, 16–25.

Pak, C. Y. C., Stewart, A., Kaplan, R., Bone, H., Notz, C., and Browne, R. (1975). Photon absorptiometric analysis of bone density in primary hyperparathyroidism. *Lancet* **2**, 7–8.

Papanicolaou, D. A., Wilder, R. L., Manolagos, S. C., and Chrousos, G. P. (1998). The pathophysiologic roles of interleukin-6 in human disease. *Ann. Intern. Med.* **128**, 127–137.

Parfitt, A. M., and Duncan, H. (1982). Metabolic bone disease affecting the spine. *In* "The Spine" (R. Rothman, ed.), 2nd ed., pp. 775–905. Saunders, Philadelphia.

Pietschmann, F., Breslau, N. A., and Pak, C. Y. C. (1992). Reduced vertebral bone density in hypercalciuric nephrolithiasis. *J. Bone Miner. Res.* **7**, 1383–1388.

Pignon, J.-M. (1997). C-kit mutations and mast cell disorders. A model of activating mutations of growth factor receptors. *Hematol. Cell Ther.* **39**, 114–116.

Raisz, L. G., and Simmons, H. A. (1985). Effects of parathyroid hormone and cortisol on prostaglandin production by neonatal rat calvaria *in vitro. Endocr. Res.* **11**, 59–74.

Rao, D. S., and Honasoge, M. (1996). Metabolic bone disease in gastrointestinal and biliary disorders. *In* "Primer on the Metabolic Bone Diseases and Disorders of Mineral Metabolism" (M. J. Favrus, ed.), 3rd ed., pp. 306–311. American Society for Bone and Mineral Research, Kelseyville. CA.

Resch, H., Pietschmann, P., Woloszczuk, W., Krexner, E., Bernecker, P., and Willvonseder, R. (1992). Bone mass and biochemical parameters of bone metabolism in men with spinal osteoporosis. *Eur. J. Clin. Invest.* **22**, 542–545.

Riggs, B. L., and Melton, L. J., III (1986). Involutional osteoporosis. *N. Engl. J. Med.* **314**, 1676–1686.

Ritzel, H., Amling, M., Minne, H. W., and Delling, G. (1997). Characteristic histopathological features in mastocytosis-mediated osteoporosis demonstrate uncoupling. *J. Bone Miner. Res.* **12**(S1), S167.

Roodman, G. D. (1997). Mechanisms of bone lesions in multiple myeloma and lymphoma. *Cancer (Philadelphia)* **80**, 1557–1563.

Ross, D. (1994). Hyperthyroidism, thyroid hormone therapy and bone. *Thyroid* **4**, 319–326.

Seeman, E. (1993). Osteoporosis in men: Epidemiology, pathophysiology and treatment possibilities. *Am. J. Med.* **95**, 225–285.

Seeman, E., and Melton, L. J., III (1983). Risk factors for spinal osteoporosis in males. *Am. J. Med.* **75**, 977–983.

Shane, E., Mancini, D., Aaronson, K., Silverberg, S. J., Seibel, M. J., Addesso, V., and McMahon, D. J. (1997). Bone mass, vitamin D deficiency, and hyperparathyroidism in congestive heart failure. *Am. J. Med.* **103**, 197–207.

Sheth, R. D., Wesolowski, C. A., Jacob, J. C., Penney, S., Hobbs, G. R., Riggs, J. E., and Bodensteiner, J. B. (1995). Effect of carbamazepine and valproate on bone mineral density. *J. Pediatr.* **127**, 256–262.

Sivri, A., Kilinc, S., Gokce-Kutsal, Y., and Ariyurek, M. (1996). Bone mineral density in ankylosing spondylitis. *Clin. Rheumatol.* **15**, 51–54.

Slemenda, C. W., Christian, J. C., Reed, T., Reister, T. K., Williams, C. J., and Johnston, C. C., Jr. (1992). Long-term bone loss in men: Effects of genetic and environmental factors. *Ann. Intern. Med.* **117**, 286–291.

Slemenda, C. W., Longcope, C., Zhou, L., Hui, S. L., Peacock, M., and Johnston, C. C. (1997). Sex steroids and bone mass in older men. Positive associations with serum estrogens and negative associations with androgens. *J. Clin. Invest.* **100**, 1755–1759.

Soreide, J. A., van Heerden, J. A., Grant, C. S., Yau Lo, C., Schleck, C., and Ilstrup, D. M. (1997). Survival after surgical treatment for primary hyperparathyroidism. *Surgery* **122**, 1117–1123.

Spotila, L. D., Constantinos, C. D., Sereda, L., Ganguly, A., Riggs, B. L., and Prockop, D. J. (1991). Mutation in a gene for type I procollagen (COL1A2) in a woman with postmenopausal osteoporosis: Evidence for phenotypic and genetic overlap with mild osteogenesis imperfecta. *Proc. Natl. Acad. Sci. U.S.A.* **88**, 5423–5427.

Smith, E. P., Boyd, J., Frank, G. R., Takahashi, H., Cohen, R. M., Specker, B., Williams, T. C., Lubahn, D. B., and Korach, K. S. (1994). Estrogen resistance caused by a mutation in the estrogen-receptor gene in a man. *N. Engl. J. Med.* **331**, 1056–1061.

Smith, L. H. (1989). The medical aspects of urolithiasis. *J. Urol.* **141**, 707–710.

Stepan, J. J., and Lachman, M. (1989). Castrated men with bone loss: Effect of calcitonin on biochemical indices of bone remodelling. *J. Clin. Endocrinol. Metab.* **69**, 523–527.

Tamatani, M., Morimoto, S., Nakajima, M., Fukuo, K., Onishi, T., Kitano, S., Niinobu, T., and Ogihara, T. (1998). Decreased circulating levels of vitamin K and 25-hydroxyvitamin D in osteopenic elderly men. *Metab., Clin. Exp.* **47**, 195–199.

Tenover, J. S. (1992). Effects of testosterone supplementation in the aging male. *J. Clin. Endocrinol. Metab.* **75**, 1092–1098.

Thiebaud, D., Burckhardt, P., Costanza, M., Sloutskis, D., Gilliard, D., Quinodoz, F., Jacquet, A. F., and Burnand, B. (1997). Importance of albumin, 25(OH)-vitamin D and IGFBP-3 as risk factors in elderly women and men with hip fracture. *Osteoporosis Int.* **7**, 457–462.

Townsend, M. F., Sanders, W. H., Northway, R. O., and Graham, S. D., Jr. (1997). Bone fractures associated with luteinizing hormone-releasing hormone agonists used in the treatment of prostate cancer. *Cancer (Philadelphia)* **79**, 545–550.

Travis, W. D., Li, C.-Y., Bergstralh, E. J., Yam, L. T., and Swee, R. G. (1988). Systemic mast cell disease. Analysis of 58 cases and literature review. *Medicine (Baltimore)* **67**, 345–368.

Vanderscheueren, D., Van Herck, E., De Coster, R., and Bouillon, R. (1996). Aromatisation of androgens is important for skeletal maintenance of aged male rats. *Calcif. Tissue Int.* **59**, 179–183.

Veldhuis, J. D., Lizarralde, G., and Iranmanesh, A. (1992). Divergent effects of short-term glucocorticoid excess on the gonadotrophic and somatotrophic axes in normal men. *J. Clin. Endocrinol. Metab.* **74**, 96–102.

Vogel, J. M., Davis, J. W., Nomura, A., Wasnich, R. D., and Ross, P. D. (1997). The effects of smoking on bone mass and the rates of bone loss among elderly Japanese-American men. *J. Bone Miner. Res.* **12**, 1495–1501.

Weide, R., Ehlenz, K., Lorenz, W., Walthers, E., Klausmann, and Pfluger, K.-H. (1996). Successful treatment of osteoporosis in systemic mastocytosis with interferon alpha-2b. *Ann. Hematol.* **72**, 41–43.

Will, R., Palmer, R., Bhalla, A. K., Ring, F., and Calin, A. (1989). Osteoporosis in early ankylosing spondylitis: A primary pathological event? *Lancet* **2**, 1483–1485.

Wolinsky-Friedland, M. (1995). Drug-induced metabolic bone disease. *Endocrinol. Metab. Clin. North Am.* **24**, 395–420.

Zerwekh, J. E., Sakhaee, K., Breslau, N. A., Gottschalk, F., and Pak, C. Y. C. (1992). Impaired bone formation in male idiopathic osteoporosis: Further reduction in the presence of concommitant hypercalciuria. *Osteoporosis Int.* **2**, 128–134.

Chapter 24

Philip D. Ross
Antonio Lombardi
Debra Freedholm
Merck & Co., Inc.
Rahway, New Jersey

The Assessment of Bone Mass in Men

I. Introduction

Although the majority of osteoporotic fractures occur among women, fractures among elderly men are also quite common and will become increasingly frequent as life expectancy increases. In fact, one study estimated that 29% of men and 56% of women will experience fractures during their remaining lifetime, if they are currently 60 years old and receive no preventive measures (Jones *et al.*, 1994). With the advent of nonhormonal therapies for prevention and treatment of osteoporosis, it is now appropriate to use BMD for evaluating fracture risk among men to assist with patient management decisions.

Bone mineral density (BMD) is widely used to identify which female patients should be given therapy for prevention or treatment of osteoporosis and also to monitor the efficacy of treatment. However, many physicians are uncertain about how to interpret BMD in men. This chapter summarizes the

Osteoporosis in Men
Copyright © 1999 by Academic Press. All rights of reproduction in any form reserved.

505

clinical application of BMD measurements, including a review of measurement techniques, comparison of age-related bone loss patterns in men and women, and discussion of the association between low BMD and increased fracture risk.

II. Clinical Interpretation of BMD

Maximum (peak) levels of BMD occur around age 30, or sooner; although this is fairly well-established for women, there are fewer data for men. Elderly men and women have low BMD, and a high risk of fractures. Therefore, it is not very useful to compare current BMD measurements for older people to average BMD values among people of similar age. Instead, the results are often expressed relative to peak BMD, as T scores. The T-score represents the number of standard deviations (SD) above or below the mean for young healthy people; positive numbers represent higher values, and negative numbers represent BMD below the average for young people.

The World Health Organization (WHO) has developed criteria for interpreting BMD which are used widely (Kanis *et al.*, 1994). In this system, patients with BMD that is at least 2.5 SD below the young adult mean (T-score < -2.5) have osteoporosis, and those with BMD between 1 and 2.5 SD below the young adult mean ($-2.5 < T$-score < -1.0) are classified as having low bone mass (or osteopenia). The goal of therapy when treating osteoporosis (patients with T-scores of -2.5 or less) is to increase BMD, or at least maintain current BMD levels. For patients with low bone mass (T-scores between -1.0 and -2.5), the goal is to prevent further declines in BMD, or to at least slow bone loss considerably.

The standardization and interpretation of BMD measurements has been complicated by the variety of skeletal sites that can be measured and by differences in calibration between manufacturers. Nevertheless, as will be shown later, most measurements are able to predict spine and nonspine fracture risk to a similar extent. One exception is hip BMD, which is somewhat better than other measurements for predicting hip fractures. However, hip fractures account for less than 10% of all nonviolent fractures among the elderly, and certain other fracture types, such as wrist and spine, often occur prior to hip fractures. Thus, most measurements are probably suitable for basing treatment decisions. The spine and hip (especially the trochanter) appear to be superior for measuring treatment response; however, the need for such monitoring is still controversial.

Perhaps the best hip BMD reference data for the United States were derived from the third National Health and Nutrition Examination Survey (NHANES III) (Looker *et al.*, 1995). Although the WHO BMD cutoffs for defining osteoporosis and osteopenia based on the female and male reference ranges differ only slightly (Table I), the estimated prevalence of male osteo-

TABLE I   Mean Femoral BMD of 20- to 29-Year-Old Non-Hispanic White Men and Women, and Cutoff Values for Osteopenia and Osteoporosis, Using WHO Definitions

| | | | BMD *cutoffs for* | |
Region	Mean (g/cm²)	Standard deviation (g/cm²)	Osteopenia	Osteoporosis
Men				
Femur neck	0.93	0.137	0.59–0.79	<0.59
Trochanter	0.78	0.118	0.49–0.66	<0.49
Total femur	1.04	0.144	0.68–0.90	<0.68
Women				
Femur neck	0.86	0.120	0.56–0.74	<0.56
Trochanter	0.71	0.099	0.46–0.61	<0.46
Total femur	0.94	0.122	0.64–0.82	<0.64

BMD was measured using Hologic model QDR-1000 machines. Modified from Looker *et al.*, *J. Bone Miner. Res.* 1997; **12**, 1761–1768, with permission of the American Society for Bone and Mineral Research.

penia is twice as high if the male cutoff is used instead of the female cutoff (Looker *et al.*, 1997). However, because the relative distributions of BMD are different in men and women, the number of men with osteoporosis is essentially the same regardless of whether male or female cutoffs are used (Looker *et al.*, 1997). Using the male cutoffs, approximately 3–6% (1–2 million) of U.S. men 50 years and older are estimated to have osteoporosis and 28–47% (8–13 million) to have osteopenia. For comparison, 13–18% (4–6 million) and 37–50% (13–17 million) women ages 50 and older have osteoporosis and osteopenia, respectively (Looker *et al.*, 1997). A European study yielded similar estimates; the prevalence of osteoporosis was 6% in men and 23% for women, ages 50 years and older (Kanis *et al.*, 1994). The greater peak BMD, slower rate of loss, and shorter life expectancy in men probably contribute to the lower prevalence of osteoporosis, relative to women.

III. Techniques for Measuring Bone Mineral Density ⎯⎯⎯⎯⎯

There are numerous technologies for measuring BMD; all are applicable to both men and women (Table II). In addition, quantitative ultrasound (QUS) provides an estimate of bone density and may also provide some information about bone structure or other aspects of bone quality. These methods for measuring bone mass are relatively safe, with low radiation exposures compared to standard x-ray techniques (there is no ionizing radiation for QUS). For example, a typical DXA scan represents less than 0.1% of the annual radiation exposure from natural sources (Rizzoli *et al.*, 1995).

TABLE II Characteristics of Methods for Evaluating Bone Density and Quantitative Ultrasound

Abbreviation	Method	Routine measurement sites	Precision (%)	Examination duration (min)	Cost
SPA	Single-photon (isotope) absorptiometry	Wrist, calcaneus	1–2	10	$25–70
SXA	Single-energy x-ray absorptiometry	Wrist, calcaneus	1–2	10	$25–70
DPA	Dual-photon (isotope) absorptiometry	Spine (A/P)	1–2	20–30	$75–150
		Hip	2–3	20–30	
		Total body	1–2	45	
DXA	Dual-energy x-ray absorptiometry	Spine (A/P)	1–2	5–10	$75–150
		Spine (lateral)	3–4	10–15	
		Hip	2–3	5–10	
		Total body	1–2	10	
QCT	Quantitative computed tomography	Spine	2–5	10–20	$100–300
pQCT	Peripheral quantitative computed tomography	Wrist	1–2	15	$30–80
RA	Radiographic absorptiometry	Phalanges, wrist, metacarpal	1–3	1–10	$20–80
QUS	Quantitative ultrasound	Calcaneus	1–5	1–10	$20–70

Characteristics of these techniques are summarized in Table II and discussed in greater depth later.

Bone mass measured with absorptiometry is usually reported as BMD (g/cm²), which is the measured bone mass in grams divided by the area of the bone region of interest; bone mineral content (BMC) is sometimes reported in units of grams, or as grams per centimeter. The QCT technique provides a measure of true volumetric density (g/cm³), whereas rectilinear techniques do not (because the bone is scanned in only two dimensions). Nevertheless, the term bone density is often used when referring to either grams per cubic centimeter or grams per square centimeter measurements.

Measurements such as the spine, hip, and wrist represent skeletal sites where osteoporotic fractures commonly occur; a variety of other sites can also be measured, depending on the technique and equipment manufacturer. Most measurement sites, but not all, contain a substantial proportion of trabecular bone. The rate of turnover in trabecular bone is usually greater than that in cortical bone; as a result, disturbances in bone balance generally produce larger changes in predominantly trabecular sites.

The procedures to acquire and analyze bone scans are relatively simple. Many densitometers display an image of the bone, and indicate the Region of Interest (ROI) within which the bone mass is measured; a small amount of operator judgment and manual intervention is required. It is very important that the manufacturer's instructions be followed carefully when choosing or changing ROIs. This is especially important when monitoring changes over time, because subtle differences in ROI placement can alter the results by several percent, or more, which is comparable in magnitude to the average BMD changes over 1 to 2 years. It is also important to watch for artifacts which may cause measurement errors and to perform quality control procedures daily to verify proper calibration and watch for measurement drifts. For these reasons, formal training or certification of operators is recommended.

A. Dual-Photon Absorptiometry and Dual-Energy X-Ray Absorptiometry

Dual-energy x-ray absorptiometry (DXA) is considered by some to be the current "gold standard" for measurement of BMD. It replaces an older, similar method, dual-photon absorptiometry (DPA), in which the photon source of the dual-energy beam is gamma radiation from gadolinium (^{153}Gd); DXA thus obviates the expense and difficulty of working with radioactive isotopes (Genant et al., 1993; Glüer et al., 1990). The largest manufacturers worldwide are Hologic (Waltham, Massachusetts, USA) and Lunar (Madison, Wisconsin, USA), with fewer instruments being produced by Norland (Ft. Atkinson, Wisconsin, USA) and Sopha (Buc, France). Although these machines have some different features, they are very similar in their basic principles of operation. To some extent, normal ranges differ between manufacturers (Arai *et al.*, 1990; Pocock *et al.*, 1992). For example, spine BMD measured with Lunar densitometers is approximately 16% higher than that using machines from other manufacturers.

1. Spine BMD

A commonly measured BMD site is the postero-anterior (PA) lumbar spine. Increases in bone density during treatment with antiresorptive agents are generally greatest at the spine. The precision of spine BMD measurements using DXA is excellent, with a coefficient of variation (CV) of approximately 1–2% (Lees and Stevenson, 1992). However, a number of factors including osteoarthrosis, osteosclerosis, and aortic calcification can introduce significant measurement errors causing spine BMD to be overestimated; these sources of interference increase with age and are common after age 65 (Genant *et al.*, 1996; Dawson-Hughes and Dallal, 1990).

Lateral spine BMD measurements have been developed to exclude the posterior spinous elements (which consist predominantly of cortical bone), thereby limiting measurements to the vertebral bodies, which contain a higher component of trabecular bone. The supine position is preferred because of its superior reproducibility compared to the earlier decubitis position (Genant *et al.*, 1996; Mazess *et al.*, 1991). However, lateral spine BMD is limited by overlapping ribs and pelvis in many patients.

2. Hip BMD

Treatment effects are generally smaller at the hip than the spine, possibly because the proportion of cortical bone is higher for the hip. Also, the precision of BMD measurements at the hip (CV of approximately 2%) is not as good as for the spine, which has a CV about 1% (Genant *et al.*, 1996; Wilson *et al.*, 1991). The hip is subdivided into several regions of interest: femoral neck, trochanter, intertrochanteric area, and Ward's triangle. Total hip BMD (combined femoral neck, trochanter, and intertrochanteric areas) is also available on some machines. Ward's triangle is a small (approximately 1 cm^2) subregion located near the base of the femoral neck; the precision of this measurement is not as good as the other hip sites. As noted earlier, the ability to predict fracture risk is similar for most sites, but the trochanter may be better than other hip sites with regard to measuring changes over time.

3. Total Body BMD

Measurement of total body BMD is usually confined to research. As the name indicates, it measures BMD of the entire skeleton. For example, one research application has been to confirm that increases in BMD at a specific site (e.g., spine) during antiresorptive treatment are not simply caused by a redistribution of bone mineral from one region to another within the skeleton but that increases occur throughout the skeleton (Hosking *et al.*, 1998). Total body BMD has better precision (short-term *in vivo* CV of about 0.5–1%) than most other sites (Genant *et al.*, 1996). However, the skeleton consists predominantly (>80%) of cortical bone (Parfitt, 1980). Because of the low rate of bone turnover at cortical sites (approximately 3% per year compared to 20–30% per year in trabecular bone), smaller changes in BMD are typically seen for total body BMD, compared to the spine (Parfitt, 1980).

4. Peripheral BMD

Heel (calcaneus) and distal (wrist) and mid-forearm bone density measurements using SPA and SXA have been used in many studies during the past 20 years. The forearm represents nonweight-bearing bone, in contrast to the heel, spine, and hip. The one-third forearm site is located at one-third the ulnar length, from the wrist, and the mid-forearm is located halfway; both are predominantly cortical bone, whereas ultradistal measurements (at the distal end of the radius) contain a substantial proportion of trabecular bone. Total forearm measurements are also available on some machines, representing a larger region from the wrist to the middle of the forearm. Forearm BMD measurements sometimes include both the radius and ulna, or only the radius. The heel and forearm sites are easily accessible and have little covering soft tissue so that single- (rather than dual-) energy absorptiometry is adequate and provides precise estimates of bone density (Weinstein *et al.*, 1991). Precision (CV) is generally around 1–2%. Response to treatment is often small at peripheral sites, especially in the mid- or one-third radius sites, which are almost completely (>95%) cortical bone (Schlenker and VonSeggen, 1976). The heel is predominantly trabecular bone; as with the spine and hip, large changes are observed during bed rest and disuse.

5. Radiographic Absorptiometry

Radiographic absorptiometry (RA) uses a radiographic film image, usually of the hand or fingers, to measure bone mass by comparing the optical density of the region of interest (bone) to a calibration standard (such as an aluminum wedge), which is included in the exposure field (Yates *et al.*, 1995; Ross, 1997). Some RA methods use existing radiographic facilities to obtain images on film, which are then analyzed on-site using an optical analyzer, or mailed to a central lab. Other methods acquire the bone image digitally, and provide density results within minutes without any film. Typical measurement sites are the phalanges (mixed cortical and trabecular regions), metacarpal (cortical), and radius (cortical). The precision (CV) ranges from good (2%) to excellent (1%).

6. Single-Energy X-Ray Absorptiometry

Like RA, single-energy x-ray absorptiometry (SXA) offers the potential of cheaper and more accessible bone mass measurement relative to DXA. Also, like RA, SXA is limited to peripheral sites, such as the forearm and heel, because it generally requires immersion in water to provide a uniform soft-tissue equivalent. Advantages of machines dedicated to peripheral measurements (either DXA or SXA) are their smaller size and cost, compared to large DXA machines required for measuring spine and hip.

7. Quantitative Computed Tomography

Quantitative computed tomography (QCT) can provide information on vertebral body bone density measurement that is similar to DXA, or it can be used to measure true volumetric (g/cc) trabecular bone density inside the vertebral body (excluding the cortical shell). For example, this technique has been used in research to investigate the relative contributions of trabecular bone versus cortical bone to the overall strength of the vertebral body. Peripheral QCT (pQCT) has also been used to measure trabecular and cortical volumetric (g/cc) bone density at peripheral sites, such as the radius and tibia.

8. Quantitative Ultrasound

Quantitative bone ultrasound measurements correlate with bone density measurements and may also measure aspects of bone quality which are independent of bone density (Faulkner *et al.*, 1994). Heel ultrasound appears to be equivalent to measurements of BMD for predicting the risk of spine and nonspine fractures (Huang *et al.*, 1999; Ross *et al.*, 1995; Gregg *et al.*, 1997). There is very little data on the usefulness of ultrasound for monitoring treatment effects or other changes over time. The precision of most QUS techniques are not as good as the better BMD methods, but recent improvements have put the CV for some QUS machines in the range of 1–2%. As with other peripheral measurements, the small size and low cost are attractive features.

IV. Age-Related Changes in Bone Mass —————————

Both cortical and trabecular bone mass decline with age in men and women. We recognize that (with the exception of QCT) densitometry techniques are not able to measure either cortical or trabecular bone exclusively, but have summarized cortical and trabecular bone separately to the extent possible, because there appear to be some differences related to these two types of bone, such as the rate of change, and response to treatment.

A. Cortical Bone

Men have approximately 7–10% (about 0.5–0.7 *T*-score) (Looker *et al.*, 1995, 1997) higher femoral bone density in early adulthood (ages 20–29) compared to women of the same race (Table I and Figure 1). Some studies have reported that cortical bone mass begins to decline in the third decade of

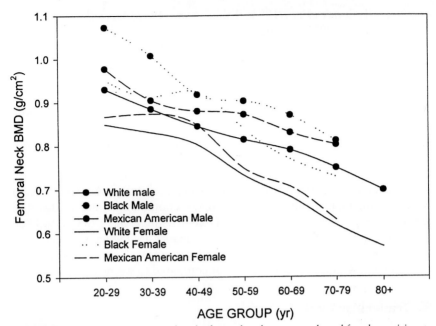

FIGURE 1   Mean BMD measured at the femoral neck among male and female participants in the third U.S. National Health and Nutrition Examination Survey, 1988–1991. Data from Looker *et al.*, 1995, with permission.

life and that this decline continues at a relatively steady rate throughout the remainder of life in both men and women (Looker *et al.*, 1995; Hannan *et al.*, 1992; Steiger *et al.*, 1992; Davis *et al.*, 1991; Gotfredsen *et al.*, 1987). However, most of those studies were cross-sectional, and other studies (including prospective studies) have indicated that bone loss at cortical sites is faster soon after menopause in women and may accelerate after about age 60 or 70 in both men and women (Ensrud *et al.*, 1995; Wishart *et al.*, 1995; Jones *et al.*, 1994; Tobin *et al.*, 1993; Garn *et al.*, 1992; Orwoll *et al.*, 1990; Mazess *et al.*, 1990; Blunt *et al.*, 1994; Orwoll and Klein, 1995; Riggs *et al.*, 1981; Davis *et al.*, 1991).

Compared to women, most studies have reported that the rate of cortical bone loss is slower in men, leading to progressively larger gender differences in cortical bone mass with age (Davis *et al.*, 1991; Blunt *et al.*, 1994; Orwoll and Klein, 1995; Riggs *et al.*, 1981; Kalender *et al.*, 1989). However, other studies (longitudinal and cross-sectional) found little difference between men and women in the pattern of decline in femoral bone density after age 60 (Hannan *et al.*, 1992; Jones *et al.*, 1994). Furthermore, data from more recent, longitudinal studies have consistently shown that the rate of cortical bone loss in men may be considerably more rapid (0.5–1% per year) (Davis et al., 1991; Jones et al., 1994; Tobin et al., 1993; Orwoll et al., 1990; Slemenda et al., 1992) than previously estimated from earlier, cross-sectional studies (0.1–0.3% per year) (Hannan et al., 1992; Mazess et al., 1990; Blunt et al., 1994; Orwoll and Klein, 1995; Riggs et al., 1981; Kalender et al., 1989). Cross-sectional studies may not yield accurate estimates of bone loss rates because peak bone density may have been different for older generations than later generations; thus, the longitudinal data are probably more reliable. Among Caucasians, femoral BMD is approximately 25% lower among men and 33% lower among women at ages 80–85, compared to peak BMD for men and women at ages 20–29, respectively (Figure 1) (Looker et al., 1995).

A number of structural factors influence the ability of long bones to withstand forces, including the length, cross-sectional shape, and the distribution of mineral relative to the applied force (Melton et al., 1988; Mosekilde and Mosekilde, 1990). The combination of smaller declines in bone mass and larger bone size in men may explain to a large extent the lower risk of fractures in men, which is typically half that compared to women of similar age.

B. Trabecular Bone

Spinal trabecular bone density (g/cm^3) measured by QCT is similar for young men and women. Spinal areal BMD (g/cm^2) measured by DXA is greater for men than women, partly because this measure does not fully account for the larger bone size of men, and possibly also because it includes a substantial amount of cortical bone (Orwoll and Klein, 1996; Genant et al., 1994). Vertebral bone density declines with age, possibly beginning as early as the third decade of life, both in men and in women (Orwoll et al., 1990; Riggs et al., 1981; Meier et al., 1984). Trabecular connectivity and the number and thickness of trabecular struts are decreased among older men, similar to postmenopausal women (Aaron et al., 1987; Mosekilde, 1989). These histologic findings, coupled with evidence of increased bone turnover, suggest that the pathophysiologic mechanism underlying age-related osteoporosis in men is similar to that in postmenopausal women (Orwoll and Klein, 1995).

Some cross-sectional studies reported that spine BMD did not decline after age 70 (or after age 50 in one study) among men (Mazess et al., 1990; Blunt et al., 1994). This is most likely an artifact caused in part by selection bias (men with poor health at older ages may not participate) and by overestimation of BMD at older ages related to osteoarthritis and other degenerative changes (Dawson-Hughes and Dallal, 1990). For example, a cross-sectional study of postmenopausal women found that the rates of BMD decreases with age were similar at almost all sites examined (including predominantly cortical sites such as the metacarpal and mid-radius and predominantly trabecular sites such as the calcaneus), with the exception of the spine, which exhibited the smallest difference with age (Ross *et al.*, 1995). Moreover, cross-sectional studies using QCT measurements of the spine, which selectively measure trabecular bone, reported that spinal trabecular bone density declines with age among men (Meier *et al.*, 1984; Cann and Genant, 1982). Progressive declines with age were also demonstrated among men with longitudinal measurements of predominantly trabecular calcaneus BMD; in fact, the rate of decline appeared to increase after age 75 (Davis *et al.*, 1991).

The age-related reduction in vertebral BMD measured by DXA appears to be greater in women than men. This may be partly because DXA measures both cortical and trabecular bone, and cortical bone loss is more rapid in women. One study reported that spine BMD decreased by 14% in men and 47% in women from youth to old age (Riggs *et al.*, 1981). However, as noted earlier, measurement errors and selection bias may have caused these data to underestimate the true declines. When measured by QCT, trabecular bone loss at the spine was similar in men and women (minus 37 and 48%, respectively), corresponding to a yearly rate of 0.72% per year decline for men (Genant *et al.*, 1988). A different study using QCT found even greater lifetime decreases of more than 50%, or 1.2% per year (Meier *et al.*, 1984). Although single-energy QCT may overestimate the reduction in spine BMD (Seeman, 1993), the finding of similar trabecular spinal bone loss in men and women measured by QCT is also consistent with the available histomorphometric data (Mosekilde and Mosekilde, 1990).

As with the spine, the age-related decrease in iliac crest trabecular volume is only marginally greater in women than in men, as measured by histomorphometric data (Aaron *et al.*, 1987; Parfitt *et al.*, 1983) and by QCT measurements (Kalender *et al.*, 1989; Meier *et al.*, 1984). Also, in the Framingham study cohort, the rate of bone loss at the largely trabecular femoral trochanter site was only slightly slower among men, compared to women (−0.45% per year and −0.53% per year, respectively) (Hannan *et al.*, 1992). In contrast, rates of bone loss at the trabecular calcaneus appear to be approximately twice as great among women as men (Davis *et al.*, 1991; Cheng *et al.*, 1997).

In summary, there is a large body of evidence showing that both cortical and trabecular bone loss occurs with age in both men and women. Declines in spinal trabecular bone appear to be similar for both genders, amounting to about 50% over a lifetime. Declines in BMD at cortical sites and the trabecular calcaneus are somewhat less for men than for women, amounting to approximately 25% for men and 33% for women at the femoral neck (Looker *et al.*, 1995). Even so, these figures may underestimate true declines in bone mass among untreated patients if participants in epidemiologic studies tend to be healthier than the general elderly population.

V. Relation between BMD and Fracture Risk _____

Both cross-sectional and prospective studies have demonstrated the importance of BMD for predicting fracture risk in women. Osteoporosis tends to be associated with low bone mass throughout the skeleton, so that bone mass at a given site, such as the hand or the forearm, can provide information concerning the status of the skeleton as a whole. Consequently, BMD at numerous skeletal sites (including spine, hip, forearm, phalanges, and calcaneus) have been demonstrated to predict fracture risk (Marshall et al., 1996; Mussolino et al., 1997; Mussolino, 1998; Ross et al., 1995; Huang et al., 1999). There is less information for men, but the data available are all consistent with those for women; studies in both genders are summarized here.

A. Hip Fracture Risk

Studies of hip fracture in men are mostly cross-sectional and show that, as seen in women, BMD is reduced at the hip, spine, and forearms, compared to age-matched controls (Greenspan et al., 1994a,b; Chevalley et al., 1991; Johnell and Nilsson, 1984). In a prospective study of 2879 white men and 1559 white women aged 45 to 74 who were followed for up to 16 years, the risk of hip fracture increased 1.7 to 1.9 times for each SD decrease in phalangeal BMD measured by RA (Mussolino, 1998; Mussolino et al., 1997). Another prospective study of men reported that the relative risk of hip fractures increased by 3.9 times (95% CI 1.3–11.6) for each 1 SD decrease in forearm BMD (Nyquist et al., 1998). However, it does not appear that this analysis was adjusted for age, which would probably reduce the magnitude of the association.

B. Risk of All Types of Fractures

The Dubbo Osteoporosis Epidemiology Study (DOES) invited all men and women aged 60 years and older living in the Dubbo region of Australia; follow-up was approximately 3 years (38 months). The overall incidence of nonviolent fractures was 1.9% per year in men and 3.3% per year in women. Each 1 SD decrease in femoral neck BMD increased the risk of fractures by 2.0 times (95% CI 1.5–2.6), after adjusting for muscle strength and balance (Nguyen et al., 1993). The 25% of men with the lowest femoral neck BMD (≤ 0.82 g/cm^2) had almost three times greater fracture incidence (3.3% per year) than the 25% of men with the highest BMD (incidence = 1.2% per year) (Nguyen et al., 1993). A later publication from the same study reported a weaker association; the risk increased 1.4 times (95% CI = 1.2–1.6) for each 1 SD decrease in BMD (Nguyen et al., 1996).

In another prospective study, baseline forearm bone mineral content was lower in Scandinavian men who went on to sustain osteoporotic fractures (hip, pelvis, forearm, proximal humerus, vertebra, and tibial condyle) during 11 years of follow-up (Gardsell *et al.*, 1990). The incidence of fractures was approximately six times higher in the 20% of men with the lowest distal forearm BMC, compared to the highest 20% (Gardsell *et al.*, 1990). Another Scandinavian study of men found similar results; each 1 SD decrease in forearm BMD increased the risk of all fractures by 1.8 (95% CI 1.1–2.8) times during 7 years of follow-up (Nyquist *et al.*, 1998). Cheng *et al.* (1997) reported that the incidence of new fractures (at any site) increased progressively with declining levels of baseline calcaneus BMD and that fracture risk is comparable for both men and women at a given level of BMD. The same report demonstrated that decreases in calcaneus BMD during follow-up were associated with increased risk of nonspine fractures among women; a lack of association among men was attributed to the smaller number of fractures.

C. Vertebral Fracture Risk

Cross-sectional studies have shown that men with vertebral fractures have reduced mean levels of bone mass at several skeletal sites, including the spine (Orwoll *et al.*, 1990; Riggs *et al.*, 1981; Resch *et al.*, 1995; Vega *et al.*, 1994; Mann *et al.*, 1992; Odvina *et al.*, 1988; Cann *et al.*, 1985), hip (Vega *et al.*, 1994; Mann *et al.*, 1992; Francis *et al.*, 1989), and total body (Hamdy *et al.*, 1992). For example, the prevalence of vertebral deformities was 6.7 times higher among men with a femoral neck BMD more than 1 SD below the normal mean, compared to those with BMD more than 1 SD above the mean (Mann *et al.*, 1992). The number of vertebral deformities was also negatively correlated with both spine and femoral neck BMD. Other large, population-based, cross-sectional studies have also reported that the prevalence of vertebral deformity is increased when BMD is low at the spine or hip, among men and women ages 50 and older (Lunt *et al.*, 1997; Jones *et al.*, 1996).

A prospective study of BMD and vertebral fracture incidence was conducted in the population-based Hawaii Osteoporosis Study (HOS) (Kim, 1996; Heilbrun *et al.*, 1991). The HOS men (mean age 68 years) were several years older than the women (mean age 63 years) at baseline, and the mean follow-up was 9.6 years for women and 6.4 years for men. New vertebral fractures were defined as vertebral height decreases of more than 15% on serial spine radiographs; 151 of 964 women and 41 of 1008 men experienced new vertebral fractures during follow-up. The rate of new vertebral fractures was approximately three times greater among women than men in each age group (Figure 2). Accordingly, the age-adjusted fracture rate among women was 2.8 (95% CI = 1.9, 4.0) times higher, compared to men.

Bone density (BMD and BMC) was a significant predictor of vertebral fractures in both HOS men and women (Table III). The risk of having a new fracture during follow-up increased by 1.5 to 2.0 times for each successive

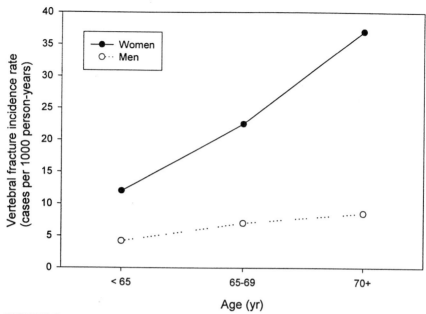

FIGURE 2   Incidence of new vertebral fractures (1981–1994) among men and women in HOS, by age group.

TABLE III   Associations of Baseline Bone Density with New Vertebral Fractures

Gender	Measurement site	Units	Relative risk[a] (95% CI)
Women	Distal radius	BMC (g/cm)	1.66 (1.40, 1.97)
	Distal radius	BMD (g/cm²)	1.58 (1.33, 1.87)
	Proximal radius	BMC (g/cm)	1.63 (1.37, 1.93)
	Proximal radius	BMD (g/cm²)	1.53 (1.31, 1.80)
	Calcaneus	BMD (g/cm²)	1.83 (1.53, 2.19)
	Lumbar spine (L1–4)	BMD (g/cm²)	1.83 (1.39, 2.41)
Men	Distal radius	BMC (g/cm)	1.69 (1.22, 2.35)
	Distal radius	BMD (g/cm²)	1.61 (1.17, 2.20)
	Proximal radius	BMC (g/cm)	1.65 (1.18, 2.31)
	Proximal radius	BMD (g/cm²)	1.51 (1.12, 2.04)
	Calcaneus	BMD (g/cm²)	1.97 (1.43, 2.70)

A separate proportional hazards model was used for each measurement, including age as a covariate.
[a]Relative risk for each BMD decrease of 1 SD. SD values were 0.133 g/cm, 0.065 g/cm², 0.113 g/cm, 0.088 g/cm², 0.065 g/cm², and 0.164 g/cm² for the distal radius (BMD and BMC), proximal radius (BMD and BMC), calcaneus, and spine in women. SD values were 0.188 g/cm, 0.083 g/cm², 0.147 g/cm, 0.083 g/cm², 0.077 g/cm², and 0.164 g/cm² for the distal radius (BMD and BMC), proximal radius (BMD and BMC), and calcaneus in men.
95% CI, 95% confidence interval.

1 SD decrease in baseline BMD for both women and men, depending on the BMD measurement site. When the incidence of new fractures was examined as a function of calcaneus BMD (Figure 3), men and women had equivalent risks of fractures for a given level of BMD. Similar results were observed for the distal and proximal radius BMD measurements.

In contrast to BMD, there were substantial differences in fracture risk between men and women at similar levels of BMC; men had *greater* risk than women for a given level of BMC. This is probably because men have larger bones, and the mineral would be distributed over a larger bone area for men, resulting in weaker bone strength (compared to an equivalent amount of mineral in a smaller bone size for women). Fortunately, the larger bones of men are accompanied by greater amounts of bone mineral than women, on average. Adjusting for body size reduced the differences in fracture risk between men and women for a given level of BMC, yielding results similar to those for BMD. Thus, BMC values do not appear to account for differences in body size between men and women. These data suggest that using BMD allows evaluation of vertebral fracture risk using a single scale for both genders. However, it is not known whether this would also hold true for fracture risk at nonvertebral sites.

The relationship between *changes* in BMD and fracture risk were also examined in the HOS. For these analyses, rates of change in BMD were

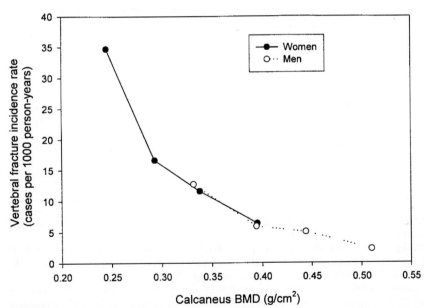

FIGURE 3   Incidence of new vertebral fractures (1981–1994) among men and women in the HOS, by quartiles of baseline calcaneus BMD.

calculated up to the end of follow-up or time of the first fracture (whichever came first). Adjusting for bone loss rate did not measurably alter the associations between BMD and fracture risk shown in Table III. Furthermore, changes in BMC and BMD were significant predictors of new vertebral fractures after adjusting for baseline bone density (Table IV), indicating that initial bone density and bone loss rate both contribute independently to fracture risk. The results indicate that faster declines in bone density are associated with increased risk of subsequent fractures. The magnitude was similar for both men and women, but did not attain statistical significance for men, probably because of the smaller sample size for men. The single exception was spine BMD; increases in spine BMD during follow-up (rather than decreases as observed for other bone density measurements) were associated with higher risk of fractures (spine BMD data were available for women only). As mentioned earlier, the increases in spine BMD probably do not reflect true changes in bone density, but rather the effects of arthritis and other health problems.

Prevalent (preexisting) vertebral fractures are an important predictor of future vertebral fractures, independent of BMD (Ross *et al.,* 1991). The prevalence of vertebral fractures (defined as vertebrae with height dimensions more than 3 SD below the normal range) increased with age in both

TABLE IV   Associations of Changes in Bone Density with New Vertebral Fractures

Gender	Measurement site	Units	Relative risk[a] (95% CI)
Women	Distal radius	BMC (g/cm)	1.40 (1.15, 1.71
	Distal radius	BMD (g/cm²)	0.94 (0.78, 1.14)
	Proximal radius	BMC (g/cm)	1.19 (1.05, 1.36)
	Proximal radius	BMD (g/cm²)	1.23 (1.04, 1.46)
	Calcaneus	BMD (g/cm²)	1.44 (1.22, 1.71)
	Lumbar spine (l1–4)	BMD (g/cm²)	0.62 (0.53, 0.73)
Men	Distal radius	BMC (g/cm)	1.13 (0.79, 1.60)
	Distal radius	BMD (g/cm²)	1.45 (1.04, 2.04)
	Proximal radius	BMC (g/cm)	1.13 (0.91, 1.41)
	Proximal radius	BMD (g/cm²)	1.18 (0.84, 1.66)
	Calcaneus	BMD (g/cm²)	1.18 (0.84, 1.65)

Analyses were adjusted for age and baseline bone density.
A separate proportional hazards model was used for each measurement, including age and baseline bone density as covariates.
[a]Relative risk for each SD of change in bone density. SD values were 0.0102 g/cm/yr, 0.0057 g/cm²/yr, 0.0090 g/cm/yr, 0.0073 g/gm²/yr, 0.00360 g/cm²/yr, and 0.0301 g/cm²/yr for the distal radius (BMD and BMC), proximal radius (BMD and BMC), calcaneus, and spine in women. SD values were 0.0122 g/cm/yr, 0.0059 g/cm²/yr, 0.0110 g/cm/yr, 0.0079 g/cm²/yr, and 0.00389 g/cm²/yr for the distal radius (BMD and BMC), proximal radius (BMD and BMC), and calcaneus in men.
95% CI, 95% confidence interval.

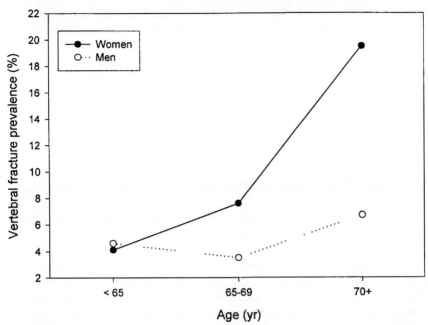

FIGURE 4   Prevalence of vertebral fractures at baseline among men and women in the Hawaii Osteoporosis Study, by age group.

men and women, but the increases with age were greater among women (Figure 4). The risk of new vertebral fractures increased progressively with the number of prevalent fractures existing at baseline, for both men and women in the HOS (Table V). The magnitude was somewhat stronger for women than men, but the confidence intervals overlap. The smaller magnitude for men may be a statistical artifact related to the smaller number of

TABLE V   Associations of Preexisting Vertebral Fractures[a] with New Vertebral Fractures

Gender	Age-adjusted relative risk	Age- and BMD-adjusted relative risk
Women	3.27 (2.42, 4.44)	2.42 (1.76, 3.32)
Men	2.39 (1.06, 5.40)	2.18 (0.94, 5.02)

[a]Categorized as no fractures, one fracture, and two or more fractures at baseline. Relative risks indicate the increase in fracture risk for each increment in baseline fracture status (i.e., comparing the risk of new vertebral fractures during follow-up for women with one fracture to those with no fractures, or comparing women with two or more fractures to those with one fracture at baseline). All analyses were adjusted for age.

fracture cases, or it may be a real effect if some of the fractures existing at baseline were caused by violent forces in the past (such as occupational injuries), and therefore do not represent true osteoporotic fractures. The higher vertebral fracture prevalence prior to age 65 among men than women in the HOS (Figure 4) has also been reported by others, and suggests that vertebral fractures among men at younger ages are related to violent causes. Adjusting for BMD did not meaningfully alter the magnitudes of associations for prevalent fractures (Table 5), indicating that BMD and prevalent fractures provide complementary information about fracture risk.

VI. Future Research Directions

Additional research is warranted to determine the extent to which reference ranges for men may differ between geographic localities and ethnic groups, as have been reported for women (Looker *et al.*, 1995; Dequeker *et al.*, 1995; Flicker *et al.*, 1995). Further research is also needed to evaluate the usefulness of BMD measurements for monitoring individual responses to therapy, because few data are available in this regard for men. Nevertheless, BMD can accurately be measured in men, and low BMD levels are associated with increased fracture risk. It follows that identifying men with low BMD, and prevention of declines in BMD are important goals in the prevention of osteoporotic fractures among men.

References

Aaron, J. E., Makins, N. B., and Sagreiy, K. (1987). The microanatomy of trabecular bone loss in normal aging men and women. *Clin. Orthop. Relat. Res.* 215, 260–271.

Arai, H., Ito, K., Nagao, K., and Furutachi, M. (1990). The evaluation of three different bone densitometry systems: XR-26, QDR-1000, and DPX. *Image Technol. Inf. Display* 22(18), 1–6.

Blunt, B. A., *et al.* (1994). Sex differences in bone mineral density in 1653 men and women in the sixth through tenth decades of life: The Rancho Bernardo Study. *J. Bone Miner. Res.* 9, 1333–1337.

Cann, C. E., and Genant, H. K. (1982). Cross-sectional studies of vertebral mineral using quantitative computed tomography. *J. Comput. Assist. Tomogr.* 6, 216–217.

Cann, C. E. *et al.* (1985). Quantitative computed tomography for prediction of vertebral fracture risk. *Bone* 6, 1–7.

Cheng, S., Suominen, H., *et al.* (1997). Calcaneal bone mineral density predicts fracture occurrence: A five-year follow-up study in elderly people. *J. Bone Miner. Res.* 12, 1075–1082.

Chevalley, T., *et al.* (1991). Preferential low bone mineral density of the femoral neck in patients with a recent fracture of the proximal femur. *Osteoporosis Int.* 1, 147–154.

Davis, J. W. *et al.* (1991). Age-related changes in bone mass among Japanese-American men. *Bone Miner.* 15, 227–236.

Dawson-Hughes, B., and Dallal, G. E. (1990). Effect of radiographic abnormalities on rate of bone loss from the spine. *Calcif. Tissue Int.* 46, 280–281.

Dequeker, J., *et al.* (1995). Dual x-ray absorptiometry—cross-calibration and normative reference ranges for the spine: Results of a European community concerted action. *Bone* 17, 247–254.

Ensrud, K. E., Palermo, L., Black, D. M., Cauley, J. A., Jergas, M., Orwoll, E. S., Nevitt, M. C., Fox, K. M., and Cummings, S. R. (1995). Hip and calcaneal bone loss increase with advancing age: Longitudinal results from the study of osteoporotic fractures. *J. Bone Miner. Res.* **10**, 1778–1787.

Faulkner, K. G., McClung, M. R., Coleman, L. J., *et al.* (1994). Quantitative ultrasound of the heel: Correlation with densitometric measurements at different skeletal sites. *Osteoporosis Int.* **4**, 42–47.

Flicker, L., *et al.* (1995). Do Australian women have greater spinal bone density than North American women? *Osteoporosis Int.* **5**, 63–65.

Francis, R. M., Peacock, M., Marshall, D. H., Horsman, A., and Aaron, J. E. (1989). Spinal osteoporosis in men. *Bone Miner.* **5**, 347–357.

Gardsell, P., Johnell, O., and Nilsson, B. E. (1990). The predictive value of forearm bone mineral content measurements in men. *Bone* **11**, 229–232.

Garn, S. M., Sullivan, T. V., Decker, S. A., Larkin, F. A., and Hawthorne, V. M. (1992). Continuing bone expansion and increasing bone loss over a two-decade period in men and women from a total community sample. *Am. J. Hum. Biol.* **4**, 57–67.

Genant, H. K., Faulkner, K. G., Glüer, C. C., and Engelke, K. (1993). Bone densitometry: Current assessment. *Osteoporosis Int., Suppl.* **1**, S91–S97.

Genant, H. K., Glüer, C. C., and Lotz, J. C. (1994). Gender differences in bone density, skeletal geometry, and fracture biomechanics. *Radiology* **190**, 636–640.

Genant, H. K., *et al.* (1988). Quantitative computed tomography in assessment of osteoporosis. *In* "Osteoporosis: Etiology, Diagnosis and Management" (B. L. Riggs and L. J. Melton, III, eds.), pp. 221–250. Raven Press, New York.

Genant, H. K., Engelke, K., Fuerst, T., Gluer, C. C., Grampp, S., harris, S. T., Jergas, M., Lang, T., Lu, Y., Majumdar, S., Mathur, A., and Takada, M. (1996). Noninvasive assessment of bone mineral and structure: State of the art. *J. Bone Miner. Res.* **11**, 707–730.

Glüer, C. C., Steiger, P., Selvidge, R., *et al.* (1990). Comparative assessment of dual-photon absorptiometry and dual-energy radiography. *Radiology* **174**(1), 223–228.

Gotfredson, A., *et al.* (1987). Total body mineral in healthy adults. *J. Lab. Clin. Med.* **110**, 362–368.

Greenspan, S. L., *et al.* (1994a). Trochanteric bone mineral density is associated with type of hip fracture in elderly. *J. Bone Miner. Res.* **9**, 1889–1894.

Greenspan, S. L. *et al.* (1994b). Fall severity and bone mineral density as risk factors for hip fracture in ambulatory elderly. *JAMA, J. Am. Med. Assoc.* **271**, 128–133.

Gregg, E. W., *et al.* (1997). The epidemiology of quantitative ultrasound: A review of the relationships with bone mass, osteoporosis, and fracture risk. *Osteoporosis Int.* **7**, 89–99.

Hamdy, R. C., *et al.* (1992). Osteoporosis in men: Prevalence, biochemical parameters. *J. Bone Miner. Res.,* Suppl 1.

Hannan, M. T., Felson, D. T., and Anderson, J. J. (1992). Bone mineral density in elderly men and women: Results from the Framingham Osteoporosis Study. *J. Bone Miner. Res.* **7**, 547–553.

Heilbrun, L. K., Ross, P. D., Wasnich, R. D., *et al.* (1991). Characteristics of respondents and nonrespondents in a prospective study of osteoporosis. *J. Clin. Epidemiol.* **44**(3), 233–239.

Hosking, D., Chilvers, C. E. D., Christiansen, C., *et al.* (1998). Prevention of bone loss with alendronate in postmenopausal women under 60 years of age. *N. Engl. J. Med.* **338**(8), 485–492.

Huang, C., Ross, P. D., Yates, A. J., and Wasnich, R. D. (1999). Prediction of fracture risk by radiographic absorptiometry and quantitative ultrasound: A prospective study. In press.

Johnell, O., and Nilsson, B. (1984). Bone mineral content in men with fractures of the upper end of the femur. *Int. Orthop.* **7**, 229–231.

Jones, G., Nguyen, T. V., Sambrook, P. N., Kelly, P. J., and Bisman, J. A. (1994). Progressive femoral neck bone loss in the elderly: Longitudinal findings from the Dubbo Osteoporosis Epidemiology Study. *Br. Med. J.* **309**, 691–695.

Jones, G., White, C., Nguyen, T., Sambrook, P. N., Kelly, P. J., and Eisman, J. A. (1996). Prevalent vertebral deformities: Relationship to bone mineral density and spinal osteophytosis in elderly men and women. *Osteoporosis Int.* **6**, 233–239.

Kalender, W. A., Felsenberg, D., Louis, O., Lopez, O., Lopez, P., Klotz, E., Osteaux, M., and Fraga, J. (1989). Reference values for trabecular and cortical vertebral bone density in single and dual-energy quantitative computed tomography. *Eur. J. Radiol.* **9**, 75–80.

Kanis, J. L., *et al.* (1994). The diagnosis of osteoporosis. *J. Bone Miner. Res.* **9**, 1137–1141.

Kim, S. (1996). Prediction of incident vertebral fractures among Japanese-American men and women. Doctoral Thesis, University of Hawaii, Honolulu.

Lees, B., and Stevenson, J. C. (1992). An evaluation of dual-energy x-ray absorptiometry and comparison with dual-photon absorptiometry. *Osteoporosis Int.* **2**, 146–152.

Looker, A. C., Wahner, H. W., Dunn, W. L., Calvo, M. S., Harris, T. B., Heyse, S. P., Johnston, C. C., J., and Lindsay, R. L. (1995). Proximal femur bone mineral levels of U.S. adults. *Osteoporosis Int.* **5**, 389–409.

Looker, A. C., Orwoll, E. S., Johnston, C. C., Lindsay, R. L., Wahner, H. W., Dunn, W. L., Calvo, M. S., Harris, T. B., and Heyse, S. P. (1997). Prevalence of low femoral bone density in older U.S. adults from NHANES III. *J. Bone Miner. Res.* **12**, 1761–1768.

Lunt, M., Felsenberg, D., Reeve, J., Benevolenskaya, L., Cannata, J., Dequeker, J., Dodenhof, C., Falch, J. A., Masaryk, P., Pols, H. A. P., Poor, G., Reid, D. M., Soheidt-Nave, C., Weber, K., Verlow, J., Kanis, J. A., O'Neill, T. W., and Silman, A. J. (1997). Bone density variations and its effects on risk of vertebral deformity in men and women studied in thirteen European centers: The EVOS Study. *J. Bone Miner. Res.* **12**, 1883–1894.

Mann, T., Oviatt, S. K., Wilson, D., Nelson, D., and Orwoll, E. S. (1992). Vertebral deformity in men. *J. Bone Miner. Res.* **7**, 1259–1265.

Marshall, D., Johnell, O., and Wedel, H. (1996). Meta-analysis of how well measures of bone mineral density predict occurrence of osteoporotic fractures. *Br. Med. J.* **312**, 1254–1259.

Mazess, R. B. *et al.* (1990). Influence of age and body weight on spine and femur bone mineral density in U.S. white men. *J. Bone Miner. Res.* **5**, 645–652.

Mazess, R. B., Gifford, C. A., Bisek, J. P., *et al.* (1991). DEXA measurement of spine density in the lateral projection. I: Methodology. *Calcif. Tissue Int.* **49**, 235–239.

Meier, D. E., *et al.* (1984). Marked disparity between trabecular and cortical bone loss with age in healthy men: Measurement by vertebral computed tomography and radial photon absorptiometry. *Ann. Intern. Med.* **101**, 605–612.

Melton, L. J., III, Chao, E. Y. S., and Lane, J. (1988). Biomechanical aspects of fractures. *In* "Osteoporosis: Etiology, Diagnosis, and Management" (B. L. Riggs and L. J. Melton, III, eds.), pp. 111–131. Raven Press, New York.

Mosekilde, Li. (1989). Sex differences in age-related loss of vertebral trabecular bone mass and structure—biomechanical consequences. *Bone* **10**, 425–432.

Mosekilde, Li., and Mosekilde, Le. (1990). Sex differences in age-related changes in vertebral body size, density, and biomechanical competence in normal individuals. *Bone* **11**, 67–73.

Mussolino, M. E. (1998). Risk factors for hip fracture in white men: The NHANES I Epidemiologic Follow-Up Study. *J. Bone Miner. Res.* **13**, 918–924.

Mussolino, M. E., Looker, A. C., Madans, J. H., *et al.* (1997). Phalangeal bone density and hip fracture risk. *Arch. Intern. Med.* **157**, 433–438.

Nguyen, T., Sambrook, P., Kelly, P., Jones, G., Lord, S., Freund, J., and Bisman, J. (1993). Prediction of osteoporotic fractures by postural instability and bone density. *Br. Med. J.* **307**, 1111–1115.

Nguyen, T. V., Eisman, J. A., Kelly, P. A.,and Sambrook, P. N. (1996). Risk factors for osteoporotic fractures in men. *Am. J. Epidemiol.* **144**, 255–263.

Nyquist, F., Gardsell, P., Sernbo, I., Jeppsson, J. O., and Johnell, O. (1998). Assessment of sex hormones and bone mineral density in relation to occurrence of fracture in men: A prospective population-based study. *Bone* **22**, 147–151.

Odvina, C. V. *et al.* (1988). Relationship between trabecular vertebral bone density and fractures. *Metab., Clin. Exp.* **37**, 221–228.

Orwoll, E. S., and Klein, R. F. (1995). Osteoporosis in men. *Endocr. Rev.* 16, 87–116.

Orwoll, E., and Klein, R. F. (1996). Osteoporosis in men: Epidemiology, pathophysiology, and clinical characterization. *In* "Osteoporosis" (R. Marcus, D. Feldman, and J. Kelsey, eds.), pp. 745–784. Academic Press, San Diego, CA.

Orwoll, E. S., Oviatt, S. K., McClung, M. R., Deftos, L. J., and Sexton, G. (1990). The rate of bone mineral loss in normal men and the effects of calcium and cholecalciferol supplementation. *Ann. Intern. Med.* 112, 29–34.

Parfitt, A. M. (1980). Morphologic basis of bone mineral measurements: Transient and steady state effects of treatment in osteoporosis. *Miner. Electrolyte Metab.* 4, 273–287.

Parfitt, A. M., Mathews, H. E., Villanueva, A. R., Kleerekoper, M., Frame, B., and Rao, D. S. (1983). Relationships between surface, volume, and thickness of iliac trabecular bone in aging and in osteoporosis. *J. Clin. Invest.* 72, 1396–1409.

Pocock, N. A., Sambrook, P. N., Nguyen, T., Kelly, P. J., Freund, J., and Eisman, J. A. (1992). Assessment of spinal and femoral bone density by dual x-ray absorptiometry: Comparison of lunar and Hologic instruments. *J. Bone Miner. Res.* 7(9), 1081–1084.

Resch, A., Schneider, B., Bernecker, P. *et al.* (1995). Risk of vertebral fractures in men: Relationship to mineral density of the vertebral body. *Am. J. Roentgenol.* 164, 1447–1450.

Riggs, B. L., Wahner, H. W., Dunn, W. L., Mazess, R. B., Offord, K. P., and Melton, L. J., III (1981). Differential changes in bone mineral density of the appendicular and axial skeleton with aging. *J. Clin. Invest.* 67, 328–335.

Rizzoli, R., Slosman, D., and Bonjour, J.-P. (1995). The role of dual-energy x-ray absorptiometry of lumbar spine and proximal femur in the diagnosis and follow-up of osteoporosis. *Am. J. Med.* 98(Suppl. 2A), 33S–36S.

Ross, P. D. (1997). Radiographic absorptiometry for measuring bone mass. *Osteoporosis Int.* 7(Suppl. 3), 103–108.

Ross, P. D., Davis, J. W., Epstein, R., and Wasnich, R. D. (1991). Pre-existing fractures and bone mass predict vertebral fracture incidence. *Ann. Intern. Med.* 114, 919–923.

Ross, P., Huang, C., Davis, J., *et al.* (1995). Predicting vertebral deformity using bone densitometry at various skeletal sites and calcaneus ultrasound. *Bone* 16, 325–332.

Schlenker, R. A., and VonSeggen, W. W. (1976). The distribution of cortical and trabecular bone mass along the lengths of the radius and ulna and the implications for in vivo bone mass measurements. *Calcif. Tissue Res.* 20, 41–52.

Seeman, E. (1993). Osteoporosis in men: Epidemiology, pathophysiology, and treatment possibilities. *Am. J. Med.* 95 (Suppl. 5A), 22S–28S.

Slemenda, C. W., Christian, J. C., Reed, T., Reister, T. K., Williams, C. J., and Johnston, C. C., Jr. (1992). Long-term bone loss in men: Effects of genetic and environmental factors. *Ann. Intern. Med.* 117, 286–291.

Steiger, P., *et al.* (1992). Age-related decrements in bone mineral density in women over age 65. *J. Bone Miner. Res.* 7, 625–631.

Tobin, J. D., *et al.* (1993). Bone density changes in normal men: A 4–19 year longitudinal study. *J. Bone Miner. Res.* 8, 102.

Vega, E., Ghiringhelli, G., Mautalen, C., Rey-Valzacchi, G., Scaglia, H., and Zylberstein, C. (1998). Bone mineral density and bone size in men with primary osteoporosis and vertebral fractures. *Calcif. Tissue Int.* 62, 465–469.

Weinstein, R. S., New, K. D., and Sappington, L. J. (1991). Dual-energy x-ray absorptiometry versus single photon absorptiometry of the radius. *Calcif. Tissue Int.* 49, 313–316.

Wilson, C. R., Fogelman, I., Blake, G. M., and Rodin, A. (1991). The effect of positioning on dual energy x-ray bone densitometry of the proximal femur. *J. Bone Miner. Res.* 13, 69–76.

Wishart, J. M., Need, A. G., Horowitz, M., Morris, H. A., and Nordin, B. E. C. (1995). Effect of age on bone density and bone turnover in men. *Clin. Endocrinol. (Oxford)* 42, 141–146.

Yates, A. J., Ross, P. D., Lydick, E., and Epstein, R. S. (1995). Radiographic absorptiometry in the diagnosis of osteoporosis. *Am. J. Med.* 98(2A), 41S–417.

Chapter 25

Eric S. Orwoll

Bone and Mineral Unit
Oregon Health Sciences University
and the Portland VA Medical Center
Portland, Oregon

The Clinical Evaluation of Osteoporosis in Men

I. Introduction

The most appropriate approach for the evaluation of osteoporosis in men has not been systematically developed or tested (a situation that still exists with respect to women as well). Previous recommendations have been reasonable (Jackson and Kleerekoper, 1990; Orwoll and Klein, 1995), but until recently there has been little information upon which to firmly base clinical algorithms. Fortunately, the fund of knowledge about osteoporosis in men has recently expanded, and those recommendations can be revised with somewhat more confidence. Nevertheless, until these clinical approaches are subject to rigorous evaluation, they must remain founded primarily in judgment and experience.

The critical issues to be considered in devising diagnostic algorithms include several key epidemiological characteristics and clinical manifesta-

Osteoporosis in Men
527

tions of the disorder, and the utility of available testing procedures in predicting disease impact and response to therapy.

II. Characteristics of Men at Risk _____

A. Age

The incidence of all fractures is higher in men than women early in life (Garraway *et al.*, 1979; Donaldson *et al.*, 1990). It has long been assumed that this gender difference is the result of serious trauma. In fact, there are some data that strongly suggest that some early life fractures are the result of impaired skeletal fragility, and the belief that fracture in younger men is a function of trauma has probably impeded the investigation of the true prevalence of bone fragility in young and middle-aged men. For instance, middle-aged men who suffer radial or tibial fractures appear to be at considerably higher risk of subsequent hip and other classic osteoporotic fractures (Owen *et al.*, 1982; M. Karlsson *et al.*, 1993; Mallmin *et al.*, 1993). In a large Norwegian population, it was noted that fractures in the non-weight-bearing skeleton were actually less common in more active individuals (those in whom the risk of trauma might be higher), perhaps because of the effects of activity on skeletal strength (Joakimsen *et al.*, 1998). Although high activity was found to be associated with vertebral deformity in the European Vertebral Osteoporosis Study (EVOS) population, bone mineral density was also lower in those with fractures (Lunt *et al.*, 1997). All this suggests that young adult men who sustain fractures should be the subject of clinical suspicion for bone fragility. The causes of fragility may be quite heterogeneous and could include low bone density, small bone size or vulnerable shape (e.g., long hip axis length), heritable disorders of bone metabolism, and so on. For examples, military recruits who sustain stress fractures have smaller bone size and are presumably less able to withstand the rigors of strenuous training (Beck *et al.*, 1996).

At about age 50 years, fractures in general (but in particular those of the pelvis, humerus, forearm, and femur) become much more common in women. Nevertheless, the incidence of fractures (particularly hip and spine) also increases rapidly with aging in men (Donaldson *et al.*, 1990) (Fig. 1), reflecting an increasing prevalence of skeletal fragility. In older men many fractures cannot be attributed to trauma and are probably osteoporotic. Recently, the Dubbo Osteoporosis Epidemiology Project (Nguyen *et al.*, 1996) raised the possibility that low trauma fracture rates in older men may be greater than previously recognized. Data from that study suggest that the lifetime risk of an atraumatic fracture is about 25% in an average 60-year-old man. In older men, the prevalence of low bone mass is high (Looker *et al.*, 1997), and those with fractures are more commonly osteopenic and have

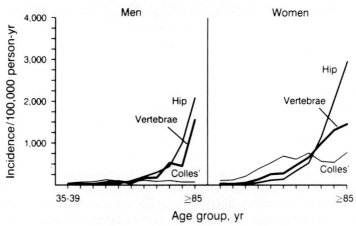

FIGURE I   Age-specific incidence rates of hip, vertebral, and Colle's fracture in Rochester, Minnesota, men and women. From Cooper and Melton (1992), with permission.

conditions associated with falling (Nguyen *et al.,* 1992; Mussolino *et al.,* 1998). Thus, fracture in men over the age of 50 years should clearly prompt the concern that low bone mass and/or other factors related to fracture risk (e.g., falls) may be present and should stimulate an appropriate evaluation. In addition, the prevalence of low bone mineral density in older men, the relationship of bone density to fracture, the high incidence of fracture, and the important personal and societal impact of fracture all suggest that screening for low bone mass in appropriate populations of men may be useful.

B. Ethnicity

Racial differences in the incidence of hip fracture in men are substantial. For instance, African-American men experience hip fractures at a rate much less than that of Caucasians (Jacobsen *et al.,* 1990). There are not extensive comparative data concerning other races, but one study clearly suggests a lower rate of hip fracture in Japanese compared to Caucasian men from the United States (Ross *et al.,* 1991). In a review of fractures attributable to osteoporosis, Melton *et al.* (1997) concluded that, in men, Caucasians have a considerably higher risk of hip fracture than do other ethnicities.

C. Falls

In addition to bone mass, the risk of falling is a major determinant of fracture in women. In men, there are few prospective data that directly relate fall propensity to subsequent fractures, but a variety of factors indirectly related to risk of falling are associated with fracture. For instance, Nguyen *et al.* (1993) found that men who had experienced a nontraumatic fracture exhibit more body sway and lower grip strength (as well as lower bone density) than nonfracture controls. Similarly, in a retrospective study of men with hip fractures (Grisso *et al.*, 1991), a number of factors associated with falls were found to be more prevalent than in controls. These included neurological disease, confusion, "ambulatory problems," and alcohol use. As in women, the use of several classes of psychotropic drugs is associated with hip fracture risk (Ray *et al.*, 1987, 1989). Finally, men with hip fracture are of lower weight, have lower fat and lean body mass, and more commonly live alone than control subjects (M. K. Karlsson *et al.*, 1993). These differences suggest a body habitus and lifestyle more conducive to falls and injury, as well as the possibility that there are other interacting risk factors (nutritional deficiencies, comorbidities), impressions that were recently substantiated in an epidemiological study of the factors associated with hip fracture in men (Poor *et al.*, 1995a) (Table I). An assessment of the propensity to fall should be an integral part of the evaluation of osteoporosis risk in men.

D. Medical Conditions

There is strong evidence that fractures in men are much more common in those with conditions that predispose to abnormalities in bone biology or fall propensity (Poor *et al.*, 1995a; Burger *et al.*, 1998; Mussolino *et al.*, 1998; Tromp *et al.*, 1998). Moreover, the risk of death, which is greater in men than in women following a hip fracture, seems to be related to the presence of comorbid conditions (Poor *et al.*, 1995b). From a clinical perspective, the appreciation of fracture risk in patients with these conditions is vital and should prompt a more aggressive approach to osteoporosis evaluation.

E. Previous Fractures

The risk of fracture is considerably higher in women who have already experienced fracture, and the same relationship is present in men (M. Karlsson *et al.*, 1993; Mallmin *et al.*, 1993; Silman, 1995; Fujiwara *et al.*, 1997; Mussolino *et al.*, 1998; Tromp *et al.*, 1998). A wide variety of fractures (Eastell and Riggs, 1980; Lane and Vigorita, 1984) are associated with low bone mass in women (Seeley *et al.*, 1991). In men there are fewer data, but the reports that have examined the relationships between bone mass, bone structure, mechanical strength, and fracture in men suggest similar associations (Mosekilde, 1989; Gardsell *et al.*, 1990). Even incidentally discovered vertebral deformities have been associated with low bone mass (Mann *et al.*, 1992) and should raise the suspicion of metabolic bone disease. Thus, the history of a previous fracture, particularly in older men or with little trauma, should prompt further evaluation.

TABLE I   Some Factors Associated with Hip Fractures in Men

Metabolic disorders	Thyroidectomy
	Gastrectomy
	Pernicious anemia
	Chronic respiratory diseases
Disorders of movement and balance	Hemiparesis/hemiplegia
	Parkinsonism dementia
	Other neurological diseases
	Vertigo
	Alcoholism
	Anemia
	Blindness
	Use of cane or walker

F. Genetics

A major part of the determination of adult bone mass is under genetic control. The nature of the relationship is not well established in either sex, and the primary evidence comes from studies of bone mass and fracture prevalence in related individuals. Longitudinal twin studies document a substantial heritability of bone mass in men (Christian *et al.*, 1989; Slemenda *et al.*, 1992). Men who have osteoporotic parents have bone mineral density levels less than control subjects (Evans *et al.*, 1988; Soroko *et al.*, 1994), and in the European Vertebral Osteoporosis Study (EVOS) maternal history of hip fracture increased the risk of vertebral fracture in men (odds ratio 1.3, 95% confidence intervals 1.00–1.8) (Diaz *et al.*, 1997). Similarly, the siblings and offspring of osteoporotic men have reduced bone density (Cohen-Solal *et al.*, 1998). Although not extensively examined, some data indicate that there is not a significant effect of gender on the heritability of bone mass, suggesting that the effect (whatever genes it may be due to) is equally strong in men and women (Smith *et al.*, 1973; Krall and Dawson-Hughes, 1993; Gueguen *et al.*, 1995). The relationship of family history to fracture risk has not been established in prospective trials, and verification of the importance of family history in the determination of fracture risk in men should await those results.

There has also been no specific gene(s) convincingly associated with bone mass or fracture in men, and so the mechanism by which family history influences bone mass or fracture risk in men is unknown. Several genes have been suggested to be of importance, including the vitamin D receptor (Morrison *et al.*, 1994; Spolita *et al.*, 1996), as of yet unknown genes on chromosome 11 (Johnson *et al.*, 1997), and type I collagen (Spolita *et al.*, 1996; Langdahl *et al.*, 1998), but not all these results are reproducible (Uitterlinden *et al.*, 1996). Despite the absence of distinct genes associated with disease (and of molecular diagnostic methods), the presence of a positive family history indicates higher risk and the need for a more vigilant approach.

III. The Clinical Approach to Osteoporosis in Men

Guidelines for the most efficient, cost-effective approach for the evaluation of the patient with osteoporosis, or the patient suspected of having osteoporosis, are poorly validated for either sex. Recommendations are therefore based on existing knowledge of disease epidemiology and clinical characteristics (discussed earlier) (Eastell and Riggs, 1980; Lane and Vigorita, 1984) rather than upon models that have been carefully tested in prospective studies. Within these constraints, it is possible to formulate an approach to the male osteoporotic (Fig. 2).

There are several clinical situations in which the presence of osteoporosis should be considered likely. These include the occurrence of fractures with little trauma, the radiographic finding of low bone mass or vertebral deformity, and the presence of conditions known to be associated with osteoporosis. In these circumstances further diagnostic steps are appropriate.

- Men with fractures. The diagnosis of osteopenic metabolic bone disease should be strongly suspected in men with a history of low trauma fractures in the absence of any evidence of a focal process (e.g., malignancy, infection, Paget's disease). The presence of significant trauma should lessen but not eliminate concern, especially in men over 50 years.
- Radiographic evidence of reduced bone mass. Radiographic signs of reduced bone mass, even in the absence of a fracture, is of concern and should be verified by a quantitative assessment of bone mass.
- Clinical conditions associated with osteoporosis. There is a spectrum of secondary causes of osteoporosis in men, including glucocorticoid excess, alcoholism, and hypogonadism (Garraway et al., 1979; M. K. Karlsson et al., 1993) (Table II).

The presence of one, or particularly several, of these conditions should prompt the consideration for a diagnostic evaluation. Specifically, a careful history and physical exam should be performed with the goal of uncovering conditions that may predispose the patient to fractures. A measure of bone mass should be obtained.

A. The Use of Bone Mass Measurements

In men who present with findings that suggest the presence of metabolic bone disease (low trauma fractures, radiographic criteria indicating the pres-

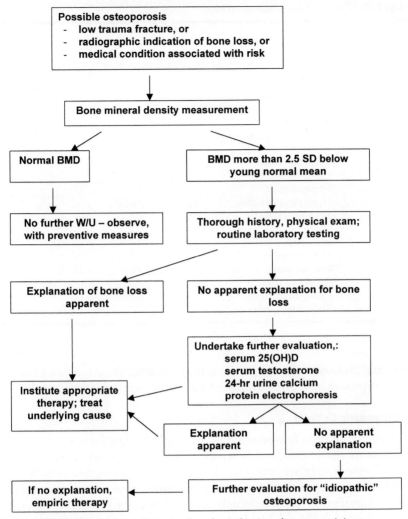

FIGURE 2   Schematic approach to the evaluation of osteoporosis in men.

ence of a reduction in bone mass, or conditions associated with bone loss), the measurement of bone mass should be strongly considered. Bone mass determinations in men can be useful in several ways, including cementing the diagnosis of osteoporosis (or other demineralizing conditions), gauging severity, and serving as a baseline from which to judge progression/improvement of the disease. Although this contention is derived from studies in women, its basic underpinnings should be applicable in men as well. Specifically, (1) bone mass is related to fracture risk (2) bone mass can be accurately and conveniently

TABLE II Causes of Osteoporosis in Men

I. Primary	Aging
	Idiopathic
	Genetic—connective tissue disorders, homocystinuria, hypophosphatasia, others
II. Secondary	Hypogonadism
	Glucocorticoid excess
	Alcoholism
	Gastrointestinal disorders/malabsorption
	Hepatic insufficiency
	Renal insufficiency
	Cystic fibrosis
	Hypercalciuria
	Hyperparathyroidism
	Anticonvulsants
	Thyrotoxicosis
	Immobilization
	Hemochromatosis
	Systemic mastocytosis
	Neoplastic diseases
	Eating disturbance
	Rheumatoid arthritis

measured (3) knowledge of bone mass may influence the diagnostic or therapeutic approach, and (4) treatment of osteoporosis affects fracture risk.

I. Diagnostic Criteria

There have been few prospective attempts to relate bone mass to eventual fracture risk in men, and hence the prognostic implications of a specific level of bone density are uncertain. The World Health Organization (WHO) (1994) has proposed that in women *osteopenia* should be identified when density is more than 1.0 standard deviations below the young normal mean, and *osteoporosis* should be identified when the density is more than 2.5 standard deviations below. Whether a similar approach can be taken in the diagnosis of osteopenia and osteoporosis in men is unknown.

A key issue in this regard is whether it is more appropriate to use gender-specific normative values of bone mass in the evaluation of osteoporosis in men or whether the same level of absolute bone mass should determine diagnostic categorization in both men and women. This issue is currently quite unclear, and technical, pathophysiologic, and public health considerations influence the decision.

From a technical perspective, gender differences may arise from the application of two-dimensional bone density measurement methods (e.g., dual-energy x-ray absorptiometry) to bones with intrinsic differences in three-dimensional shape and size. Geometric differences can lead to artifacts which result in apparently higher bone mineral density levels in those with larger bones (i.e., men) (Carter *et al.*, 1992). How these geometric influences on bone density measures relate to fracture risk prediction is unclear.

The pathophysiology of fracture is complex and is influenced by several factors in addition to true bone mass or density. These include some variables with clear gender differences, such as bone size and shape, structure (e.g., cortical thickness), muscle strength, and fall character. These variables may influence the relationship between bone density and fracture risk. For instance, with the same bone density, an individual with larger bones (i.e., a man) may have a substantially lower fracture risk.

The public health implications of any diagnostic criteria must be carefully considered. Looker *et al.* (1995) recently attempted to apply the -1 and -2.5 standard deviation WHO criteria with the "young, normal" mean levels derived from a male reference population to identify what proportion of the overall U.S. male population would have osteopenia or osteoporosis. They found that 47% of men aged 50 or more would have osteopenia at the femoral neck measurement site and 6% would have osteoporosis. Using the young, normal mean values derived from a female reference population (hence with lower absolute bone density levels), they found that approximately the same number of men would be found to be osteoporotic, but that the number identified with osteopenia would be considerably greater. The choice of reference population (men or women) thus would have profound public health and cost implications.

There are some experimental data that may be helpful in approaching the problem of what diagnostic criteria to use, but they are by no means conclusive. Cross-sectional studies indicate that men who experience fractures have greater absolute levels of bone density than do women with comparable fractures (Chevalley *et al.*, 1991; M. Karlsson *et al.*, 1993; Greenspan *et al.*, 1994), and reveal that the use of gender specific reference data yield osteoporosis prevalence figures in concert with observed fracture rates (Melton *et al.*, 1998). In the large EVOS study of vertebral fracture, the risk of having a vertebral deformity was higher in men than in women after adjusting to the same bone mineral density (BMD) (Lunt *et al.*, 1997). Hence most, but not all (De Lait *et al.*, 1997), cross-sectional trials support the use of gender-specific reference values.

The most effective approach to the resolution of this problem would be via prospective trials in men of the relationship between measures of bone density or mass and future fracture risk. Those are becoming available, and to date they suggest that gender-specific diagnostic criteria may not be appropriate. For instance, Cheng *et al.* (1997) and Ross *et al.* (Chapter 24) found that calcaneal bone mass predicts fracture risk in both men and women and that the relationship between absolute levels of bone density and fracture risk was not gender-specific. The available prospective trials are still few and do not yet adequately settle the controversy. Unfortunately, because the influence of factors such as technical artifact and bone geometry vary according to the type of assessment methods being used, the issue of whether to use gender-specific reference values may have to be examined for each bone mass measurement technique individually.

Until prospective trials provide a definitive answer, the use of gender-specific reference values seems most appropriate. That approach yields reasonable numbers of men who would require some form of diagnostic and therapeutic intervention. The adoption of female reference values would greatly limit the number of men that meet threshold levels for intervention and may deprive some of appropriate care.

B. Screening for Men at High Fracture Risk

In addition to those men who evince clinical evidence of skeletal fragility, a broader strategy to identify those at risk may be useful. Bone mass measures are currently recommended in all postmenopausal women (National Osteoporosis Foundation). This approach is based on the availability of safe and effective measurement techniques as well as effective preventive and treatment options, even though the cost-effectiveness of screening in women is unproven. In men, bone density measures are certainly safe and appear to have a similar level of predictive value for fracture, but there are no well-validated treatment modalities. Bone mass screening strategies in men have not been widely discussed. Nevertheless, the magnitude of the problem posed by fractures in men is huge, and the potential savings to be accrued from fracture prevention are large in both personal and economic terms. Should preventive and treatment strategies prove effective in men, screening for fracture risk in selected populations should be considered.

General fracture-risk screening in men may be useful at and above approximately age 65–70 years. The incidence of fracture begins to rise quickly approximately then (Fig. 1), and intervention may be quite effective. An appropriate screening strategy should include measures of bone mass as well as simple assessments of fall propensity (e.g., chair stand). The usefulness of this or similar strategies certainly must be subject to specific evaluation.

IV. Differential Diagnosis

If a man is found to be osteopenic or osteoporotic, an evaluation should be considered to determine the cause of the disorder with reasonable certainty. In women with low trauma fractures, the vast majority have histological osteoporosis, but a small proportion is found to be osteomalacic (Aaron *et al.*, 1974; Campbell *et al.*, 1984; Hordon and Peacock, 1990). Similarly, a portion of men with fracture have osteomalacia (Aaron *et al.*, 1974;

Campbell *et al.*, 1984; Hordon and Peacock, 1990). Osteomalacia is estimated to be present in <4–47% of men with femoral fractures, with most reports being ≤20% (Aaron *et al.*, 1974; Sokoloff, 1978; Campbell *et al.*, 1984; Wilton *et al.*, 1987; Hordon and Peacock, 1990). Because food is fortified with vitamin D, occult osteomalacia may be less frequent in the United States than in other areas (e.g., Northern Europe). Increasing age is associated with a greater prevalence of osteomalacia (Hordon and Peacock, 1990). Some have suggested that women with femoral fracture are more frequently osteomalacic than men (Aaron *et al.*, 1974; Campbell *et al.*, 1984), but others report no distinction (Hordon and Peacock, 1990). Thus far, the only patients who have been carefully surveyed are those with femoral fractures, and it is not known whether populations with other fractures (e.g., vertebral) would include similar proportions of osteoporotic and osteomalacic individuals. Although the exact magnitude of the problem presented by osteomalacia in men is uncertain, it is clear that the differential diagnosis of low bone mass and fractures in men must consider the possibility. This becomes particularly imperative because the treatment for osteomalacia differs considerably from that of osteoporosis (Marel *et al.*, 1986).

V. Initial Evaluation of Osteoporosis: History, Physical, and Routine Biochemical Measures _____

The history, physical, and routine biochemical profile can be very helpful in directing a focused evaluation of a man with low bone mass, and is usually successful in revealing major causes of fragility. A variety of approaches for the differential diagnosis of low bone mass have been suggested using standard clinical and biochemical information (Campbell *et al.*, 1984; Johnston *et al.*, 1991; Looker *et al.*, 1995). The goals of this stage of the evaluation should be to determine the specific diagnosis (what is the cause of the low bone mass—osteoporosis or osteomalacia?) and to identify contributing factors in the genesis of the disorder. Of particular importance in the history and physical, therefore, are clinical signs of genetic (osteogenesis imperfecta, Ehlers Danlos, Marfans, etc.), nutritional/environmental, social (alcohol or tobacco), medical, or pharmacological factors that may be present to aid in these goals. Routine laboratory testing should include levels of serum creatinine, calcium, phosphorus, alkaline phosphatase, and liver function tests as well as a complete blood count. If, on the basis of these tests, there is evidence for medical conditions associated with bone loss (alcoholism, hyperparathyroidism, malignancy, Cushing's syndrome, thyrotoxicosis, malabsorption, etc.) a definitive diagnosis should be pursued with appropriate testing.

The choice of more focused laboratory testing should be designed to uncover other factors that commonly contribute to the etiology of osteoporosis in men. In view of their relatively low cost and the frequency with which they may yield useful data not uncovered in the initial history, physical, and laboratory evaluation, the following can be considered a routine part of the evaluation of men with reduced bone mass. Once again, the validation that these recommendations are cost-effective is not available.

- 24-hour urine calcium and creatinine. Hypercalciuria is common in men and has been linked to osteopenia. It should be suspected as a factor if 24-hour urine calcium excretion is >300 mg on a routine diet. Hypocalciuria (<100 mg) should raise the suspicion of markedly reduced dietary calcium absorption (due to vitamin D deficiency, bowel disease, or malnutrition).
- Serum 25-hydroxyvitamin D level. Vitamin D insufficiency is common and is easily correctable.
- Serum testosterone (free or total). Clearly low testosterone levels suggest hypogonadism, a treatable condition associated with low bone mass. Unfortunately, borderline low values are also common, but the success of androgen replacement has not been evaluated in those patients. Because testosterone concentrations fluctuate, it may require more than a single determination to reflect average levels adequately. Although recently linked to bone mass in men, there has been inadequate study to suggest estrogen determinations are clinically useful.
- Serum protein electrophoresis (in those >50 years, particularly when anemic, to exclude multiple myeloma).

VI. Evaluation of the Patient with Unexplained Osteoporosis

In men with reduced bone mass and in whom no clear pathophysiology is identified by the routine methods just described, it has been considered appropriate to be diagnostically aggressive, primarily because the potential for occult "secondary" causes of osteoporosis may be higher in men. However, the incidence of occult causes of osteoporosis in men, or whether it is greater than in women, is poorly studied. The diagnostic yield and cost-effectiveness of extensive biochemical studies in the man with apparently "idiopathic" osteoporosis is thus unknown. Nevertheless, lacking this information, a reasonable evaluation of the man without a clear etiology for osteoporosis might include:

- 24-hour urine cortisol.
- Serum thyroid stimulating hormone level.
- Indices of histamine metabolism (urinary N'-methylhistamine) (Golkar and Bernhard, 1997). Mastocytosis is an uncommon cause of

bone loss and is particularly of concern in the presence of typical skin lesions and symptoms.
- Biochemical marker of bone remodeling. The rate of remodeling can be useful in constructing a differential diagnosis. In the presence of evidence of high remodeling (and the absence of any apparent cause), bone biopsy may be appropriate to determine if bone marrow pathology is present.

Should all these steps be unrewarding, the diagnosis of idiopathic osteoporosis can be confirmed. At that point, therapy must be empirical.

VII. Falls

Falls are a major determinant of fracture, and it is important to recognize patients at risk. There are a variety of quantitative techniques to estimate balance and fall propensity, but semiquantitative approaches are probably quite appropriate in most clinical settings. A simple observation of strength and gait can reveal unsteadiness and impaired mobility. In women, the chair stand has been useful in identifying those at risk for fracture (Cummings *et al.*, 1995). The recognition that falling is likely should lead to appropriate intervention (safety aids, physical therapy, exercise, etc.).

VIII. Discussion of Diagnostic Measures of Particular Interest

A. Biochemical Markers of Mineral Metabolism

Bone mass is, of course, intimately linked to mineral metabolism. On that basis, prominent relationships between indices of mineral homeostasis and metabolic bone disease should be expected. In fact, in men as in women, gross derangements in mineral physiology are associated with skeletal disorders. For instance, men with hyperparathyroidism, vitamin D deficiency, malignancies, hypercalciuria, and so on are at risk for osteopenia and fractures (Orwoll and Klein, 1995), and the differential diagnosis of osteopenic disorders should include the consideration of these diseases (discussed later). Certainly, the prevalence of vitamin D insufficiency appears to be high in both sexes and should be of particular concern to clinicians (Thomas *et al.*, 1998).

The issue of whether the immense increase in fracture rates that occur with aging in men is related to concomitant alterations in mineral metabolism is more difficult to resolve. Increasing age is associated with slight but significant increases in parathyroid hormone levels and declines in 25(OH)D levels (Orwoll and Meier, 1986), and these changes have been linked to the gradual decrease in bone mass that accompanies aging (Orwoll and Meier, 1986; Riggs and Melton, 1986; Gallagher *et al.*, 1998). Declines in calcium absorption have also been reported to occur in older men, possibly related to reductions in the ability to produce 1,25(OH)2D in the kidney (Riggs and Melton, 1986). This fall in 1,25(OH)2D levels seems to be limited to those that have more severe reductions in renal function (Orwoll and Meier, 1986; Halloran *et al.*, 1990). Although there are no definite gender differences in these age-related changes, there have been some reports that older men have higher 25(OH)D levels than women (Dawson-Hughes *et al.*, 1997; Gallagher *et al.*, 1998; Thomas *et al.*, 1998). Nevertheless, an improvement in bone mass is seen in normal older men with modest calcium and vitamin D supplementation (Dawson-Hughes *et al.*, 1997), suggesting that alterations in mineral metabolism may contribute to age-related increases in fractures.

In view of the prevalence of vitamin D deficiency (particularly in northern latitudes) and the relationship of vitamin D deficiency to osteopenia and fractures, the assessment of 25(OH)D levels should be considered useful. In patients with quite low levels of 25(OH)D (<15 ng/mL), routine amounts of supplementation (400–800 IU/d) may be inadequate to achieve optimal nutrition, and higher doses can be used. Repeat 25(OH)D levels can be used to monitor the success of therapy. The measurement of 1,25(OH)2D levels in routine clinical situations, and the use of PTH measures in patients with normal serum calcium concentrations, are of unclear usefulness.

B. Biochemical Markers of Bone Remodeling

The unequivocal decline in bone mass that occurs with aging in men is undoubtedly the result of trends in the remodeling process that result in a relative excess of bone resorption. Histological evaluations of cancellous bone indicate that there is trabecular plate thinning and dropout and that these changes have expected biomechanical consequences (Mosekilde, 1989). In men this process is similar to that which occurs in women, with the exception that at menopause women experience a particularly rapid rate of trabecular plate perforation and loss (Eriksen, 1986; Mosekilde, 1989; Mosekilde and Mosekilde, 1990). In cortical bones, aging men also are affected by bone resorption, loss of bone mass, and an increase in fragility. At endocortical sites, bone resorption occurs and results in cortical thinning. Whereas this happens to some extent in both men and women, the biomechanical consequences are somewhat lessened in men by a simultaneous increase in periosteal bone accretion that yields larger bones more fracture resistant (Martin and Atkinson, 1977).

The specific remodeling imbalance which is responsible for the age-related decline in bone mass in men is unclear. The postmenopausal period in women appears to be associated with an increase in bone remodeling rates with a particular excess of resorption; however, there is no counterpart in men. The decline in bone mass may be less the result of absolute increases in bone resorption than reduction in the rate of osteoblastic bone formation (Nordin *et al.*, 1984; Marie *et al.*, 1991; Clarke *et al.*, 1996). Of course, disruptions of remodeling may be accelerated in overt disease states (hyperparathyroidism, immobilization, glucocorticoid excess, etc.), leading to more rapid bone loss and increasing fracture risk.

The histomorphometric changes in bone metabolism that are associated with bone loss in men would be expected to be reflected in alterations in biochemical indices of bone remodeling. The available literature is modest and somewhat inconsistent. Unfortunately, all studies to date in men are cross-sectional. Delmas *et al.* (1993) reported that there was a gradual increase in pyridinoline excretion with age in men starting in middle age, and Orwoll and Deftos (1990) found an increase in osteocalcin levels with aging in normal men. Similar findings have been reported for bone alkaline phosphatase (Garnero and Delmas, 1993). On the other hand, Wishart *et al.* (1995) described a fall in several markers of bone formation and resorption was associated with increasing age in men. Orwoll *et al.* (1998) recently examined urinary N-telopeptide levels in a large group of men and found no change after the age of 30 years (Fig. 3). Although there was a tendency for N-telopeptide excretion to increase in the oldest men, the trend was not

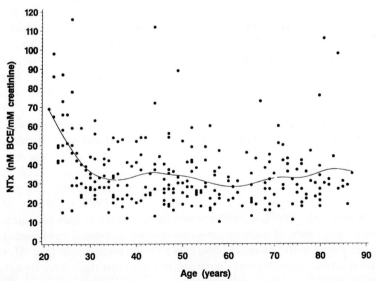

FIGURE 3   Urinary NTX/creatinine in normal men by age. Individual subject values are plotted as a function of age. The solid line is fit to the data using a cubic spline method. Reproduced from Orwoll *et al.* (1998). Collagen N-telopeptide excretion in men. *J. Bone Miner. Res.* **83**, 3930–3935, © The Endocrine Society, with permission.

significant. In studies that concentrated on older men (rather than a spectrum of young to old), two groups have reported that there is a slight increase in biochemical indices with age (Schneider and Barrett-Connor, 1997; Gallagher et al., 1998). If a consensus can be reached from the existing literature, it is that there is little change in biochemical indices of resorption in men until the later stages of life, when slight increases occur. Markers of bone formation may increase with age.

An important finding reported by two groups is that markers of bone remodeling are higher in men during the third decade than they are in the rest of adult life (Wishart et al., 1995; Orwoll et al., 1998) (Fig. 3). This is apparently a continuation of the process of peak bone mass development since markers of remodeling are known to be increased during growth and adolescence (Hanson et al., 1992; Rico et al., 1992). From a clinical perspective, it is important to recognize the phenomenon when attempting to use biochemical indices during this period of life. Another important finding has been the description of a diurnal variation in markers of bone metabolism in men and women (Lakatos et al., 1995; Greenspan et al., 1996), which may be to some extent related to the diurnal variation in cortisol secretion (Nielsen et al., 1992).

The relationship between biochemical indices of remodeling and bone health is not well understood in men. Whereas in women there are longitudinal data that support the usefulness of measuring biochemical indices as predictors of change in bone mass or of fracture risk, no such data are available in men. However, urinary level of collagen N-telopeptide are apparently correlated with levels of bone mass in men (as in women) (Fig. 4) (Schneider and Barrett-Connor, 1997), and higher levels of serum osteocalcin are associated with higher parathyroid hormone concentrations (Gallagher et al., 1998). Some have described differences in indices of remodeling between normal and osteoporotic men (Resch et al., 1992), and low bone mass was related to high bone turnover in male long distance runners (Hetland et al., 1993). Again, all these studies have been cross-sectional, and longitudinal trials are necessary to understand the real value of biochemical measures in men.

One area in which a reasonable experience with biochemical markers has accumulated is in the treatment of hypogonadal men with androgens. Hypogonadism in men is associated with an acceleration in bone remodeling and increases in biochemical indices (Stepan et al., 1989; Goldwray et al., 1993; Guo et al., 1997), a phenomenon quite similar to that seen in postmenopausal women. In a variety of recent studies, androgen replacement has been associated with changes in markers of bone metabolism (Fig. 5), with concomitant increases in bone density. Although most trials have reported a decline in both formation and resorption markers (Katznelson et al., 1996; Guo et al., 1997), some have described an increase in formation parameters and have suggested that androgens increase osteoblastic activity while reducing resorption (Morley et al., 1993; Wang et al., 1996). Similarly, in normal

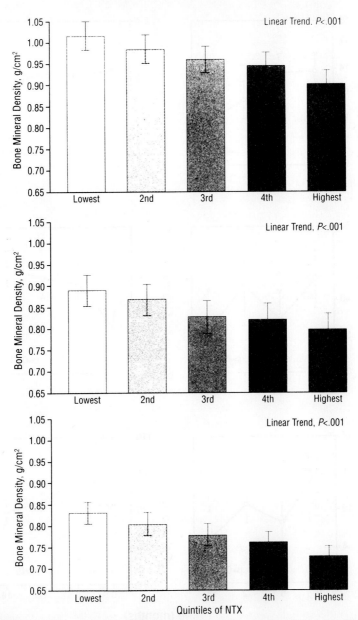

FIGURE 4   Total hip mean bone mineral density levels by quintiles of N-telopeptide (NTX) levels in 374 men (top), 223 estrogen users (center), and 364 nonestrogen users (bottom). The figures are adjusted for age, body mass index, total daily calcium, current smoking, alcohol use 3 or more days per week, exercise 3 or more times per week, limited physical health, non-insulin-dependent diabetes mellitus, and current use of thiazide diuretics, thyroid hormone, and corticosteroids. Reproduced from Schneider and Barrett-Connor (1997), *Arch. Intern. Med.* **157,** 1241–1245, Copyright 1997, American Medical Association, with permission.

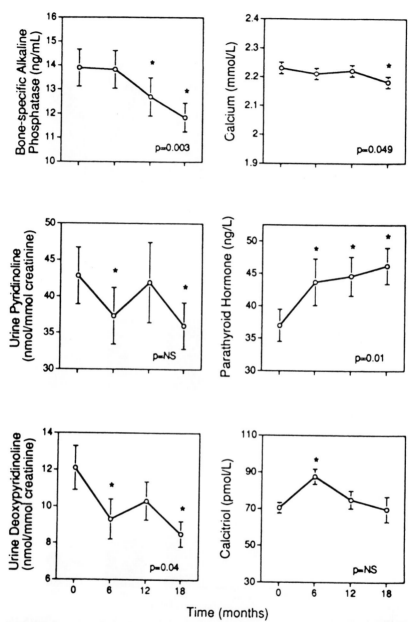

FIGURE 5 Indexes of bone turnover, calcium regulatory hormones, and calcium in hypogonadal men receiving testosterone replacement therapy. Data are expressed as the mean ± SEM. Statistical significance for analysis of the mean slope is shown in the bottom right-hand corner of each figure. * $p < 0.05$ compared to the baseline value, by paired t test analysis. Reproduced from Katznelson *et al.* (1996). Increase in bone density and lean body mass during testosterone administration in men with acquired hypogonadism. *J. Clin. Endocrinol. Metab.* **81,** 4358–4365, © The Endocrine Society, with permission.

older men or eugonadal men with osteoporosis, treatment with testosterone has been noted to reduce indices of resorption with smaller changes in markers of formation (Tenover, 1992; Anderson *et al.*, 1997). These are interesting findings, but the meaning of the biochemical changes remains uncertain. It would be helpful to have a direct measure of bone remodeling in these situations to document authentic relationships between markers of formation and resorption and their respective morphological counterparts.

C. Histomorphometric Characterization

Transiliac bone biopsy is a safe and effective means of assessing skeletal histology and remodeling characteristics (Klein and Gunness, 1992). Some have suggested that a transiliac bone biopsy is indicated in those men in whom a thorough biochemical evaluation has failed to reveal an etiology for osteoporosis (Jackson and Kleerekoper, 1990). The rationale for this approach is based on the need to accomplish several objectives: (1) ensure that occult osteomalacia is not present; (2) identify unusual causes of osteoporosis that may be revealed only by a histological analysis, such as mastocytosis (Chines *et al.*, 1991, 1993), and (3) to yield information concerning the remodeling rate, which in turn may further direct the differential diagnosis (e.g., unappreciated thyrotoxicosis or secondary hyperparathyroidism suggested by the presence of increased turnover) or may be helpful in designing the most appropriate therapeutic approach. On the other hand, considerable histological heterogeneity exists among men with osteoporosis, and whether distinct histological patterns represent different stages of a single disease entity, separate subtypes of the disease, or simply an arbitrary subdivision of a normal distribution of remodeling rates is unknown. Realistically, the cost and invasiveness of a bone biopsy, coupled with the uncertain likelihood of detecting useful information (in addition to that available from noninvasive testing) has relegated the procedure to only the most unusual situations.

A more reasonable approach in men with idiopathic osteoporosis may be to use the advantages of biochemical markers of bone turnover. The presence of an increase in biochemical indices of remodeling may indicate a condition associated with higher bone turnover. On the other hand, the presence of normal or low levels of markers is probably common in men with "idiopathic" osteoporosis and does not suggest the presence of one of the less common forms of metabolic bone disease.

D. Growth Factors and Cytokine Measures

Growth factors must be important in the regulation of bone metabolism in men as well as women (Chapter 9), but there is little information concerning the specific nature of their roles or their usefulness in the clinical situation. Growth factors (Johansson *et al.*, 1994; Kurland *et al.*, 1997) (Fig. 6)

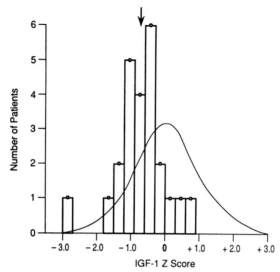

FIGURE 6   Distribution of IGF-1 Z scores in men with idiopathic osteoporosis. The graph shows the mean Z score -0.75 is significantly lower ($p = 0.0002$) than the theoretical Gaussian distribution of the normal population (mean Z = 0). Reproduced from Kurland *et al.* (1997). Insulin-like growth factor-I in men with idiopathic osteoporosis. *J. Clin. Endocrinol. Metab.* **82,** 2799–2805, © The Endocrine Society, with permission.

or one of the growth factor binding proteins (IGFBP-3) (Johansson *et al.,* 1997) have been reported to be related to bone mass in normal men, and in those with idiopathic osteoporosis evidence has recently arisen suggesting insulin-like growth factor 1 (IGF-1) may be reduced (Ljunghall *et al.,* 1992; Kurland *et al.,* 1997). These studies found that mean levels of IGF-1 were lower than in control populations but were nevertheless within the expected normal ranges. These data are intriguing in view of the association between growth hormone deficiency and low bone mass in men (Inzucchi and Robbins, 1996), a relationship that may primarily reflect growth hormone deficiency during peak bone mass development (Toogood *et al.,* 1997).

The etiologic role of growth factors in the genesis of osteoporosis in men is of great interest but clearly must be further examined. Unless there is other evidence of growth hormone deficiency, the measurement of growth factor levels cannot be considered a routine part of the evaluation of osteoporosis in men.

IX. Summary

In view of the limited information concerning the disorder, the evaluation of osteoporosis in men is a clinical challenge. Nevertheless, it is becoming more apparent that principles developed for the approach to osteoporosis in women are probably useful in approaching similar problems in men. Men at highest risk (and who therefore deserve most diagnostic attention) are older, Caucasian, have medical conditions associated with low bone mass or falls, have a positive family history of osteoporosis, and have had previous fractures. A primary goal should be to understand the factors that contribute to fracture risk, and the most important aspect of the evaluation is the initial history, physical examination, and routine laboratory testing. Bone mass measures are very useful in identifying those at increased fracture risk, but diagnostic criteria are still not well formulated in men. Unfortunately, in a large fraction of men (particularly younger patients), no obvious etiology will be identified (idiopathic osteoporosis).

There is a clear need for additional information concerning the determinants of osteoporotic fracture risk in men and the relationship of measures of skeletal integrity to fracture risk. That information will provide the design of rational diagnostic schemes. Objective testing of the utility and cost-effectiveness of diagnostic paradigms is of particular importance.

References

Aaron, J. E., Stasiak, L., Gallagher, J. C., Longton, E. B., Nicholson, M., Anderson, J., and Nordin, B. E. C. (1974). Frequency of osteomalacia and osteoporosis in fractures of the proximal femur. *Lancet* **1**, 229–233.

Anderson, F. H., Francis, R. M., Peaston, R. T., and Wastell, H. J. (1997). Androgen supplementation in eugonadal men with osteoporosis: Effects of six months' treatment on markers of bone formation and resorption. *J. Bone Miner. Res.* **12**, 472–478.

Beck, T. J., Ruff, C. B., Mourtada, F. A., Shaffer, R. A., Maxwell-Williams, K., Kao, G. L., Sartoris, D. J., and Brodine, S. (1996). Dual-energy x-ray absorptiometry derived structural geometry for stress fracture prediction in male U.S. marine corps recruits. *J. Bone Miner. Res.* **11**, 645–653.

Burger, H., de Laet, C. E. D. H., van Daele, P. L. A., Weel, A. E. A. M., Wittman, J. C. M., Hofman, A., and Pols, H. A. P. (1998). Risk ractors for increased bone loss in an elderly population. *Am. J. Epidemiol.* **147**, 871–879.

Campbell, G. A., Hosking, D. J., Kemm, J. R., and Boyd, R. V. (1984). How common is osteomalacia in the elderly? *Lancet* **2**, 386–388.

Carter, D. R., Bouxsein, M. L., and Marcus, R. (1992). New approaches for interpreting projected bone densitometry data. *J. Bone Miner. Res.* **7**, 137–145.

Cheng, S., Suominen, H., Sakari-Rantala, R., Laukkanen, P., Avikainen, V., and Heikkinen, E. (1997). Calcaneal bone mineral density predicts fracture occurrence: A five-year follow-up study in elderly people. *J. Bone Miner. Res.* **12**, 1075–1082.

Chevalley, T., Rizzoli, R., Nydegger, V., Slosman, D., Tkatch, L., Rapin, C.-H., Vasey, H., and Bonjour, J.-P. (1991). Preferential low bone mineral density of the femoral neck in patients with a recent fracture of the proximal femur. *Osteoporosis Int.* **1**, 147–154.

Chines, A., Pacifici, R., Avioli, L. V., Teitelbaum, S. L., and Korenblat, P. E. (1991). Systemic mastocytosis presenting as osteoporosis: A clinical and histomorphometric study. *J. Clin. Endocrinol. Metab.* **72**, 140–144.

Chines, A., Pacifici, R., Avioli, L. A., Korenblat, P. E., and Teitelbaum, S. L. (1993). Systemic mastocytosis and osteoporosis. *Osteoporosis Int.* **1**, S147–S149.

Christian, J. C., Yu, P.-L., Slemenda, C. W., and Johnston, C. C. J. (1989). Heritability of bone mass: A longitudinal study in aging male twins. *Am. J. Hum. Genet.* **44**, 429–433.

Clarke, B. L., Ebeling, P. R., Jones, J. D., Wahner, H. W., O'Fallon, W. M., and Fitzpatrick, L. A. (1996). Changes in quantitative bone histomorphometry in aging healthy men. *J. Clin. Endocrinol. Metab.* **81**, 2264–2270.

Cohen-Solal, M. E., Baudoin, C., Omouri, M., Kuntz, D., and de Vernejoul, M. C. (1998). Bone mass in middle-aged osteoporotic men and their relatives: Familial effect. *J. Bone Miner. Res.* **13**, 1909–1914.

Cooper, C., and Melton, L. J. III. (1992). Epidemiology of osteoporosis. *Trends Endocrinol. Metab.* **3**, 224–229.

Cummings, S. R., Nevitt, M. C., Browner, W. S., Stone, K., Fox, K. M., Ensrud, K. E., Cauley, J., Black, D., and Vogt, T. M. (1995). Risk factors for hip fracture in white women. *N. Engl. J. Med.* **332**, 767–773.

Dawson-Hughes, B., Harris, S. S., Krall, E. A., and Dallal, G. E. (1997). Effect of calcium and vitamin D supplementation on bone density in men and women 65 years of age or older. *N. Engl. J. Med.* **337**, 670–702.

De Lait, C. E. D. H., van Hout, B. A., Burger, H., Hofman, A., and Pols, H. A. P. (1997). Bone density and risk of hip fracture in men and women: Cross sectional analysis. *Br. Med. J.* **315**, 221–225.

Delmas, P. D., Gineyts, E., Bertholin, A., Garnero, P., and Marchand, F. (1993). Immunoassay of pyridinoline crosslink excretion in normal adults and in Paget's disease. *J. Bone Miner. Res.* **8**(5), 643–648.

Diaz, M. N., O'Neill, T. W., and Silman, A. J. (1997). The influence of family history of hip fracture on the risk of vertebral deformity in men and women: The European Vertebral Osteoporosis Study. *Bone* **20**, 145–149.

Donaldson, L. J., Cook, A., and Thomson, R. G. (1990). Incidence of fractures in a geographically defined population. *J. Epidemiol. Commun. Health* **44**, 241–245.

Eastell, R., and Riggs, B. L. (1980). Diagnostic evaluation of osteoporosis. *Endocrinol. Metab. Clin. North Am.* **17**, 547–571.

Eriksen, E. F. (1986). Normal and pathological remodeling of human trabecular bone: Three dimensional reconstruction of the remodeling sequence in normals and in metabolic bone disease. *Endocr. Rev.* **7**, 379–408.

Evans, R. A., Marel, G. M., Lancaster, E. K., Kos, S., Evans, M., and Wong, S. Y. P. (1988). Bone mass is low in relatives of osteoporotic patients. *Ann. Intern. Med.* **109**, 870–873.

Fujiwara, S., Kasagi, F., Yamada, M., and Kodama, K. (1997). Risk factors for hip fracture in a Japanese cohort. *J. Bone Miner. Res.* **12**, 998–1004.

Gallagher, J. C., Kinyamu, H. K., Fowler, S. E., Dawson-Hughes, B., Dalsky, G. P., and Sherman, S. S. (1998). Calciotropic hormones and bone markers in the elderly. *J. Bone Miner. Res.* **13**, 475–482.

Gardsell, P., Johnell, O., and Nilsson, B. E. (1990). Thre predictive value of forearm bone mineral content measurements in men. *Bone* **11**, 229–232.

Garnero, P., and Delmas, P. D. (1993). Assessment of the serum levels of bone alkaline phosphatase with a new immunoradiometric assay in patients with metabolic bone disease. *J. Clin. Endocrinol. Metab.* **77**, 1046–1053.

Garraway, W. M., Stauffer, R. N., Kurland, L. T., and O'Fallon, W. M. (1979). Limb fractures in a defined population. I. Frequency and distribution. *Mayo Clin. Proc.* **54**, 701–707.

Goldwray, D., Weisman, Y., Jaccard, N., Merdler, C., Chen, J., and Matzkin, H. (1993). Decreased bone mineral density in elderly men treated with the gonadotropin-releasing hormone agonist decapeptyl (D-trp6-GnRH). *J. Clin. Endocrinol. Metab.* **76**, 288–290.

Golkar, L., and Bernhard, J. D. (1997). Mastocytosis. *Lancet* **349**, 1379–1385.

Greenspan, S. L., Myers, E. R., Maitland, L. A., Kido, T. H., Krasnow, M. B., and Hayes, W. C. (1994). Trochanteric bone mineral density is associated with type of hip fracture in the elderly. *J. Bone Miner. Res.* **9**, 1889–1894.

Greenspan, S. L., Dresner-Pollack, R., Parker, R. A., London, D., and Ferguson, L. (1996). Diurnal variation of bone mineral turnover in elderly men and women. *Calcif. Tissue Int.* **60**, 419–423.

Grisso, J. A., Chiu, G. Y., Maislin, G., Steinmann, W. C., and Portale, J. (1991). Risk factors for hip fractures in men: A preliminary study. *J. Bone Miner. Res.* **6**, 865–868.

Gueguen, R., Jouanny, P., Guillemin, F., Kuntz, C., Pourel, J., and Siest, G. (1995). Segregation analysis and variance components analysis of bone mineral density in healthy families. *J. Bone Miner. Res.* **10**, 2017–2022.

Guo, C.-Y., Jones, H., and Eastell, R. (1997). Treatment of isolated hypogonadotropic hypogonadism effect on bone mineral density and bone turnover. *J. Clin. Endocrinol. Metab.* **82**, 658–665.

Halloran, B. P., Portale, A. A., Lonergan, E. T., and Morris, R. C. J. (1990). Production and metabolic clearance of 1,25-dihydroxyvitamin D in men: Effect of advancing age. *J. Clin. Endocrinol. Metab.* **70**, 318–323.

Hanson, D. A., Weis, M. A. E., Bollen, A.-M., Maslan, S. L., Singer, F. R., and Eyre, D. R. (1992). A specific immunoassay for monitoring human bone resorption: Quantitation of Type I collagen cross-linked n-telopeptides in urine. *J. Bone Miner. Res.* **7**, 1251–1258.

Hetland, M. L., Haarbo, J., and Christiansen, C. (1993). Low bone mass and high bone turnover in male long distance runners. *J. Clin. Endocrinol. Metab.* **77**, 770–775.

Hordon, L. D., and Peacock, M. (1990). Osteomalacia and osteoporosis in femoral neck fracture. *Bone Miner.* **11**, 247–259.

Inzucchi, S. E., and Robbins, R. J. (1996). Growth hormone and the maintenance of adult bone mineral density. *Clin. Endocrinol. (Oxford)* **45**, 665–673.

Jackson, J. A., and Kleerekoper, M. (1990). Osteoporosis in men: Diagnosis, pathophysiology, and prevention. *Medicine (Baltimore)* **69**, 137–152.

Jacobsen, S. J., Goldberg, J., Miles, T. P., Brody, J. A., Stiers, W., and Rimm, A. A. (1990). Hip fracture incidence among the old and very old: A population-based study of 745,435 cases. *Am. J. Public Health* **80**, 871–873.

Joakimsen, R. M., Fonnebo, V., Magnus, J. H., Stormer, J., Tollan, A., and Sogaard, A. J. (1998). The Tromo Study: Physical activity and the incidence of fractures in a middle-aged population. *J. Bone Miner. Res.* **13**, 1149–1157.

Johansson, A., Forslund, A., and Hambraeus, L. (1994). Growth-hormone-dependent insulin-like growth factor binding protein is a major determinant of bone mineral density in healthy men. *J. Bone Miner. Res.* **9**, 915–921.

Johansson, A. G., Eriksen, E. F., Lindh, E., Langdahl, B., Blum, W. F., Lindahl, A., Ljunggren, O., and Ljunghall, S. (1997). Reductions in serum levels of the growth hormone-dependent insulin-like growth factor binding protein and a negative bone balance at the level of individual remodeling units in idiopathic osteoporosis in men. *J. Clin. Endocrinol. Metab.* **82**, 2795–2798.

Johnson, M. L., Gong, G., Kimberling, W., Recker, S. M., Kimmel, D. B., and Recker, R. R. (1997). Linkage of a gene causing high bone mass to human chromosome 11 (11q12-13). *Am. J. Hum. Genet.* **60**, 1326–1332.

Johnston, C. C., Jr., Slemenda, C. W., and Melton, L. J., III (1991). Clinical use of bone densitometry. *N. Engl. J. Med.* **324**, 1105–1109.

Karlsson, M., Hasserius, R., and Obrant, E. J. (1993). Individuals who sustain nonosteoporotic fractures continue to also sustain fragility fractures. *Calcif. Tissue Int.* **53**, 229–231.

Karlsson, M. K., Johnell, O., Nilsson, B. E., Sernbo, I., and Obrant, K. J. (1993). Bone mienral mass in hip fracture patients. *Bone* **14**, 161–165.

Katznelson, L., Finkelstein, J. S., Schoenfeld, D. A., Rosenthal, D. I., Anderson, E. J., and Klibanski, A. (1996). Increase in bone density and lean body mass during testosterone administration in men with acquired hypogonadism. *J. Clin. Endocrinol. Metab.* **81**, 4358–4365.

Klein, R. F., and Gunness, M. (1992). The transiliac bone biopsy: When to get it and how to interpret it. *Endocrinologist* **2**, 158–168.

Krall, E. A., and Dawson-Hughes, B. (1993). Heritable and life-style determinants of bone mineral density. *J. Bone Miner. Res.* **8,** 1–9.

Kurland, T. S., Rosen, C. J., Cosman, F., McMahon, D., Chan, F., Shane, E., Lindsay, R., Dempster, D., and Bilezikian, J. P. (1997). Insulin-like growth factor-I in men with idiopathic osteoporosis. *J. Clin. Endocrinol. Metab.* **82,** 2799–2805.

Lakatos, P., Blumsohn, A., Eastell, R., Tarjan, G., Shinoda, H., and Stern, P. H. (1995). Circadian rhythm of *in vitro* bone-resorbing activity in human serum. *J. Clin. Endocrinol. Metab.* **80,** 3185–3190.

Lane, J. M., and Vigorita, V. J. (1984). Osteoporosis. *Orthop. Clin. North Am.* **15,** 711–728.

Langdahl, B. L., Ralston, S. H., Grant, S. F. A., and Eriksen, E. F. (1998). An Sp1 binding site polymorphism in the COL1A1 gene predicts osteoporostic fractures in both men and women. *J. Bone Miner. Res.* **13,** 1384–1389.

Ljunghall, S., Johansson, A. G., Burman, P., Kampe, O., Lindh, E., and Karlsson, F. A. (1992). Low plasma levels of insulin-like growth factor 1 (IGF-1) in male patients with idiopathic osteoporosis. *J. Intern. Med.* **232,** 59–64.

Looker, A. C., Johnston, C. C., Wahner, H. W. J., Dunn, W. L., Calvo, M. S., Harris, T. B., Heyse, S. P., and Lindsay, R. L. (1995). Defining low femur bone density levels in men. *17th Annu. Meet. Am. Soc. Bone Miner. Res.*

Looker, A. C., Orwoll, E. S., Johnston, C. C., Lindsay, R. L., Heinz, W. W., Dunn, W. L., Calvo, M. S., Harris, T. B., and Heyse, S. P. (1997). Prevalence of low femoral bone density in older U.S. adults from NHANES III. *J. Bone Miner. Res.* **12,** 1761–1768.

Lunt, M., Felsenberg, D., Reeve, J., Benevolenskaya, L., Cannata, J., Dequeker, J., Dodenhof, C., Falch, J. A., Masaryk, P., Pols, H. A. P., Poor, G., Reid, D. M., Scheidt-Nave, C., Weber, K., Varlow, J., Kanis, J. A., O'Neill, T. W., and Silman, A. J. (1997). Bone density variation and its effects on risk of vertebral deformity in men and women studied in thirteen European centers: The EVOS Study. *J. Bone Miner. Res.* **12,** 1883–1894.

Mallmin, H., Ljunghall, S., Persson, I., Naessen, T., Krusemo, U. B., and Bergstrom, R. (1993). Fracture of the distal forearm as a forecaster of subsequent hip fracture: A population-based cohort study with 24 years follow-up. *Calcif. Tissue Int.* **52,** 269–272.

Mann, T., Oviatt, S. K., Wilson, D., Nelson, D., and Orwoll, E. S. (1992). Vertebral deformity in men. *J. Bone Miner. Res.* **7,** 1259–1265.

Marel, G. M., McKenna, M. J., and Frame, B. (1986). Osteomalacia. *In* "Bone and Mineral Res/4" (W. A. Peck, ed.), Vol. 4, pp. 335–413. Elsevier, Amsterdam.

Marie, P. J., de Vernejoul, M. C., Donnes, D., and Hott, M. (1991). Decreased DNA synthesis by culture osteoblastic cells in eugonadal osteoporotic men with defective bone formation. *J. Clin. Invest.* **88,** 1167–1172.

Martin, R. B., and Atkinson, P. J. (1977). Age and sex-related changes in the structure and strength of the human femoral shaft. *J. Biomech.* **10,** 223–231.

Melton, L. J., Thamer, M., Ray, N. F., Chan, J. K., Chesnut, C. H., Einhorn, T. A., Johnston, C. C., Raisz, L. G., Silverman, S. L., and Siris, E. S. (1997). Fractures attributable of osteoporosis: Report from the National Osteoporosis Foundation. *J. Bone Miner. Res.* **12,** 16–23.

Melton, L. J., Atkinson, E. J., O'Connor, M. K., O'Fallon, W. M., and Riggs, B. L. (1998). Bone density and fracture risk in men. *J. Bone Miner. Res.* **13,** 1915–1923.

Morley, J. E., Perry, H. M., III, Kaiser, F. E., Kraenzel, D., Jensen, J., Houston, K., Mattammal, M., and Perry, H. M., Jr. (1993). Effects of testosterone replacement therapy in old hypogonadal males: A preliminary study. *J. Am. Geriatr. Soc.* **41,** 149–152.

Morrison, N. A., Qi, J. C., Tokita, A., Kelly, P. J., Crofts, L., Nguyen, T. V., Sambrook, P. N., and Eisman, J. A. (1994). Prediction of bone density from vitamin D receptor alleles. *Nature (London)* **367,** 284–287.

Mosekilde, L. (1989). Sex differences in age-related loss of vertebral trabecular bone mass and structure—biomechanical consequences. *Bone* **10,** 425–432.

Mosekilde, L., and Mosekilde, L. (1990). Sex differences in age-related changes in vertebral body size, density and biomechanical competence in normal individuals. *Bone* **11,** 67–73.

Mussolino, M. E., Looker, A. C., Madans, J. H., Langlois, J. A., and Orwoll, E. S. (1998). Risk factors for hip fracture in white men: The NHANES I Epidemiologic Follow-up Study. *J. Bone Miner. Res.* **13**, 918–924.

Nguyen, T. V., Sambrook, P. N., Kelly, P. J., Lord, S., Freund, J., and Eisman, J. A. (1992). Body sway and bone mineral density are predictors of fracture prevalence: The DUBBO Osteoporosis Epidemiology Study. *J. Bone Miner. Res.* **7**(1), S112.

Nguyen, T., Sambrook, P., Kelly, P., Jones, G., Lord, S., and Freund, J. (1993). Prediction of osteoporotic fractures by postural instability and bone density. *Br. Med. J.* **307**, 1111–1115.

Nguyen, T. V., Eisman, J. A., Kelly, P. J., and Sambrook, P. N. (1996). Risk factors for osteoporotic fractures in elderly men. *Am. J. Epidemiol.* **144**, 258–261.

Nielsen, H. K., Brixen, K., Kassem, M., Charles, P., and Mosekilde, L. (1992). Inhibition of the morning cortisol peak abolishes the expected morning decrease in serum osteocalcin in normal males: Evidence of a controlling effect of serum cortisol on the circadian rhythm in serum osteocalcin. *J. Clin. Endocrinol. Metab.* **74**, 1410–1414.

Nordin, B. E. C., Aaron, J., Speed, R., Francis, R. M., and Makins, N. (1984). Bone formation and resorption as the determinants of trabecular bone volume in normal and osteoporotic men. *Scott. Med. J.* **29**, 171–175.

Orwoll, E. S., and Deftos, L. J. (1990). Serum osteocalcin (BGP) levels in normal men: A longitudinal evaluation reveals an age-associated increase. *J. Bone Miner. Res.* **5**(3), 259–262.

Orwoll, E. S., and Klein, R. F. (1995). Osteoporosis in men. *Endocr. Rev.* **16**, 87–116.

Orwoll, E. S., and Meier, D. E. (1986). Alterations in calcium, vitamin D, and parathyroid hormone physiology in normal men with aging: Relationship to the development of senile osteopenia. *J. Clin. Endocrinol. Metab.* **63**, 1262–1269.

Orwoll, E. S., Bell, N. H., Nanes, M. S., Flessland, K. A., Pettinger, M. B., Mallinak, J. S., and Cain, D. F. (1998). Collagen N-telopeptide excretion in men: The effects of age and intrasubject variability. *J. Bone Miner. Res.* **83**, 3930–3935.

Owen, R. A., Melton, L. J., Ilstrup, D. M., Johnson, K. A., and Riggs, B. L. (1982). Colles' fracture and subsequent hip fracture risk. *Clin. Orthop.* **171**, 37–43.

Poor, G., Atkinson, E. J., O'Fallon, W. M., and Melton, J. L. (1995a). Predictors of hip fractures in elderly men. *J. Bone Miner. Res.* **10**, 1902–1905.

Poor, G., Atkinson, E. J., O'Fallon, W. M., and Melton, L. J. (1995b). Determinants of reduced survival following hip fractures in men. *Clin. Orthop. Relat. Res.* **319**, 260–265.

Ray, W. A., Griffin, M. R., Schaffner, W., Baugh, D. K., and Melton, L. J., III (1987). Psychotropic drug use and the risk of hip fracture. *N. Engl. J. Med.* **316**, 363–370.

Ray, W. A., Griffin, M. R., and Downey, W. (1989). Benzodiazepines of long and short elimination half-life and the risk of hip fracture. *JAMA, J. Am. Med. Assoc.* **262**, 3303–3307.

Resch, H., Pietschmann, P., Woloszczuk, W., Krexner, E., Bernecker, P., and Willvonseder, R. (1992). Bone mass and biochemical parameters of bone metabolism in men with spinal osteoporosis. *Eur. J. Clin. Invest.* **22**, 542–545.

Rico, H., Revilla, M., Hernandez, E. R., Villa, L. F., and Alvarez del Buergo, M. (1992). Sex differences in the acquisition of total bone mineral mass peak assessed through dual-energy x-ray absorptiometry. *Calcif. Tissue Int.* **51**, 251–254.

Riggs, B. L., and Melton, L. J. III. (1986). Medical progress: Involutional osteoporosis. *N. Engl. J. Med.* **314**, 1676–1686.

Ross, P. D., Norimatsu, H., Davis, J. W., Yano, K., Wasnich, R. D., Fujiwara, S., Hosoda, Y., and Melton, L. J., III (1991). A comparison of hip fracture incidence among native Japanese, Japanese Americans, and American Caucasians. *Am. J. Epidemiol.* **133**, 801–809.

Schneider, D. L., and Barrett-Connor, E. L. (1997). Urinary N-telopeptide levels discriminate normal, osteopenic and osteoporotic bone mineral density. *Arch. Intern. Med.* **157**, 1241–1245.

Seeley, D. G., Browner, W. S., Nevitt, M. C., Genant, H. K., Scott, J. C., and Cummings, S. R. (1991). Which fractures are associated with low appendicular bone mass in elderly women? *Ann. Intern. Med.* **115**, 837–842.

Silman, A. J. (1995). The patient with fracture: The risk of subsequent fractures. *Am. J. Med.* **98** (Suppl. 2A), 12S–16S.

Slemenda, C. W., Christian, J. C., Reed, T., Reister, T. K., Williams, C. J., and Johnston, C. C., Jr. (1992). Long-term bone loss in men: Effects of genetic and environmental factors. *Ann. Intern. Med.* **117**, 286–291.

Smith, D. M., Nance, W. E., Kang, K. W., Christian, J. C., and Johnston, C. C. (1973). Genetic factors determining bone mass. *J. Clin. Invest.* **52**, 2800–2808.

Sokoloff, L. (1978). Occult osteomalacia in America (USA) patients with fracture of the hip. *Am. J. Surg. Pathol.* **2**, 21–30.

Soroko, S. B., Barrett-Connor, E., Edelstein, S. L., and Kritz-Silverstein, D. (1994). Family history of osteoporosis and bone mineral density at the axial skeleton: The Rancho Bernardo Study. *J. Bone Miner. Res.* **9**, 761–769.

Spolita, L. D., Caminis, J., Devoto, M., Shimoya, K., Sereda, L., Ott, J., Whyte, M. P., Tenenhouse, A., and Prockop, D. J. (1996). Osteopenia in 37 members of seven families: Analysis based on a model of dominant inheritance. *Mol. Med.* **2**, 313–324.

Stepan, J. J., Lachman, M., Zverina, J., Pacovsky, V., and Baylink, D. J. (1989). Castrated men exhibit bone loss: Effect of calcitonin treatment on biochemical indices of bone remodeling. *J. Clin. Endocrinol. Metab.* **69**, 523–527.

Tenover, J. S. (1992). Effects of testosterone supplementation in the aging male. *J. Clin. Endocrinol. Metab.* **75**, 1092–1098.

Thomas, M. K., Lloyd-Jones, D. M., Thadhani, R. I., Shaw, A. C., Deraska, D. J., Kitch, B. T., Vamvakas, E. C., Dick, I. M. A., Prince, R. L., and Finkelstein, J. S. (1998). Hypovitaminosis D in medical inpatients. *N. Engl. J. Med.* **338**, 777–783.

Toogood, A. A., Adams, J. E., O'Neill, P. A., and Shalet, S. M. (1997). Elderly patients with adult onset growth hormone deficiency are not osteopenic. *J. Clin. Endocrinol. Metab.* **82**, 1462–1466.

Tromp, A. M., Smit, J. H., Deeg, D. J. H., Bouter, L. M., and Lips, P. (1998). Predictors for falls and fractures in the Longitudinal Aging Study of Amsterdam. *J. Bone Miner. Res.* **13**, 1932–1939.

Uitterlinden, A. G., Pols, H. A. P., Burger, H., Huang, Q., Van Daele, P. L. A., Van Duijn, C. M., Hofman, A., Birkenhager, J. C., and Leeuwen, J. P. T. M. (1996). A large-scale population-based study of the association of vitamin D receptor gene polymorphisms with bone mineral density. *J. Bone Miner. Res.* **11**, 1241–1248.

Wang, C., Eyre, D. R., Clark, D., Kleinberg, C., Newman, C., Iranmanesh, A., Veldhuis, J., Dudley, R. E., Berman, N., Davidson, T., Barstow, T. J., Sinow, R., Alexander, G., and Swerdloff, R. S. (1996). Sublingual testosterone replacement improves muscle mass and strength, decreases bone resorption, and increases bone formation markers in hypogonadal men—A Clinical Research Center Study. *J. Clin. Endocrinol. Metab.* **81**, 3654–3662.

Wilton, T. J., Hosking, D. J., Pawley, E., Stevens, A., and Harvey, L. (1987). Osteomalacia and femoral neck fractures in the elderly patient. *J. Bone Jt. Surg., Br. Vol.* **69-B**, 388–390.

Wishart, J. M., Need, A. G., Horowitz, M., Morris, H. A., and Nordin, B. E. C. (1995). Effect of age on bone density and bone turnover in men. *Clin. Endocrinol. (Oxford)* **42**, 141–146.

World Health Organization (1994). "Assessment of Fracture Risk and its Application to Screening for Postmenopausal Osteoporosis," Report of a WHO Study Group. World Health Organization, Geneva.

Chapter 26

Eric S. Orwoll

Bone and Mineral Unit
Oregon Health Sciences University
and the Portland VA Medical Center
Portland, Oregon

The Prevention and Therapy of Osteoporosis in Men

I. Introduction

The prevention and therapy of osteoporotic disorders in men is virtually unexplored. No substantial controlled trials of any regimen are currently available. In the United States, there are no approved pharmacological therapies for osteoporosis in men. As a result of this dirth of information, recommendations must come from assumptions based on the current understanding of bone biology and pathophysiology and from the much larger experience in women.

Because of gender differences, the preventative and therapeutic strategies developed in women may have unexpected results when used in men. For instance, most therapeutic experience available is in postmenopausal women, a group that has developed osteoporosis through etiological mechanisms probably quite distinct from those affecting most men with the disorder. Morever, osteoporotic postmenopausal women may have bone remodeling dynamics that are distinct from those in similarly aged osteoporotic men and very different from young men with osteoporosis. On another level, there are differences in bone architecture between men and women that could influence the relative merits of the available pharamacological approaches. For instance, since bone strength in men may more heavily depend on periosteal bone accretion during aging, the relative merits of drugs that affect periosteal bone dynamics could be altered. Finally, the endocrine milieu is considerably different in men and women, and the effects of therapeutic agents may be different as a result. The most obvious example of gender-related endocrine differences is the contrast in sex hormone concentrations, but other endocrine distinctions exist as well (Pfeilschifter et al., 1996; Burman et al., 1997; Barrett-Connor and Goodman-Gruen, 1998). For all these reasons, preventive and treatment methods should be specifically tested in men. Until those trials are available, approaches must be derived from reasoned but untested assumptions.

II. Prevention

The prevention of osteoporotic fracture should be a routine part of the care of men, especially those over age 50 years. The use of preventive strategies should also be incorporated into the management of men who have already developed osteoporosis so as to minimize the chance of further progression of the disease.

A. Conditions Associated with Osteoporosis— A Major Concern

Of paramount importance in the prevention and management of osteoporosis in either gender is the recognition and correction of the factors that may be contributing to the disorder. Consideration should be given to conditions that may affect both bone fragility and the likelihood of falls. Excessive thinness should be avoided because men with low weight, especially if further weight loss occurs, are at higher fracture risk (Mussolino et al., 1998). The benefit to be derived from the betterment of conditions associated with osteoporosis depends on the situation but can be dramatic. For instance, the successful treatment of hyperparathyroidism, glucocorticoid excess, vitamin D deficiency, hypogonadism, and renal disease have been associated with substantial gains in bone mass (Martin et al., 1986; Pocock et al., 1987; Hermus et al., 1995; Guo et al., 1996; Katznelson et al., 1996; Abdelhadi and Nordenstrom, 1998). The importance of ameliorating these and other conditions is so great that they should usually be addressed, and the resulting benefits assessed (at least in the short term), before specific anti-osteoporosis drugs are used. Moreover, the use of certain therapies may be relatively contraindicated in the face of remodeling abnormalities associated with some disorders. For instance, antiresorptive drugs (which reduce overall rates of bone remodeling) may not be appropriate in the face of vitamin D deficiency.

At present there are no indications that men with conditions associated with skeletal disorders should be approached differently than are women in similar situations.

B. Exercise

Exercise is comprehensively considered in Chapter 8. Whereas an exercise prescription is difficult to generate with currently available information, activity is probably beneficial in several ways. Reductions in strength and coordination contribute to fracture via an increased risk of falling (Rubenstein and Josephson, 1992). In addition, inactivity is associated with bone loss, and exercise may increase or maintain bone mass (Fujimura et al., 1997). Specific exercise regimens to accomplish these goals have not been established in men or women, although strength can be dramatically increased and risk of falls can be reduced in the elderly with reasonable levels of exercise (Rubenstein and Josephson, 1992). That fracture rates are lower in elderly men who exercise modestly buttresses this contention (Paganini-Hill et al., 1991).

C. Calcium/Vitamin D

An area of obvious interest is the influence of calcium and vitamin D nutrition (Chapter 11). Calcium intake is probably important in the achievement of optimal peak bone mass in boys (Johnston et al., 1992), as well as the prevention and therapy of osteoporosis later in life. Calcium absorption declines with aging in men as in women, particularly after the age of 60, and well-documented changes in mineral metabolism occur concomitantly with age in men (Chapter 10). These data suggest that both optimal levels of calcium intake may change with age and that inadequate calcium nutrition can have an adverse effect on skeletal mass. However, the level of calcium intake that should be recommended is unclear, as few prospective studies have addressed this issue.

No bone density benefit was observed from calcium/vitamin D supplementation in a very well-nourished population (mean dietary calcium intake >1000 mg/day) (Orwoll et al., 1990), and no antifracture benefit was observed in a large trial of vitamin D supplementation in older men and women with relatively high baseline intakes (Lips et al., 1996). Dietary calcium intake was not found to be related to fracture rate in the men followed as part of the Health Professionals Follow-up Study (Owusu et al., 1997). On the other hand, an improvement in bone density was noted in healthy older men in response to a calcium and vitamin D supplement, whereas placebo-treated men lost bone (Dawson-Hughes *et al.,* 1997). On the basis of the available information, and the likelihood of a high degree of safety, the U.S. Institute of Medicine recently recommended that men should have a calcium intake of 1200 mg/day and a vitamin D intake of 800 IU. A reasonable approach, therefore, is to suggest a calcium intake of at least 1200 mg/day in both preventative and therapeutic situations. A NIH Consensus Development Conference has suggested the somewhat higher calcium intake of 1500 mg/day in men after 65 years (National Institutes of Health, 1994).

Although these recommendations for supplemental calcium and vitamin D are reasonable, some attention to individual differences is probably important. For instance, the use of an invariant level of vitamin D supplementation (e.g., 800 IU/day) may result in inadequate effects in some patients, especially those who have low levels of vitamin D at baseline. In a study of the effects of vitamin D (and calcium supplementation) in men, Orwoll *et al.* (1988) found that the average increase in 25(OH) vitamin D levels in response to 25 μg (1000 IU) per day of cholecalciferol was 30 nmol/L (12 ng/ dL). However, the increase was no greater in those who started with reduced 25(OH) vitamin D levels (Fig. 1), with the result that men who start with low vitamin D levels could be inadequately treated with conventional amounts of supplement. Certainly vitamin D insufficiency is common in older men

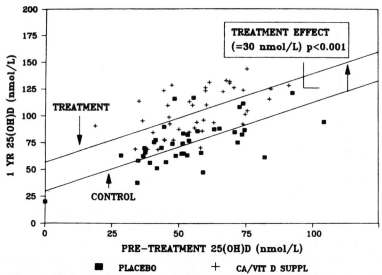

FIGURE I   The relationship between baseline and follow-up 25(OH)D levels in normal men treated with 25 μg (1000 IU) per day of cholecalciferol or placebo for 1 year. The regression line for each group is shown. Reproduced from Orwoll *et al.* (1988). *Am. J. Clin. Nutr.,* American Society for Clinical Nutrition, with permission.

(Lips *et al.*, 1987; Delvin *et al.*, 1988; van der Wielen *et al.*, 1995; Thomas *et al.*, 1998), and thus adjustments in the dose of supplements based on initial vitamin D levels may be useful. Moreover, the use of follow-up vitamin D levels should provide assurance that adequate vitamin D levels have been achieved. Similarly, in some special situations (e.g., glucocorticoid excess and malabsorption), dietary calcium requirements may be somewhat increased over those routinely recommended. At a given level of sodium excretion, elderly men were found to have a greater calcium excretion than women (despite similar dietary calcium intakes) (Dawson-Hughes *et al.*, 1996), suggesting that excess dietary sodium intake should be especially avoided in men at risk for osteoporosis.

One theoretical concern regarding dietary calcium/vitamin D supplementation has been the precipitation of calcium renal stones in susceptible individuals. Recent data, though, suggest that dietary calcium intake actually correlated negatively with the risk of nephrolithiasis in men (Curhan *et al.*, 1993), potentially by increasing gastrointestinal oxalate binding. The Institute of Medicine recommendations indicate that intakes below 2000 mg/day are safe.

III. Therapy

The identification of men who would benefit from pharmacological therapy cannot currently be based on prospectively derived evidence. Nevertheless, some judgments can be made concerning those likely to improve. A reasonable approach is summarized in Fig. 2. Essentially, men with bone density in a range associated with substantially increased fracture risk (more than 2 to 2.5 standard deviations below the young normal reference mean) should be considered therapeutic candidates. In addition, those with bone density levels less dramatically reduced, but in whom there are other indications that fracture risk may be increased (e.g., previous low-trauma fractures and conditions associated with rapid bone loss), should be considered for early treatment. Finally, men who have been managed with preventive measures (e.g., exercise and calcium/vitamin D) but have continued to lose bone density should be considered for early pharmacological intervention.

Virtually all available therapeutic agents (with the exception of androgens) were initially developed for the treatment of osteoporosis in postmenopausal women. Efforts have recently been made to evaluate those approaches in men, and initial results are encouraging.

A. Androgens

The role of androgens and other sex steroids in bone metabolism in men, and the usefulness of androgen replacement therapy in the prevention and

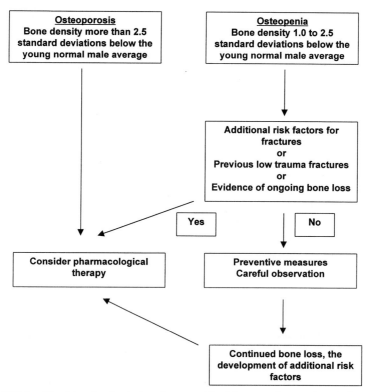

FIGURE 2   Algorithm for the choice of men at risk of fracture who may benefit from pharmacological therapy.

treatment of osteoporosis, are discussed in Chapter 13. Clearly, androgen replacement has a role in the therapy of men with hypogonadism, and there is emerging information concerning the usefulness of androgen administration in older men with borderline testosterone concentrations.

B. Calcitonin

There has been one trial of calcitonin therapy in a small group of men with idiopathic osteoporosis (Agrawal *et al.*, 1981) in which total body calcium tended to increase during a 24-month treatment interval (100 IU administered subcutaneously each day with a calcium and vitamin D supplement). However, the change was not significantly different from that observed in the control groups (receiving calcium plus vitamin D supplements or vitamin D alone), and there were no changes in radial bone mass. In another uncontrolled, 12-month trial of subcutaneously administered cyclical calcitonin (100 IU three times per week for three months, followed by three months without calcitonin) in men with vertebral osteoporosis, small benefits were noted in spinal and proximal femoral bone density (compared to baseline) (Erlacher *et al.*, 1997). Men have been included in several other trials of calcitonin therapy, but the results in men are not separable from those in women subjects. There are no published studies of the effectiveness of intranasal calcitonin in men. Although there are few data, from a theoretical perspective calcitonin should be useful in reducing osteoclastic activity in at least some patients with osteoporosis, or in those at risk of continuing bone loss.

Pain following vertebral fracture has been reported to be alleviated with calcitonin, and some reports of this benefit have included men (Lyritis *et al.*, 1997). Whether men can be expected to respond differently than women is unknown.

C. Bisphosphonates

There have been few trials of bisphosphonates performed exclusively in men, and many have been reported only in preliminary form (Eastell *et al.*, 1998). Nevertheless, there is no conceptual barrier to the use of bisphosphonates in men, and initial reports describe positive results. Additional results of longitudinal controlled trials performed specifically in men should be available soon.

Male patients with osteoporosis have been included in mixed patient populations and have seemed to experience beneficial effects on calcium balance and lumbar spine bone density during treatment with pamidronate (Valkema *et al.*, 1989). Men were specifically reported to benefit (increased vertebral bone density, with no change in femoral density) from etidronate treatment in a 12-month study (Orme *et al.*, 1994). An uncontrolled observational experience with intermittent cyclical etidronate (with calcium supplementation) in men with idiopathic osteoporosis and vertebral fractures (Anderson *et al.*, 1997) recently found small increases in lumbar spine and proximal femoral bone mass (3.2% and 0.7% per year, respectively) (Fig. 3), but no data were presented concerning fracture occurrence. There were no changes in alkaline phosphatase levels. In another uncontrolled trial, Geusens *et al.* (1997) reported a somewhat more robust response to cyclical etidronate in osteoporotic men (Fig. 4).

Bisphosphonates have also been examined in men with secondary causes of osteoporosis, especially in the context of glucocorticoid therapy. Men were included in some studies that indicated a positive effect of etidronate in glucocorticoid-treated patients (Pitt *et al.*, 1998), but the results were not described by gender. In a large trial of alendronate in men receiving glucocorticoids, positive effects were noted in lumbar spine bone mineral density (BMD) (Saag *et al.*, 1998) (Table I). Gender specific results were not provided at other skeletal sites.

There are a variety of other situations in which bisphosphonates may be useful, but little experience is yet available. For instance, inhibitors of bone resorption have been considered attractive in states of immobilization and in

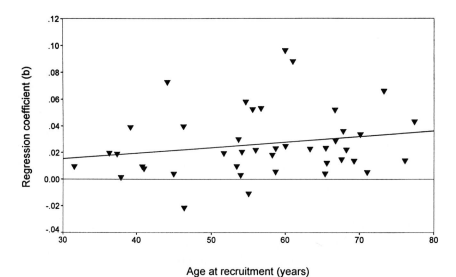

Age at recruitment (years)

FIGURE 3   Men with idiopathic osteoporosis appeared to have a positive response to therapy with intermittent cyclical etidronate, especially subjects of greater age. The scatterplot is of change in lumbar spine bone mineral density (BMD) against age at first scan. The average change in BMD per year of treatment was 0.024 g/cm², or 3.2%. From Anderson *et al.* (1997), *Age Ageing* **26**, 359–365, by permission of Oxford University Press.

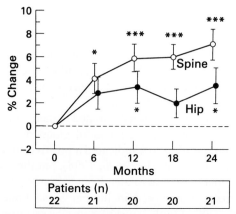

FIGURE 4   Changes in bone density in the lumbar spine and femoral neck in men with idiopathic osteoporosis treated with cyclic etidronate. The number of patients at each time point are shown. *$P < 0.05$, ***$p < 0.001$ versus baseline. Reproduced from Geusens *et al.* (1997), with permission.

TABLE I Percent Change in Lumbar Spine Bone Mineral Density in Glucocorticoid-Treated Subjects from Baseline to Week 48 According to Site, Sex, and Menopause[a]

	Placebo		5 mg of Alendronate		10 mg of Alendronate	
	No. of patients	Percent change	No. of patients	Percent change	No. of patients	Percent change
Sex and menopausal status	142	−0.4 ± 0.3	146	+2.1 ± 0.3[b,c]	145	+2.9 ± 0.3[b,c]
Men	49	−0.7 ± 0.4	40	+3.4 ± 0.6	41	+2.9 ± 0.5
Premenopausal women	35	−0.3 ± 0.7	30	+2.0 ± 0.6	29	+2.0 ± 0.6
Postmenopausal women receiving estrogen	18	−0.6 ± 0.9	27	+1.6 ± 0.7	25	+1.5 ± 0.6
Postmenopausal women not receiving estrogen	40	−0.1 ± 0.6	49	+1.5 ± 0.5	50	+4.0 ± 0.6

[a]Plus-minus values are means ± SE.

[b]$p \leq 0.001$ for the comparison with the baseline values.

[c]$p \leq 0.001$ for the comparison with placebo.

Reproduced from Saag *et al.* (1998), *New Engl. J. Med.* 339, 292–299, Copyright © 1998 Massachusetts Medical Society. All rights reserved.

inflammatory conditions (e.g., rheumatoid arthritis). Men who receive antiandrogen therapy for prostate carcinoma are at risk of bone loss, and antiresorptive therapy should provide some protection for those patients. In fact, Diamond *et al.* (1998) reported that intermittent cyclic etidronate therapy (plus calcium) reversed bone loss initially experienced in men following long-acting gonadotropin-releasing hormone agonist plus androgen antagonist therapy (Table II). Some early reports are available in other conditions (Heilberg *et al.,* 1998), and more can be expected as the effects of bisphosphonates in men are further explored.

Dose response relationships and the frequency of complications in men are currently unknown.

D. Thiazide Diuretics

Evidence supports a beneficial effect of thiazide administration on bone mass, rates of bone loss, and hip fracture risk in men (Wasnich *et al.,* 1983; LeCroix *et al.,* 1990; Morton *et al.,* 1994). For instance, in case-controlled trials the use of thiazides reduced the rate of loss in calcaneal bone density by 49% compared to controls (Wasnich *et al.,* 1990) and the relative risk of hip fracture was halved by exposure to thiazides for more than 6 years (Ray

TABLE II   Percent Change in Bone Mineral Density in Men with Prostate Carcinoma Treated with Combined Androgen Blockade Prior to and After 6 Months of Intermittent Cyclic Etidronate Therapy

BMD	Combined androgen blockade		p Value[c]
	Without ICT[a]	With ICT[b]	
Spinal QCT	−6.6% (−10 to −3.2)	7.8% (−0.8 to 16.6)	$p = 0.01$
Femoral neck	−6.5% (−9.5 to −3.5)	−2.4% (−6.6 to 1.7)	$p = 0.02$
Ward's triangle	−7.5% (−12.4 to −2.7)	1.9% (−4 to 7.9)	$p = 0.04$
Trochanter	−6.2% (−10.5 to −2)	0.6% (−6.4 to 7.7)	$p = 0.08$

BMD, bone mineral density; ICT, intermittent cyclic etidronate therapy; QCT, bone density measured by quantitative computed tomography.

Values are the mean percentage change in bone mineral density after 6 months of therapy (95% confidence interval).

[a]Mean values calculated for 11 of 12 men at 0–6 months on combined androgen blockade (one man died).

[b]Mean values calculated for 8 of 12 men at 6–12 months on combinaton of combined androgen blockade and intermittent cyclic etidronate therapy (four men died).

[c]The p values were established using the Student's t test for paired data.

Reproduced from Diamond *et al.* (1998), CANCER, Vol. 83, pp. 1561–1566. Copyright © 1998 American Cancer Society. Reprinted by permission of Wiley-Liss, Inc., a subsidiary of John Wiley & Sons, Inc.

et al., 1989). In a trial of similar design, thiazide use in men was associated with an adjusted odds ratio of femur fracture of 0.2 (95%, CI 0.1–0.7) (Herings *et al.*, 1996). Other diuretics did not seem to impart the same benefits. Unfortunately, none of the available studies has been randomized or controlled, so a confident estimate of the magnitude of the protective effect isn't possible. Moreover, the available literature doesn't allow a comparison of the relative benefits in men and women (Jones *et al.*, 1995). The mechanism for the positive effect is unclear, but it has been postulated to stem from the hypocalciuric effects of thiazides. Although not appropriately considered a primary treatment modality, a thiazide is probably the diuretic of choice in osteoporotic patients (other considerations notwithstanding).

E. Fluoride

The use of fluoride in the therapy of osteoporosis remains controversial. Consistent and sometimes dramatic increases in vertebral bone mass can be achieved with supplemental fluoride, but the effectiveness of fluoride therapy in reducing fracture rates is uncertain. Nevertheless, there is an active interest in refining the formulation and dose of fluoride in the hope of taking better advantage of its anabolic properties. In fact, a recent evaluation of cyclically administered slow-release form of fluoride was reported to increase bone mass and reduce fracture rates in older women (Pak *et al.*, 1994). As with many of the other therapies discussed, there have been few specific trials of fluoride administration in men. In some studies, osteoporotic men have been included in the treatment groups, but it is difficult to ascertain whether responses were in any way gender-specific. Ringe *et al.* (1998) recently described a 36-month controlled trial of intermittent monofluorophosphate and calcium (versus calcium alone) in a large group of men with idiopathic osteoporosis. Whereas the calcium-treated men lost bone density at the spine, radius, and proximal femur, those treated with fluoride experienced increases. The most marked change was seen at the lumbar spine ($+8.9\%$), with more modest increases at the other sites. Importantly, fewer patients experienced vertebral fractures in the fluoride-treated group (10% versus 40%, $p = 0.008$) (Fig. 5), and back pain was reduced ($p = 0.0003$). There were fewer nonvertebral fractures in the fluoride-treated men as well, but the difference was not significant. These results are similar to parallel studies in women and suggest that fluoride may have some benefit in men, particularly those at risk of vertebral fracture.

F. Emerging Therapies

Parathyroid hormone administration to osteoporotic subjects has been shown to increase trabecular bone formation and bone volume in concert with an increase in calcium balance. In a small group of men with idiopathic

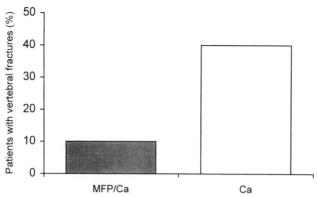

FIGURE 5   The percentage of osteoporotic men who experienced new vertebral fractures during 3 years of treatment with monofluorophosphate plus calcium (MFP/Ca) or calcium alone (Ca). Reproduced from Ringe *et al.* (1998), with permission.

osteoporosis, Slovik *et al.* (1986) found that combined parathyroid hormone (PTH) and 1,25-dihydroxyvitamin D administration increased trabecular (spinal) bone mass and improved intestinal calcium absorption. Preliminary results by Kurland *et al.* (1998b) also suggest that men with idiopathic osteoporosis obtain considerable increases in bone density (especially at the lumbar spine) with PTH therapy (plus calcium supplementation). Biochemical indices of remodeling appear to parallel the increase in bone density, and measures of some indices predicted the degree of response (Kurland *et al.,* 1998a). Although the role of PTH administration in the treatment of osteoporosis remains unclear (either alone or in concert with other agents), its potential appears similar in men and women.

  Growth hormone (or other growth factors) (Chapter 9) may have anabolic actions on the skeleton in the elderly and in subjects with osteoporosis, but the available data are inconclusive (Marcus and Hoffman, 1998). Low levels of IGF-I have reported to be present in men with idiopathic osteoporosis (Ljunghall *et al.,* 1992), and in a study of healthy older men with low IGF-I levels, Rudman *et al.* (1990) found that in addition to positive effects on lean mass, fat mass, and skin thickness, vertebral bone mass was increased slightly (1.6%) by the administration of growth hormone for 6 months. Radial and proximal femoral densities were unaffected. There are a number of reports that growth hormone administration may improve bone mass in growth hormone deficient adults (Marcus, 1997; Kotzmann *et al.,* 1998), and the treatment of adults with growth hormone provokes an increase in biochemical markers of bone remodeling. Men have been reported to be more responsive to replacement therapy with growth hormone than women (Fig. 6) (Burman *et al.,* 1997). The potential benefits of growth hormone on body composition (increased lean mass and perhaps muscle strength)

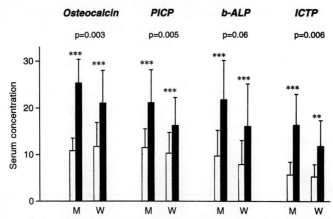

FIGURE 6   Concentrations of osteocalcin (μg/L), carboxyl-terminal cross-linked telopeptide of type I collagen (ICTP; μg/L), carboxyl-terminal propeptide of type I procollagen (PICP, μg/L × 10⁻¹) and bone specific alkaline phosphatase (b-ALP; μkat/L × 10⁻¹) in 21 men and 15 women with GHD before and after 9 months of treatment with recombinant human growth hormone. Results are shown as the mean ± SD. **, $p < 0.01$; ***, $p < 0.001$. The p values in letters refer to the difference in response to treatment between men and women. Reproduced from Burman *et al.* (1997). Growth hormone-deficient men are more responsive to GH replacement therapy than women. *J. Clin. Endocrinol. Metab.* **82**, 550–555, © The Endocrine Society, with permission.

(Rudman *et al.*, 1991) have been suggested to have additional benefits in patients with osteoporosis, but the functional importance of those changes has been questioned (Papadakis *et al.*, 1996). Despite interesting preliminary findings, the use of growth hormone is fraught with a variety of uncertainties, the benefits remain inconsistent, and experimental results have been difficult to interpret (Marcus and Hoffman, 1998). In either sex, growth hormone therapy is thus of potential but as yet unproven usefulness.

IV. Summary

The prevention and treatment of osteoporosis in men remains problematic because there are still very few controlled trials at hand to guide the use of available approaches. Without that knowledge, confident estimates of the effectiveness of available therapeutic approaches cannot be made. Nevertheless, such trials have begun, and we can look forward to the emergence of more useful information in the next several years.

In the interval, clinicians must make judgments on the basis of the meager data available. The essentials of preventive therapy that have been established for women appear to be appropriate in men (the elimination/treatment of conditions associated with bone loss or falls, safe levels of activity, adequate calcium and vitamin D nutrition). Antiresorptive therapies should be effective in men, and the emerging experience thus far supports a beneficial effect on bisphosphonates in those with idiopathic osteoporosis as well as with selected secondary causes of bone loss (e.g., glucocorticoid therapy). As of yet there is inadequate experience with other available regimens (e.g., calcitonin and fluoride). Bone forming agents also should have a role in the treatment of osteoporotic men, and early results with parathyroid hormone mirror those in women.

References

Abdelhadi, M., and Nordenstrom, J. (1998). Bone mineral recovery after parathyroidectomy in patients with primary and renal hyperparathyroidism. *J. Clin. Endocrinol. Metab.* **83,** 3845–3851.

Agrawal, R., Wallach, S., Cohn, S., Tessier, M., Verch, R., Hussain, M., and Zanzi, I. (1981). Calcitonin treatment of osteoporosis. *In* "Calcitonin" (A. Pecile, ed.), p. 237. Exerpta Medica, Amsterdam.

Anderson, F. H., Francis, R. M., Bishop, J. C., and Rawlings, D. J. (1997). Effect of intermittent cyclical disodium etidronate therapy on bone mineral density in men with vertebral fractures. *Age Ageing* **26,** 359–365.

Barrett-Connor, E., and Goodman-Gruen, D. (1998). Gender differences in insulin-like growth factor and bone mineral density association in old age: The Rancho Bernardo Study. *J. Bone Miner. Res.* **13,** 1343–1349.

Burman, P., Johansson, A. G., Siegbahn, A., Vessby, B., and Karlsson, A. (1997). Growth hormone (GH)-deficient men are more responsive to GH replacement therapy than women. *J. Clin. Endocrinol. Metab.* **82,** 550–555.

Curhan, G. C., Willett, W. C., Rimm, E. B., and Stampfer, M. J. (1993). A prospective study of dietary calcium and other nutrients and the risk of symptomatic kidney stones. *N. Engl. J. Med.* **328,** 833–838.

Dawson-Hughes, B., Fowler, S. E., Dalsky, G., and Gallagher, C. (1996). Sodium excretion influences calcium homeostasis in elderly men and women. *J. Nutr.* **126,** 2107–2112.

Dawson-Hughes, B., Harris, S. S., Krall, E. A., and Dallal, G. E. (1997). Effect of calcium and vitamin D supplementation on bone density in men and women 65 years of age or older. *N. Engl. J. Med.* **337,** 670–702.

Delvin, E. E., Imbach, A., and Copti, M. (1988). Vitamin D nutritional status and related biochemical indices in an autonomous elderly population. *Am. J. Clin. Nutr.* **48,** 373–378.

Diamond, T., Campbell, J., Bryant, C., and Lynch, W. (1998). The effect of combined androgen blockade on bone turnover and bone mineral densities in men treated for prostate carcinoma. *Cancer (Philadelphia)* **83,** 1561–1566.

Eastell, R., Boyle, I. T., Compston, J., Cooper, C., Fogelman, I., Francis, R. M., Hosking, D. J., Purdie, D. W., Ralston, S., Reeve, J., Reid, D. M., Russell, R. G. G., and Stevenson, J. C. (1998). Management of male osteoporosis: Report of the UK Consensus Group. *Q. J. Med.* **91,** 71–92.

Erlacher, L., Kettenbach, J., Kiener, H., Graninger, W., Kainberger, F., and Pietschmann, P. (1997). Salmon calcitonin and calcium in the treatment of male osteoporosis: The effect on bone mineral density. *Wien. Klin. Wochenschr.* **109,** 270–274.

Fujimura, R., Ashizawa, N., Watanabe, M., Mukai, N., Amagai, H., Fukubayashi, T., Hayashi, K., Tokuyama, K., and Suzuki, M. (1997). Effect of resistance exercise training on bone formation and resorption in young male subjects assessed by biomarkers of bone metabolism. *J. Bone Miner. Res.* **12**, 656–662.

Geusens, P., Van Hoof, J., Raus, J., Dequeker, J., Nijs, J., and Joly, J. (1997). Treatment with etidronate for men with idiopathic osteoporosis. *Ann. Rheum. Dis.* **56**, 280.

Guo, C.-Y., Thomas, W. E. G., Al-Dehaimi, A. W., Assiri, A. M. A., and Eastell, R. (1996). Longitudinal changes in bone mineral density and bone turnover in postmenopausal women with primary hyperparathyroidism. *J. Clin. Endocrinol. Metab.* **81**, 3487–3491.

Heilberg, I. P., Martini, L. A., Teixeira, S. H., Szejnfeld, V. L., Carvalho, A. B., Lobao, R., and Draibe, S. A. (1998). Effect of etidronate treatment on bone mass of male nephrolithiasis patients with idiopathic hypercalciuria and osteopenia. *Nephron* **79**, 430–437.

Herings, R. M. C., Stricker, B. H. C., de Boer, A., Bakker, A., Sturmans, F., and Stergachis, A. (1996). Current use of thiazide diuretics and prevention of femur fractures. *J. Clin. Epidemiol.* **49**, 115–119.

Hermus, A. R., Smals, A. G., Swinkels, L. M., Huysmans, D. A., Pieters, G. F., Sweep, C. F., Corstens, F. H., and Kloppenborg, P. W. (1995). Bone mineral density and bone turnover before and after surgical cure of Cushing's syndrome. *J. Clin. Endocrinol. Metab.* **80**, 2859–2865.

Johnston, C. C., Miller, J. Z., Slemenda, C. W., Reister, T. K., Hui, S., Christian, J. C., and Peacock, M. (1992). Calcium supplementation and increases in bone mineral density in children. *N. Engl. J. Med.* **327**, 82–87.

Jones, G., Nguyen, T., Sambrook, P. N., and Eisman, J. A. (1995). Thiazide diuretic and fractures: Can meta-analysis help? *J. Bone Miner. Res.* **10**, 106–111.

Katznelson, L., Finkelstein, J. S., Schoenfeld, D. A., Rosenthal, D. I., Anderson, E. J., and Klibanski, A. (1996). Increase in bone density and lean body mass during testosterone administration in men with acquired hypogonadism. *J. Clin. Endocrinol. Metab.* **81**, 4358–4365.

Kotzmann, H., Riedl, M., Bernecker, P., Clodi, M., Kainberger, F., Kaider, A., Woloszczuk, W., and Luger, A. (1998). Effects of long-term growth hormone substitution therapy on bone mineral density and parameters of bone metabolism in adult patients with growth hormone deficiency. *Calcif. Tissue Int.* **62**, 40–46.

Kurland, E. S., Cosman, F., McMahon, D. G., Shen, V., Lindsay, R., Rosen, C. J., and Bilezikian, J. P. (1998a). Changes in bone markers predict bone accrual in osteoporotic men treated with parathyroid hormone. *Bone* **23** (Suppl.), S158 (abstr.).

Kurland, E. S., Cosman, F., McMahon, D. J., Rosen, C. J., Lindsay, R., and Bilezikian, J. P. (1998b). Parathyroid hormone (PTH 1-34) increases cancellous bone mass markedly in men with idiopathic osteoporosis. *Bone* **23** (Suppl.), S158 (abstr.).

LeCroix, A. Z., Wienpahl, J., White, L. R., Wallace, R. B., Scherr, P. A., George, L. K., Cornoni-Huntley, J., and Ostfeld, A. M. (1990). Thiazide diuretic agents and the incidence of hip fracture. *N. Engl. J. Med.* **322**, 286–290.

Lips, P., van Ginkel, F. C., Jongen, M. J. M., Rubertus, F., van der Vijgh, W. J. F., and Netelenbos, J. C. (1987). Determinants of vitamin D status in patients with hip fracture and in elderly control subjects. *Am. J. Clin. Nutr.* **46**, 1005–1010.

Lips, P., Graafmans, W. C., Ooms, M. E., Bezemer, P. D., and Bouter, L. M. (1996). Vitamin D supplementation and fracture incidence in elderly persons. *Ann. Intern. Men* **124**, 400–406.

Ljunghall, S., Johansson, A. G., Burman, P., Kampe, O., Lindh, E., and Karlsson, F. A. (1992). Low plasma levels of insulin-like growth factor 1 (IGF-1) in male patients with idiopathic osteoporosis. *J. Intern. Med.* **232**, 59–64.

Lyritis, G. P., Paspati, I., Karachalios, T., Loakimidis, D., Skarantavos, G., and Lyritis, P. G. (1997). Pain relief from nasal salmon calcitonin in osteoporotic vertebral crush fractures. *Acta Orthop. Scand.* **68** (Suppl. 275), 112–114.

Marcus, R. (1997). Skeletal effects of growth hormone and IGF-1 in adults. *Endocrine* **7**, 53–55.

Marcus, R., and Hoffman, A. R. (1998). Growth hormone as therapy for older men and women. *Annu. Rev. Pharmacol. Toxicol.* **38**, 45–61.

Martin, P., Bergmann, P., Gillett, C., Fuss, M., Kinneart, P., Corvilain, J., and van Geertruyden, J. (1986). Partially reversible osteopenia after surgery for primary hyperparathyroidism. *Arch. Intern. Med.* **146**, 689–691.

Morton, D. J., Barrett-Connor, E. L., and Edelstein, S. L. (1994). Thiazides and bone mineral density in elderly men and women. *Am. J. Epidemiol.* **139**, 1107–1115.

Mussolino, M. E., Looker, A. C., Madans, J. H., Langlois, J. A., and Orwoll, E. S. (1998). Risk factors for hip fracture in white men: The NHANES I Epidemiologic Follow-up Study. *J. Bone Miner. Res.* **13**, 918–924.

National Institutes of Health (1994). *Optional Calcium Intake.* NIH Consensus Development Conference. June 6–8; 12(4), 1–34.

Orme, S. M., Simpson, M., Stewart, S. P., Oldroyd, B., Westmacott, C. F., Smith, M. A., and Belchetz, P. E. (1994). Comparison of changes in bone mineral in idiopathic and secondary osteoporosis following therapy with cyclical disodium etidronate and high dose calcium supplementation. *Clin. Endocrinol. (Oxford)* **41**, 245–250.

Orwoll, E. S., Weigel, R. M., Oviatt, S. K., McClung, M. R., and Deftos, L. J. (1988). Calcium and cholecalciferol: Effects of small supplements in normal men. *Am. J. Clin. Nutr.* **48**, 127–130.

Orwoll, E. S., Oviatt, S. K., McClung, M. R., Deftos, L. J., and Sexton, G. (1990). The rate of bone mineral loss in normal men and the effects of calcium and cholecalciferol supplementation. *Ann. Intern. Med.* **112**, 29–34.

Owusu, W., Willett, W. C., Feskanich, D., Ascherio, A., Spiegelman, D., and Colditz, G. A. (1997). Calcium intake and the incidence of forearm and hip fractures among men. *J. Nutr.* **127**, 1782–1787.

Paganini-Hill, A., Chao, A., Ross, R. K., and Henderson, B. E. (1991). Exercise and other factors in the prevention of hip fracture: The Leisure World Study. *Epidemiology* **2**, 16–25.

Pak, C. Y. C., Sakhaee, K., Piziak, V., Peterson, R. D., Breslau, N. A., Boyd, P., Poindexter, J. R., Herzog, J., Heard-Sakhaee, A., Haynes, S., Adams-Huet, B., and Reisch, J. S. (1994). Slow-release sodium fluoride in the management of postmenopausal osteoporosis: A randomized controlled trial, *Ann. Intern. Med.* **120**, 625–632.

Papadakis, M. A., Grady, D., Black, D., Tierney, M. J., Gooding, G. A. W., Schambelan, M., and Grunfeld, C. (1996). Growth hormone replacement in healthy older men improved body composition but not functional ability. *Ann. Intern. Med.* **124**, 708–716.

Pfeilschifter, J., Scheidt-Nave, C., Leidig-Bruckner, G., Woitge, H. W., Blum, W. F., Wuster, C., Haack, D., and Ziegler, R. (1996). Relationship between circulating insulin like growth factor components and sex hormones in a population-based sample of 50- to 80-year-old men and women. *J. Clin. Endocrinol. Metab.* **81**, 2534–2540.

Pitt, P., Li, F., Todd, P., Webber, D., Pack, S., and Moniz, C. (1998). A double blind placebo controlled study to determine the effects of intermittent cyclical etidronate on bone mineral density in patients on long-term oral corticosteroid treatment. *Thorax* **53**, 351–356.

Pocock, N. A., Eisman, J. A., Dunstan, C. R., Evans, R. A., Thomas, D. H., and Huq, N. L. (1987). Recovery from steroid-induced osteoporosis. *Ann. Intern. Med.* **107**, 319–323.

Ray, W. A., Griffin, M. R., Downey, W., and Melton, L. J. III. (1989). Long-term use of thiazide diuretics and risk of hip fracture. *Lancet* **1**, 687–690.

Ringe, J. D., Dorst, A., Kipshoven, C., Rovati, L. C., and Setniker, I. (1998). Avoidance of vertebral fractures in men with idiopathic osteoporosis by a three year therapy with calcium and low-dose intermittent monofluorophosphate. *Osteoporosis Int.* **8**, 47–52.

Rubenstein, L. Z., and Josephson, K. R. (1992). Causes and prevention of falls in elderly people. *In* "Falls, Balance and Gait Disorders in the Elderly" (B. Vellas, M. Toupet, L. Rubenstein, J. L. Albarede, and Y. Christen, eds.), pp. 21–36. Elsevier, Paris.

Rudman, D., Feller, A. G., Hoskote, S., Nagraj, S., Gergans, G. A., Lalitha, P. Y., Goldberg, A. F., Schlenker, R. A., Cohn, L., Rudman, I. W., and Mattson, D. E. (1990). Effects of human growth hormone in men over 60 years old. *N. Engl. J. Med.* **323**, 1–6.

Rudman, D., Feller, A. G., Cohn, L., Shetty, K. R., Rudman, I. W., and Draper, M. W. (1991). Effects of human growth hormone on body composition in elderly men. *Horm. Res.* **36** (Suppl. 1), 73–81.

Saag, K. G., Emkey, R., Schnitzer, T. J., Brown, J. P., Hawkins, F., Goemaere, S., Thamsborg, G., Liberman, U. A., Delmas, P. D., Malice, M.-P., Czachur, M., and Diafotis, A. G. (1998). Alendronate for the prevention and treatment of glucocorticoid-induced osteoporosis. *N. Engl. J. Med.* **339**, 292–299.

Slovik, D. M., Rosenthal, D. I., Doppelt, S. H., Potts, J. R. J., Daly, M. A., Campbell, J. A., and Neer, R. M. (1986). Restoration of spinal bone in osteoporotic men by treatment with human parathyroid hormone (1-34) and 1,25-dihydroxyvitamin D. *J. Bone Miner. Res.* **1**, 377–381.

Thomas, M. K., Lloyd-Jones, D. M., Thadhani, R. I., Shaw, A. C., Deraska, D. J., Kitch, B. T., Vamvakas, E. C., Dick, I. M., Prince, R. L., and Finkelstein, J. S. (1998). Hypovitaminosis D in medical inpatients. *N. Engl. J. Med.* **338**, 777–783.

Valkema, R., Vismans, F.-J. F. E., Papapoulos, S. E., Pauwels, E. K. J., and Bijvoet, O. L. M. (1989). Maintained improvement in calcium balance and bone mineral content in patients with osteoporosis treated with the bisphosphonate APD. *Bone Miner.* **5**, 183–192.

van der Wielen, R. P. J., Lowik, M. R. H., van den Berg, H., de Groot, L. C. P. G. M., Haller, J., Moreiras, O., and van Staveren, W. A. (1995). Serum vitamin D concentrations among elderly people in Europe. *Lancet* **346**, 207–210.

Wasnich, R. D., Benfante, R. J., Yano, K., Heilbrun, L., and Vogel, J. M. (1983). Thiazide effect on the mineral content of bone. *N. Engl. J. Med.* **309**, 344–347.

Wasnich, R., Davis, J., Ross, P., Vogel, J. (1990). Effect of thiazide on rates of bone mineral loss: A longitudinal study. *Br. Med. J.* **301**, 1303–1305.

Index